CHINESE PATTERNS OF BEHAVIOR

CHINESE PATTERNS OF BEHAVIOR: A SOURCEBOOK OF PSYCHOLOGICAL AND PSYCHIATRIC STUDIES

Edited by
DAVID YAU-FAI HO
JOHN A. SPINKS
and
CECILIA SIU-HING YEUNG

PRAEGER

New York
Westport, Connecticut
London

Library of Congress Cataloging-in-Publication Data

Chinese patterns of behavior.

Bibliography: p.
Includes index.
1. National characteristics, Chinese—Periodicals—Indexes. 2. Chinese—Psychology—Periodicals—Indexes. 3. Chinese—Mental health—Periodicals—Indexes. 4. National characteristics—Abstracts. 5. Chinese—Psychology—Abstracts. 6. Chinese—Mental health—Abstracts. I. Ho, David Y. F. II. Spinks, John A. III. Yeung, Cecilia Siu-Hing.
Z3108.P7C48 1989 [BF755.C5] 016.1558'4951 88-32335
ISBN 0-275-93270-2 (alk. paper)

Library of Congress Catalog Card Number: 88-32335
ISBN: 0-275-93270-2

First published in 1989

Praeger Publishers, One Madison Avenue, New York, NY 10010
A division of Greenwood Press, Inc.

Printed in the United States of America

The paper used in this book complies with the Permanent Paper Standard issued by the National Information Standards Organization (Z39.48-1984).

10 9 8 7 6 5 4 3 2 1

To our families

And to students of Chinese culture and society

CONTENTS

PREFACE

Psychological and psychiatric studies of Chinese patterns of thinking and behavior derive their significance from the simple fact that they concern more than a fifth of humankind. Yet, despite their sizable amount, collectively these studies do not comprise a coherent body of knowledge, with later investigations being built upon the refinement of earlier ones and the avoidance of their failures. Individual investigators or groups of investigators often work quite independently, each apparently uninformed about the work of others. Furthermore, research studies are too often the result of piecemeal efforts. This is obviously not the ideal fashion in which scientific knowledge is to be advanced.

Interdisciplinary, language, and political barriers have impeded the coordination of research efforts. A formidable problem is that familiarity with the relevant literature, which is quite extensive, cannot be achieved without considerable effort. The reason for this is that it derives from very diverse sources, with great variations in theoretical orientation and methodological approach, as well as in the scope, depth, and quality of analysis. It is scattered in books, monographs, and periodicals addressed to different groups of readers. The authors have diverse academic and intellectual backgrounds, the majority being psychologists, psychiatrists, anthropologists, sociologists, political scientists, and educationalists. Furthermore, a substantial portion are written in Chinese, not consulted by non- Chinese readers, or are published in books or journals which are not readily accessible to international scholars. Most of these materials would not be found in the international databases currently available. More generally, given its diversity, the literature cannot be adequately covered even from an exhaustive search of these databases.

The aim of the present editors is to bring together the diverse sources of material into a reference book. We have labored to achieve a comprehensive coverage of the literature, mostly in Chinese or English, up to 1986. The literature search was complemented by a search through DIALOG. In addition, help was solicited from numerous scholars to send relevant materials to the editors.

This book is addressed primarily to social scientists, psychologists, psychiatrists, and mental health professionals who have a special interest in cross-cultural issues in general or Chinese people, society, and culture in particular; and, of course, to sinologists. We believe that scholars will find it a useful source of information. At least three worthwhile purposes would be served. First, the book saves researchers an enormous amount of time from having to undertake the laborious task of an initial library search for materials wanted. Second, it offers a provisional solution to the problem of language barrier for non-Chinese readers. Third, we hope that it will encourage and enable greater coordination of efforts among different investigators in the field, so that a body of scientific knowledge built upon hierarchically ordered investigations will be more readily realized in the future.

Our book is the result of many years of labor. The magnitude of the task we undertook exceeded all estimates, as more and more materials were found and had to be processed. We admit, almost with a sense of embarrassment, that the collection of materials began in the late 1960s! Our labor has finally come to fruition, despite the many obstructions and difficulties which hindered our progress at different times. We feel that the end-product is a fitting tribute to researchers around the world engaged in the study of Chinese patterns of behavior, as well as to the thousands of Chinese and non-Chinese who participated as subjects. The fruit of our perseverance, we hope, will be a vital tool for these researchers in the future. As teachers at the University of Hong Kong, we are already aware of the tremendous help which this bibliographic data-base can offer to researchers and students of Chinese psychology. We sincerely hope that it will provide, not only an impetus and incentive for further and deeper study of Chinese individuals, but a basis for facilitation of this research and co-operation amongst scholars.

We wish to acknowledge the financial help we have received from the Committee on Conference and Research Grants and the Centre of Asian Studies of the University of Hong Kong. We also wish to thank Business Simulations Ltd., Scriventon House, Speldhurst, Kent, U.K., which provided the excellent PC data-base management software system, Cardbox-Plus, used for storing, editing, searching, manipulating and printing this bibliography. Further information on this system is available on request from the second editor. We would also like to thank the Computer Centre on the University of Hong Kong for their advice and support.

Numerous individuals have participated in the task of producing this book: endless searching, checking, indexing, typing, and proofreading. Among them are Chiu Chi-yue, Susanne Beard, Kan Tsi-kit, Anna Ku, Able Ho, Stewart Lam and Lenny Li. We owe them our heartfelt gratitude. Finally, we wish to thank the many scholars passing through Hong Kong, Chinese and non-Chinese alike, who have given us encouragement.

David Y. F. Ho
John A. Spinks
Cecilia S. H. Yeung

CHINESE PATTERNS OF BEHAVIOR

INTRODUCTION 1

This reference book comprises 3,548 bibliographic citations and more than half that number of abstracts of psychological and psychiatric studies pertaining to normal and abnormal behavior in Chinese culture. These materials were selected from a comprehensive search of the literature in psychology, psychiatry, and related disciplines up to the end of 1986. The literature search covered only sources in Chinese and English, although relevant publications in other languages, when identified, were also included. Most of the studies included have been published, although many are not readily accessible to international scholars.

The studies are organized into 13 chapters, partly based on the PsycINFO content classification categories. Within chapters items are arranged and numbered primarily by author(s) in an alphabetic order and secondarily by year of publication. An author index and a subject index facilitate literature searches. In addition, this introductory chapter and introductory notes to each chapter serve to introduce globally the literature to the reader.

English translations of citations from non-English sources are given when available, edited when necessary; when not available, translation is provided by the editors. Many of the abstracts, especially those from Chinese-language sources, were translated into English, extensively edited, or newly written.

SELECTION, COVERAGE, AND INDEXING

Criteria for Selection

The following criteria were established for selecting materials to be included in this reference book.

For inclusion, an item should pertain to Chinese psychology or psychiatry; to perceptions or stereotypes about China or Chinese people; or to normal or abnormal patterns of thinking and behavior in the context of Chinese society or culture, including cognition, learning, psychosocial development, social behavior or communication, personality, psychopathology, mental health, prevention and treatment of mental disorders.

Empirical studies in which Chinese have served as subjects and which have some relevance to the above may be included. All ethnic Chinese groups are included, regardless of geographical location, such as mainland China,

Taiwan, Hong Kong, Singapore, and North America. (Asian Americans or Singaporeans would not be included, unless the study states explicitly that ethnic Chinese are involved.)

Inclusion is delimited to studies which are primarily psychological or psychiatric in nature. However, studies in allied disciplines, such as anthropology, sociology, linguistics, education, and political science, may also be included if judged to be relevant. Inclusion is also delimited to published studies, although exceptions (e.g., conference papers) can be made for those judged to be important. Abstracts are to be included when available. However, if an item is judged to meet the criteria for inclusion only marginally, the available abstract would be excluded.

The term *Chinese psychology* is broadly interpreted to include the following.

1. Psychology of Chinese people(s): a body of psychological knowledge, theoretical or empirical, about patterns of thinking and behaving among Chinese people(s). Most items in this book fall within this domain.

2. Psychology in China: the history and current status of psychology, as an academic discipline or a professional specialty, within a Chinese geopolitical community.

3. A psychology created by Chinese psychologists (or psychologists in China): a new theoretical system or school of thought in psychology created by Chinese psychologists (or psychologists in China) who may be identified by their common adherence to a definite philosophical base (e.g., dialectical materialism). (No such psychology has yet developed beyond the embryonic stage.)

4. Chinese psychological thought: psychological conceptions of Chinese thinkers, both historical and contemporary, about human nature, cognition, and behavior; the goal and meaning of life; relationships between the individual and others, the family, society, nature, and the cosmos.

5. Psychology with a Chinese identity: a theoretical system or school of thought in psychology derived from methods, concepts, and principles which are rooted in, or derived from: (a) the religious- philosophical tradition, or (b) the mass culture of China. (A question arises: To what extent can these methods, concepts, principles be differentiated from those employed in other theoretical systems or schools of thought? At present, this question cannot be adequately answered, because a mature psychology with a Chinese identity has yet to emerge.)

The same broad interpretation is applied to the term *Chinese psychiatry*.

Periodicals from Mainland China, Taiwan, and Hong Kong

A special effort was made to search periodicals from the People's Republic of China (PRC), Taiwan, and Hong Kong. Most of these are not covered by PsycINFO or other databases. The following periodicals were exhaustively searched.

People's Republic of China.

1. *Acta Psychologica Sinica.* This journal is published by the Science Press. Publication began in 1956, was suspended from 1967 to 1978 on account of the Great Cultural Revolution, and was resumed in 1979. Editorial responsibility is assumed by the Chinese Psychological Society. Articles are written in Chinese, with abstracts in English. The journal has a wide circulation (30,000 copies in 1980) and has been abstracted in *Psychological Abstracts* since 1965.

2. *Chinese Journal of Neurology and Psychiatry.* This journal was published by the People's Hygiene Press, beginning from 1955. Publication was suspended during the Great Cultural Revolution, and was resumed in 1979, this time by the Chinese Medical Association. Editorial responsibility is assumed by the Chinese Society of Neurology and Psychiatry. Articles are written in Chinese, some with abstracts in English.

3. *Information on Psychological Sciences.* Previously published from 1964 till the beginning of the Great Cultural Revolution, this journal resumed publication in 1981. Editorial responsibility is assumed by the East China

Normal University in Shanghai on behalf on the Chinese Psychological Society. Articles are written in Chinese, some with abstracts in English.

4. *Journal of Psychology.* This journal started publication in 1986, by the Sichuan Institute of Education. Articles are written in Chinese.

Taiwan.

1. *Bulletin of Educational Psychology.* This bulletin has been published by the Department of Educational Psychology, National Taiwan Normal University, since 1967. It was named *Psychology and Education* from 1967 to 1971. Most articles are written in Chinese (with English abstracts), but a few are written in English.

2. *Bulletin of the Institute of Ethnology (Academia Sinica).* This bulletin has been published by the Institute of Ethnology, Academia Sinica, since 1956. Most articles are written in Chinese (with English abstracts), but some are written in Chinese. Many of the articles are of psychological or psychiatric significance.

3. *Chinese Journal of Mental Health: An Interdisciplinary Journal of Mental Health.* This journal has been published by the Chinese National Association for Mental Hygiene since 1984. Articles are written in Chinese, with abstracts in English.

4. *Chinese Journal of Psychology.* This journal has been published by the Chinese Psychological Association since 1984. From 1958 to 1983, it was named *Acta Psychological Taiwanica*, published by the Department of Psychology, National Taiwan University. Articles are in written in Chinese (with English abstracts) or English (with Chinese abstracts). The journal has been abstracted in *Psychological Abstracts* since 1958.

5. *Journal of Education and Psychology.* This journal has been published by the Graduate School of Education, National Chengchi University, since 1977. From 1977 to 1978, its English title was Research in Education and Psychology. Articles are written in Chinese, with abstracts in English.

6. *Psychological Testing.* This journal has been published by the Chinese Association of Psychological Testing since 1953. Articles are written in Chinese.

Hong Kong.

1. *Bulletin of the Hong Kong Psychological Society.* This bulletin has been published by the Hong Kong Psychological Society since 1978. Articles are written in English, although articles written in Chinese may also be accepted. The bulletin has been abstracted in *Psychological Abstracts*, *Human Resources Abstracts*, *Sage Urban Abstracts*, and *Sage Family Studies Abstracts* since 1982.

2. *Hong Kong Journal of Mental Health.* This journal has been published by the Mental Health Association of Hong Kong since 1972. Most articles are written in English, but a few are written in Chinese.

3. *Journal of the Hong Kong Psychiatric Association.* This journal has been published by the Hong Kong Psychiatric Association since 1981. Articles are written in English.

4. *New Horizons.* This journal of education is published by the Hong Kong Teachers' Association. Articles are written in English or Chinese.

Indexing

All items were indexed, using subject terms selected from the *Thesaurus of Psychological Index Terms* (American Psychological Association, 1985). We have added 15 terms which are particularly suitable for the literature. These are:

Chinese characters
Chinese medicine
Chinese thinkers
clanism
collectivism
culturocentrism
face
familism
filial piety
individualism
modernity
nepotism
relation centeredness
traditionalism
translation

For most records, 5 to 10 index terms were sufficient. The subject index was then derived from this indexing.

To facilitate efficient management and retrieval, all materials were input into a database managed by Cardbox-Plus software for bibliographic databases. Each record contained the citation, including the author(s), date(s) of publication, title, and publication information; index terms; language of publication; PsycINFO content classification category or categories (up to three); and, if available, the abstract as well as citation information on republication(s). The Cardbox-Plus software was used for all data-base management, searching, editing, sorting and listing.

PUBLICATION TRENDS

Quantitative Aspects

A statistical analysis of the database yielded some interesting data on publication trends. The data on publications are summarized in Table 1. A perusal of this table reveals the following trends and patterns.

1. The literature is really quite extensive. The present volume contains a total of 3,548 items. In this connection, it may be noted that an exhaustive compilation of the psychological literature in China from 1949 to 1982 by Nanjing University Library (1983) lists approximately 10,100 items (although most of these would not meet the criteria for inclusion in the present volume). In contrast, a computerized literature search by Domino (1985) yielded only 826 citations on psychology and psychiatry in the PRC, many of which were inaccessible, not in English, outdated, or irrelevant. The author considered 54 selected studies, published since 1970 and available in most university libraries, to be a thorough representation of what is currently known about Chinese psychology and psychiatry!

The number of publications has been increasing quite rapidly. On the average, there were fewer than 10 publications per year before 1955; in contrast, over 200 items have been published per year since 1980. The rapid increase in the volume of published materials is likely to continue. This may well be the last point in time that acquiring a comprehensive knowledge in the field is still with the grasp of scholars who are willing to make the effort. Increasingly, specialization will be forced upon scholars.

2. Frequency counts by content classification categories shows that approximately a quarter (25.8%) of the studies concern abnormal patterns of behavior--abnormal psychology and psychiatry (physical, psychological, and psychiatric disorders + treatment and prevention). Items in social (21.0%), developmental (13.4%), and educational psychology (10.2%) together comprise the bulk of studies pertaining to normal patterns of behavior. None of the remaining categories exceed 10%.

The paucity of items in applied psychology as well as in professional personnel and professional issues reflects the underdevelopment of professional (especially industrial) psychology in China. (In the cases of experimental psychology and physiological psychology, the paucity of items results largely from the criteria for selecting materials we established.)

3. Significantly, publications in English (61.0%) outnumber those in Chinese (37.4%) by a factor of 1.63. This reflects of the dominance of the English language in the world of scholarly publications. Prior to 1955, Chinese-language publications could hardly be found. (There are very few items in other languages, but this is because no special effort was made to search the literature in other languages.)

In terms of content classification, Chinese-language items exceed English-language ones in general psychology, developmental psychology, applied psychology, and especially psychometrics. The case of developmental psychology results from the fact that a large percentage of psychologists, in both the PRC and Taiwan, are in the educational-developmental field (and are employed in normal, i.e., teachers' training, colleges and universities). The case of psychometrics reflects the long-standing preoccupation Chinese psychologists in Taiwan have had with testing and measurement. Chinese-language publications are particularly deficient in the category of professional personnel and professional issues, reflecting a lack of concern with professional development. English-language items are particularly numerous in social psychology and, to a lesser extent, in abnormal psychology and psychiatry.

4. In terms of geopolitical community, the frequency ranking, in a descending order, is: PRC (25.8%), Taiwan (22.6%), and Hong Kong (12.4%). As expected, the majority of studies pertaining to both the PRC and Taiwan are conducted by Chinese researchers and are published in Chinese-language journals. Studies pertaining to Hong Kong, however, are predominantly in English; a large portion are found in international journals. Hong Kong seems to attract the attention of foreign researchers, out of proportion to its size. Perhaps this underscores Ho's (1986, p. 219) statement, "Hong Kong itself is an unprecedented sociopolitical experiment as well as a natural laboratory of cross-cultural interaction." There were, of course, no publications pertaining to the PRC prior to 1950. (The PRC came into being in 1949.) The decrease in frequency during the periods 1965-1969 and 1970-1974 reflects the destructive effects of the Great Cultural Revolution on scholarly research on the PRC, inside or outside mainland China. At any rate, the amount of research is totally inadequate, when gauged against the size and importance of the PRC as the world's largest geopolitical community. At the moment, it must be said that the lack of psychological and psychiatric studies in, and about, mainland China constitutes a serious deficiency in knowledge.

The interaction of geopolitical location and content classification reveals some interesting patterns. Items pertaining to the PRC are overrepresented in general psychology, experimental psychology, physiological psychology, communication systems, developmental psychology, and assessment, treatment, and prevention. The case of general psychology reflects the preoccupation with historical and philosophical issues by psychologists in the PRC. Underrepresentation is found in psychometrics, personality, and social psychology. It is instructive to compare these trends with a statistical analysis of articles published in the *Acta Psychological Sinica* from 1956-1984 (Guan, Wei, and Chen 1985; cf. Petzold 1986). The results show that the number of articles in educational and developmental psychology is the highest, followed by that in general psychology; relatively few articles deal with the solution of practical problems. As to Taiwan, overrepresentation is found in psychometrics, personality, and educational psychology. As stated above, the overrepresentation in psychometrics reflects the preoccupation with testing and measurement by psychologists in the Taiwan. Underrepresentation is found in physiological psychology and in professional personnel and professional issues. Hong Kong is overrepresented in physical, psychological, and psychiatric disorders, and especially in professional personnel and professional issues. The latter case reflects the fact that professional psychology, clinical psychology in particular, is far more developed in Hong Kong than in the PRC or Taiwan.

5. Chinese Americans have received considerable attention, especially since the mid-1970s, with 111 relevant citations or 3.1% of the total (according to the frequency of the subject term *Asian Americans*). This results directly from the overwhelming American superiority in manpower and material resources for research. It also reflects the enhanced consciousness about ethnicity in American society and the preoccupation of Asian Americans with issues of acculturation and ethnic identity. The majority of studies are in social psychology (40.5%) and abnormal psychology and psychiatry (28.8%).

Category	Total	Language			Geographical area			
		Chinese	English	Other	People's Republic of China	Taiwan	Hong Kong	U.S.
Language								
Chinese	1327	--	--	--	584	527	16	0
English	2166	--	--	--	318	273	422	111
Other languages	55	--	--	--	12	1	3	0
Geographical area								
People's Republic of China	914	584	318	12	--	--	--	--
Taiwan	801	527	273	1	--	--	--	--
Hong Kong	441	16	422	3	--	--	--	--
U.S. (Chinese Americans)	111	0	11	0	--	--	--	--
Content classification								
General psychology	201	112	84	5	106	8	10	1
Psychometrics	116	81	35	0	16	75	9	0
Experimental psychology	150	72	75	3	45	16	7	2
Physiological psychology	41	14	26	1	13	0	0	1
Communication systems	171	71	92	8	45	20	10	3
Developmental psychology	475	247	225	3	180	102	56	8
Personality	230	109	120	1	19	103	14	9
Social psychology	746	107	634	5	90	143	104	45
Educational psychology	361	178	178	5	77	150	40	8
Applied psychology	104	65	38	1	31	44	9	1
Physical, psychological, and psychiatric disorders	507	153	346	8	123	88	96	16
Assessment, treatment, and prevention	407	114	278	15	160	51	66	16
Professional personnel and professional issues	39	4	35	0	9	1	20	1
Total	3548	1327	2166	55	914	801	441	111

Table 1. Breakdown of bibliographic citations by language,

Time period										
1887-1939	40-44	45-49	50-54	55-59	60-64	65-69	70-74	75-79	80-84	85-86
Language (cont'd)										
11	1	1	16	110	145	101	102	219	416	205
54	11	22	32	52	82	182	387	461	648	235
1	1	0	0	0	1	5	4	15	28	0
Geographical area (cont'd)										
0	0	0	3	63	106	38	55	125	343	181
1	1	0	15	40	59	82	124	207	200	72
0	0	0	0	8	9	29	49	86	171	89
4	1	1	9	5	7	11	19	38	16	0
Content classification (cont'd)										
7	0	0	0	12	19	8	10	31	92	22
0	1	0	6	7	19	11	10	23	29	10
7	0	0	0	1	10	4	17	32	45	34
0	0	0	0	1	0	0	5	5	25	5
4	0	0	0	2	13	18	21	35	58	20
4	2	4	3	8	35	37	57	78	182	65
20	0	5	8	11	17	37	32	41	38	21
12	8	11	18	17	28	83	172	158	187	52
1	0	0	4	11	32	32	52	87	106	36
1	0	1	1	13	8	8	3	19	32	18
6	2	1	6	39	32	36	54	92	151	88
4	0	1	2	40	15	13	54	85	134	59
0	0	0	0	0	0	1	6	9	13	10
66	13	23	48	162	228	288	493	695	1092	440

geographical area, and time period.

Further insight may be gained from an examination of the subject terms used for indexing citations. These terms are grouped according to geographical area, subject population, and topic, in a descending order of frequency. (The frequency of single-word subject terms includes those of compound terms in which the single word appears. Terms with a frequency count of less than 50 are not shown.)

Sampling

591 children
495 students
271 adults
265 school age children
239 Asians
237 college students
226 adolescents
111 Asian Americans
111 preschool age children
75 junior high school students
74 high school students
66 patients
62 human females
53 psychiatric patients

Topic

411 cross cultural differences
322 personality
313 development
294 attitudes
257 psychology
244 disorders
232 sex
228 language
225 adulthood
220 health
192 history
190 perception
178 behavior
170 family
164 education
164 sociocultural factors
159 mental disorders
151 psychiatry
149 achievement
146 ethnic groups
146 learning
121 intelligence
117 cognitive development
114 age differences
106 personality traits
99 mental health
95 human sex differences
91 values
89 history of psychology
85 reading
83 treatment
82 cognitive processes
81 ability
77 philosophies
75 academic achievement
74 neurosis
73 countries
73 literature [including literature review]
70 Chinese characters
69 case report

69 epidemiology
68 adjustment
66 schizophrenia
65 sciences
64 test validity
61 socialization
59 written language
57 personnel
56 adolescence
56 stereotyped attitudes
56 teaching
54 memory
54 racial and ethnic differences
53 Chinese medicine
53 test construction
52 counseling
52 parent child relations
51 analysis
51 social change
50 mental health services

It may be seen that as many as 411 citations or 11.6% of the total involve cross-cultural comparisons; 54 citations or 1.5% involve cross-ethnic comparisons. In addition, the term *ethnic groups* is used for indexing 146 citations (4.1%), and countries for 73 citations (2.1%). This reflects both an interest in Chinese culture among foreign investigators and a high degree of importance attached to cross-cultural psychology among Chinese investigators. The term *United States* appears with a surprisingly high frequency of 127 (3.6%). This is because, when cross-cultural or cross-ethnic comparisons are made, the group with whom Chinese subjects are compared is typically American. It happens that Americans have been the most intensively studied national group--to the point where they have almost come to be taken as a standard reference group against which other national groups are compared. The point should be made, however, that the American pattern may be more atypical than typical in a world-wide perspective. This is yet another reason why other cultural or ethnic groups should be included in cross-cultural studies.

Frequencies of terms indexing subject populations indicate that children (16.7%), especially school-age children (7.5%), have most often been studied or used as research subjects--more than twice as frequently as adults (7.6%). Adolescents (6.4%) have been studied less frequently. A disproportionate amount of attention has been directed to females (1.7%) in comparison with males (0.6%). Among disordered populations, psychiatric patients (1.5%) have received the most attention. There is a heavy reliance on using students (14.0%), especially college students (6.7%), to serve as research subjects -- to the neglect of other subject populations. Apparently, researchers have been guided more by expediency than by relevance in their undertakings!

Qualitative Aspects

The present book does not purport to be an evaluation of the literature. Items were not selected or rejected on the basis of quality. Nevertheless, in the course of processing a vast amount of the relevant materials, the editors unavoidably formed impressions about their quality. A distillate of these impressions is what we would like to share with our readers.

A salient impression we have formed concerns the imbalance between quantity and quality. Too many studies lack substance or are poorly written! There is a dearth of insightful or creative theoretical formulations; methodological weaknesses abound in empirical studies. The problem sometimes goes deeper and concerns the very trustworthiness of the data presented, or of the appropriateness and accuracy of the statistical analyses performed. If quality were a criterion for inclusion, a large portion of the items in this book would be eliminated.

The literature on thought and action in Chinese culture suffers not so much from a lack of empirical data as from a lack of data quality, an inability of investigators to interpret and present findings meaningfully, and a lack of integration between evidence and theory construction. In particular, anyone who is familiar with the periodicals in the PRC or Taiwan cannot fail to notice that the amount of empirical data gathered by researchers is considerable, involving not infrequently huge sample sizes. But, alas, too often they result from unimaginative research or thoughtless replications of western studies. Or worse, they do not result from concept-driven research: attempts to answer theoretical questions on the basis of collected data; rather, they result from what appears to be instrument-driven activity: the collection of data prompted by the mere availability of measuring instruments (most of which are western in origin). Psychologists, no less than others, sometimes owe their identity to the instruments they use!

Against this background, it is gratifying to note that, in recent years, Chinese researchers have shown increasing awareness of the problem of blind copying from the west. This awareness was translated into concrete action when a conference on the sinicization of social and behavioral science research was organized in Taiwan in 1980. The conference proceedings (Yang and Wen 1982) has been published. Another volume of collected essays on modernization and sinicization (Li, Yang, and Wen 1985) has also appeared.

Another problem is the lack of communication and cooperation among researchers. Uncoordinated, rather than collaborative, efforts have characterized their activities; and compartmentalized rigidity, rather than permeability, has characterized the flow of information. Each individual or group of individuals seem to be doing their own thing. Researchers are often uninformed about the work of others, particularly those outside of their own academic discipline; and, understandably, foreign investigators are typically ignorant about studies published in Chinese. Research results are often published in journals or monographs with circulations limited largely to small inner circles. Against this background, two edited books on the psychology of Chinese people, one in English (Bond 1966) and another in Chinese (Yang 1988), represent encouraging collective efforts recently made.

People's Republic of China. As to the PRC, theoretical questions about the direction of development that psychology should take do not give rise merely to idle academic discussions. They have serious ideological implications. How can psychology serves the needs of socialist reconstruction? How can conflicting ideologies be reconciled within psychology? Will a new psychology emerge, philosophically based on dialectical materialism? Or one bearing distinctively the unique features of Chinese socialism? These questions, it should be observed, have not generated empirical research. And thus it is fair to say that no systematic position or school of thought based on an interplay between theory construction and empirical research has yet emerged.

In any case, the reinstatement of psychology and of psychiatry-- indeed, of scholarship in general--after the fall of the Gang of Four (see Ching 1980; Pan 1979) is one of the most important recent events in the world of learning. Previously information on these disciplines was extremely limited. Most published materials were written by foreigners; of these, political scientists and other social scientists interested in China predominated. Through no fault of their own, foreign researchers had to rely on methods of investigation-at-a-distance, such as content analysis of cultural products, interviews conducted with emigres, and reports from professionals who had visited China. In the last few years, a number of foreign investigators have been able to conduct research within China, but such opportunities remain limited.

Significantly, since the late 1970s, psychological articles by mainland Chinese authors have appeared in international journals, and non-Chinese authors have contributed to PRC periodicals. Presently mainland psychologists are more receptive to Western psychology than they have ever been since 1949. The influence of Russian psychology has declined. In an analysis of 595 articles published in two psychology journals since 1979, Petzold (1986) found that, of the foreign sources cited (including Russian), English citations are the most frequent. However, Chinese (PRC) sources are still cited more frequently than English sources, except in the area of physiological psychology. Public consciousness about psychology and popular demands for psychological knowledge are rapidly growing. Psychology has not only recovered from the devastation of the Great Cultural Revolution but also found a new mission -- to contribute to the Four Modernizations. It is here to stay on the academic and cultural scene!

Nevertheless, it remains the case that psychology lags behind other social sciences which, in turn, lag behind the physical sciences. (Sociology is farther behind.) And among the medical specialities, psychiatry occupies a rather low order of priority. Underdevelopment results from not only lack of quantity but also restricted scope of research. In the PRC literature, one finds a continued preoccupation with classical, often trivial, problems that absorbed the attention of academicians in the early history of scientific psychology and psychiatry, but very little exploration into new directions. This restricted scope follows from definition: Both psychology and psychiatry appear to be more narrowly defined than they are in other countries. Thus social psychology is just beginning to make its appearance (cf. Petzold 1986); as yet, social and cultural psychiatry is nowhere to be found.

Implications. We hope that our honest expression of dissatisfaction with the quality of the literature will have, nonetheless, constructive consequences. We feel that the key to redress the imbalance between quantity and quality lies in quality control in the publication machinery which, in turn, hinges on an impartial system of peer evaluation and the strict observance of editorial responsibility. In this connection, it is of significance to note that a system of blind review of submissions was instituted for the Hong Kong Journal of Mental Health in 1984 and the Bulletin of the Hong Kong Psychological Society in 1987.

It is sad to reflect on the fact that there is not a single Chinese periodical in psychology or psychiatry which is authoritative and internationally recognized. It is sadder to contemplate the probability that, if such a journal were to appear, it might be in the United States rather than in China. The Chinese-language literature in general, it has to be admitted, has had virtually no impact on contemporary mainstream thinking in psychology or psychiatry. But we look forward to the day when, with better quality control, it will assume its rightful place in the world's behavioral science and psychiatric literature. Encouraging signs in this direction can already be discerned.

REFERENCES

American Psychological Association. (1985). *Thesaurus of psychological index terms (4th ed.)*. Washington, DC: Author.

Ching, C. C. (1980). Psychology in the People's Republic of China. *American Psychologist, 35,* 1084-1089.

Bond, M. H. (Ed.). (1986). *The psychology of the Chinese people.* Hong Kong: Oxford University Press.

Domino, G. (1985). Psychology and psychiatry in the People's Republic of China: An annotated bibliography. *Professional Psychology: Research and Practice, 16,* 529-539.

Ho, D. Y. F. (1986). Psychology in Hong Kong. *International Journal of Psychology, 21,* 213-223.

Guan, L. R, Wei, M. X., and Chen, Y. M. [A statistical analysis of monographs published in "Acta Psychological Sinica", 1956- 1984]. *Acta Psychologica Sinica, 17,* 327-331. (In Chinese.)

Li, Y. Y., Yang, K. S., and Wen, C. I. (Eds.). (1982). [*Collected essays on modernization and sinicization*]. Taipei: Kuei Kuan. (In Chinese.)

Nanjing University Library (Compiler). (1983). [*Index of the psychological literature in China (1949-1982)*]. Nanjing: Nanjing University. (In Chinese.)

Pan, S. (1979). [Chinese psychology in the new period of development]. *Acta Psychologica Sinica, 11,* 1-9. (In Chinese.)

Petzold, M. (1986). Psychology in the People's Republic of China--A historical overview and quantitative analysis. *Psychologia, 29,* 57-65.

Yang, K. S. (Ed.). (1988). [*Psychology of Chinese people*]. Taipei: Kuei Kuan. (In Chinese.)

Yang, K. S., & Wen, C. I. (Eds.). (1982). [*The sinicization of social and behavioral science research in China*]. Taipei: Academia Sinica, Institute of Ethnology. (In Chinese.)

GENERAL PSYCHOLOGY 2

Frequency data on citations in this chapter, in terms of content classification subcategories, are presented in Table 2.

Table 2: *Number of Citations by Content Classification, Language, and Geographical Area*

Content classification	Total	CL	EL	OL	PRC	T	HK	US
General psychology	36	12	23	1	22	2	6	0
Parapsychology	7	1	6	0	3	0	0	0
History, philosophies, and theories	152	96	52	4	81	6	2	0
Research methods, apparatus, and computer applications	6	3	3	0	0	0	2	1
Total	201	112	84	5	106	8	10	1

Note: CL = Chinese language; EL = English language; OL = other languages. PRC = People's Republic of China; T = Taiwan; HK = Hong Kong; US = United States (Chinese Americans--according to the frequency of the subject term Asian Americans).

Subject terms used for indexing citations related to general psychology are grouped according to geographical area and topic. These are presented below, in a descending order of frequency. (The frequency of single-word subject terms includes those of compound terms in which the single word appears. Subjects terms used for indexing citations from other chapters may have been included, because some citations have more than one--up to three--content classification category. Therefore, the frequency of a subject term may exceed that used for indexing citations in the present chapter alone. Terms with a frequency of less than 10 are not shown.)

Geographical area

112	Peoples Republic of China
76	Asia
10	Hong Kong

Topic

130	psychology
99	history
70	history of psychology
57	philosophies
2	Chinese thinkers
27	organizations
27	professional organizations
24	conference proceedings
23	literature
18	sciences
13	materialism
13	theories
11	politics
10	literature review

Table 2 shows that the majority of citations (75.6%) belong to the subcategory of history, philosophies, and theories. Of these, the majority pertain to the PRC. The subject term *Chinese thinkers* appears with a notably high frequency, pointing to the great interest psychologists in the PRC have on psychological thought in the Chinese religious-philosophical tradition.

The history and status of psychology in the PRC has received considerable attention from both Chinese and foreign scholars, as can be seen from published book-length contributions (Brown 1981; Chin and Chin 1969; Gao 1985) and reviews (Executive Committee of the Chinese Psychological Society 1982; Kao 1985; Petzold 1987). A number of books (Pan 1983; Yan 1981, 1983) devoted to psychological thought in historical China have been written by psychologists in the PRC.

REFERENCES

Brown, L. B. (1981). *Psychology in contemporary China*. Oxford: Pergamon Press.

Chin, R., & Chin, A. L. S. (1969). *Psychological research in Communist China: 1949-1966*. Cambridge, MA: MIT Press.

The Executive Committee of the Chinese Psychological Society. (1982). [Retrospect and prospect of 60 years of psychology in China: In commemoration of the 60th anniversary of the founding of the Chinese Psychological Society]. *Acta Psychologica Sinica, 14*(2), 127-138. (In Chinese.)

Gao, J. F. et al. (Eds.). (1985). [*History of Chinese psychology*]. Beijing: People's Education Press. (In Chinese.)

Kao, S. R. (1985). [Psychology in Mainland China: Review and preview of research developments: (1949-1985)] [Tenth Anniversary Special Issue]. *The China Tribune, 21*(1), 137-150. (In Chinese.)

Pan, S. (Ed.). (1983). [*A study of psychological thought in ancient China*]. Nanchang, Jiangxi: People's Press. (In Chinese.)

Petzold, M. (1987). The social history of Chinese psychology. In M. G. Ash & W. R. Woodward (Eds.), *Psychology in twentieth- century thought and society* (pp. 213-231). Cambridge: Cambridge University Press.

Yan, G. C. (1981). [*A study of Pre-Qin psychological thought*]. Hunan People's Press. (In Chinese.)

Yan, G. C. (1983). [*A study of psychological thought during the Han, Wei, and the Six Dynasties*]. Hunan People's Press. (In Chinese.)

1

[A glossary of general psychological terms]. **(1935). Shanghai: Commercial Press.** (In Chinese.)

2

[A glossary of psychological terms]. **(1974). Taipei: Wen Ching Press.** (In Chinese.)

3

Anderson, E. N. (1984). "Heating and cooling" foods re-examined. *Social Science Information, 23,* **755-773.**

The history of humoral medicine, particularly the traditional Chinese classification of diseases as hot or cold and foods as heating or cooling, was reviewed. It was shown that this system involves several nutritional beliefs that are potentially beneficial. The formation of such patterns of beliefs was considered in relation to recent work in cognitive social psychology, and it was suggested that these beliefs persist not only because they are occasionally correct but also because they are easy to learn and use. The potential usefulness of these beliefs in teaching nutrition was discussed.

4

Banerjee, S. (1986). Reproduction of social structures: An artificial intelligence model. *Journal of Conflict Resolution, 30,* **221-252.**

The author argued that an enduring social structure is a pattern of action that reproduces itself by stimulating and reinforcing the schemata animating its actions. These concepts are operationalized by an artificial intelligence program written in PROLOG that takes as a knowledge base a representation of the preferences and judgments of social causality of subjects in some historical situation. This computer model of social interaction is illustrated by a simulation of T. Skocpol's analysis of China's sociopolitical structure in the 1930s and G. O'Donnell's analysis of the Latin American bureaucratic-authoritarian structure of the 1960s.

5

Basic Theory Department, Institute of Psychology, Chinese Academy of Sciences. (1985). [A general view on the development of basic-theory study in psychology both within and without China in 1970s and early 1980s]. *Information on Psychological Sciences,* **No. 2, 1-6.** (In Chinese.)

6

Blomeyer, R. (1977). [An I Ching experiment]. *Analytische Psychologie, 8,* **130-145.** (In other language.)

The I Ching, a compilation of Chinese nature philosophy, is traditionally used as an oracle. The author hypothesized that such an ambiguously worded text, applicable to a variety of situations, lends itself to the illusion that each reading corresponds to one's situation. To test this hypothesis, 5 series of 64 trials each were conducted. In the 1st series, readings were obtained by the researcher throwing dice directly before a psychotherapeutic session, posing questions about the important contents of the therapeutic hour. The researcher was impressed by the number of apparent correspondences. No matter how he varied the procedure in the following trials, however, including arbitrarily assigning readings in numerical sequence, he continued to find 20-50% apparent correspondence between the I Ching reading and the content to be predicted. It appears practically impossible not to find correspondences, given the nature of the text and the subjective readiness to construe a good fit. Psi phenomena could be neither verified nor ruled out. No criteria emerged to distinguish meaningful from chance correspondences.

7

Blowers, G., & Wong, T. (1983 - 1984). Questions of psychology [Interviews with Erik Kvan] [Special double issue]. *Hong Kong Psychological Society Bulletin,* **Nos. 11-12.**

8

Bond, M. (1980). Presidential address 1980. *Hong Kong Psychological Society Bulletin,* **No. 5, 45-48.**

9

Bond, M. H. (Ed.). (1986). *The psychology of the Chinese people.* **Hong Kong: Oxford University Press.**

This edited book contains chapters written by authors in Hong Kong and Taiwan on the psychology of Chinese people. The literature, drawn from both Chinese and English language sources, is extensively reviewed.

10

Brown, L. B. (1981). *Psychology in contemporary China.* **Oxford: Pergamon Press.**

This book not only takes a thorough look at Chinese psychology, but also includes extensive translations of excerpts from Acta Psychologica Sinica.

11

Brown, L. B. (1983). Social psychology in China. *British Journal of Social Psychology, 22,* **363-372.**

Describes the development of psychology in China from 1917 with special reference to the political constraints on accepting social psychology after the Liberation in 1949 but particularly during the Cultural Revolution. Throughout this period, Western social psychology was criticized for its bourgeois orientation and insensitivity to a class analysis. Since 1980, however, a role for social psychology has been acknowledged with respect to analysis and training in management and education.

12

Brozek, J. (1983). Study of the history of psychology around the world: Recent institutional and organizational development. *Revista de Historia de la Psicologia*, **4, 293-345.**

The present paper presented overviews on developments concerning the history, publications, professional meetings, academia, and research trends of psychology in Asia and the Pacific area, China, Europe, Czechoslovakia, East and West Germany, Great Britain, the U.S.S.R., Canada, the U.S., and South America.

13

Chai, W. X. (1981). [Thoughts of sport psychology in ancient China]. *Acta Psychologica Sinica*, *13*, **124-128.** (In Chinese.)

14

Chang, T. S. (1938). [Thought, language, and culture]. *Sociological World*, *10*. **(Translated by A. C. Li,** *Yenching Journal of Social Studies*, **1939,** *1*, **155-191. Reprinted in** *ETC: A Review of General Semantics*, **1952,** *9*, **203-226; and in G. P. Stone & H. A. Farberman (Eds.),** *Social psychology through symbolic interaction* **("A Chinese philosopher's theory of knowledge"). Toronto: Ginn-Blaisdell, 1970.)** (In Chinese.)

15

Che, W. B., & Guo, Z. J. (1979). [Thirty years of Chinese theoretical psychology]. *Acta Psychologica Sinica*, *11*, **267-280.** (In Chinese.)

Summarizes Chinese theoretical psychology during the past 30 yrs. The authors present a brief historical background, then proceed to describe some disputes in basic theoretical problems. The directions of future development of Chinese theoretical psychology are pointed out.

16

Chen, D. J. (1960). [The Second Congress of the Chinese Psychological Society]. *Acta Psychologica Sinica*, **No. 2, 128-131.** (In Chinese.)

17

Chen, D. J. (1964). [The 1963 annual meeting of the Chinese Psychological Society]. *Acta Psychologica Sinica*, **No. 1, 109-112.** (In Chinese.)

18

Chen, D. R. (1979). [Wundt's contributions to scientific psychology at Hiedelberg]. *Acta Psychologica Sinica*, *11*, **365-373.** (In Chinese.)

Reviews the psychological works of W. Wundt (1855-1874), which contributed toward making psychology a distinctive scientific discipline because of Wundt's spontaneous, naive materialism as a natural scientist. Some of his intellectual influences on today's psychology in China are considered.

19

Chen, L., & Wang, A. S. (1979). [Hold on to scientific experimentation in psychology]. *Acta Psychologica Sinica*, *11*, **10-16.** (In Chinese.)

Prior to the Great Cultural Revolution in China, articles were published that opposed psychological research, especially its experimental methods. An analysis and criticism of these articles is presented. The authors point out that the founders of Marxism-Leninism repeatedly stressed the point that psychology is a science, but psychological research has demonstrated itself to be of benefit to social practice as well.

20

Chen, T. J. (1959). [How psychology can be of service to the socialistic reconstruction]. *Acta Psychologica Sinica*, **No. 3, 142-145. (Translated by U.S. Joint Publications Research Service, No. 3,424,** *Articles on psychology in Communist China*, **pp. 3-10.)** (In Chinese.)

21

Chen, Y. G. (1982). [On Confucius' thoughts on educational psychology]. *Acta Psychologica Sinica*, *14*, **466-472.** (In Chinese.)

22

Chen, Y. H. (1960). [Learn Mao Tse-tung thought and raise the theoretical level of psychology]. *Acta Psychologica Sinica*, **No. 3, 138-144.** (In Chinese.)

23

Chen, Y. H. (1965). [Critique on modern bourgeois social psychology]. *Acta Psychologica Sinica*, *2*, **106-113.** (In Chinese.)

24

Cheng, C., & Ciao, D. (1981). [Annual Academic Conference of medical psychology yields successful results in many respects]. *Acta Psychologica Sinica*, *13*, **247.** (In Chinese.)

25

Cheng, F. M. (1970). [A summary of the recent researches on the elementary school intelligence tests]. *Psychological Testing*, *17*, **743-756.** (In Chinese.)

26

Chin, R., & Chin, A. L. S. (1969). *Psychological research in Communist China: 1949-1966.* **Cambridge, MA: MIT Press.**

27

Chin, W. (1975). The struggle between two different world outlooks in the conception of the human body. *Scientia Sinica, 18,* **412-424.**

28

Chinese Society of Neurology and Psychiatry. (1969). [*Chinese and English version of diagnostic terms in neurology and psychiatry*]. **Taipei: Author.** (In Chinese.)

29

[*Chinese translation of psychological terms*]. **(1982). Hong Kong: The Chinese University Press.** (In Chinese.)

30

Ching, C. C. (1979, September/October). [An interview]. *APA Monitor,* **pp. 21-22.**

31

Ching, C. C. (1980). Psychology in the People's Republic of China. *American Psychologist, 35,* **1084-1089.**

Describes 5 periods of the development of psychology in China: (a) the beginnings of Chinese psychology (1910-1948), (b) psychology in the early days of the People's Republic of China (1949-1957), (c) the period of growth and development (1958-1965), (d) the attack on psychology by the Gang of Four (1966-1975), and (e) the revival of psychology since 1976. Development of psychology after the founding of the People's Republic of China in 1949 is emphasized, and its disruption between 1966 and 1975, as well as the progress made in its reconstruction since 1976, is also stressed.

32

Ching, C. C. (1983). [The current state of psychological science in China]. *Psikologicheskii Zhurnal, 4,* **155-158.** (In other language.)

The modern period of development for Chinese psychology began when Chinese scientists familiarized themselves with Western psychology. The first psychology lecture took place in 1917 at Peking University: in 1921, the Chinese Psychological Society was created. Some early experiments dealt with the perception of size and distance and the connection between illumination and sight. There was also work on neurophysiological and biochemical components of memory and learning. In clinical practice, Chinese psychologists created a psychotherapeutic group that dealt with the speed of the synthetic therapy of neurasthenia. The method involved both drug and physical therapy with traditional Chinese exercises. In the 1960's, psychologists studied the human being-machine system. After the cultural revolution, psychology was directed to serve 4 areas: industry, agriculture, science and technology, and defense. Applied psychological research flourished.

33

Ching, C. C. (1984). Psychology and the four modernizations in China. *International Journal of Psychology, 19,* **57-63.**

Reviews the development of Chinese psychology from the early 1900's to the present time, with particular emphasis on the period after 1949 when Chinese psychology was faced with the task of reestablishment. Progress as well as drawbacks are described. At present, China is in the process of modernizations in industry, agriculture, science and technology, and defense. The Four Modernizations have opened up new prospects for psychological research, particularly social psychology and applied psychology, which could contribute to China's national aspirations. It is concluded that a culturally specific psychology is necessary to meet the demands of conditions in China. While the emphasis is now on the impact of psychology on Third World countries, the outcome may actually depend on the impact of Third World development on psychology.

34

Chou, S. K. (1927). Trends in Chinese psychological interests since 1922. *American Journal of Psychology, 38,* **487-488.**

35

Chou, S. K. (1927). The present status of psychology in China. *American Journal of Psychology, 38,* **664-666.**

36

Chu, C. H. (1962). [Some problems of internal contradictions in human psyche]. *Acta Psychologica Sinica, 1,* **1-8.** (In Chinese.)

37

Department of Education, Shanxi Normal University (1979). [Thirty years of Chinese psychology]. *Acta Psychologica Sinica, 11,* **255-266.** (In Chinese.)

Divides the 30 yrs development of Chinese psychology into 4 main periods: The 1st period (1949-1958) has been characterized by the learning of Marxism-Leninism, Pavlov's theory and Soviet psychology, the criticism of bourgeois psychology, and some preliminary experimental research. The 2nd period (1959-1965) was that of rapid development and proliferation of psychology. In the 3rd period (1966-1976) Chinese psychology was at a halt due to the interference of the "Gang of Four". With the victory over the Gang of Four begins the 4th period (1976-1979) in which Chinese psychology enters an era of vigorous development.

38

Department of Education, Shanxi Normal University. (1980). [Thirty years of Chinese child and educational psychology]. *Acta Psychologica Sinica, 12,* **127-134.** (In Chinese.)

39

Domino, G. (1985). Psychology and psychiatry in the People's Republic of China: An annotated bibliography. *Professional Psychology: Research and Practice, 16,* **529-539.**

The author summarized 54 studies, published since 1970 and available in most university libraries, that represent a thorough analysis of what is currently known about Chinese psychology and psychiatry. The bibliography was selected from a computerized literature search yielding 826 citations, much of which were inaccessible, not in English, totally irrelevant, or outdated.

40

DuBois, P. H. (1964). A test-dominated society: China, 1115 B.C.-1905 A.D. In A. Anastasi (Ed.), *Testing problems in perspective: 25th Anniversary volume of topical readings from the Invitational Conference on Testing Problems* **(pp. 29-36). (Reprinted in W. L. Barnette, Jr. (Ed.),** *Readings in psychological tests and measurements* **(pp. 249-255). New York: Dorsey Press, 1976.)**

41

Ebon, M. (1981). Parapsychology in contemporary China. *Parapsychology Review, 12,* **1-5.**

Discusses the efforts made in China since 1979, as part of the "four modernizations", to develop theory and research in parapsychology. The ways that the Chinese have fitted parapsychology into a Marxist framework are outlined; recent research on children who seemed to be able to "read with their ears" is described; and some predictions about the future of parapsychology in China are presented.

42

Editorial Office of Acta Psychologica Sinica. (1983). [Psychology should enthusiastically serve the construction of socialistic modernization]. *Acta Psychologica Sinica, 15,* **241-243.** (In Chinese.)

43

[*English-Chinese Dictionary of Psychology*]. **(1981). Beijing: Science Press.** (In Chinese.)

44

Fan, Y. C. (1969). [The discontinuation of psychological testing by the Examination Yuan: Dedicated to the memory of the late presidents of the CAPT, Joseph W. Ai and F. K. Wang]. *Psychological Testing, 16,* **565-566.** (In Chinese.)

45

Gao, J. F. (1984). Brief history of the historiography of psychology in China [Essays in honor of Prof. Joseph Brozek, Monograph]. *Revista de Historia de la Psicologia* **(Valencia),** *5,* **183-185.**

The historiography of psychology in China was outlined from its beginnings in the 1920s to the publication of a history of modern Western psychology in 1982.

46

Gao, J. F. et al. (Eds.). (1985). [History of Chinese psychology]. Beijing: People's Education Press. (In Chinese.)

47

Gardner, H. (1980). China's born-again psychology. *Psychology Today, 14,* **45-50.**

48

Gilbert, A. R. (1973). An essay on the history of Asian psychology. *Proceedings of the 81st Annual Convention of the American Psychological Association, 8,* **937-938.**

49

Guan, L. R. (1981). [The delegation of American psychologists visiting China]. *Acta Psychologica Sinica, 13,* **243-245.** (In Chinese.)

50

Guan, L. R., Wei, M. X., & Chen, Y. M. (1985). [A statistical analysis of monographs published in "Acta Psychologica Sinica", 1956-1984]. *Acta Psychologica Sinica, 17,* **327-331.** (In Chinese.)

Analysis shows that the number of publications concerning educational and developmental psychology is the highest, followed by those on general psychology. The authors mainly come from research institutions, but those from universities have increased recently. The bulk of contributors are from Beijing, Shanghai, and Hangzhou. Papers dealing with the solutions to practical problems are relatively few.

51

Han, L. (1981). [The 1st Annual Conference of the CPA Division of General & Experimental Psychology]. *Acta Psychologica Sinica, 13,* **246.** (In Chinese.)

52

Heider, J. (1982). The leader who knows how things happen. *Journal of Humanistic Psychology*, *22*, **33-39.**

The author presents 12 of the original 181 chapters of Lao Tzu's sixth-century BC Chinese text Tao Te Ching, on how to rule a kingdom and lead a wise life. This text has been adapted for use by group leaders and humanistic educators. These particular chapters deal with the characteristics of a wise leader.

53

Ho, D. Y. F. (1972). Field studies in foreign cultures: A cautionary note on methodological difficulties. *Psychologia*, *15*, **15-21.**

The present paper argued for the necessity of a thorough consideration of certain methodological issues as a precondition for sound field research in foreign cultures. A detailed case study illustrated how a failure in dealing with these issues can lead to difficulties in both the observation and interpretation of events. Observational reports in foreign studies are to be viewed as accounts of the interaction between members of different cultures -- as it is perceived and related by the foreign investigator. Accordingly, a study of how members of different cultures interact is propaedeutic to these research undertakings. Several aspects of this interactional process were discussed: (a) The difficulties in communications, (b) the perceptions of the investigator as a function of ethnocentric bias and social distance from the indigenous people, and (c) the disturbance of the very phenomenon under investigation resulting from the observation itself.

54

Ho, D. Y. F. (1978). The conception of man in Mao Tse-tung Thought. *Psychiatry*, *41*, **391-402.**

Discusses the philosophic assumptions about human nature embodied in Mao Tse-tung Thought, the guide to action in the Chinese revolution, and how these assumptions are linked to Mao's political ideology. The relevance of Mao's conception of human nature for contemporary psychology is explained.

55

Ho, D. Y. F. (1978). Reflections on the development of psychology in Hong Kong society: Students, teachers, and academic institutions. In M. Akita (Ed.), *Proceedings of the 1st Planning Committee for a Pan-Asian Conference of Psychology* **(pp. 75- 89), Kyoto, Japan. (Republished in** *Philippine Journal of Psychology*, **1980,** *13*, **34-39.)**

This paper reviews the development of psychology in Hong Kong society, focusing especially on the academic sphere. Encouraging achievements are noted, although serious problems arising from the transplantation of Western psychology into foreign soil may be discerned. Remarks by psychology teachers, made in private, reflect their concern that there is a basic incompatibility between the conceptual approach and values of Western psychology, as they are taught to students, and the readiness with which students are willing or able to integrate them into their lives. The remarks also point to a remarkable encapsulation and retreat from self-knowledge among students. It is argued that a radical change in the approach to psychology in Hong Kong is needed: to help students to relate psychology to life and, more generally, to work toward a creative synthesis of Eastern and Western ideas--to create a new psychology, one which has indigenous roots and which will not leave the individual with a sense of alienation from his culture.

56

Ho, D. Y. F. (1982). Asian psychology. *International Psychologist*, *23*, **21-22.**

57

Ho, D. Y. F. (1982). Asian concepts in behavioral science. *Psychologia: An International Journal of Psychology in the Orient*, *25*, **228-235. (Republished in** *Bulletin of the Hong Kong Psychological Society*, **1983,** *10*, **41-49.)**

Reviews the use of six key concepts in behavioral science from three Asian cultures: the Chinese concepts of filial piety, ^jen^, and face; the Japanese concepts of ^amae^ and ^on^ ; and the Filipino concept of ^utang-la-loob^. The relational character of Asian concepts, in contrast to the individualistic character of Western concepts (e.g., self, ego, and actor) is discussed. It is argued that these concepts provide powerful conceptual tools that promise to free behavioral science from its overreliance on Western individualistic concepts.

58

Ho, D. Y. F. (1983). Comment on "Analogy and mysticism and the structure of culture". *Current Anthropology*, *24*, **169.**

59

Ho, D. Y. F. (1986). Psychology in Hong Kong. *International Journal of Psychology*, *21*, **213-223.**

Western psychology has had only a brief history in Hong Kong. However, it has grown considerably in the last two decades and is now firmly established academically and professionally. Currently, the Hong Kong Psychological Society has about 200 members and affiliates. Postgraduate training in research and in professional (clinical and educational) psychology is offered on a limited scale. Academic psychologists are active in research and in international bodies. Among practitioners, clinical psychologists number about 60 and educational psychologists about 20--already among the largest in Asia. Two considerations are paramount in discussing future directions: to develop a psychology with indigenous roots, and to face the challenge of changing sociopolitical realities posed by the return of Hong Kong to China's sovereignty in 1997.

60

Hsiao, S. (1977). Psychology in China. *American Psychologist, 32,* **374-376.**

Based on meetings with Chinese psychologists, a report is presented indicating that psychologists in the People's Republic of China are engaged in research concerning theory, Chinese language, child development, vision, audition, and areas of physiological psychology including acupuncture, pain, memory, and CNS functioning. The Institute of Psychology within the Chinese Academy of Sciences represents the center for psychological research.

61

Hsu, L. (1978). Some psychological investigations in the People's Republic of China. *Australian Psychologist, 13,* **359-367.**

This article presents an overview of research projects carried out by the Institute of Psychology of the Chinese Academy of Sciences. These projects were listed under four major categories: (a) sensory and perceptual processes, (b) physiological psychology, (c) genetic psychology, and (d) acupuncture anesthesia.

62

Hu, W. K. (1961). [The discussion of some psychological problems in the light of dialectical materialism]. *Acta Psychologica Sinica,* **No. 1, 1-12.** (In Chinese.)

63

Huang, C. H., Du, W. D., & He, W. B. (1984). [Psychohygienic ideas in the Nei Jing]. *Information on Psychological Sciences,* **No. 6, 34-37.** (In Chinese.)

64

Hwang, K. K. (1985). [The development of psychology in Taiwan over a forty-year period] [Tenth Anniversary Special Issue]. *The China Tribune, 21,* **120-136.** (In Chinese.)

65

Institute of Psychology, Academica Sinica. (1979). [The division of basic psychological theories in the Psychological Society of China was set up in Beijing]. *Acta Psychologica Sinica, 11,* **252-254.** (In Chinese.)

66

Iwahara, S. (1963). Oriental psychology. In M. H. Marx and W. A. Hillix (Eds.), *Systems and theories in psychology* **(pp. 456-72). New York: McGraw-Hill.**

67

Iwahara, S. (1977). Asia: Psychology. In B. B. Wolman (Ed.), *International encyclopedia of psychiatry, psychology, psychoanalysis, and neurology* **(Vol. 2, pp. 152-154). New York: Aesculapius.**

68

Jung, C. G. (1958). Forward to the I Ching. In H. Read, M. Fordham, & G. Adler (Eds.), *The collected works of C. G. Jung* **(Vol. 11). London: Routledge & Kegan Paul.**

69

Jung, C. J. (1967). Commentary on "The Secret of the Golden Flower". In H. Read, M. Fordham, G. Alder, & W. McGuire (Eds.), *The collected works of C. G. Jung: Vol. 13. Alchemical studies* **(pp. 1-56). London: Routledge & Kegan Paul.**

70

Kao, S. R. (1985). [Psychology in Mainland China: Review and preview of research developments: (1949-1985)] [Tenth Anniversary Special Issue]. *The China Tribune, 21,* **137-150.** (In Chinese.)

71

Kelman, H. (1958). Communing and relating: Vol. 2. The mind structure of East and West. *American Journal of Psychoanalysis, 18,* **158-170.**

The guiding principle in the mind structure of the East is juxtaposition and identity whereas in the West it is unity and variety. "By mind structure is meant an inherent guiding principle that shapes the perception of people in how they see the world and live in it, and ask and answer all the big questions, such as Who am I? What am I? What is life? What is death?" Time has entirely different functions in the East and West. Eastern cognition is interested in consciousness itself. Western cognition is interested in the object of consciousness. Eastern and Western civilizations are descendants of the magic world. The magic world is one of dynamic experiencing in which causality has no place.

72

Kelman, H. (1960). Psychoanalytic thought and eastern wisdom. In J. H. Masserman (Ed.), *Psychoanalysis and human values: Vol. 3. Of science and psychoanalysis* **(pp. 124-139). New York: Grune & Stratton.**

73

Kiang, T. (1982). Sighted hands: A report on experiments with 4 Chinese children to test their ability to see colour pictures and symbols with their hands. *Journal of the Society for Psychical Research, 51,* **304-308.**

Conducted 3 experiments in which 4 children (aged 10-12 yrs) were able to describe accurately familiar and unfamiliar characters and symbols contained within a sealed box. The author concludes that these Ss did have "sighted" hands and that this faculty did not depend on a recent knowledge of the content of the test sample. A 4th experiment in which the Ss were to have been not allowed to touch the boxes was uncompleted. These negative results indicate that extrasensory functioning depends critically on the S's mental and physical state.

74

King, A. Y. C., & Bond, M. H. (1985). The Confucian paradigm of men: A sociological view. In W. S. Tseng & D. Y. H. Wu (Eds.), *Chinese culture and mental health* **(pp. 29-45). Orlando, Fl: Academic Press.**

75

Klein, S. (1983). Analogy and mysticism and the structure of culture. *Current Anthropology, 24,* **151-180.**

76

Knowles, M. C. (1982). The 1981 conference of the Chinese Psychological Society. *Australian Psychologist, 17,* **119-127.**

Describes the growth of the Chinese Psychological Society (CPS) and discusses the 1981 conference to which overseas delegates were asked for the first time. The growth of the CPS is closely linked to the development of psychology in China, which in turn is inseparable from the country's long cultural heritage. In addition, other social and political events have left unmistakable and perhaps indelible marks on the society.

77

Kong, K. L., Tsoi, T. S., & Chu, S. M. (1983). [A syllable recognition system based on peak and latency measures]. *Acta Psychologica Taiwanica, 25,* **49-60.** (In Chinese.)

The validity of a new concept of feature extraction was tested in a syllable recognition system consisting of an analog speech terminal and a minicomputer (PDP MINC-23). The entire Cantonese phoneme vocabulary were used as recognition items. Spectral analysis was carried out by a bank of 20 bandpass filters. The rectified and low-pass-filtered output was sampled at the beginning, the end, and for the whole duration of the syllable. Using analog peak-hold detectors, the amplitude in each channel (response peak), and the maximum voltage difference between adjacent channels (latency) were measured. A recognition item was represented by a series of these voltage measurements. The three most probable vocabulary items given a series of voltages was computed. For one speaker using his own reference templates, the cumulative percentages of correct recognition for the three responses were 77.4, 92.5 for yun mu's; 91.2, 96.5, and 99.1 for consonants; and 75.2, 98.1, and 99.4 for tones. These results are encouraging. The system is particularly suitable for automatic recognition of the Chinese language at the acoustic level and its advantages compared to other systems were discussed.

78

Krueger, J. R. (1961). An early instance of conditioning from the Chinese dynastic histories. *Psychological Reports, 9,* **117.**

79

Kuo, Y. Y. (1976). China. In U. S. Sexton & H. Misiak (Eds.), *Psychology around the world* **(pp. 72-90). Monterey, CA: Brooks/Cole.**

80

Kvan, E. (1981). Doing psychology in Hong Kong. *Hong Kong Psychological Society Bulletin,* **No. 6, 23-31.**

81

Lee, C. (1984). Personal reflections on Qigong. *PSI Research, 3,* **84-90.**

Describes the ancient Chinese practice of qigong (a form of breathing/relaxation exercise), its theoretical aspects and history, and its relevance for parapsychology.

82

Lei, Y. H., & Li, J. B. (1982). [On the psychological thought of Han Fei]. *Acta Psychologica Sinica, 14,* **311-317.** (In Chinese.)

83

Li, J. C. (1974). A criticism of Lin Piao's theory "innate genius"--His theoretical program for usurping party leadership and seizing state power. *Scientia Sinica, 17,* **439-445.**

84

Li, L. J. (1986). [In promotion of the reform and development of psychology: Reviewing notes on psychology]. *Information on Psychological Sciences,* **No. 4, 62-63.** (In Chinese.)

85

Lin, Y. H. L. (1939). Confucius on interpersonal relations. *Psychiatry, 2,* **475-481.**

86

Lin, Z. X. (1985). [The Fifth National Conference of the Chinese Psychological Society]. *Acta Psychologica Sinica, 17,* **216-223.** (In Chinese.)

This is a report on the Fifth National Conference of the Chinese Psychological Society. It includes four parts: general orientation, group activities, election of the standing committee and organization of branch committees, and a summary.

87

Luo, Z. S. (1981). [Xun Zi's materialistic psychological thoughts]. *Acta Psychologica Sinica, 13,* **3-10.** (In Chinese.)

Studies the works of Xun Zi, an ancient Chinese philosopher, regarding his thoughts about the relationships between humans and nature, human nature and false appearance, and mind and body. Also explored were his comments on the processes of recognition, cognition and behavior, moods and desires, consciousness, personality, and learning. It is thought that Zi's philosophies comprised a salient trend of materialism.

88

MacHovec, F. J. (1975). Hypnosis before Mesmer. *American Journal of Clinical Hypnosis, 17,* **215-220.**

89

Masson-Oursel, P. (1916). La sophistique: Etude de philosophie comparee. *Revue de Metaphysique et de Morale, 25,* **353-362.** (In other language.)

90

Mental Health Association of Hong Kong (1983). *Index of published articles, up to and including December, 1982.* **Hong Kong: Author.**

91

Miao, H. C. (1961). [Report on 1960 Psychology Conference, Chinese Psychological Association, Shanghai Branch]. *Acta Psychologica Sinica,* **No. 3, 216-218.** (In Chinese.)

92

Miller, M. H., Tseng, K. H., & Lau, T. (1977). Asia: Mental health and psychiatry. In B. B. Wolman (Ed.), *International encyclopedia of psychiatry, psychology, psychoanalysis, and neurology* **(Vol. 2, pp. 144-152). New York: Aesculapius.**

93

Mirabito, J. J. (1980). Chinese and Western man: A challenge to the assumption of an inherent nature to human beings. *Dissertation Abstracts International, 40,* **B4985-4986.**

94

Munro, D. J. (1977). *The concept of man in contemporary China.* **Ann Arbor: University of Michigan Press.**

95

Murphy, G., & Murphy, L. B. (Eds.) (1968). *Asian psychology.* **New York: Basic Books.**

96

Nakamura, H. (1960). *Ways of thinking of eastern peoples.* **Tokyo: Japanese National Commission for UNESCO, Government of Japan.**

97

Nakamura, H. (1964). [*Ways of thinking of eastern peoples: India, China, Tibet, Japan.*] **(Philip P. Wiener, Trans.) Honolulu, Hawaii: East-West Center Press.** (In other language.)

98

Nanjing University Library (Compiler). (1983). [*Index of the psychological literature in China from 1949 to 1982*]. **Nanjing University.** (In Chinese.)

An exhaustive compilation of the psychological literature in Chinese, covering journals in psychology and related disciplines, essay collections, conference papers, and books. There are approximately 10,000 items.

99

Needman, J. (1956). *Science and civilization in China: Vol. 2. History of scientific thought.* **Cambridge: Cambridge University Press.**

100

Otis, L. P., & Kuo, E. C. (1984). Extraordinary beliefs among students in Singapore and Canada. *Journal of Psychology, 116,* **215-226.**

Investigated the extent of belief in a wide variety of extraordinary phenomena among 113 university students in a Western-developed country--Canada--and 76 undergraduates in an Eastern-developed country--Singapore. A questionnaire that included 34 items on extraordinary belief (beliefs dealing with traditional religion, luck, fortune-telling, psychic phenomena, spirits, and strange sightings) was completed by Ss. Canadian Ss were found to be significantly more skeptical than their Singapore peers and were particularly skeptical regarding religious beliefs and beliefs about spirits. However, both groups shared quite similar views concerning psychic and other extraordinary phenomena. Singapore Ss of Chinese, Indian, and Malay descent differed mainly with respect to their religious views. The results are discussed in terms of the presumed relationship between technological advancement and level of extraordinary belief.

101

Over, R. (1980). Impressions of psychology in the People's Republic of China. *Australian Psychologist*, *15*, **486-493.**

Outlines continuities and discontinuities in the development of psychology in China over the last 60 yrs and identifies trends in teaching, research, and practice. Psychology has been reestablished following disruption to the discipline during the Cultural Revolution. The Institute of Psychology, Chinese Psychological Society, and colleges and universities are discussed in the context of observations made by the author in 1979 while working in the Institute under the sponsorship of the Chinese Academy of Sciences.

102

Over, R. (1980). Chinese psychologists trained in the United Kingdom. *Bulletin of the British Psychological Society*, *33*, **130-131.**

103

Pan, S. (1956). [Use collective energy to develop scientific psychology for the socialist construction of our country]. *Acta Psychologica Sinica*, *1*, **1-10.** (In Chinese.)

104

Pan, S. (1958). [A general review of psychology in China]. *Acta Psychologica Sinica*, *2*, **3-9.** (In Chinese.)

The author introduced the general conditions of psychology in China in historical order. A brief retrospective account of the introduction of Western psychology to China in the early 20's was given. In the later period of the reactionary rule of Kuomintang, psychological activities in China were completely suspended, so the main context of the article narrates the development of psychology after the founding of New China. This development includes the correct leadership of and strong support from the Communist Party, the enlargement of the team of psychological workers and the establishment of the Chinese Psychological Association, the achievements in reforming thoughts and profession by psychological workers, the unison of psychological science with socialistic constructions in the 12-year plan, the present activities of Chinese psychological profession and some practical problems in existence.

105

Pan, S. (1959). China's recent research work on psychology. *Psychologia*, *2*, **193-201.**

106

Pan, S. (1960). [Responding to the big leap scaling the peaks of psychological science]. *Acta Psychologica Sinica*, **No. 2, 63-66.** (In Chinese.)

107

Pan, S. (1960). [Learning Mao Tse-tung thought & raising the scientific level of psychology]. *Acta Psychologica Sinica*, **No. 3, 135-137.** (In Chinese.)

108

Pan, S. (1963). A letter to Professor Koji Sato. *Psychologia*, *6*, **175.**

109

Pan, S. (1981). [Some suggestions as to how to develop the science of psychology under the present situation in China]. *Acta Psychologica Sinica*, *13*, **373-379.** (In Chinese.)

110

Pan, S. (1982). [A summary of 60 years of experience, open a new stage of development in psychology in China - Opening speech of the Third Representative Assembly and Academy Conference in Commemoration of 60 years of the founding of the Chinese Psychological Society]. *Acta Psychologica Sinica*, *14*, **139-142.** (In Chinese.)

111

Pan, S. (1983). [The reconstruction of psychology to serve the new situation of socialist modernization]. *Information on Psychological Sciences*, **No. 2, 5-8.** (In Chinese.)

112

Pan, S. (Ed.). (1983). [*A study of psychological thought in ancient China*]. **Nanchang, Jiangxi: People's Press.** (In Chinese.)

113

Pan, S. (1984). [Contending views in ancient Chinese psychology]. *Acta Psychologica Sinica*, *16*, **103-112.** (In Chinese.)

114

Pan, S. (1985). [On the reform of China's psychological work - Opening speech at the Fifth National Academic Conference of the Chinese Psychological Society]. *Information on Psychological Sciences*, **No. 1, 1-3.** (In Chinese.)

115

Pan, S. (1986). [Strive to open a new phase in China's psychological studies through reform]. *Information on Psychological Sciences*, **No. 1, 1-5.** (In Chinese.)

An excerpt is given from a report delivered by Professor Pan Shu at the 1985 annual meeting of the Committee of Basic Theory Specialties of the Chinese Association of Psychology. It expounded the possibility and urgency of opening up a new phase in China's psychological studies through reform. Some aspects of reform and psychological studies in China were discussed.

116

Pan, S., & Chen, D. J. (1959). [Ten years' developments in Chinese psychology]. *Acta Psychologica Sinica*, **No. 4, 191-203.** (In Chinese.)

In describing ten years' of developments in Chinese psychology, the authors have divided the whole decade into three main periods. The preliminary efforts of the first period (1949-1952) in washing off the academic thoughts of bourgeois psychology ended in victory, and the policies concerning the reformation and reconstruction of psychology upon the basis of Marxism and Pavlov's theory were firmly established. In the second period (1952-1957) the reformation and rebuilding of psychology were actually tested for the first time, and the plans for the development of psychology were made. The third period (1957-1959) has been characterized by thorough scholastic debates of psychological problems, the close alliance of psychological practice with the Socialistic reconstruction and a great advancement on the road of active reconstruction of psychology upon the dialectic Materialism. The directions of the future developments of psychology in China are pointed out.

117

Pan, S., Chen, L., Wang, J. H., & Chen, D. R. (1980). [Wilhelm Wundt and Chinese psychology]. *Acta Psychologica Sinica*, *12*, **367-376.** (In Chinese.)

Demonstrates that although only one Chinese scholar ever attended Wundt's lectures in Leipzig in 1908-1911, Wundt's psychological research and theories had an observable impact on Chinese scientific psychology. The influence of some materialistic and dialectic elements in Wundt's work is noted.

118

Pan, S., & Gao, J. F. (1983). [Organize and excavate the treasures of psychological thoughts in ancient China]. *Acta Psychologica Sinica*, *15*, **138-143.** (In Chinese.)

119

Pei, L. (1981). [A brief introduction of the inaugural meeting of the CPA Division of Physiological Psychology and its academic activities]. *Acta Psychologica Sinica*, *13*, **248.** (In Chinese.)

120

Pei, W. (1980). [Centennial Meeting of the Foundation of Wundt's Psychological Laboratory in Beijing]. *Acta Psychologica Sinica*, *12*, **482.** (In Chinese.)

121

Peng, F. (1979). [Historical lessons should be borne in mind: Analysis of the 1958 campaign to criticize psychology]. *Acta Psychologica Sinica*, *11*, **17-21.** (In Chinese.)

Argues that the campaign in China to criticize psychology launched by Peking Normal University in 1958 was completely wrong in orientation and practice. Some useful lessons must be drawn from this campaign: (1) It is important to promote scientific democracy and adhere to the legal system; (2) Academic problems should not be settled as political ones; and (3) the roles of intellectuals must be evaluated correctly.

122

Perry, J. W. (1985). Individuality: A spiritual task and societal hazard. *ReVISION*, **8(1), 53-58.**

The author discussed the historical development of the imagery of a spiritual center that was prominent in both the ancient practices and in the experiences of people today, arguing that it is in the spiritual center where the clearest evidence of the step-by-step evolution of individuality can be found. This image of a spiritual center is what Jung has called the archetype of the self, characteristically represented as a quadrated circle or mandala that combines, unites, or reconciles the opposites. A history of myth and rituality was presented to illustrate the evolution of the concept of individuality. It was contended that the problems faced by society today grow out of a definition of individuality that has come to mean mere self-seeking and a democracy that has altogether lost its meaning. Immense numbers of people grow up without any sense of belonging to a community and so lack feelings of loyalty and caring.

123

Petzold, M. (1979, August). Pink Freud in China? Mao's Erben enfdecken die Psychologie. *Psychologie Heute*, *6*, **66-75.**

124

Petzold, M. (Ed). (1980). Psychology in contemporary China. *Chinese Sociology and Anthropology*, *12*, **1-123.**

125

Petzold, M. (1981). Psychologische Forschung in China, Geschichte und gegenwartige Entwicklungen [Psychological research in China: History and contemporary trends]. *Berichte des Bundesinstituts fur ostwissenschaftliche und internationale Studien,* **No. 9.** (In other language.)

126

Petzold, M. (1985). The social history of Chinese psychology. In M. G. Ash & W. R. Woodward (Eds.), *Psychology in twentieth century thought and society.* **Cambridge, MA: Cambridge University Press.**

127

Petzold, M. (1986). Psychology in the People's Republic of China--A historical overview and quantitative analysis. *Psychologia, 29,* **57-65.**

The history of psychology in the People's Republic of China was reviewed. Roots of Chinese psychology go back to the last century when modern Western psychology was introduced into China. Chinese psychology was established as an academic discipline in the 1920s. After the revolution in 1949 psychology was strongly oriented toward Soviet psychology and was hindered by several political campaigns, especially the Great Cultural Revolution. In the late 1970s psychology was reestablished as a science. Research is active especially in developmental and educational psychology. A quantitative analysis of the two leading psychology journals yielded the rank order of different areas in current research. An analysis of citations showed that, although there is a strong reference to English language sources, Chinese psychologists are citing respective Chinese authors more frequently.

128

Ratner, C. (1979). Psychology in the People's Republic of China. *Eastern Horizon, 18,* **13-17.**

129

Ratner, C. (1984). The Chinese psychology convention, 1984. *New Ideas in Psychology, 3,* **229-232.**

130

[Resolution adopted by the Second Congress of the Chinese Psychological Society]. (1960). *Acta Psychologica Sinica,* **No. 2, 67.** (In Chinese.)

131

Rychlak, J. F. (1976). *Dialectic: Humanistic rationale for behavior and development: II. Contributions to human development.* **Basel, Switzerland: S. Karger.**

In an effort to publicize the "currently underestimated and often misunderstood" concept of dialectic in psychological theorizing, this volume compiles 12 papers which illustrate the application of this concept to the study of human behavior and development. Among topics discussed are the dialectic as an approach to psychological aesthetics, Freud as a dialectician, dialectical aspects of moral development, Chinese dialectical thought and character, and dialectic man as a subject in psychological research.

132

Science for the people (1974). *China: Science walks on two legs.* **New York, NY: Avon.**

Presents the observations of a group of American scientists on the status of scientific research and thought in China, and how Chinese scientists and workers, specialists and nonspecialists interact to work for common goals. The effects of a revolutionary society on the processes of science and the status of mental health programs are also considered.

133

Shen, D. C. (1983). [Why do Chinese psychologists pay attention to the study of the history and theory of psychology]. *Information Psychological Sciences,* **No. 2, 33-35.** (In Chinese.)

134

Shen, D. C. (1986). [Psychology and introspection]. *Acta Psychologica Sinica, 18,* **227-234.** (In Chinese.)

135

Shen, D. C., & Wang, Q. (1981). [Congratulatory article to Prof. Tang Yue, for sixty years of hardwork in the research and teaching of psychology]. *Acta Psychologica Sinica, 13,* **370-372.** (In Chinese.)

136

Shum, J. C. (1982). Psychology, East and West. *Bulletin of the British Psychological Society, 35,* **273-274.**

Comments on C. C. Ching's (1981) article outlining his tour of Britain and France. Ching's thought-provoking comments and observations about his British and French colleagues and their work are presented.

137

Simon, H. A. (1983). [Developmental course and prospect of psychology]. *Acta Psychologica Sinica, 15,* **375-380.** (In Chinese.)

Describes the translation into Chinese of J. Haven's (1857) Menthal Philosophy. This translation was one of the first introducing Western psychology to China; the translation was published in China in 1889.

138

[Sixty years of Chinese psychology: Retrospect and prospect (abstract)]. (1982). *Information on Psychological Sciences,* **No. 4, 1-4.** (In Chinese.)

139

Ssu, M. F. (1965). [The principles of class analysis must be applied in the research on psychology of moral education]. *Acta Psychologica Sinica*, **No. 2, 114-120.** (In Chinese.)

140

Steffy, J., & Vilenskaya, L. (1984). Some comparisons of psychic healing in the USSR, Eastern and Western Europe, North America, China and Brazil. *PSI Research*, *3*, **29-52.**

Contends that psychic healers throughout the world determine the condition of the patient and nature of the disease or disorder in several ways that include the patient's description, clairvoyant means, and looking to the field around the person. They heal by centering themselves, using the sensitivity of the hand to assess the energy field, mobilizing areas in the field that are sluggish, congested, or static, and directing excess body energies to assist in healing. There have been a number of instances of successful healings at a distance, but some healers believe they can only be effective when they lay their hands on patients. Some believe that healing abilities are inborn while others feel everyone has these abilities waiting to be noticed. It is a common belief that many traditional systems of spiritual development lead to the development of an individual's potential to heal. Soviet researchers are optimistic about psychic healing, while Western researchers have remained cautious about its role in medical science and society at large. Ancient healing techniques of India, China, and American Indians offer benefits to contemporary medical science.

141

Su, H. Y. (1958). [Development of psychology in China in the last decade]. *Acta Psychologica Taiwanica*, **No. 1, 112-115.** (In Chinese.)

142

Su, H. Y. (1965). The psychological research in the department of psychology at National Taiwan University since 1948. *Acta Psychologica Taiwanica*, **7, 1-9.**

143

Sun, Y. (1959). [A review of literatures on criticisms of Freudian psycho-analysis]. *Acta Psychologica Sinica*, **No. 4, 264-270.** (In Chinese.)

144

Tang, T. (1975). A preface to experimental psychology in China. *Psychologia: An International Journal of Psychology in the Orient*, *18*, **30-34.**

Notes that, except for conflicting interview reports as to whether or not psychology exists as a science or as an institution, little is known outside the People's Republic of China (PRC) about contemporary psychology in China. Recently, however, psychologists visiting China reported seeing excellent psychology libraries and many English and Chinese editions of R. Woodworth and H. Schlosberg's Experimental Psychology. The preface to the Chinese edition of Experimental Psychology is translated and presented here, because it is regarded as denotative information on the nature of experimental psychology in China. This preface provides a delineation of the theoretical position of PRC psychology. Its contents and wide circulation within China suggest that psychology is both a science and a viable institution in that nation.

145

[The Chinese Psychological Delegation Present at the XXIIth International Congress of Psychology]. (1981). *Acta Psychologica Sinica*, *13*, **115-116.** (In Chinese.)

146

The Executive Committee of the Chinese Psychological Society. (1982). [Retrospect and prospect of 60 years of psychology in China: In commemoration of the 60th anniversary of the founding of the Chinese Psychological Society]. *Acta Psychologica Sinica*, *14*, **127-138.** (In Chinese.)

Reviews the development of psychology in China and summarizes major research results. Emphasis is placed on the need to hold Marxist philosophy as the guiding principle in psychology, to expand theoretical and applied research, and to promote the training of students in psychology.

147

[The First Congress of Psychologists and Symposium held by Fuchian (Fujian) Psychological Society]. (1961). *Acta Psychologica Sinica*, **No. 4, 289-290.** (In Chinese.)

148

[The Psychological Congress of Kuangsi Chuang (Guangxi Zhuang) Autonomous Region held in Kueilin (Guilin)]. (1960). *Acta Psychologica Sinica*, **No. 4, 269.** (In Chinese.)

149

[Theoretical problems of psychology in the realization of class struggles: A discussion by the psychological workers of Hsi-An (Xian)]. (1959). *Acta Psychologica Sinica*, **No. 2, 129. (Translated by U.S. Joint Publications Research Service, No. 3,424, 1-2).** (In Chinese.)

150

Ting, T. (1959). [How to develop medical psychology in China]. ***Acta Psychologica Sinica*, No. 3, 148-150. (Translated by U.S. Joint Publications Research Service, No. 3,424, pp. 11-17.)** (In Chinese.)

The author asserts the importance of medical psychology in medical and prophylactic works during the establishment of socialism in China. Criticisms are given against the traditional viewpoint which looks upon the human being as a mere biological organism but overlooks man's psychological activities. Remarks are made on the so-called "psycho-somatic medicine" developed in medical circles in capitalistic nations. From the historical facts of scientific development a solution is given to the problems of psychic nature and psychosomatic relationship achieved in the light of the philosophy of Marxism and Leninism and of the scientific theories of Pavlov. The author states that extremely superior conditions exist today in China for establishing and developing medical psychology. Finally, the author introduces the present condition of medical psychology in China and its applications in researches.

151

Tseng, W. S. (1972). Psychiatric study of shamanism in Taiwan. ***Archives General Psychiatry*, *26*, 561-565.**

152

Tsoi, M. M., & Pryde, N. A. (1985). Clinical psychology services in Hong Kong. In Special Issue: Clinical Psychology Abroad. *Newsletter of Division of Clinical Psychology, British Psychological Society*, *49*, **13-15.**

153

Turtle, A. M., & Blowers, G. H. (1984). Historiography of modern psychology in Asia, Southeast Asia and the South Pacific: Activities, aspects and prospects [Essays in honor of Prof. Joseph Brozek, Monograph]. *Revista de Historia de la Psicologia^ (Valencia), **5**, 367-374.*

The authors presented a list of general textbooks on the history of psychology; publications dealing with the subject in India, Indonesia, Japan, Korea, Malaysia, Pakistan, People's Republic of China, the Philippines, and Thailand; sources of contemporary reference; and institutional development. It was suggested that in the countries considered, psychology is developing under conditions differing from its development in the West (including Australia and New Zealand).

154

Wang, J. S. (1980). [On the modernization of psychology in China: Fundamental theoretical viewpoint and methodology]. Acta Psychologica Sinica, 12, *30-36. (In Chinese.)*

Comments on Chinese psychological research during the last 30 yrs, highlighting the investigation of conditioned reflexes and class analysis. The author suggests the establishment of a completely new system of psychology possessing 5 distinguishing traits: (a) theories guided by dialectic materialism, (b) national peculiarities, (c) contemporary features, (d) the integration of natural and social sciences, and (e) the combination of theory and practice. New methodologies more suitable to the special characteristics of psychology also need to be created.

155

Wang, J. S. (1984). [On psychological methodology in China]. Information on Psychological Sciences, *No. 2, 33-38. (In Chinese.)*

The composition of psychological methodology consists of the two aspects of strategy and tactics; the perceptual method and the logical thinking method; and the method of philosophy, the common method of science, and the special method of psychology. Psychology in China has paid attention to the tactics of methodology, the perceptual method, and the common method of science; but it has not to the strategy of methodology, the method of logical thinking, and the special method of psychology. The present author holds that the unity of the subjective method and the objective method and of the perceptual method and the logical thinking method should be emphasized; and that attention should be paid to research on the special method of psychology. The present author proposes a synthetic method for psychological research.

156

Wang, M. Q. (1984). [On yingyang, personality and health theories in Huang Di Nei Jing]. Information on Psychological Sciences, *No. 3, 33-37. (In Chinese.)*

157

Wang, S. H. (1979). Parapsychology in the Republic of China. Parapsychology Review, 10, *17-18.*

The national psi organization in China is the Society for Parapsychological Studies of the Republic of China (SPSROC), founded in Taipei in 1977. SPSROC has 305 members, publishes a bimonthly journal (Parapsychology), and maintains a reading room. The Society frequently invites parapsychologists to lecture; their topics are listed, as are research projects being conducted by members.

158

Wei, M. R. (1981). [On the psychological point of view of Dai Zhen--An 18th century Chinese thinker]. Acta Psychologica Sinica, 13, *386-393. (In Chinese.)*

159

Wei, M. X., & Shi, S. H. (1981). [Famous psychologists offer suggestions on research and teaching of psychology in China]. Acta Psychologica Sinica, 13, *464-468. (In Chinese.)*

160

Weiss, M. S. (1977). The research experience in a Chinese-American community. Journal of Social Issues, 33, *120-132.*

Describes field experience with a Chinese community in an American city. It is suggested that the anthropologist's ability to maintain a low profile during such field experience depends not only upon his/her desire for uninvolved objectivity but also upon the community's willingness to accept and tolerate an uncommitted stranger.

161

Wolman, B. B. (1979). International directory of psychology: A guide to people, places, and policies. *New York: Plenum.*

162

Wright, A. F., & Twitchett, D. (1962). Confucian personalities. *Stanford: Stanford Univeristy Press.*

163

Wu, T. T. (1980). [Some problems in compiling a text of psychology for teachers' college students]. Acta Psychologica Sinica, 12, *267-271. (In Chinese.)*

This paper has two purposes. The first is to enumerate some principles guiding the work of compiling a psychology text for a required course for non-education department students of the teachers college. The second purpose is to clarify some theoretical problems as follows: (1) the classification of mental activities, (2) the nature of such a course of psychology, (3) the evaluation of Pavlov's theory of higher nervous activity, (4) the integration of basic psychological theories and educational practices, (5) the class character of mental phenomena.

164

Xu, L. C. (1978). [Thirty years of Chinese psychology]. Nature^ (Peoples' Republic of China). (In Chinese.)

165

Xu, L. C. (1979). [Psychology in the service of the Four Modernizations]. *Acta Psychologica Sinica, 11,* **22-28.** (In Chinese.)

In this paper, the author explains the four main tasks of Chinese psychologists toward the realization of the four modernizations. First, in order to make China a modern socialist country, psychologists need to educate and train a great many experts. They should make their contributions to education. Second, psychologists should make every effort to increase labor productivity. Third, psychological tasks in the medical front are examined within the context of pollution, the environment, and family changes. Behavior modification and counseling are likewise emphasized. Fourth, social psychology studies should help to resolve questions of how to mobilize the initiative of the masses, and to produce more effective measures for the investigation of public opinion, social attitudes toward various policies and events. Finally, the author emphasizes the importance of fundamental theoretical research.

166

Xu, L. C. (1979). [The road is tortuous, but the prospects are bright--30 years' development of Chinese psychology]. *Nature Journal Yearbook, 1,* **136-143.** (In Chinese.)

167

Xu, L. C., Ching, C. C., & Over, R. (1980). Recent developments in psychology within the People's Republic of China. *International Journal of Psychology, 15,* **131-144.**

Discusses the state of psychology in the context of trends, continuities, and discontinuities over the last 60 yrs. The work of psychologists was disrupted between 1966 and 1976 by the activities of the "gang of four". In the Institute of Psychology, research is being done in perception, in physiological and developmental psychology, and in theories and systems. The Chinese Psychological Society resumed activities in 1977, and Acta Psychologica Sinica reappeared in 1979.

168

Xu, Q. D. (1980). [A study of psychological thoughts in the ancient Chinese writer Wang Chong's work]. *Acta Psychologica Sinica, 12,* **377-384.** (In Chinese.)

169

Yan, G. C. (1981). *A study of Pre-Qin psychological thought.* **China: Hunan People's Press.** (In Chinese.)

170

Yan, G. C. (1982). [A comment on the psychological thought of Huai Nan-zi]. *Acta Psychologica Sinica, 14,* **285-293.** (In Chinese.)

171

Yan, G. C. (1982). [Some theories of feeling in ancient China]. *Information on Psychological Sciences,* **No. 6, 34-38.** (In Chinese.)

172

Yan, G. C. (1983). *A study of psychological thought during the Han, Wei, and the Six Dynasties.* **China: Hunan People's Press.** (In Chinese.)

173

Yan, G. C. (1984). [On Wang Anshi's materialistic views on psychology]. *Acta Psychologica Sinica, 16,* **113-120.** (In Chinese.)

174

Yan, G. C. (1985). [Basic ideas about volition in ancient China]. *Information on Psychological Sciences,* **No. 3, 45-48.** (In Chinese.)

175

Yan, G. C. (1986). [A study of the psychological thoughts of Lao and Zhuang's Taoist school]. *Information on Psychological Sciences,* **No. 4, 1-9.** (In Chinese.)

This article consisted of five parts: (1) With regard to the relationship between the "shape" and the "spirit," Lao generally believed in dualism, whereas Zhuang dealt with this problem on the basis of cosmogony. (2) Lao divided the cognitive process into three stages, investigation, clarity, and total comprehension; Zhuang divided it into two stages, contact and consideration. (3) Both Lao and Zhuang regarded emotion and desire as harmful to moral integrity, and advocated stoicism. (4) Concerning the psychology of learning, both advocated modesty, gradual accumulation, limit to speciality, and concentration. (5) Zhuang proposed nine methods of knowing people which are similar to modern psychological ideas.

176

Yan, L. S., & Li, C. H. (1984). [Ancient Chinese thinkers on individual differences]. *Information on Psychological Sciences,* **No. 6, 8-14.** (In Chinese.)

177

Yang, H. N. (1974). A criticism of the reactionary theory of "innate genius" in the light of the origin and development of thinking. *Scientia Sinica, 17,* **293-302.**

178

Yang, K. S. (1982). [Sinicization of psychological research in Chinese society: Directions and issues]. In K. S. Yang & C. I. Wen (Eds.), [*Sinicization of research in social and behavioral sciences*] **(pp. 153-187). Taipei: Academia Sinica, Institute of Ethnology.** (In Chinese.)

179

Yang, K. S., & Wen, C. I. (Eds.). (1982). [*The sinicization of social and behavioral science research in China*]. **Taipei: Academia Sinica, Institute of Ethnology.** (In Chinese.)

180

Yang, X. H. (1983). [Some opinions of the study of the history of Chinese psychology]. *Acta Psychologica Sinica, 15,* **289-293.** (In Chinese.)

Proposes that there is an urgent need to study the history of Chinese psychology and stresses the importance of incorporating Chinese characteristics into psychology. The basic principles and methods in the study of the history of Chinese psychology are discussed. Proposals are presented to facilitate research, and the formation of a nationwide psychological cooperative and the building of research institutions are suggested.

181

Yang, X. H. (1984). [On Wang Tingxiang's materialistic approach to psychology]. *Acta Psychologica Sinica, 16,* **124-131.** (In Chinese.)

182

Yang, X. H. (1984). [The study of the history of Chinese psychology: Its history and present]. *Information on Psychological Sciences,* **No. 4, 54-57.** (In Chinese.)

183

Yang, Y. M. et al. (1979). [We should pay attention to the ancient Chinese literature on psychology]. *Shanxi Teachers' College Journal,* **No. 3.** (In Chinese.)

184

Yang, Y. M., & Guo, Z. Y. (1985). [A tentative study of Shangyang's and Hanfei's psychological ideas]. *Information on Psychological Sciences,* **No. 1, 21-26.** (In Chinese.)

185

Yao, S. C. (1974). The theory of "innate genius"--The theoretical program of Lin Piao's "Restoring the Rites". *Scientia Sinica, 17,* **133-136.**

186

Yee, A. H. (1973). Psychology in China bows to the Cultural Revolution. *APA Monitor, 4,* **1-4. (Reprinted as "China revisited" in** *International Exchange And Cultural Exchange,* **1973,** *9,* **1-8.)**

187

Yu, C. C. (1939 - 1940). [Psychological concepts of Chu-tze and Shun-tze]. *Chinese Journal of Psychology, 4.* (In Chinese.)

188

Zeng, L. G. (1980). [A research into the psychological thoughts of an ancient Chinese writer Xunzi]. *Acta Psychologica Sinica, 12,* **385-389.** (In Chinese.)

189

Zhang, B. Y. (1979). [A symposium on medical psychology sponsored by Beijing Psychological Society]. *Acta Psychologica Sinica, 11,* **373-374.** (In Chinese.)

190

Zhang, J. T. (1984). [CAS-NAS Joint Psychology Conference on issues in cognition held in America]. *Acta Psychologica Sinica, 16,* **347-348.** (In Chinese.)

191

Zhang, R. J., & Zhu, Y. X. (Eds.). (1984). [*A dictionary of personalities in psychology*]. **Tianjin: Tianjin People's Press.** (In Chinese.)

192

Zhao, B. R. (1982). [Thirty years of philosophical research in Chinese psychology]. *Information on Psychological Sciences,* **No. 6, 40-44.** (In Chinese.)

193

Zhao, L. R. (1979). [The Second Annual Meeting of the Chinese Psychological Society]. *Acta Psychologica Sinica, 11,* **137-142.** (In Chinese.)

194

Zhao, L. R. (1980). [Third academic annual meeting of the Chinese psychological association]. *Acta Psychologica Sinica, 12,* **244-250.** (In Chinese.)

195

Zhao, L. R. (1980). [The past and present status of the Chinese Psychological Association and its activities]. *Acta Psychologica Sinica, 12,* **473-481.** (In Chinese.)

196

Zhao, L. R. (1981). [An introduction to psychology in Taiwan province]. *Acta Psychologica Sinica, 13,* **364-368.** (In Chinese.)

197

Zhao, L. R., & He, G. C. (1980). [In Chinese Psychological Association and its local societies]. *Acta Psychologica Sinica, 12,* **116-123.** (In Chinese.)

198

Zhu, Y. X. (1982). [Research on the thoughts of Cheng-ying and Cheng-yi]. *Acta Psychologica Sinica, 14,* **473-479.** (In Chinese.)

199

Zhu, Y. X. (1983). [On Wang Ting-xiang's psychological thoughts]. *Information on Psychological Sciences,* **No. 2, 18-23.** (In Chinese.)

Wang Ting-xiang (1474-1544 A.D.) was a Chinese philosopher and scientist. His psychological thoughts dealt with relationships between mind and body and between mind and object, as well as other problems, such as human nature, recognition, emotion, and desires. He made a penetrating analysis of many psychological questions, and exerted a great influence on Wang Fu-zhi's (1619-1692 A.D.) materialistic psychological thoughts.

200

Zou, D. Y. (1983). [A comment on the psychological thought of Fan Zhen]. *Acta Psychologica Sinica, 15,* **150-155.** (In Chinese.)

201

Zou, D. Y. (1984). [A commentary on Gong Zizhen's Psychological thought]. *Acta Psychologica Sinica, 16,* **121-123.** (In Chinese.)

The following references are also relevant to this chapter:

425, 473, 504, 577, 942, 1202, 1294, 1337, 2375, 2429, 2634, 3465.

PSYCHOMETRICS 3

Frequency data on citations in this chapter, in terms of content classification subcategories, are presented in Table 3.

Table 3: *Number of Citations by Content Classification, Language, and Geographical Area*

Content classification	Total	CL	EL	OL	PRC	T	HK	US
Psychometrics	9	4	5	0	0	5	2	0
Test construction and validation	106	77	29	0	16	70	7	0
Statistics and mathematics	1	0	1	0	0	0	0	0
Total	116	81	35	0	16	75	9	0

Note: CL = Chinese language; EL = English language; OL = other languages. PRC = People's Republic of China; T = Taiwan; HK = Hong Kong; US = United States (Chinese Americans--according to the frequency of the subject term Asian Americans).

Subject terms used for indexing citations related to psychometrics are grouped according to geographical area, subject population, and topic. These are presented below, in a descending order of frequency. (The frequency of single-word subject terms includes those of compound terms in which the single word appears. Subjects terms used for indexing citations from other chapters may have been included. Terms with a frequency of less than 10 are not shown.)

Geographical area

92 Taiwan
23 Asia
22 Peoples Republic of China

Subject population

27	children
25	students
13	school age children
11	adults
10	college students

Topic

42	test construction
41	test validity
36	intelligence
36	personality
25	intelligence measures
21	cross cultural differences
18	test reliability
16	testing
14	personality measures
13	adulthood
13	analysis
12	language
12	test standardization
11	psychodiagnosis
11	test norms
10	measurement

Table 3 shows that the overwhelming majority of citations (91.4%) belong to the subcategory of test construction and validation. Of these, the majority pertain to Taiwan. As noted in the Introduction, psychologists in Taiwan have a special preoccupation with psychological testing and measurement. An inspection of the frequencies of subject terms indicates that intelligence and personality are the psychological attributes most frequently tested or measured.

202

Ai, J. W. (1954). [The standardization of silent reading diagnostic tests in elementary schools]. *Psychological Testing, 2,* **140-142.** (In Chinese.)

203

Ai, J. W. (1954). [The standardization of arithmetic diagnostic tests in elementary schools]. *Psychological Testing, 2,* **143-145.** (In Chinese.)

204

Bryson S., Mononen, L. J., & Yu, L. (1980). Procedural constraints on the measurement of laterality in young children. *Neuropsychologia, 18,* **243-246.**

Conducted 2 experiments with 60 4-, 7-, and 10-yr-old Chinese males to investigate ear-asymmetry in children from different cultural and linguistic backgrounds. Right-ear superiority on dichotic listening was demonstrated in the 4-yr-olds with self-paced intertrial-intervals (ITIs) but not with standard 5-sec ITIs. It is concluded that methodological problems associated with ear-asymmetry measurement in young children may generate spurious false-negative estimates of laterality.

205

Chan, D. W. (1985). The Chinese version of the General Health Questionnaire: Does language make a difference? *Psychological Medicine, 15,* **147-155.**

The English and Chinese versions of the General Health Questionnaire (GHQ) was administered to 72 bilingual undergraduates to evaluate the equivalence of the two versions. Thirty-seven subjects received the English version followed by the Chinese version of the GHQ; the remaining subjects received the two measures in the opposite order. Item, reliability, and factor analyses revealed that, although discrepancies were observed at the item level, the two versions were found to be comparable at the scale level. Evidence was provided for the relative robustness of the symptom dimensions as assessed by the two versions of the GHQ.

206

Chan, D. W. O. (1984). Factor analysis of the HK-WISC at 11 age levels between 5 and 15 years. *Journal of Consulting & Clinical Psychology, 52,* **482-483.**

The Hong Kong Wechsler Intelligence Scale for Children (HK-WISC), a Cantonese version of the WISC--R, was factor analyzed across 11 age groups (5-15 yrs) in the standardization sample of Chinese children (N = 1,100). The 3 factors--Verbal Comprehension, Perceptual Organization, and Freedom From Distractibility--identified in the WISC-R also emerged. The distractibility factor appeared to be less stable across age levels. Departure from the hypothesized Arithmetic/Digit Span/Coding triad of loadings for this factor was apparent at ages 5, 10, 13, and 15 yrs.

207

Chan, D. W. O., & Chan, T. S. C. (1983). Reliability, validity and the structure of the General Health Questionnaire in a Chinese context. *Psychological Medicine, 13,* **363-371.**

The 30-item General Health Questionnaire (GHQ), Self-Reporting Questionnaire (SRQ), and MMPI were administered to 225 English-speaking Chinese undergraduates. The GHQ was found to have high internal consistency as a scale and assessed 5 dimensions of psychopathology: anxiety, inadequate coping, depression, insomnia, and social dysfunctioning. As a brief screening instrument, it correlated 0.49 with the SRQ. In the "case-noncase" classification, it yielded a concordance rate of above 75% with the SRQ. Using the MMPI modal profiles derived from classification research as criterion measures, sensitivity, specificity, and correct classification rates were above 70%.

208

Chan, F., Hua, M. S., Ju, J. J., & Chow S. L. (1984). Factorial structure of the Chinese scale of attitudes towards disabled persons: A cross-cultural validation. *International Journal of Rehabilitation Research, 7,* **317-319.**

An attitude-toward-the-disabled scale was administered to 80 Chinese college students from Hong Kong, Singapore, and Taiwan. Results showed that the Chinese students had moderately positive attitudes toward people with disabilities but had some reservations about rehabilitation programs. The authors attributed this finding to cultural factors, because in China a person with a disability is not expected to be productive or independent and is automatically cared for by the family.

209

Chan, J. (1984). Raven's progressive matrices tests in Hong Kong. *New Horizons,* **No. 25, 43-49.**

210

Chan, Y. H. (1964). [A study of the Bell Adjustment Inventory, student form]. *Psychological Testing, 11,* **39-59.** (In Chinese.)

211

Chen, C. M., & Cheng, F. M. (1974). [A study of the Horn Art Aptitude Inventory]. *Psychological Testing, 21,* **18-38.** (In Chinese.)

212

Chen, M. C. et al. (Eds.). (1985). [A compilation of educational and psychological tests in China] (2 vols.). Kao Hsiung, Taiwan: Fu Hua. (In Chinese.)

213

Chen, M. J., Braithwaite, V., & Huang, J. T. (1982). Attributes of intelligent behavior: Perceived relevance and difficulty by Australian and Chinese students. *Journal of Cross-Cultural Psychology, 13,* **139-156.**

Examined the cross-cultural generalizability of 2 Western intelligence tests--the Stanford-Binet and the WAIS--in a non-Western culture. 976 Australian and 1,003 Chinese university and high school students participated in a rating task. Items from the 2 tests were rated on the aspects of relevance and difficulty. On relevance ratings, the underlying 3-factor structure of the Chinese sample correlated well with that of the Australian, suggesting a basic common structure for the concept of intelligence across cultures. The 3 factors were Spatial-Mechanical, Verbal, and Memory. Results also show that both cultures consider spatial-mechanical items most important and memory items least important. The two samples differed, however, in mean difficulty scores on the 3 dimensions. These differences were attributed to possible cultural differences in nurturing and providing opportunities to practice the different skills. It is concluded that the concept of intelligence is comparable between Australian and Chinese cultures, and that, for both cultures, the 2 tests are legitimate measures of the intelligence construct.

214

Chen, Y. H. (1964). [Construction of the General Ability Test (Form A)]. *Psychological Testing, 11,* **79-95.** (In Chinese.)

215

Chen, Y. H., Lu, C. M., Wang, J. D., & Kuo, W. F. (1979). [A report on the first Chinese revision of WISC]. *Bulletin of Educational Psychology, 12,* **89-98.** (In Chinese.)

The first Chinese revision of the WISC was attempted for use with Chinese children aged 6 through 15 years in Taiwan. The standardization sample included 100 children in each of 10 age groups, ranging from 6 1/2 through 15 1/2 years. The total sample contained 1,000 cases, with 500 boys and 500 girls. Psychometric properties were summarized as follows: (1) The spilt-half coefficient for the Full Scale was .94. (2) The stability coefficients of Full Scale IQs were .91 for the 9 1/2 age group and .95 for the 12 1/2 age group. (3) The coefficients of correlation betweem WISC Full Scale IQs and Stanford-Binet IQs were .83 for the 8 1/2 age group and .89 for the 13 1/2 age group.

216

Chen, Z. G. et al. (1983). [Item analysis of Eysenck Personality Questionnaire tested in Beijing-district]. *Acta Psychologica Sinica, 15,* **211-218.** (In Chinese.)

Tested a sample of 643 Chinese Ss on the Eysenck Personality Questionnaire (EPQ) in an attempt to modify the EPQ for use with the Chinese. It is suggested that, with further testing and analysis, the EPQ may be applicable to the Chinese culture.

217

Cheng, F. M. (1953). [The construction and analysis of a Job Knowledge Test for the Chinese Air Force]. *Psychological Testing, 1,* **9-24.** (In Chinese.)

218

Cheng, F. M. (1954). [Validity of the Chinese Air Force General Classification Test]. *Psychological Testing, 2,* **83-101.** (In Chinese.)

219

Cheng, F. M. (1960). [The reliability of achievement tests for the qualification examination]. *Psychological Testing, 8,* **549-556.** (In Chinese.)

220

Cheng, F. M. (1962). [The construction of the elementary school verbal intelligence tests]. *Psychological Testing, 9,* **604-617.** (In Chinese.)

221

Cheng, F. M. (1977). [An analysis of the results of the revised Bennet Mechanical Comprehension tests]. *Psychological Testing, 24,* **41-45.** (In Chinese.)

222

Cheng, F. M., & Lin, M. J. (1969). [Standardization of the Revised Minnesota Paper Form Board Test]. *Psychological Testing, 16,* **584-616.** (In Chinese.)

223

Cheng, F. M., & Lu, C. Y. (1978). [Follow-up studies on the Fourth Chinese Revision of Binet-Simon Scale]. *Psychological Testing, 25,* **1-4.** (In Chinese.)

224

Cheng, F. M., & Tsai, Y. H. (1971). [A study of the Group Personality Projective Test]. *Psychological Testing, 18,* **869-894.** (In Chinese.)

225

Cheng, F. Y. (1954). [Revision of the Kuhlmann-Anderson Test and its application]. *Psychological Testing, 2,* **105-111.** (In Chinese.)

226

Cheung, F. M. C. (1985). Cross-cultural considerations for the translation and adaptation of the Chinese MMPI in Hong Kong. In J. N. Butcher & C. D. Spielberger (Eds.), *Advances in personality assessment* **(Vol. 4, pp. 131-158). Hillsdale, NJ: Lawrence Erlbaum Associates.**

227

Chi, W. H. (1971). [Standardization of the Cattell Culture Fair Intelligence Test (Scale 2) in China]. *Psychological Testing, 18,* **921-942.** (In Chinese.)

228

Chia, F. M. (1969). [Construction of the General Ability Test (Form A)]. *Psychological Testing, 16,* **567-572.** (In Chinese.)

229

Chia, F. M. (1970). [Evaluation of the General Ability Test for Junior High School Students (Form A)]. *Psychological Testing, 17,* **757-766.** (In Chinese.)

230

Chia, F. M. (1971). [The construction of five aptitude tests used in junior high schools]. *Psychological Testing, 18,* **849-868.** (In Chinese.)

231

Chien, M. F., & Tsay, S. L. (1978). [A preliminary report on the construction of the Elementary School Achievement Test]. *Psychological Testing, 25,* **64-74.** (In Chinese.)

232

Chin, W. C. (1970). [The revision of an art aptitude test for use in Chinese elementary schools]. *Psychological Testing, 17,* **795-811.** (In Chinese.)

233

Chinese Behavioral Sciences Corporation. (Ed.). (1978). *[Introduction to Chinese psychological tests: A compilation]*. **Taipei: Author.** (In Chinese.)

234

Chiu, L. H. (1978). A Chinese version of the children's form of the Manifest Anxiety Scale. *Psychological Testing, 25,* **94-102.**

A Chinese translation of the Manifest Anxiety Scale (CMAS) was administered to 613 Chinese fourth- and fifth-grade children. The results showed that an overall frequency distribution was comparable to that obtained for American children, except that the former was more symmetrical. Girls scored significantly higher than boys, and the fourth graders significantly higher than the fifth graders. As to the L scale, a tendency was noted for girls to have higher scores than boys, but this difference did not reach statistical significance. No significant difference in lie scores was found between the fourth and the fifth graders. Odd-even reliabilities showed that both Anxiety and L scales were internally consistent. Significant negative correlations were found between these two scales.

235

Dai, X. Y. et al. (1986). [The "Changsha-Wechsler Intelligence Scale for Young Children" "C-WISYC"]. *Information on Psychological Sciences,* **No. 2, 23-30.** (In Chinese.)

236

Doerr, H. O., & Storrie, M. C. (1982). Neuropsychological testing in the People's Republic of China: The Halstead-Reitan Seattle/Changsha project. *Clinical Neuropsychology, 4,* **49-51.**

Discusses the 1st author's visit to China and subsequent collaboration with colleagues at Hunan Medical College in setting up a neuropsychology laboratory and adapting the Halstead-Reitan Neuropsychological Test Battery for use with the Chinese population. A description of the modifications in the translated version are presented. In addition to the obvious clinical utility, data collected in such collaborative efforts could provide the basis for an investigation of cultural and educational factors impacting neuropsychological test performance.

237

Domino, G. (1980). Chinese tangrams as a technique to assess creativity. *Journal of Creative Behavior, 14,* **204-213.**

To develop a test of creativity that is interesting and easily administered, does not draw on other abilities, and may be statistically analyzed, the puzzle known as tangrams was employed. A tangram is made up of 7 pieces, each of which is a simple shape. In this application, the task of the S is to assemble the pieces to create original pictures. The designs created by a sample of 32 children in a 3rd-grade class for the gifted were shown to be significantly higher on Fluency, Flexibility, and Originality than those produced by a comparable sample of children enrolled in a standard class. Performance of 57 undergraduates on the tangrams, scored on the same 3 variables, was shown to correlate significantly with 4 of 5 tests of creativity. A correlation of .62 was found between human movement responses on the Holtzman Inkblot Test and on the tangrams, for a sample of 26 students enrolled in an advanced design course. For each of the S groups, correlations were computed between indices of academic achievement and performance on the tangrams. Of a total of 72 such correlations, only 2 were significant. It is concluded that the initial validity data presented are encouraging.

238

Driver, J. S. (1982). The dimensionality of cross-cultural cognition: personality (cognitive motivation as measured by the General Environmental/Personal Life Indices (GE/PLIS) (a multivariate instrument), sex and alcohol-related behaviors). *Dissertation Abstracts International, 43,* **B1235-1236.**

239

Eysenck, H. J. et al. (1984). A new Visual Aesthetic Sensitivity Test: 4. Cross-cultural comparisons between a Chinese sample from Singapore and an English sample. *Personality & Individual Differences, 5,* **599-600.**

The authos administered the Visual Aesthetic Sensitivity Test to 1,097 Chinese (aged 9-40 years) and 784 English students and children (aged 10-17 years) to study the possible influence of cultural factors. The data showed that there were few between-group differences. It was noted that the Chinese sample actually scored slightly better than the European sample on a test designed in the European tradition. Difficulty levels of the items were similar for subjects from two cultures.

240

Fong, K. C., & Lin, H. T. (1963). [A simplification of Canata's Intelligence Test (Form B)]. *Psychological Testing, 10,* **804-811.** (In Chinese.)

241

Gerr, S. (1982). A possible analogy between contours in mathematics--as exemplified by Cauchy's integral formula--and contours in the arts. *Perception, 11,* **483-490.**

Presents an analogy between contour drawing and a particular mathematical theorem that depends on the fact that both methods use definite values along a contour to imply a totality of values within the contour. The author uses a hypothetical "gestalt-like integration" in the case of the art contour and the usual process of mathematical integration in the case of Cauchy's formula. The traditional Chinese philosophy of painting is invoked in support of the analogy, and applications of this analogy to the psychology of art and mathematics are discussed.

242

Gong, Y. X. et al. (1983). [Revision of Wechsler's Adult Intelligence Scale in China]. *Acta Psychologica Sinica, 15,* **362-370.** (In Chinese.)

A Chinese version of the WAIS was validated by administering it to a representative Chinese sample (2,029 urban and 992 rural Ss). The reliability of this version of the WAIS, as assessed by the split-half procedure, subtest intercorrelations, and test-retest correlations, was supported. High educational attainment and young age correlated with high test scores, thus supporting the validity of the scale. Separate norms are presented for rural and urban standardization samples.

243

Gong, Y. X. (1984). [The Eysenck Personality Questionnaire revised in China]. *Information on Psychological Sciences,* **No. 4, 11-18.** (In Chinese.)

This study comprises two parts: a comparison of Eysenck Personality Questionnaire (EPQ) scores among Chinese, English, and Greeks, and item selection from original versions of the EPQ. A Chinese sample of 2,517 adults and 3,441 junior high school students were tested in 1981 and 1982. The results were compared with those of English and Greek samples. From the Chinese sample, scores of 1,000 adults and 1,000 students were used for factor analysis. These subjects represented various ages, sexes, educational levels, and geographic regions. Eighty-eight items for adults and 88 items for students were selected, and the EPQ age norms were established.

244

Gong, Z. X., & Guo, D. (1984). [An intelligence screening test for preschool and primary school-children--Picture Vocabulary Test]. *Acta Psychologica Sinica, 16,* **392-401.** (In Chinese.)

The Peabody Picture Vocabulary Test was revised and applied to 764 children aged 3-1/2 to 8 years in Shanghai. The results obtained were: test-retest reliability = .945; interscorer reliability = .913; split-half reliability = .945; standard error of measurement = 4.5. Intertest validity coefficients were: for "Item 50," r = .478; for Draw a man, r = .466; for the Full Scale IQ of WPPSI, r = .427; for Chinese exam r = .652; and for math exam, r = .609. This test has been applied to more than 5,000 children, and has proved to be a simple and convenient general intelligence screening test in pediatrics and child education.

245

[Grade norms for public junior high school students on the Army General Classification Test]. (1972). *Psychological Testing, 19,* **1044-1054.** (In Chinese.)

246

Hou, F. (1954). [A report on the development of a new non-verbal intelligence test]. *Psychological Testing, 2,* **78-82.** (In Chinese.)

247

Hsiao, H. H. (1941). [Hsiao's revision of Personal Data Sheet]. *Educational Bulletin, 4.* (In Chinese.)

248

Hsu, C. W. (1957). [Construction of the Chinese Army Aptitude Test Battery]. *Psychological Testing, 5,* **344-349.** (In Chinese.)

249

Hsu, C. W. (1963). [The construction of the Comprehensive Aptitude Test for middle schools]. *Psychological Testing, 10,* **769-775.** (In Chinese.)

250

Hwang, K. Y., Choug, S. C., & Fu, C. H. (1978). [A first report on the revision of the Lorge-Thorndike Nonverbal Intelligence Test]. *Psychological Testing, 25,* **75-84.** (In Chinese.)

251

Jin, Y., & Zhu, J. X. (1984). [Report on the application of the WISC-R to a group of second graders in Shanghai]. *Information on Psychological Sciences,* **No. 4, 19-23.** (In Chinese.)

252

Kao, L. Y. (1962). [The standardization of a Chinese version of the Thurstone Temperament Schedule]. *Psychological Testing, 9,* **35-48.** (In Chinese.)

253

Kau, L. J., Yeh, E. K., Lin, M. Y., Chu, T. F., Chou, M. H., & Li, S. I. (1981). [A study with the revised Chinese version of Brayman's comprehensive occupational therapy evaluation scale]. *Acta Psychologica Taiwanica, 23,* **1-7.** (In Chinese.)

To evaluate the behavior of psychiatric patients in occupational therapy settings, the authors translated into Chinese and revised Brayman's Comprehensive Occupational Therapy Evaluation (COTE) Scale. The Chinese version pertains to 20 behaviors that occur frequently in occupational therapy situations. Four occupational therapists simultaneously observed and rated separately the behavior of 55 patients at the Taipei City Psychiatric Center from July to October, 1980. The main findings were: (1) Interrater reliability coefficients ranged between .61 to .94. (2) Internal consistency coefficients ranged from .83 to .85, the average being .84. (3) A validity study showed that the revised scale predicted relapse within three months after discharge from hospital. The results of the study also showed that the revised version of the COTE scale was sensitive to the nature and extent of deviant behaviors and indicated changes over a period of time.

254

Keyes, S. (1984). Measuring sex-role stereotypes: Attitudes among Hong Kong Chinese adolescents and the development of the Chinese Sex-Role Inventory. *Sex Roles, 10,* **129-140.**

Data from 79 13-yr-olds and 83 16-yr-olds enrolled in an Anglo-Chinese secondary school in Hong Kong were used to construct a Chinese Sex-Role Inventory following the procedures used by S. Bem to construct the Bem Sex-Role Inventory. All Ss were ethnically Chinese. Ss were presented with a probe questionnaire, a definitional rating scale was constructed from responses, and Ss' responses to the scale determined final selection of terms. Results show that the 51-item Chinese Sex-Role Inventory could be divided into several sections: 27 items dealt with quality-of-character terms; other sections dealt with school subjects and minimum level of education wished to be achieved. It is concluded that there is value in obtaining from Ss themselves the attributes used to define masculinity and femininity.

255

Knudsen, A. K., Gorham, D. R., & Moseley, E. C. (1966). Universal popular responses to inkblots in five cultures: Denmark, Germany, Hong Kong, Mexico and United States. *Journal of Projective Techniques and Personality Assessment, 30,* **135-142.**

256

Ko, Y. H. (1972). The Bender-Gestalt Test as a test for visual-verbal coordination. *Acta Psychologica Taiwanica, 14,* **52-66.**

The Bender-Gestalt Test used as a test for visual-verbal coordination requires the subject to make a detailed oral description of each of the first five Bender figures. In the present study, this method of using the Bender Gestalt Test was used with 50 subjects. The results showed that the method could yield information highly valid for the assessment of subjects' intelligence. It was suggested that the test could play an important role in the measurement of intelligence. The results also showed that this new use of the Bender-Gestalt Test can yield materials unobtainable from other tests but capable of assisting the clinician to assess his client's attentional disposition, thought processes, and personality traits. Possible methods of establishing valid systems for scoring these psychological processes are discussed.

257

Ko, Y. H. (1975). [A study of the reliability and the validity of the Ko's Mental Health Questionnaire]. *Psychological Testing, 22,* **42-45.** (In Chinese.)

258

Ko, Y. H., Yang, S. K., & Tsai, Y. L. (1964). [Validity of the Ko Mental Health Questionnaire]. *Psychological Testing, 11,* **34-38.** (In Chinese.)

259

Koh, Y. H. (1957). [A scoring system for the Bender Gestalt Test and its relation to intelligence]. *Psychological Testing, 5,* **356-361.** (In Chinese.)

260

Koo, C. W. (1958). [The construction and administration of the Recruit Qualification Test]. *Psychological Testing, 6,* **424-432.** (In Chinese.)

261

Ku, C. W. (1963). [A report on the Non-verbal Elementary School Intelligence Test]. *Psychological Testing, 10,* **781-793.** (In Chinese.)

262

Kuo, H. K., & Marsella, A. J. (1977). The meaning and measurement of Machiavellianism in Chinese and American college students. *Journal of Social Psychology, 101,* **165-173.**

Although there has been considerable cross-cultural research on Machiavellianism in recent years, researchers have failed to examine the conceptual equivalence of the concept across cultural boundaries. Measures of Machiavellianism (Mach IV) have been used which were derived from Western concepts and which may not have similar meanings when applied to non-Western groups. The present study examined the factorial structure of the Mach IV scale in matched samples (age, sex, education, and social desirability) of 128 male and female Chinese and American college students. It was hypothesized that the groups would differ with respect to the factorial structure of the Mach IV because of ethnocultural differences in meaning of the factorial terms and in their behavioral referents, correlates, and functional implications. Results support the hypothesis. It is concluded that researchers must exercise considerable care in cross-cultural personality research, since constructs may lack conceptual and behavioral equivalence.

263

Lao, R. C. (1978). Levenson's IPC (Internal-External Control) Scale: A comparison of Chinese and American students. *Journal of Cross-Cultural Psychology, 9,* **113-124.**

To examine further the cross-cultural feasibility of the internal-external control of reinforcement construct, one part of the present study was conducted in Taiwan, using 517 Chinese college students, and the other part consisted of 423 American college students. H. Levenson's (1972) IPC Scale (Internal, Powerful Others, and Chance Scale) and an information questionnaire were used to compare the 2 groups. After translating the materials into Chinese for the Chinese Ss, comparisons of the locus of control concept between the 2 cultures and between sexes were made. In general, similar patterns between males and females on the IPC were found for both American and Chinese students, and I, P, and C were also found to correlate with a similar number of confidence and expectancy variables for the 2 cultures. Results, taken together and compared with data from previous studies, suggest that the locus of control variable may be tapping some basic psychological dimension common to both cultures.

264

Leu, W. H., Ko, Y. H., & Chen, W. Y. (1966). A preliminary report of the tryout of MMPI on the freshmen of National Taiwan University. *Acta Psychologica Taiwanica, 8,* **79-84.**

The Chinese form of the Minnesota Multiphasic Personality Inventory (MMPI) was administered to 704 freshmen in National Taiwan University. The scores showed large differences from those of the Minnesota normative groups, including L and F scores. The possible explanations of these differences in terms of translational distortion and cultural difference suggest the necessity to have a further intensive study of the applicability of the MMPI to Chinese culture.

265

Li, A. K. F. (1964). The use of ability tests in Hong Kong. *International Journal of Experimental Research in Education,* **1, 2.**

266

Li, A. K. F. (1966). The Cantonese semantic differential scales. *Journal of Education* **(University of Hong Kong), No. 23, 23-27.**

267

Li, D. et al. (1983). [Preliminary test results on the WISC-R in the Shanghai metropolitan area]. *Information on Psychological Sciences,* **No. 4, 10-20.** (In Chinese.)

This research is an attempt to adapt the Wechsler Intelligence Scale for Children-Revised for use in China. Preliminary data on 352 children 6-16 years old in the Shanghai metropolitan area are reported.

268

Lin, C. T. (1980). [A sketch on the methods of mental testing in ancient China]. *Acta Psychologica Sinica, 12,* **75-80.** (In Chinese.)

Asserts that the Chinese anticipated many aspects of Western psychology by as much as 2,000 yrs. The imperial examination system is stated to be an early means of intelligence and personality assessment, and the distraction, shape analysis, and antithetical phrase tests developed by Chinese philosophers and literary figures parallel tests developed in the West in the 20th century.

269

Lin, M. H., & Chu, C. P. (1975). [A revision of Torrance Test of creative thinking: The verbal form]. *Psychological Testing, 22,* **80-87.** (In Chinese.)

270

Lin, P. C. (1970). [A revision of Cattell's Culture Fair Intelligence Test]. *Psychological Testing, 17,* **814-842.** (In Chinese.)

271

Lin, P. C. (1978). [The factor structure of the least preferred scale and its relationship with stereotyping and self concept]. *Acta Psychologica Taiwanica, 20,* **41-52.** (In Chinese.)

499 Chinese school administrators and teachers completed the Least Preferred Co-Worker Scale (LPCS). Results show the following: (a) There are 3 dimensions (not 1) in the LPCS. (b) Approximately 25% of the Ss had not rated a real person on the scale, but had, instead, rated a stereotyped object. (c) Stereotypes obtained lower LPCS scores than nonstereotypes. (d) There were differential effects of sex, age, and position (administration vs teaching) on the LPCS scores of the 2 groups.

272

Lindgren, H. C. (1976). Measuring need to achieve by nAch--nAff Scale: A forced-choice questionnaire. *Psychological Reports, 39,* **907-910.**

To measure the need to achieve (nAch), a questionnaire was constructed which required the S to make a forced choice on each of 30 pairs of adjectives. Items were derived from the Adjective Check List's Achievement and Affiliation scales. When the questionnaire was scored for nAch, differences between sex and age groupings of 469 college students were nonsignificant, but scores for males were positively and significantly correlated with grades on midterms and GPA, whereas correlations for females were low and significant only at the .10 level. 27 bank tellers' nAch scores correlated positively with supervisors' ratings and were significantly lower than those of college students. Nine expectant mothers had the lowest scores on nAch while male Chinese-speaking immigrants under age 30 scored the highest. Results are consistent with previous research and with expectations based on everyday impressions.

273

Ling, W. Q. (1985). [Factor analysis of the Test Anxiety Scale (TAI) of Chinese university students]. *Acta Psychologica Sinica, 17,* **137-143.** (In Chinese.)

The Test Anxiety Scale TAI was given to Chinese university students. The results indicated that test anxiety was higher in females than in males. A factor analysis resulted in five factors, four of which were common to both sexes. Worrying About the Examination Results was a factor unique to female students, and Disliking and Criticizing Examinations was unique male students.

274

Liu, I. M., Chang, B. H., & Yang, Y. T. (1979). [Constructing a word-construction test]. *Acta Psychologica Taiwanica, 21,* **85-90.** (In Chinese.)

Third and fifth graders were presented with a set of 30 word fragments, and were instructed to construct words by combining two or more fragments. The words constructed were analyzed by word characteristics (numbers of fragments used and frequency counts) and output intervals. From the obtained results, it could be inferred that children depended first on external fragments to generate words in order to compare and check them with internal word models, and then on internally generated word models based on the partial cues of word fragments. This view is consistent with the results obtained from the second administration of the test (for a reliability measure) and also with a word-chain test used for test validation.

275

Lo, M. Y., & Chien, M. F. (1964). [Validity of the Maudsley Personality Inventory and its relation to social desirability]. *Psychological Testing, 11,* **29-33.** (In Chinese.)

276

Lu, C. M. (1977). [The Chinese Language Achievement Test for senior high school students]. *Psychological Testing, 24,* **52-59.** (In Chinese.)

277

Lu, C. M. (1978). [A report on the revision of the Gordon Personal Inventory]. *Psychological Testing, 25,* **54-63.** (In Chinese.)

278

Lu, C. M., & Chien, M. F. (1968). [A preliminary report on the revision of WAIS for the Chinese people]. *Psychology and Education, 2,* **138-149.** (In Chinese.)

The main purpose of this research was to develop a Chinese version of the Wechsler Adult Intelligence Scale. The form of the original scale was preserved, but the contents of test items were revised according to cultural and social conditions. The sample consisted of 348 men and 205 women--553 inhabitants of northern Taiwan. The result indicated that the revised scale was an adequate instrument for measuring adult intelligence in Taiwan. There were expected differences among six age groups, making it necessary to establish different norms. However, sex differences were negligible. The reliability coefficients were satisfactorily high for both the Verbal and the Performance scales. Full Scale IQs had a correlation of .73 with the General Classification Test, and .78 with Raven's Progressive Matrices.

279

Lu, C. Y. (1956). [The construction and application of the Naval Basic Test Battery]. *Psychological Testing, 4,* **264-271.** (In Chinese.)

280

Lu, C. Y. (1957). [Preliminary research on unifying the grades of the Chinese Naval General Classification Test]. *Psychological Testing, 5,* **332-335.** (In Chinese.)

281

Lu, C. Y. (1963). [Some notes on the revision of Binet-Simon Scale]. *Psychological Testing, 10,* **734-737.** (In Chinese.)

282

Lu, C. Y. (1965). [A preliminary report on the revision of the MMPI]. *Psychological Testing, 12,* **132-143.** (In Chinese.)

283

Lu, C. Y. (1968). [Construction of the Adolescent Personality Inventory]. *Psychological Testing, 15,* **453-463.** (In Chinese.)

284

Lu, C. Y. (1969). [An intelligence test for junior high school students]. *Psychology and Education, 3,* **39-47.** (In Chinese.)

Since the extension of the public education program, educational and vocational guidance has been greatly emphasized in public junior high schools in Taiwan. Consequently the need for psychological tests has become very pressing. This paper reports the preparation of an intelligence test for junior high school students. Preliminary results indicated that its validity was satisfactory. Percentile norms were established.

285

Lu, C. Y. (1975). [A Report on the revision of the Gordon Personal Profile]. *Bulletin of Educational Psychology, 8,* **1-9.** (In Chinese.)

Reports on the translation of the Gordon Personal Profile into Chinese, and its standardization with data from 1,928 high school and university students. Reliability and validity data are provided.

286

Lu, C. Y. (1977). [A report on the Fourth Chinese Revision of the Binet Scale]. *Psychological Testing, 24,* **1-10.** (In Chinese.)

287

Lu, C. Y. (1978). [The development of the primary battery of the school and college ability test]. *Bulletin of Educational Psychology, 11,* **1-8.** (In Chinese.)

One battery in the whole series of the School College Tests contains three distinct subtests: comprehension (general information), picture vocabulary, and size and number. These short subtests measure verbal and quantitative skills important in assessing readiness for school work. In the present study. the battery was standardized on a sample of 279 children from 19 kindergartens and 20 primary schools. Two types of norms were provided: age norms reported in terms of raw scores converted to deviation IQs, and grade norms in terms of percentile ranks. Both reliability and validity were very satisfactory.

288

Lu, C. Y., Hwang, C. H., & Tseng, L. C. (1960). [A preliminary report on the third Chinese revision of the Binet-Simon Scale]. *Psychological Testing, 8,* **537-548.** (In Chinese.)

289

Lubin, B., & Collins, J. F. (1985). Depression Adjective Check Lists: Spanish, Hebrew, Chinese and English versions. *Journal of Clinical Psychology, 41,* **213-217.**

Data were presented on the translation, reliability, concurrent validity, and norms of the Spanish, Hebrew, and Chinese versions of three equivalent forms of the Depression Adjective Check Lists as compared to the English version. Reliability estimates (split-half, alternate form and internal consistency) for the 4 versions were quite similar in magnitude. Concurrent validity was determined in each case by means of correlations with translated versions of a series of scales.

290

Maykovich, M. K. (1980). Social distance between the Chinese and Americans. *Acta Psychologica Taiwanica, 22,* **1-12.**

Tested the validity of the Yang-Lee-Yu Social Distance Scale (a modified version of the Bogardus Social Distance Scale) and measured social distance as perceived by Chinese students and farmers toward Americans. The scale was administered to 240 university students and 204 farmers. Ss were asked their willingness to engage in various types of social interaction (e.g., marriage, intimate friendship, sharing a taxi) with White, Black, and Chinese-Americans. With regard to validity, the Guttman coefficient of reproducibility was improved when 2 items were interchanged. The new scale now lists 3 items in the order (1) marriage, (2) becoming a close kin by marriage, and (3) becoming an intimate friend. Results show the following: (1) The perception of Sino-American social distance was affected by international events such as the US derecognition of the Republic of China; (2) Chinese students felt closer to Chinese-Americans than to Whites, and most distant toward Blacks; and (3) farmers were either uncertain of their sentiment toward Americans or did not wish to have any transactions with them.

291

National Coordination Group of MMPI (1982). **[The revision, employment and evaluation of MMPI in China].** *Acta Psychologica Sinica, 14,* **449-458.** (In Chinese.)

Results of revision, evaluation, and use of the MMPI in China show that the reliability and validity of the inventory was high. It is suggested that the results be carefully analyzed in combination with the norms of the Chinese people.

292

Nishimoto, R. H. (1986). Measurement equivalence across cultures: Langner's twenty-two item index of psychiatric symptoms. *Dissertation Abstracts International, 46,* **A2443.**

293

[Psychological tests developed in Taiwan]. (1968). *Psychological Testing, 15,* **539-564.** (In Chinese.)

294

[Recent developments of psychological testing in China]. (1970). *Psychological Testing, 17,* **735-739.** (In Chinese.)

295

Shyu, M. S. (1976). [The Chinese revision of California Test of Personality (Elementary Level)]. *Psychological Testing, 23,* **71-77.** (In Chinese.)

296

Simpson, R. F. (1963). I. Q. in Hong Kong: Some views on intelligence and its measurement Hong Kong. *Journal of Education^ (University of Hong Kong),* **21,** *22-30.*

297

Smilkstein, G., Ashworth, C., & Montano, D. (1982). Validity and reliability of the Family APGAR as a test of family function. Journal of Family Practice, 15, *303-311.*

Supports the use of the Family APGAR (Adaptation, Partnership, Growth, Affection, Resolve) index as a reliable, validated, utilitarian instrument to measure an S's satisfaction with 5 components of family function. Mean total Family APGAR scores for several population groups are reported along with associated validity and reliability studies. A study from Taiwan (C. C. Hsu, 1973) supports the use of the Family APGAR in student populations 10 yrs of age and older.

298

Steinberg, A. R. (1985). Content analysis of naturally occurring events: An alternative approach to traditional personality assessment. Dissertation Abstracts International, 46, *B993.*

299

Stetson, D., & Wagner, E. E. (1980). A note on the use of the Hand Test in cross-cultural research: Comparison of Iranian, Chinese and American students. Journal of Personality Assessment, 44, *603.*

Administered the Hand Test to 30 Taiwanese and 30 Iranian male university students, who were matched separately with American students for age and year in school. Five variables discriminated between the Iranian and the American Ss, with the Iranians scoring higher on Dependence, Average Initial Response Time, and High-Low scores and lower on Active and Environmental scores. Four variables discriminated between the Chinese and American Ss; the Chinese had higher Communication, Interpersonal, Average Initial Response Time, and High-Low scores.

300

Sun, C. W. (1963). [Construction and analysis of the General Classification Test]. Psychological Testing, 10, *794-803. (In Chinese.)*

301

Sun, K. K. (1960). [A Battery of Achievement Tests for elementary school children]. Psychological Testing, 8, *557-568. (In Chinese.)*

302

Tang, S. C., & Yang, Y. W. (1959). [A general intelligence test for freshmen students in Tunghai University]. Psychological Testing, 7, *491-493. (In Chinese.)*

303

The Cooperation Group for the Construction of the "Clinical Memory Test" (Institute of Psychology, Academia Sinica). (1986). [The construction of the "Clinical Memory Test"]. Acta Psychologica Sinica, 18, *100-108. (In Chinese.)*

A battery of the Clinical Memory Test was designed and constructed to suit the need for memory assessment in practice and research. It consists of 5 subtests. Two matched forms, A and B, were simultaneously composed. For standardization of the test, 2161 literate subjects and 1149 illiterate subjects were selected. The test result of the two standardization samples appeared in normal distribution, and the correlation ratio between forms A and B in replication test was 0.85. The relationship between memory assessment and learning performance, or between memory assessment and age, was consistent with experience. The application of this test to brain tumor patients showed that the recognition of meaningless figures was related with the function of the right hemisphere while the paired-association learning with that of the left hemisphere, a result in accordance with our prediction. These results indicated the qualified reliability and validity of the test.

304

Tsoi, M. M., & Tam, W. Y. K. (1983). A Chinese visual analogue mood scale for rating subjective feelings. Acta Psychologica Taiwanica, 25, *67-74.*

Sixteen visual analogue mood scales were translated from English to Chinese and the two versions attained significantly high correlation when completed by 42 bilingual university students. The Chinese version of the scale was administered to over 170 university students. Three factors were abstracted from the scale, namely, Alertness, Contentedness and Friendliness. The Alertness factor replicated the first factor in the English factor analysis study (Bond & Lader, 1974) of the mood scale. However, Chinese subjects perceived scales describing feelings of contentment as related to relaxation and tranquillity while western subjects associated contentment with being sociable and gregarious. Hence, the Friendliness factor was isolated as the third factor in this study in contrast to the Calmness factor which was isolated as the third factor in the original English study. A further factor analysis was performed with a four-factor solution. Once again, an Alertness factor and a Friendliness factor were obtained. The Contentedness factor broke down into a Contentedness factor and a Calmness factor. The four-factor solution can be adopted to provide four subscales of the analogue scale. This Chinese Visual Analogue Mood Scale is recommended for use in research on arousal, pain research and psychophysiological studies in general.

305

Turner, S. M., & Mo, L. L. (1984). Chinese adolescents' self-concept as measured by the Offer Self-image Questionnaire. Journal of Youth & Adolescence, 13, *131-143.*

Examined self-image among 426 Taiwanese 9th graders and adolescent factory workers, using Chinese translation of the Offer Self-Image Questionnaire for Adolescents. It was found that Chinese subjects scored significantly lower than norms for Americans on the Psychological Self dimension. Chinese scores were slightly higher on morals and lower on social relationships and vocational-educational goals than Americans. The biggest difference between the groups was in sexual attitudes, in which the Chinese were much more conservative. Female adolescents working in factories scored lower than other subjects on self-image; this may be due to the paternalism and the monotonous assembly-line work that contributed to a negative, nonsupportive environment. The effects of different socialization practices in the two cultures on cultural attitudes were discussed.

306

Wang, F. K. (1959). [Psychological testing programs in Taiwan today]. Psychological Testing, 7, *466-467. (In Chinese.)*

307

Wang, F. K. (1963). [Recent developments of psychological testing in China]. Psychological Testing, 10, *708-712. (In Chinese.)*

308

Wang, H., & Chu, C. P. (1975). [A revision of Torrance Test of creative thinking: The figural form]. Psychological Testing, 22, *88-94. (In Chinese.)*

309

Wang, M. J. (1969). Report on the revision of the Thematic Apperception Test. Acta Psychologica Taiwanica, 11, *24-41.*

The revision of the Thematic Apperception Test (TAT) in the Test Revision Project started with the purpose of adapting it and making it applicable to the Chinese culture. A new set of TAT cards, drawn by a Chinese artist according to the criteria for designing such a series, was substituted for the original TAT cards. Two preliminary tests were performed to determine a final set of TAT cards. In the first test 27 TAT picture slides were presented to 83 university students. The stimulus value of each picture was analyzed and the picture modified and redrafted, until a series of satisfactory pictures evolved for use. The second preliminary test secured 20 subjects' individual responses to the TAT cards. These responses were analyzed into four categories of need; achievement, affiliation, power and aggression. A measure of ambiguity was applied to each card, and modifications were made until the final set of TAT cards was obtained for Chinese use. This new set of TAT cards was administered to 120 university subjects and 20 schizophrenic patients equally divided in terms of sex and educational level. Their protocols were analyzed in terms of the four need categories. Intrascore reliabilities based on 20 subjects were .93, .82, .86, and .95 for achievement, affiliation, power, and aggression respectively.

310

Wang, X. L., & Hu, X. R. (1986). [An attempt at the making of a teacher's professionalism scale]. Information on Psychological Sciences, *No. 3, 27-31. (In Chinese.)*

311

Wu, W. T., & Chen, Y. H. (1977). [The Diagnostic Mathematics Test]. Psychological Testing, 24, *60-73. (In Chinese.)*

312

Yamamoto, J. et al. (1982). The Psychiatric Status Schedule for Asian Americans. American Journal of Psychiatry, 139, *1181-1184.*

Translated the Psychiatric Status Schedule into Chinese, Japanese, and Korean and devised an audiovisual version of the measure. The audiovisual version was validated by comparing computer diagnoses by mental health professionals (MHPs) who used the translated version, with the computer diagnoses of MHPs and volunteers who used the audiovisual version. 60 Chinese, Japanese, and Korean Ss were diagnosed. Moderate reliability was found between the standard translated and the audiovisual versions.

313

Yang, K. S., Su, C., Hsu, H. H., & Huang, C. H. (1962). [Rorschach responses of normal Chinese adults: Vol. 1. The normal details]. Acta Psychologica Taiwanica, *No. 4, 78-103. (In Chinese.)*

314

Yang, K. S., Tzuo, H. Y., & Wu, C. Y. (1963). Rorschach responses of normal Chinese adults: Vol. 2. The popular responses. Journal of Social Psychology, 60, *175-186.*

Ten Rorschach responses were determined as popular for normal Chinese adults, based on a sample of 347 responses. A set of 6 sample statistics of number and percentage was calculated for the weighted and nonweighted popular responses. In addition, some intra- and cross-cultural comparisons were made between the list obtained by the present authors and those of other authors. At least one popular response, Card VI W Turtle, can be considered as unique to normal Chinese adults.

315

Yang, P. H. L., & Lin, L. H. (1975). [A study of the predictive validity of the California Test of Mental Maturity (Level V)]. Psychological Testing, 22, *64-72. (In Chinese.)*

316

Zhang, D. X. (1983). [The construction and application of tests of creative potentials in thinking]. Acta Psychologica Sinica, 15, *19-28. (In Chinese.)*

To explore children's creative potentials in thinking, a battery of tests has recently been constructed, using subtests such as association, generalization, reasoning, number series, mathematical comprehension, problem-solving, and moral judgment. All these tests involve both convergent and divergent thinking; the former emphasizes mathematical questions and the latter questions concerning self-expressions. These tests were administered repeatedly with different forms to 224 school children. Evidence for validity could be seen in the obtained high correlations with mathematics achievement and other cognitive measures.

317

Zhu, Y. M. et al. (1984). [The WPPSI and its trial application in Shanghai Proper]. Information on Psychological Sciences, *No. 5, 22-29. (In Chinese.)*

The following references are also relevant to this chapter:

579, 630, 706, 848, 906, 1173, 1206, 1288, 1295, 1313, 1317, 1323, 1371, 1712, 2206, 2268, 2426, 2649, 2777, 2884, 2887, 3165, 3221, 3245, 3248, 3427.

EXPERIMENTAL PSYCHOLOGY 4

Frequency data on citations in this chapter, in terms of content classification subcategories, are presented in Table 4.

Table 4: *Number of Citations by Content Classification, Language, and Geographical Area*

Content classificntion	Total	CL	EL	OL	PRC	T	HK	US
Experimental psychology	7	1	6	0	1	1	0	0
Perception & motor processes	14	11	3	0	11	1	0	0
Visual perception	29	16	13	0	11	2	1	0
Auditory & speech perception	7	4	3	0	11	2	1	0
Cognitive processes	51	19	31	1	6	4	6	1
Learning & memory	34	19	13	2	12	5	0	1
Motivation & emotion	4	1	3	0	0	3	0	0
Attention & consciousness states	4	1	3	0	1	0	0	0
Total		150	72	75	3	45	16	72

Note: CL = Chinese language; EL = English language; OL = other languages. PRC = People's Republic of China; T = Taiwan; HK = Hong Kong; US = United States (Chinese Americans--according to the frequency of the subject term Asian Americans).

Subject terms used for indexing citations related to experimental psychology are grouped according to geographical area, subject population, and topic. These are presented below, in a descending order of frequency. (The frequency of single-word subject terms includes those of compound terms in which the single word appears. Subjects terms used for indexing citations from other chapters may have been included. Terms with a frequency of less than 10 are not shown.)

Geographical area

60	Peoples Republic of China
19	Taiwan

Subject population

33	children
22	students
19	school age children
13	adults
10	college students

Topic

54	perception
35	language
35	learning
27	memory
25	reading
18	cross cultural differences
18	adulthood
17	Chinese characters
17	cognitive processes
16	visual perception
15	short term memory
13	written language
12	human information storage
11	foreign languages
11	pictorial stimuli
10	age differences
10	discrimination
10	time
10	words (phonetic units)

Table 4 shows that most citations concern cognitive processes (56.7%--inclusive learning and memory), and perceptual (especially visual) and motor processes (33.3%). Among subject terms indexing topics, *perception* appears with the highest frequency, followed by language and learning. As shown by terms indexing geographical areas, the PRC predominates over Taiwan.

318

Adams, F. M., & Osgood, C. E. (1973). A cross-cultural study of the affective meanings of color. *Journal of Cross-Cultural Psychology, 4,* **135-156.**

319

Bahrick, H. P. (1970). Discriminative and associative aspects of retroactive inhibition. *Quarterly Journal of Experimental Psychology, 22,* **565-573.**

Followed original learning of paired drawings of meaningful objects or of modified Chinese characters by interpolated learning in which details of drawings were changed in 1 of 2 degrees with or without rearrangement of the original pairings. 5 groups of 10 undergraduates each were tested for accuracy of identification of the original drawings and for associative matching of the original pairs. Identification errors were attributed jointly to confusion between original and interpolated drawings, and to unlearning of those features of original drawings which were in conflict with comparable features of interpolated drawings. Rearrangement of pairs during interpolated learning produced associative interference on the matching test, and additional discriminatory interference on the identification test. Effects of associative and discriminative interference on individual drawings were uncorrelated for meaningful material and only slightly correlated for meaningless material.

320

Ball, O. E., & Torrance, E. P. (1978). Culture and tendencies to draw objects in internal visual perspective. *Perceptual & Motor Skills, 47,* **1071-1075.**

100 Ss from each of 9 countries representing 3 cultures--Eastern (Japan, China, and India), European (France, Norway, and West Germany), and Western (US, Canada, and the Virgin Islands)--were compared on their ability to visualize objects from an unusual (internal) visual perspective on Activity 3 of the Torrance Tests of Creative Thinking, Form B. Intercultural and intracultural differences were found; Ss from Eastern cultures demonstrated a significantly greater frequency of internal visualizations than did European and Western cultures when a streamlined scoring procedure was used.

321

Baron, J., & Strawson, C. (1976). Use of orthographic and word-specific knowledge in reading words aloud. *Journal of Experimental Psychology: Human Perception & Performance, 2,* **386-393.**

Words that conform to spelling-sound correspondence rules (e.g., sweet) are read aloud more quickly than words that do not conform (e.g., sword). This suggests that the rules are used in reading a word, in spite of past learning of the association between the word and its entire pronunciation. This effect is larger in Ss who rely heavily on the rules, as determined by independent tests. Two experiments were conducted, the 1st with 30 college students and the 2nd with 16 college students, 8 of whom were Chinese and 8 Phoenician. In addition, mixing case affects reading of nonconforming words more than of conforming ones, suggesting that word-specific associations use units larger than single letters.

322

Bennion, R. B. (1974). Response mode and memory coding strategies: A study in learning of Chinese-English pairs. *Dissertation Abstracts International, 35,* **A3505.**

323

Bertino, M., Beauchamp, G. K., & Jen, K. L. C. (1983). Rated taste perception in two cultural groups. *Chemical Senses, 8,* **3-15.**

Examined intensity and pleasantness ratings of various concentrations of sucrose, caffeine, and NaCl in 42 undergraduates (aged 17-31 yrs) of European descent born in the US, and in 28 undergraduates (aged 23-33 yrs) of Chinese descent born in Taiwan. A subsample of Ss from each group was retested similarly with cookies containing varying levels of sucrose. The Taiwanese Ss rated sucrose as tasting sweeter regardless of whether it was in solution or cookies. Taiwanese Ss assigned higher sweetness ratings to sucrose in solution when compared to US Ss. When the sucrose was in cookies, the Taiwanese group assigned higher pleasantness ratings at the lower sucrose concentrations. At the higher sucrose concentrations, the US group assigned higher pleasantness ratings. There was no significant ethnic effect upon rated bitterness or pleasantness of caffeine. Taiwanese rated low concentrations of salt as tasting saltier and high concentrations of salt as tasting less salty when compared to US Ss. The Taiwanese generally rated the NaCl solutions as tasting more pleasant. It is suggested that these group differences may be related to the way sucrose and salt are used in the 2 cultures.

324

Besner, D., Daniels, S., & Slade, C. (1982). Ideogram reading and right hemisphere language. *British Journal of Psychology, 73,* **21-28.**

Reports 2 experiments on the identification of ideographs. In Exp I, 16 British, right-handed undergraduates showed a right visual field advantage when reporting Arabic numerals. A right field advantage was also obtained in Exp II when 8 Chinese and Japanese students reported numbers presented in Arabic and Kanji formats. Results are discussed in the context of the literature, which shows a left visual field advantage for the identification of single ideographs in Chinese and Japanese, and a right visual field advantage for items in alphabetic and syllabic scripts. It is suggested that it is not the direct mapping between ideographs and the morphemes of a language that yields a left visual field advantage, but associated incidental stimulus characteristics that make demands on preprocessing operations that are carried out more efficiently in the right hemisphere. It is argued that the literature does not address the question of whether alphabetic, syllabic, and ideographic scripts are processed by dissociable mechanisms.

325

Biederman, I., & Tsao, Y. C. (1979). On processing Chinese ideographs and English words: Some implications from Stroop-test results. *Cognitive Psychology, 11,* **125-132.**

When 16 Chinese graduate and undergraduate students tried to name the color of characters that represented conflicting color words, they showed markedly greater interference than did 16 English speaking students performing an English version of the same task. This effect cannot be attributed to bilingualism among the Chinese Ss since bilinguals in other languages show smaller Stroop-interference than monolingual controls. Instead, there may be some fundamental differences in the perceptual demands of reading Chinese and English, which can have widespread implications for human information processing.

326

Binnie-Dawson, J. L., & Choi, P. P. (1982). A study of perceptual and cultural cues in Chinese and Western paintings. *Psychologia: An International Journal of Psychology in the Orient, 25,* **18-31.**

Analyzed the aesthetic value of Chinese and Western paints by employing the eye-movement x-y plotter and by comparing differences in pictorial perception among 19 Chinese and 2 Western undergraduates. Ss were also administered a rod-and-frame test and a semantic differential. Results show that Chinese Ss responded to Chinese landscape paintings with cultural rather than perceptual cues and that the Chinese paintings were more culturally meaningful to Chinese Ss than were Western paintings. Sex differences in scanning behavior were also noted, and those Chinese who were field-independent responded to Chinese paintings with increased eye movements and analytical scanning as compared to field-dependent Chinese Ss.

327

Boey, K. W. (1978). Cognitive complexity and rigidity measured under task-oriented and ego-involved conditions. *Journal of Sociology & Psychology* **(A joint publication of Singapore Sociology Society and Nanyang University Sociology and Psychology Society),** ***1,*** **9-17.**

328

Borresen, C. R., & Wolf, M. (1976). Autokinetic movement as a function of symbolic meaning of target shape. *Perceptual & Motor Skills, 42,* **723-726.**

Measured the autokinetic movement responses of 10 American, 10 Chinese, and 10 Iranian male 18-32 yr old students to religious symbols and control stimuli. The hypothesis of differential direction response as a function of the target shapes was supported. Iranian Ss gave significantly more "down" responses than the American and Chinese Ss.

329

Carlson, E. R. (1962). Generality of order of concept attainment. *Psychological Reports, 10,* **375-380.**

330

Carr, W. K., & Francke, A. W. (1976). Culture and the development of vision. *Journal of the American Optometric Association, 47,* **14-41.**

Used Chinese ethnographic data, to predict a model of a style ("inwardizing") of visual performance. Inwardizing is defined as a style of visual performance in which the viewer builds his space world inward from an object and where objects are less important than the relationships between the objects and the viewer. A 21-point optometric examination was performed on 8 Chinese Ss, and the results are compared with a control group of American Ss. Throughout the optometric examination the Chinese Ss displayed the predicted pattern of inwardizing visual performance. That physiologically measurable patterns of visual performance could be predicted on the basis of ethnographic data gives experimental support to the anthropological assumption of reciprocity between biology and culture. Suggestions are presented for the direction of future studies by various professions on the culturally determined pattern of visual performance.

331

Chang, C. H., & Kuo, S. Y. (1973). [The relationships between verbal complexity and paired-associate learning and retention in elementary school children]. *Bulletin of Educational Psychology, 6,* **1-13.** (In Chinese.)

Studied 100 normal 4th and 5th graders equally divided by sex. Verbal fluency was determined by the number of freely recalled associations in 2 min for each of 20 words. The learning material consisted of 12 paired associate unrelated Chinese characters. Ss were trained to the criterion of 2 correct responses using the method of adjusted learning, which controls for the effect of overlearning. Retention was measured after 1 day and 10 days. Results indicate that (a) verbal fluency was negatively correlated with level of intelligence; (b) verbal fluency was negatively correlated with speed of learning, but positively correlated with speed of forgetting; and (c) there was no difference between boys and girls in learning or retention. Findings are discussed in terms of the interference learning theory proposed by B. J. Underwood and L. Postman.

332

Chang, S. S., Lin, S. J., Wu, C. H., & Yeh, C. H. (1962). Manipulation and learning in children. *Acta Psychologica Taiwanica*, **No. 4, 1-10.**

333

Chang, S. S., & Yang, K. S. (1960). A preliminary study on the manipulation motives of young children. *Acta Psychologica Taiwanica*, **No. 2, 33-42.**

334

Chang, S. S., & Yang, K. S. (1961). The manipulation motive of young children. *Acta Psychologica Taiwanica*, **No. 3, 1-17.**

335

Chao, C. H., & Liu, I. M. (1983). Common and specific features being dissociable or nondissociable as affecting analogical reasoning. *Acta Psychologica Taiwanica*, *25*, **1-12.**

This study investigated how manipulating dissociable or nondissociable common and specific features in pictorial analogies affected analogical reasoning. There were four experimental paradigms: (1) A Person : B Person :: C Person : D1 Person, D2 Person (Paradigm 1); (2) A Cat : B Cat :: C Cat : D1 Cat, D2 Cat (Paradigm 2); (3) A Person : B Person :: C Cat : D1 Cat, D2 Cat (Paradigm 3); (4) A Cat : B Cat :: C Person : D1 Person, D2 Person (Paradigm 4). It was found that when the condition of a small specific feature change from the A to the B term and a large specific feature change from the C to the D (D1 and D2) term was pitted against the condition of a large specific feature change from the A to the B term and a small specific feature change from the C to the D term, the latter condition produced longer solution times, supporting Liu's model (1981) that the feature changes from the C to the D term serve as reference feature changes for extracting the feature changes that go from the A to the B term. It was also found that whether the common and specific features were dissociable or nondissociable interacted to affect solution times. Moreover, the subject was able to disregard the dissociable specific feature changes from the C to the D term but unable to disregard the nondissociable specific feature changes for Paradigms 3 and 4.

336

Chen, H. C. (1985). Reading Chinese text in sequential display format: Effects of display size. *Perceptual & Motor Skills*, *61*, **595-598.**

The author investigated the comprehension of 40 native-Chinese-speaking undergraduates of rapid, serial presentations of Chinese text displayed on a computer monitor. Ten passages in Chinese were presented as sequences of text segments, ranging from 1-13 characters in length, to a fixed location on the computer screen at rates of 230 and 460 characters per minute. Subjects were better able to answer questions in slow than in fast display conditions. Comprehension was maximal for display sizes of about 9 characters regardless of display rates.

337

Chen, H. C., & Juola, J. F. (1982). Dimensions of lexical coding in Chinese and English. *Memory & Cognition*, *10*, **216-224.**

Assessed the effects of the differences in the phonology-orthography relationship between English and Chinese in a study of the roles of phonemic, graphemic, and semantic information on lexical coding and memory for Chinese logographs and English words. The natural confounding between phonemic and graphemic information in English was matched in the Chinese words used. A scaling study indicated that this attempt to equate degree of phonemic-graphemic confounding was successful. A 2nd study used a recognition memory task for English and Chinese words with 48 college students who were native speakers of 1 of the 2 languages. Ss selected 1 of 2 test words that was phonemically, graphemically, or semantically similar to a word on a previously studied list. Differences in the dimensions of lexical coding in memory were demonstrated in significant Stimulus Type by Decision Type interactions in the recognition data. Chinese Ss responded most rapidly and accurately in the graphemic recognition task, whereas performance was generally equivalent in all 3 tasks for the English-speaking Ss. Alphabetic and logographic writing systems apparently activate different coding and memory mechanisms such that logographic characters produce significantly more visual information in memory, whereas alphabetic words result in a more integrated code involving visual, phonological, and semantic information.

338

Chen, H. P., & Chou, S. K. (1935). General versus specific color preferences of Chinese students. *Journal of Social Psychology*, *6*, **290-314.**

339

Chen, K. S. (1964). [Rate of forgetting in the recitation of poems and essays]. *Acta Psychologica Sinica*, **No. 1, 84-93.** (In Chinese.)

An experimental study on memory was carried out with poems and essays, selected from junior middle school reading material. The results showed: (1) Initially, forgetting proceeded faster for essays than for poems, with the reverse occurring later; (2) Differences in the components of materials forgotten, which were related to the difference in rate of forgetting, between poems and essays were observed. Omissions and alterations occurred more frequently in essays than in poems, whereas displacements and reversals occurred more frequently in poems than in essays.

340

Chen, M. J. (1982). Sequential response tendencies and reading habits: A study with Chinese readers. *Australian Journal of Psychology*, *34*, **103-115.**

Studied the sequential response tendencies of 64 Chinese college students in a naming task with unrelated Chinese characters. Two modes of reading Chinese were identified: Mode A was the same as reading English; Mode B started at the top-rightmost corner of a page, descended vertically, and read from right-to-left, column-by-column. All Ss were familiar with both reading modes and perhaps had greater experience with Mode B. However, when given an option, Ss tended to respond predominantly in Mode A. Results could not be accounted for by reading habits alone and are attributed to the manifestation of a hypothetical sequencing mechanism.

341

Chen, S. Y., Yang, B. M., & Han, Z. (1986). [The dependence of reaction and movement time upon responding members and athletic training]. *Acta Psychologica Sinica*, *18*, **1-7.** (In Chinese.)

The simple auditory reaction time (RT) and movement time (MT) of 60 amateur athletes and 20 nonathletes were determined through their hand and foot responses. The results were: (1) The RT for the hand was reliably faster than that for the foot, but the MT for the hand was slower than that for the foot. (2) The relationships between hand and foot responses in RT, MT and RT + MT were all positive and significant. (3) There was no significant difference in RT between athletes and nonathletes. The existence of differences in MT and RT + MT between the two categories of subjects depended on the athletic events undertaken. (4) Although a significant and positive correlation between simple RT and MT was obtained, it was too small for effective prediction.

342

Chen, Y. M., He, B. Y. et al. (1979). [A serial study on the relative spectral luminosity among Chinese people: Vol. I. Photopic relative spectral luminosity]. *Acta Psychologica Sinica*, *11*, **221-227.** (In Chinese.)

Examined the relative spectral luminosity in 50 Chinese adults either below or above 30 yrs of age using the flicker method. The average maximum spectral sensitivity of Ss was 555nm and that most Ss had a maximum value at 555 or 560nm, indicating that it is considerably concentrated. A comparison of the 2 age groups revealed a variation with age in the short-wave end of the spectrum such that the value smoothly decreased as age increased. Findings also indicate that there is probably no significant difference between White and Asian races with respect to the relative spectral luminosity curve.

343

Cheng, C. M. (1978). [Speech recoding and word decoding of the Chinese characters in short-term memory]. *Acta Psychologica Taiwanica*, *20*, **39-43.** (In Chinese.)

344

Cheng, C. M., & Chen, C. S. (1982). Speech recoding: An involuntary control. *Acta Psychologica Taiwanica*, *24*, **127-140.**

Speech syllable production was examined in 2 experiments. In Experiment I, 36 undergraduate students were visually presented with an English consonant and asked to quickly name a syllable consisting of the consonant and either an I or A, depending on the color in which the consonant was printed. Results indicated that naming speed was faster when the resulting syllable sound matched the consonant name than when it did not match. Involuntary speech recoding was evaluated in Experiment II (16 undergraduates), with 2 memory conditions being compared. On each trial, a list of consonants embedded in a vowel environment was auditorially presented to the subject, and the subject was required to name each consonant. The subject was told to name the consonants in either the form in which they were acoustically presented or in a vowel environment different from the one in which they were auditorially embedded. Results indicated that when articulatory information about memory items was not suppressed but remained available in a form incongruent with its input auditory form, short-term recall was impaired.

345

Cheng, P. W., & Holyoak, K. J. (1985). Pragmatic reasoning schemas. *Cognitive Psychology*, *17*, **391-416.**

It was proposed that people typically reason about realistic situations using knowledge structures that the authors have termed pragmatic reasoning schemas, which are generalized sets of rules defined in relation to classes of goals. Three experiments with 82 undergraduates enrolled in a Hong Kong university and 184 undergraduates from an American university were designed to investigate the impact of a permission schema on deductive reasoning. Experiment I demonstrated that by evoking the permission schema it was possible to facilitate performance in P. C. Wason's selection paradigm for subjects who have had no experience with the specific content of the problems. Experiment II showed that a selection problem worded in terms of an abstract permission elicited better performance than one worded in terms of a concrete but arbitrary situation, providing evidence for an abstract permission schema that is free of domain-specific content. Experiment III indicated that evocation of a permission schema affected not only tasks requiring procedural knowledge but also a linguistic rephrasing task requiring declarative knowledge.

346

Ching, C. C., & Jiao, S. L. (1981). Sensory and perceptual studies in the People's Republic of China. *Psychologia: An International Journal of Psychology in the Orient*, *24*, **133-145.**

Reviews research in China relating to sensory and perceptual processes from the early 1960's through the present. Some basic studies from which fundamental laws of sensation and perception were obtained and others that had direct bearing on Chinese industrial applications are cited, including those on visual sensitivity, color vision, figural perception, spatial perception, audition, and other sensory processes.

347

Chou, S. K. (1936). Some comments on color preference of Chinese students. *Journal of Social Psychology*, *7*, **119-121.**

348

Chou, Y. Y. (1965). [Features of thinking in pupils from the 2nd term of the first grade of elementary school as revealed in mistakes in solving arithmetic problems]. *Acta Psychologica Sinica*, *30*, **38-49.** (In Chinese.)

349

Chuang, C. J. (1972). [Effects of associative structure in verbal learning]. *Acta Psychologica Taiwanica*, *14*, **67-91.** (In Chinese.)

Investigated the influence of interword association, interitem association strength, (IAS) and mutual frequency (MF) index on verbal learning in 3 experiments with Taiwanese university students. In Exp. I, Ss were given 198 Chinese verbs and instructed to give meaningfully-related verbs for 10 sec/word. In Exp. II, Ss were given 2 16-item serial learning lists with high or low IAS. Results were attributed to correlated increases in response recall as a function of degree of IAS. In Exp. III, 2 lists of 20 stimulus-response pairs with high or low MF index were used. Results indicate that the paired associate list with high MF index was learned faster than the one with low MF index.

350

Chuang, C. J. (1975). [Effects of mental imaginability in paired-associate learning]. *Acta Psychologica Taiwanica*, *17*, **145-150.** (In Chinese.)

Conducted 2 experiments with a total of 220 university students. In Exp I, 200 Chinese nouns were scaled for mental imaginability by 200 Ss. In Exp II, the effect of mental imaginability on paired-associate learning was investigated. 2 word lists with different imaginability were learned by 20 Ss in this experiment. The effect of high and low imaginability was then compared. Results indicate that the list with high imaginability was learned faster than the one with low imaginability.

351

Chuang, C. J. (1982). [Effects of inter-word and inter-line space on reading Chinese]. *Acta Psychologica Taiwanica*, *24*, **121-126.** (In Chinese.)

The purpose of this study was to evaluate effects of interword and interline space on reading Chinese. It was found that interword and interline space had no effects on reading common words (Experiment 1). However, when the reading materials were sentences, it was found that interword and interline space had significant effects on the detection of incorrect words embedded in sentence contexts (Experiment 2).

352

Craham, V. T. (1926). The intelligence of Chinese children in San Francisco. *Journal of Comparative Psychology*, *6*, **43-71.**

353

Fang, L. L., Yu, J. S., Jing, G., & Gao, J. (1980). [A measurement of the visual depth differential limen among Chinese male young people: Vol. 2]. *Acta Psychologica Sinica*, *12*, **303-306.** (In Chinese.)

Examined the dynamic-depth limen (DL) and the interrelation between static-depth DL and dynamic-depth DL in 435 Ss. Results indicate that the mean of dynamic-depth DL is 4.46 sec(arc) and that there exists a positive correlation between static- and dynamic-depth DL.

354

Fang, Z., Shen, Y., & Wang, S. X. (1979). [Assessment of hearing of standard colloquial Chinese]. *Acta Psychologica Sinica*, *11*, **304-312.** (In Chinese.)

355

Freeman, R. D. (1980). Visual acuity is better for letters in rows than in columns. *Nature*, *286*, **62-64.**

Tested the visual acuity of 11 American adults using letters presented pseudo-randomly with different inter-letter spacings, in rows or columns. Ss were required to identify letters from left to right or from top to bottom in each isolated row or column. Significantly more errors were made for letters in columns than for those in rows. The effect did not depend on order or direction of letter presentation, and it was not found when acuity determinations were made using a nonletter test symbol. To explore the conjecture that the effect could be associated with previous experience, 2 additional groups of Ss were tested. First, 5 bilingual

Chinese, whose 1st language is read in both horizontal and vertical arrays, were tested using Chinese characters and English letters. Second, acuity determinations were made with 5 4-6 yr old American children who could identify letters but did not read. In each case, acuity was not significantly different for horizontal or vertical presentations, a finding consistent with the notion that learning may influence the development of visual resolution.

356

Gandour, J. (1983). Tone perception in Far Eastern languages. *Journal of Phonetics, 11,* **149-175.**

50 undergraduate or graduate student listeners from each of 4 Oriental tone languages (Cantonese, Mandarin, Taiwanese, Thai) and 50 listeners from a nontone language (English) were asked to make direct paired-comparison judgments of tone dissimilarity. Stimuli consisted of 19 fundamental frequency trajectories (5 level, 4 rising, 4 falling, 3 falling-rising, 3 rising-falling) superimposed on a synthetic speechlike monosyllable. The dissimilarities data were organized into 250 dissimilarity matrices and analyzed by the INDSCAL multidimensional scaling model. Analysis revealed 2 dimensions that were interpreted primarily as "height" and "direction". The relative importance of these dimensions varied systematically across Ss, based on language group membership. The direction dimension was relatively more important to listeners of a tone language than a nontone language and to Thai listeners in comparison to Chinese. Discriminant analysis revealed that listeners of tone languages vs a nontone language, Thai listeners vs Chinese, and Cantonese listeners vs Mandarin and Taiwanese can be correctly classified into their respective language groups on the basis of their pattern of dimension weights. Hierarchical clustering analysis indicated that differences in clustering of the stimulus tones could be related to abstract structural properties of listeners' phonological systems.

357

Glenn, F. A. (1978). The roles of orthography and speech coding in fluent reading. *Dissertation Abstracts International, 38,* **B3434.**

358

Goldstein, A. G., Knight, P., Bailis, K. L., & Conover, J. (1981). Recognition memory for accented and unaccented voices. *Bulletin of the Psychonomic Society, 17,* **217-220.**

Laboratory research has established that face recognition memory performance for own-race faces is better than for other-race faces. Three studies are reported exploring the possibility that the other-race effect will generalize to voice recognition memory. Recognition memory performance for nonnative American speakers speaking both English and their native languages (Chinese and Spanish) was compared with memory for native American speakers. A total of 46 male and 129 listeners participated. With relatively long speech samples, accented voices were no more difficult to recognize than were unaccented voices; reducing the speech sample duration decreased recognition memory for accented and unaccented voices, but the reduction was greater for accented voices.

359

Goodnow, J. J. (1969). Cultural variations in cognitive skills. In D. R. Price-Williams (Ed.), *Cross-cultural studies.* **Penguin. (Reprinted in W. W. Lambert & R. Weisbrod (Eds.),** *Comparative perspectives on social psychology.* **Boston: Little-Brown, 1971.)**

360

Guan, L. R., Gao, J., & Xu, L. C. (1986). [Perceptible distance of a road sign varies with the car speed]. *Acta Psychologica Sinica, 18,* **185-189.** (In Chinese.)

The study showed that to a driver, the perceptible distance of a road sign was inversely proportional to the speed of his car. The higher the speed, the shorter the perceptible distance. Compared with walking pace, a car travelling at 100 kilometers an hour cut down the perceptible distance by 35-45%. The results indicated that this was possibly caused by the driver's psychophysiological stress when driving at high speed.

361

Han, K., & Lin, Z. X. (1983). [Discrimination of size by sight and touch in preschool children]. *Acta Psychologica Sinica, 15,* **329-335.** (In Chinese.)

The experiment investigated whether the accuracy of size discrimination involving only either sight or touch differs from that made using both senses. The subjects were 80 preschool children aged 3-6 years of age. They were tested under four perceptual conditions: sight-sight, touch-touch, sight-touch, and touch-sight. The results indicated significant differences among these four conditions. The most accurate size discrimination was found under the sight-sight condition, followed by the touch-touch condition. The least accurate was found under the cross-modal conditions. The accuracy of discrimination under the sight-sight and touch-touch conditions increased with age. Peak accuracy under cross-modal conditions was found at 5 years of age.

362

Hao, Y. T. (1924). The memory span of 600 Chinese school children in San Francisco. *School and Society, 20,* **507-510.**

363

Hardyck, C., Tzeng, O. J., & Wang, W. S. Y. (1977). Cerebral lateralisation effects in visual half-field experiments. *Nature, 269,* **705-707.**

Investigated behavioral differences in cerebral hemispheres in 6 experiments with right-handed adults. Ss fixated on a reference point in a 3-field tachistoscope; stimuli were shown to the right visual field projecting to the left hemisphere, the left visual field projecting to the right hemisphere, or with one member of a stimulus pair projected to each visual field. Two experiments, which differed from the others in their ratio of trials to experimental stimuli, found significant hemisphere function differences. In one study, 8 Ss made judgments of same-different stimulus pairs made up of 4 Chinese characters and 4 English words presented over 200 trials, and in the other study, 8 Ss made same-different judgments of 6 pairs of figures from the Primary Mental Abilities Test over 200 trials. In the 2 studies an ANOVA of reaction time and an analysis of response accuracy, respectively, showed significant hemisphere differences. An explanation that lateralization effects reflect hemispheric differences in memory storage location is consistent with these results. A review of other studies indicated that in those reporting no hemispheric differences equal numbers of stimuli and trials were used, while those finding significant differences had unequal numbers. It is suggested that to obtain cerebral lateralization effects, a condition that allows judgments to be made from memory must be produced. It is concluded that active cognitive processes are not lateralized and interpretative models which view active cognitive processing as being lateralized are not correct.

364

Harrison, A. A., & Zajonc, R. B. (1970). The effects of frequency and duration of exposure on response competition and affective ratings. *Journal of Psychology,* **75, 163-169.**

Initially novel stimuli (Chinese ideographs) were shown to 66 female undergraduates in the frequencies of 0, 1, 2, 5, 10, and 25 exposures. 1/2 were presented for 2 sec/exposure, the remainder for 10 sec/exposure. Consistent with earlier findings, response competition decreased (.001) and affective ratings were enhanced (.025) as exposure frequency was increased. Extended exposure duration reduced response competition (.05) but enhanced affective ratings only when they were collected prior to the response competition assessment. It is suggested that when ratings are collected afterwards, the response competition assessment task contributes to the stimulus rating.

365

He, B. Y., Ma, M. C., Chen, Y. M., Xu, Z. H., Ji, G. P., Zhang, J. T., Zhang, Z. H., & Wang, H. L. (1979). [A systematic study on the relative spectral luminosity among Chinese people]. *Acta Psychologica Sinica, 11,* **39-46.** (In Chinese.)

Results from a study of the relative spectral luminosity among Chinese people indicate that both photopic and scotopic relative spectral luminosity coincided with or were very similar to those of the International Commission on Illumination. These findings in turn support opinions that suggest that a significant ethnological difference in this respect is unlikely. Both photopic and scotopic relative spectral luminous efficiency functions increased with age on the short wave side of the spectrum. Under the conditions of 4 sizes of visual angle, results show that as the size of visual field increased, relative luminous efficiencies heightened for short wavelength S. Under the conditions of 4 luminosity levels, the relative luminous efficiency curves became slender when the luminosity rose.

366

Hong, G. K., Skiba, A. H., Yepes, E., & O'Brien, R. M. (1982). Effects of ethnicity of hypnotist and subject on hypnotic susceptibility. *International Journal of Clinical & Experimental Hypnosis, 30,* **23-31.**

Examined the effect of ethnic similarity of hypnotist and hypnotic S on hypnotic susceptibility. The 1st part of the study compared the performance of 16 16-37 yr old Anglo vs 16 Chinese hypnotists on 16 Anglo vs 16 Chinese Ss. In the 2nd half of the study, 16 Anglo and 32 Hispanic Ss and hypnotists were compared using the same Anglo hypnotist-S control group. Ss were administered the Stanford Hypnotic Susceptibility Scale, Form A. A 2 * 2 ANOVA was performed on the data for each part of the study. Ethnic similarity of hypnotist and S was found not to enhance hypnotic susceptibility. Results are discussed in relation to the assumed superiority of homoethnicity in psychotherapy.

367

Hoosain, R., & Osgood, C. E. (1983). Processing times for English and Chinese words. *Perception & Psychophysics, 34,* **573-577.**

In Exp I, 18 US undergraduates and 20 Hong Kong Chinese undergraduates were asked to judge the positive/negative affective polarity of 30 word pairs in their respective languages. Response times were significantly quicker for Chinese, although there was no difference in latencies in simply pronouncing "positive" and "negative" in the 2 languages. However, in Exp II, with 3 English-speaking and 4 Cantonese-speaking Ss, pronunciation durations for the English test words were shorter than those for Chinese. Results are related to the alphabetic vs morphemic nature of English and Chinese and to their difference in the requirement for phonological recoding in word processing.

368

Hsiung, J. C. (1969). Chinese ways of thinking and Chinese language. *Journal of the Chinese Language Teachers' Association, 4,* **41-54.**

369

Hsu, C. C. (1971). [Chinese children's responses to Raven's Colored Progressive Matrices: A 3-year longitudinal study on the first graders in an urban elementary school]. *Journal of Formosan Medical Association, 70,* **579-593.** (In Chinese.)

370

Huang, J. T. (1979). [Time-dependent and separability hypothesis of Chinese words association]. *Acta Psychologica Taiwanica, 21,* **41-48.** (In Chinese.)

Two experiments tested the hypothesis that the previously documented correlation of word frequency with word associations may not occur with respect to Chinese 2-character words; it was postulated that when an S is required to associate as many words as possible in response to a presented word without a time restriction, the S may first generate words as a response to the stimulus word, and then may generate words by considering each constituent as a stimulus if he or she runs out of associations. Therefore, no correlation would exist between word frequency and word association with Chinese 2-character words according to this time-dependent separability hypothesis. In Exp I, which presented and mixed 2-character and single-character Chinese words, Ss were instructed to respond to as many associates as possible to each word. Exp II, in which 5 groups of Ss were used, varied frequency counts of 2-character words and of their constituent characters. Results show that the differential responding rate between low- and high-frequency single-character words was not significantly different from that of 2-character words and that Ss produced associations by initially responding to the 1st constituent of 2-character words.

371

Huang, J. T., & Liu, I. M. (1978). [Paired-associate learning proficiency as a function of frequency count, meaningfulness, and imagery value in Chinese two-character ideograms]. *Acta Psychologica Taiwanica, 20,* **5-17.** (In Chinese.)

Attempted to establish the normative frequency count (F), meaningfulness (M), and imagery value (I) of 239 Chinese 2-character words; and assessed the differential effect of F, M, and I, respectively, by manipulating only 1 of the 3 attributes and keeping the other 2 constant, on the learning proficiency in an alternate study-recall paired-associate learning (PAL) paradigm. Exp I shows the significant correlation between F and M and between M and I, which are in accord with their alphabetic equivalents. The nonsignificant correlation between F and I is partly attributed to the biased selection of high-frequency abstract and low-frequency concrete words. Exp II shows (a) a significant F effect on response (R) and an interaction of stimulus vs response units (S * R) in PAL; and (b) the significant I effect on all 3 sources of variation, namely, S, R, S * R.

372

Huang, Y. H. (1976). [The effects of anxiety relief and intelligence on syllogistic argument]. *Bulletin of Educational Psychology, 9,* **33-42.** (In Chinese.)

It was hypothesized that, when habit strength was kept constant and the drive state reduced, the response tendency would be a function of intelligence. In this experiment, subjects' reasoning in each of four figure-moods without error was the criterion for controlling habit strength. The independent variables were anxiety and intelligence. Anxiety was aroused by instructing subjects that test results of syllogistic reasoning would be used in midterm evaluation; however, it was relieved by permitting the subjects to consult the text during testing. It was found that, in terms of valid syllogistic arguments made, there were no significant interactions between anxiety and intelligence, and no significant differences between the high-anxiety and the low-anxiety subjects within the same range of intelligence. However, there were highly significant differences between the high-intelligence and the middle-intelligence subjects, and between the high-intelligence and the low-intelligence subjects, irrespective of their anxiety levels. As predicted, under the condition of anxiety relief, deductive reasoning was determined by the subjects' intelligence when habit strength was kept under control.

373

Hull, C. L. (1920). Quantitative aspects of the evolution of concepts: An experimental study. *Psychological Monographs, 28,* **85.**

374

Ji, G. P., He, B. Y. et al. (1980). [A serial study on the relative spectral luminosity among Chinese people: Vol. 3. The effect of the different visual fields on V(lambda)]. *Acta Psychologica Sinica, 12,* **307-310.** (In Chinese.)

Five experienced adult Ss with normal vision completed a visual experiment using the flicker method. Four visual fields were used with a constant level of luminance, and test points of wavelength were selected in the 420-700 nm range. Results indicate that in all visual fields, the V(lambda) values were similar in the long-wave region of the spectrum but systematically increased with the increment of the visual field in the short-wave region.

375

Jin, Q. C., & Chiao, S. L. (1983). [Sensory and perceptual studies in the People's Republic of China]. *Information on Psychological Sciences*, **No. 1, 7-14.** (In Chinese.)

376

Just, M. A., & Carpenter, P. A. (1975). Comparative studies of comprehension: An investigation of Chinese, Norwegian, and English. *Memory & Cognition, 3*, **465-473.**

Compared the processing of complex embedded sentences in Chinese, Norwegian, and English to determine if the underlying mental operations are similar in these diverse languages. Ss were 12 university students and staff who were native Chinese speakers. The task involved reading a sentence like "It's true that the dots aren't red" and deciding whether it was true or false according to an accompanying picture. The verification latencies were analyzed in terms of a model based on 1 central mental operation. Results for all 3 languages conformed to the predictions of the model and showed similar processing rates. Moreover, the Norwegian study with 12 Norwegian university students expanded the analysis to include quantification in sentences like "It's true that many of the dots aren't red". The studies suggest that certain fundamental operations may be universally implicated in language processing.

377

Kao, H. S. (1980). [A psychological analysis of the stylistic variations in Chinese calligraphy]. *Acta Psychologica Taiwanica, 22*, **51-68.** (In Chinese.)

The concept of progressive motive variability (PMV) identifies an increased motor instability as a function of the progress of a control task, with a peak approaching the later or terminal segments of the task performance. In the present study, the concept of PMV is extended within an analysis of the stylistic variations in Chinese calligraphy. Four specific stylistic variations as a function of the progress of calligraphic writing are suggested for calligraphic performance: (1) progressive enlargement of the characters, (2) progressive trend toward increasing scriptiveness of the characters, (3) deviant character column alignment, and (4) enlargement of the between-column spacing. A review of some classic pieces of Chinese calligraphy has shown evidence for all four PMV-based expectations regarding the calligraphic variations in Chinese brush writing. A total of 20 photos of such pieces of calligraphy are used to discuss these unique characteristics. Suggestions are offered for a direction of future research on Chinese calligraphy.

378

Kao, H. S. R., Lam, P. W., & Shek, D. T. L. (1985). Different modes of handwriting control: Some psychophysiological evidence. *Chinese Journal of Psychology, 27*, **49-63.**

The present study is an attempt to investigate the behavioral and psychophysiological components involved in different modes of handwriting in Chinese calligraphy. In terms of the information processing perspective, it is suggested that the various modes of handwriting control might place different demands on the various aspects of the information processing system. Twelve subjects forming four groups of three subjects each traced with a brush pen 20 randomly presented Chinese characters after a practice session of 5 minutes. One group consisted of novices; the others were subjects with an average of, respectively, 39, 30, and 25 years of experience in calligraphy. The writing tasks included tracing, copying, and freehand writing of the Chinese characters. Heartrate and behavioral (writing time) responses were recorded as the dependent variables. The results showed that these various modes of control (especially tracing and freehand modes) can be differentiated in terms of writing time and heartrate responses. Separate analysis of discrete heartrate responses following the onset of the writing task showed that heartrate deceleration is greatest for tracing as compared to other modes of handwriting. The meaning and functional significance of such behavioral and psychophysiological components associated with these modes of handwriting control is discussed in terms of the information processing perspective.

379

Kitao, N. et al. (1977). [Concreteness, hieroglyphicity and familiarity of kanji (Japanese form of Chinese characters)]. *Japanese Journal of Psychology, 48*, **105-111.** (In other language.)

To investigate psychological attributes of 881 kanji characters, 1,000 Ss were required to make a dichotomous choice in terms of concreteness (C), and to rate the characters on a 7-point scale in terms of hieroglyphicity (H) and in terms of familiarity (F). There was high positive correlation between C and H values; however, the F value yielded negligible correlations with the other 2 values. To test the validity of these results, recognition as a function of C value (high or low) was examined; only the F value remained constant. Results reveal that the ease of recognition was positively related to the degree of concreteness.

380

Klein, T. W. (1972). Individual and racial differences in sensitivity to flickering light. *Dissertation Abstracts International, 32*, **B7342-7343.**

381

Kuehn, G. B. (1986). Discrimination and identification of Chinese and English infant vocalizations. *Dissertation Abstracts International, 46,* **B2475.**

382

Kvan, E. (1983). Reflections on doing psychological research in Hong Kong: A reply to Ripple. *Hong Kong Psychological Society Bulletin,* **No. 10, 24-27.**

Critiques R. Ripple's paper on conducting psychological research in Hong Kong and comments that Ripple did not adequately prove that developmental regularities are the same everywhere. Ripple also failed to discuss the idea of indigenous psychology in detail.

383

Lau, S., & Ho, S. F. (1980). [Efficiency in reading Chinese written from right to left and from left to right]. *Acta Psychologica Taiwanica, 22,* **29-31.** (In Chinese.)

In studying the accuracy and speed of reading horizontally written Chinese words, it was found that reading was much superior when words were written from left to right vs from right to left.

384

Li, H. Z., Hu, R. X. et al. (1983). [Experimental study on the stability of intentional attention in 5-6 years old children]. *Acta Psychologica Sinica, 15,* **178-184.** (In Chinese.)

385

Li, X. T. (1983). [The distribution of left and right handedness in Chinese people]. *Acta Psychologica Sinica, 15,* **268-276.** (In Chinese.)

There is so far no scientific data on the distribution of left- and right-handedness in China. A survey of 18,593 healthy people and 1,748 neuropsychiatric patients was conducted throughout the country. The sample of healthy people consisted of kindergarten, primary school, middle school, and college students; monozygotic and dizygotic twins; and various kinds of professionals. The handedness of seven minorities besides the Hans was also surveyed. It was found that the percentage of left-handedness was only 0.23%, far lower than in Western countries.

386

Liang, B. Y., & Xu, L. G. (1986). [An experimental study of visual fatigue under different lightings]. *Acta Psychologica Sinica, 18,* **25-34.** (In Chinese.)

Using accommodation and convergence time of the eye, brightness discrimination and subjective estimations of fatigue as indicators of visual fatigue, eight lightings at two levels of lighting power and four color temperatures of light were compared. The results were: (1) When the nature of lighting was under control, visual fatigue was more marked under 2-nit lightings than under 10-nit lightings. (2) With the same level of lighting power, the visual fatigue under red lightings was more marked than that under white lightings. The differences among white lightings at the three different color temperatures were not significant. (3) The differences between the 10-nit red lightings and the 32-nit white lightings were also not significant.

387

Liang, K. C., & Liu, I. M. (1977). [Process of verifying multi-attribute sentences against pictures]. *Acta Psychologica Taiwanica, 19,* **39-47.** (In Chinese.)

Previous sentence-picture verification experiments indicate that a decrease in the difference between true affirmative reaction times (RTs) and false affirmative RTs was obtained for the sentences and pictures depicting objects of multiple attributes, and that false negative RTs were longer than true negative RTs. The finding was hypothesized (Liu and Liang, 1977) to be due to a difficulty in retrieving the negative polarity marker when an object described in a sentence contained more than one attribute. In Experiment 1 the number of attributes was increased to three. In Experiment 2 a negative polarity marker was placed before each of the sentence elements describing attributes of an object. The results of two experiments support the retrieval hypothesis. It was further noted that subjects tended to reduce "multi-attribute" sentences to single-attribute sentences in the course of the verification process. A tentative theory was briefly outlined.

388

Lin, C. S. (1973). [The classical conditioning of GSR to visual verbal-stimuli: Development of word meaning]. *Bulletin of Educational Psychology, 6,* **57-76.** (In Chinese.)

Presented a list of 12 nonsense Chinese characters to 30 college students in a learning task. The characters were randomly divided into 3 categories. Words in E category were continuously paired with an aversive stimulus (electric shock) and those in S category with an appetitive stimulus (the sound of a music bell). No stimulus was given for words in N category. The emotional word meaning elicited by the words was measured by asking Ss to rate them on a 7-point semantic differential scale. Results indicate that (a) the magnitude of the conditioned GSR elicited by E words and S words was significantly larger than that elicited by N words; (b) the conditioned GSR elicited by E words was significantly larger than that elicited by S words; (c) when the rating responses on scales of semantic differential before and after conditioning session were compared, the meaning of E words tended to move toward the negative evaluative poles, where that of S words tended to move toward the positive evaluative pole.

389

Lin, C. S. (1985). [Empirical studies based on Witkin's theory of psychological differentiation]. *Bulletin of Educational Psychology, 18,* **39-56.** (In Chinese.)

390

Lin, C. S. (1986). [An experiment on the hemispheric differences in the perception of visual stimuli and the validation of tests and scales hypothetically measuring cerebral laterality]. *Bulletin of Educational Psychology, 19,* **37-54.** (In Chinese.)

Part one of this study investigated the hemispheric asymmetries in the perception of visual stimuli. Four kinds of visual materials (Chinese characters, English syllables, latticed squares, and gestalt closure), were tachistoscopically exposed in the left visual field (LVF) and right visual field (RVF) of 71 college students, through visual half-field presentation. The results were: (1) English syllables presented in RVF to left hemisphere (LH) were more accurately identified than if they were presented in LVF to right hemisphere (RH). (2) No significant laterality differences were found in regard to the recall scores of Chinese characters. (3) Contradictory to what was predicted, subjects yielded significantly more accurate responses to the latticed square items when they were exposed to the LH than the RH. There was no lateral superiority for the gestalt closure items. The hypothesis that the RH is superior for holistic or simultaneous information processing was supported in this case. Part two described the results of the study on validation of tests and scales hypothesized to measure cerebral laterality.

391

Lin, Z. X. et al. (1986). [An experimental research of the effects of different ways of information influx on the location of objects at right and various slanting angles]. *Information on Psychological Science,* **No. 5, 34-39.** (In Chinese.)

392

Lin, Z. X., & Sun, X. R. (1986). [Factors affecting the accuracy of depth perception and distance judgment]. *Acta Psychologica Sinica, 18,* **257-263.** (In Chinese.)

Some factors affecting the accuracy of depth discrimination and distance judgment were studied in this experiment. The results showed that depth discrimination and distance judgment were most accurate under normal binocular observation at zero degrees. Errors increased in binocular observation at 45 degrees sideways, and the largest errors occurred when using one eye only. To compare the accuracy of relative distance judgments, it was found that judgment of the relative distance of 2/4 was more accurate than that of the 1/4 and 3/4 distances. The coordinative movement of both eyes in binocular observation was a very important factor affecting depth discrimination and distance judgment.

393

Lin, Z. X., & Zhi, F. (1980). [Thirty years' developments in Chinese experimental psychology]. *Acta Psychologica Sinica, 12,* **9-15.** (In Chinese.)

Describes the development of experimental psychology in China since the revolution.

394

Liu, F., & Kong, W. Y. (1959). [An analysis of relationship between the practice in productive labor and the acquisition of theorctical knowledge in middle school students]. *Acta Psychologica Sinica,* **No. 5, 279-292.** (In Chinese.)

This study investigated the relationship between the practice of industrial productive work and the acquisition of theoretical knowledge of physics in middle school students. It was observed that when students did productive work, their interest, understanding and memory of theoretical knowledge (of physics) was facilitated. This, in turn, helped students understand the process of labor work, thereby promoting the efficiency of work. Under such circumstances, students' knowledge was broadened. The authors considered that the changes in students' attitude toward learning and the raising of efficiency in learning resulting from their practice of productive work is itself a reflection of labor processes, and that such laws of reflection could be applied in increasing the efficiency of teaching.

395

Liu, I., & Hsu, M. (1974). [Measuring creative thinking in Taiwan by the Torrance test]. *Testing and Guidance, 2,* **108-109.** (In Chinese.)

396

Liu, I. M. (1977). [Application of imagery mnemonics: Acquisition of English vocabulary by senior high school students]. *Acta Psychologica Taiwanica, 19,* **31-38.** (In Chinese.)

The keyword method originally proposed by Atkinson and Raugh (1975) as a mnemonic aid for vocabulary learning was found to be not applicable to the first-year high school students (Experiment 1). Some variants of the keyword method intended for separating the information-processing stage in the keyword method were also ineffective (Experiments 2 and 3). The experimental results, however, indicated that this ineffectiveness was primarily due to the intrinsic mediators aroused by presenting new foreign words to the trained subjects. Theoretical implications of the present study for paired-associate learning in general were briefly discussed.

397

Liu, I. M. (1978). [Effect of sentence context on the acquisition of word meaning]. *Acta Psychologica Taiwanica, 20,* **29-37.** (In Chinese.)

In acquiring the meanings of new words, the sentence context within which new words are embedded undoubtedly plays an important role. According to the results of Experiments 1 and 2, mere repetitions of new words in sentence contexts resulted in meaning acquisition. This phenomenon merely reflected the performance component (how to express meanings of words) of meaning acquisition. The results of Experiments 3 and 4 showed that the acquisition of word meaning should include not only the meaning of new words per se but the function of these new words in their sentence contexts. Only when the subjects acquired meanings of new words in their sentence contexts could they efficiently utilize the newly acquired words. Although the mean number of new words acquired was lower in the context of sentences than without context, the acquired new words tended to be resistant to forgetting in the former rather than in the latter condition.

398

Liu, I. M., & Chang, S. L. (1981). [Short-term memory of affirmative and negative sentences]. *Acta Psychologica Taiwanica, 23,* **131-136.** (In Chinese.)

399

Liu, K. S., & Shen, H. M. (1977). [Effects of language structure and intertrial interval on the speed of silent reading]. *Acta Psychologica Taiwanica, 19,* **57-59.** (In Chinese.)

Tested 40 Chinese and German college students to investigate the effects of language structure and intertrial interval (ITI) on the speed of silent reading. Ss read silently from 1 to 100 under the 2 conditions of ITIs of 10 sec and 60 sec. Results show that the speed of silent reading was slower when using German than when using Chinese. Under the condition of 10-sec ITI, the speed of silent reading was found to decrease as the number of trials increased.

400

Lung, S. S., & Fan, C. (1960). [Determination of the normal threshold of hearing of young people 16-25 years of age: Vol. 2. The normal threshold of hearing]. *Acta Psychologica Sinica,* **No. 2, 109-114.** (In Chinese.)

Audiometric data on the normal threshold of hearing for nine different frequencies (from 125 to 8,000) were obtained. The threshold curves were compared with those obtained by different investigators abroad.

401

Lung, S. S. & Wang, D. A. (1960). [A determination of the normal threshold of hearing of young people 16-25 years of age: 1. Equivalent curve by artificial ear calibration of earphones]. *Acta Psychologica Sinica,* **No. 1, 54-61.** (In Chinese.)

The first part of a work measuring the normal threshold of hearing is reported. Usable results were obtained from 1843 young people 16-25 years of age. Common electromagnetic earphones were used. The calibration was done on a Bruel and Kjaer artificial ear. During the test, subjects were seated in a soundproof chamber. An "equivalent curve" was plotted from the overall arithmetic means for different frequencies. Calculating the means separately for the male and female sexes and for the right and left ears, revealed no significant differences.

402

Lyczak, R. A. (1979). The effects of exposure to a language on subsequent learning. *Language & Speech, 22,* **81-88.**

Exposed 32 Chinese undergraduates, over a period of 4 days, to 3 hrs of recorded Thai conversation, Japanese conversation, or music. On the 5th day all Ss learned to recognize (translate) 10 Thai sentences in a paired associate type task. Type of exposure had no effect on response latency or rate of learning. In a postcriterion task Ss were provided translations and asked to produce the Thai sentences. Ss exposed to Thai produced more words than those exposed to music or Japanese; Ss exposed to Japanese produced words from fewer sentences than those exposed to music or Thai. Results are discussed in terms of perceptual learning theory and subvocal rehearsal.

403

Ma, M. C., He, B. Y. et al. (1981). [A serial study on the relative spectral luminosity among Chinese people: Vol. 4. Influence of the luminance levels on the relative spectral luminosity]. *Acta Psychologica Sinica, 13,* **186-191.** (In Chinese.)

Utilizing the flicker method and the just-noticeable-difference technique, luminosity curves at 4 luminance levels--7.62, 76.2, 762, and 7,620 td--were obtained. Results show that the mu curves become slender when luminosity rises (i.e., as luminance levels increase, the sensitivity to the 2 ends of the visible spectrum decreases while the sensitivity to the middle of the spectrum remains relatively invariable).

404

Ma, M. C., & Wang, P. Z. (1981). [Empirical tests for feature selection based on a psychological rule of recognizing ambiguously shaped Chinese characters]. *Acta Psychologica Sinica, 13,* **311-316.** (In Chinese.)

Suggests a rule of recognition that contains relations between physical variables (line extension) and perceived attributes. Three psychological measurements--identification, confidence, and goodness scales--were used. Results demonstrate that each of the psychological paradigms gave the same rule; this rule can be expressed with fuzzy sets and is a dynamic property when ambiguously shaped Chinese characters are presented in different directions. Findings suggest that the fuzzy relation is the reason for the difference between a machine and a human observer for recognizing handwritten Chinese characters.

405

Ma, M. C., Zhang, L. F., Wu, X. Y., & Jiang, S. Z. (1986). [A fuzzy set approach to the estimation of respiratory sensation]. *Acta Psychologica Sinica, 18,* **8-14.** (In Chinese.)

Psychological magnitude associated with respiratory resistive load was considered as a fuzzy one in this study. A fuzzy set approach called Multistage Evaluation Scale (MES) was adopted to reveal a possibility distribution of this fuzzy magnitude, and a formula for treatment of the data was used to estimate psychological magnitude associated with respiratory resistive load. Thirty-seven healthy young male subjects experienced six levels of suprathreshold added resistance, loaded at different phases of the breathing cycle. The results revealed that the relationship between resistive load and perceived magnitude could be expressed by psychophysical power function. The severity of the sensory experience caused by equal resistive intensity differed significantly when loaded at different phases of the breathing cycle, but the speed of sensory growth did not manifest significant change. The physical and physiological magnitudes were correlated to each sensory category grade of the scale, which may be useful for establishing resistive standards for respiratory protective equipment.

406

Mao, Y. Y., Kung, W. Y., & Chen, P. L. (1965). [Relation between the structure of arithmetic problems, their formulation (by pupils), and pupils' psychological activity in the process of problem-solving]. *Acta Psychologica Sinica, 4,* **291-298.** (In Chinese.)

407

Marsella, A. J. (1978). Thoughts on cross-cultural studies on the epidemiology of depression. *Culture, Medicine & Psychiatry, 2,* **343-357.**

408

McClain, L., & Huang, J. Y. (1982). Speed of simple arithmetic in bilinguals. *Memory & Cognition, 10,* **591-596.**

Four types of bilinguals (10 with Chinese as preferred language and English as a 2nd language, 10 with English as preferred and Chinese as 2nd, 20 with Spanish as preferred and English as 2nd, and 20 with English as preferred and Spanish as 2nd language) solved simple addition problems that were auditorily presented in their preferred language, the language in which they 1st learned arithmetic, or in their nonpreferred language. Ss responded in the language in which the problems were presented. Solution time averaged .227 sec faster in the preferred language and was an increasing linear function of the number of addition operations required. The intercepts of the preferred and nonpreferred language functions significantly differed, but the slopes did not. The preferred language advantage was attributed to faster encoding and/or response times in the preferred language. When bilinguals used only one of their languages in a given experimental session, encoding/response times in the 2 languages were equivalent and the preferred language advantage was eliminated.

409

Mo, L. (1986). [An experiment about the encoding mode of short-term memory]. *Acta Psychologica Sinica, 18,* **166-173.** (In Chinese.)

In this experiment, research was made on the encoding mode of short-term memory in signal detection, using Chinese characters as material. The result showed that generally speaking, Chinese characters were encoded mainly according to their forms. This result differs from that using English letters as material. Moreover, the encoding mode changed in some degree with different Chinese characters committed to short-term memory. This supported the hypothesis that the encoding mode of short-term memory varies with situations.

410

Moran, L. J., & Huang, I. N. (1975). Note on cognitive dictionary structure of adult Chinese and on a Piagetian semantic universal. *Psychological Reports, 36,* **180.**

Studied the free-word associations of 74 Chinese 4-6 yr olds and 35 Chinese 18-24 yr olds. Results extend previous findings that the cognitive structure (as opposed to content) of Japanese and North American adults does not serve as a model for the child's early cognitive dictionary. The associations of all 3 groups of children were mainly enactive (e.g., apple-eat).

411

Mou, L. C., & Anderson, N. S. (1981). Graphemic and phonemic codings of Chinese characters in short-term retention. *Bulletin of the Psychonomic Society, 17,* **255-258.**

Investigated the effect of phonemic or graphemic similarity on recoding of Chinese words using 22 Chinese undergraduates enrolled at an American university. The introduction of acoustic and visual similarity within the list using a retroactive interference design for memory of items showed that both intralist variables were factors causing reduction in recall, with acoustic similarity being more detrimental to short-term retention. An auditory interference task also had a more severe effect than a visual interference task. Results suggest that dual encoding processes are involved in reading and remembering Chinese.

412

Murakami, Y. (1980). [On the memory unit within kana-letter and kanji-letter words in the tip of the tongue phenomena]. *Japanese Journal of Psychology, 51,* **41-44.** (In other language.)

300 students were read definitions of 20 words represented by Kana letters (Japanese alphabet) and Chinese characters. 222 partial reports were treated as though in the tip-of-the-tongue state and analyzed by D. C. Rubin's method. Results indicate that major clusters were composed of 1-3 Kana letters or 1 Chinese character. In addition to partially supporting Rubin's conclusion, the findings suggest the possibility that the memory unit for the Japanese word is not the morpheme but the "pseudo-letter morpheme".

413

National Academy of Sciences, & Chinese Academy of Sciences. (1984). *Issues in cognition: Proceedings of a Joint Conference in Psychology.* **Washington, DC: National Academy of Sciences and American Psychological Association.**

414

Peng, D. L., Guo, D. J., & Zhang, S. L. (1986). [The retrieval of information in Chinese characters in making similarity judgment under recall conditions]. *Acta Psychologica Sinica, 18,* **264-271.** (In Chinese.)

Following the paper "The retrieval of information in Chinese characters in making similarity judgment under recognition conditions," the authors conducted this experiment which dealt with the same problem under recall conditions. Main results showed that the reaction time of form-similarity judgments was the shortest, followed by that of phonetic-similarity judgments, and finally that of semantic-similarity judgments. Significant differences were found between form-similarity and semantic-similarity judgments and between phonetic-similarity and semantic-similarity judgments. The results indicated an increase in the effect of phonetic recoding under recall conditions as compared with that under recognition conditions.

415

Peng, D. L., Orchard, L. N., & Stern, J. A. (1983). Evaluation of eye movement variables of Chinese and American readers. *Pavlovian Journal of Biological Science, 18,* **94-102.**

Recorded eye movements of 20 competent American readers of English and 23 competent readers of Chinese as they read in their respective languages. No important differences in oculometric patterns of fixation pause durations were found for Chinese and English readers, suggesting that cognitive aspects of reading are more important than perceptual ones in determining eye movement patterns and fixation pauses of competent readers. An analysis of undershoot saccades associated with return of the eyes from the end of one line to the beginning of the next suggested that these occur more frequently during reading than during the performance of similar eye movements that are more perceptually determined. However, the amount of undershoot did not discriminate between readers of alphabetic and logographic texts. Results suggest that the perceptual "habits" built up during the development and perfection of reading skills are not a limiting cause in the reading of English by Chinese individuals.

416

Peng, R. X., Sun, X. R., Lin, Z. X., Dong, H. Y., Gu, W. K., & Liu, Y. X. (1980). [A study of preferred colors of familiar objects in transparencies]. *Acta Psychologica Sinica, 12,* **415-423.** (In Chinese.)

60 observers made category judgments in evaluating color samples: Chinese skin hue, blue sky, and yellow-green uniform. Results are presented in the form of preferred chromaticities and color ranges for familiar objects. The preferred Chinese skin color was found to be more reddish, but the purity was the same as the natural skin color. The purity of the blue-sky color was appreciably greater than any of the other sky colors evaluated, while the purity of the preferred uniform color was much lower than the "natural" color.

417

Peng, R. X., & Zhang, W. T. (1984). [Some characteristics in tachistoscopic recognition of Chinese characters]. *Acta Psychologica Sinica, 16,* **49-54.** (In Chinese.)

A tachistoscopic study of the recognition of Chinese characters and 2-character words revealed several common patterns in recognizing characters with different structures. Characters with a symmetrical structure were easier to recognize than were those with half-enclosed structures. Some similarities between adults and children were noted with respect to the extraction of character features in recognition. The lower-right quarter was frequently extracted for characters separated vertically, while the upper-right quarter was extracted for half-encircled characters. Possible implications for teaching Chinese characters are noted. The machine recognition of characters is also discussed.

418

Phizicky, H. (1972). Effect of censure, ego involvement, and rivalry on letter-cancellation performance by Chinese and North Americans. *Psychonomic Science, 28,* **219-221.**

Investigated the hypothesis that Chinese students would be motivated best through ego involvement and North Americans through social competitiveness. 9 Chinese, born in Hong Kong, and 9 native North Americans, all English-speaking male undergraduates, performed a letter-cancellation task under each of 3 conditions: after an ego-involving comment, after a comment inspiring competition, and after no comment. Analysis indicates a significant main effect of condition (p.05) and a significant Condition * Race interaction (p.025). Scheffe tests confirmed the hypothesis.

419

Potter, M. C., So, K. F., von Eckardt, B., & Feldman, L. B. (1984). Lexical and conceptual representation in beginning and proficient bilinguals. *Journal of Verbal Learning & Verbal Behavior, 23,* **23-38.**

In a paper presented at a symposium on concepts and their surface representations, held by the Eastern Psychological Association in New York in April 1981, the present authors discuss 2 hypotheses--word association and concept mediation--about the association between the equivalent words in a bilingual's 2 languages. The word association hypothesis proposes that a direct association is established between words in the 2 languages. During 2nd-language acquisition, that association is used to understand and produce words in the 2nd language by retrieving a word in the 1st language. The concept mediation hypothesis proposes that the only connection between the 2 languages is via an underlying, amodal conceptual system, one to which pictured objects also have access. The hypotheses make different predictions about the time to name pictures in the 2nd language relative to the time to translate 1st-language words into the 2nd language. Two experiments with 24 college-age proficient Chinese-English bilinguals and 28 nonfluent English-French bilingual American high school students were conducted. Ss read words aloud, named pictures, and translated words; one Chinese-English group categorized pictures and words. Results are consistent with the concept mediation hypothesis and contradicted predictions of the word association hypothesis. There was no evidence for a direct association between words in the 2 languages in either bilingual group.

420

Ripple, R. (1983). Reflections on doing psychological research in Hong Kong. *Hong Kong Psychological Society Bulletin,* **No. 10, 7-23.**

The author describes experiences as a psychological researcher in Hong Kong with respect to culture and language. Also discussed are the cross-cultural aspects of life-span development of 3 divergent thinking abilities--fluency, flexibility, and originality--the relative magnitude of such creative thinking among Hong Kong Chinese, and the effect of language on the expression of the 3 divergent thinking abilities.

421

Russell, J. A. (1983). Pancultural aspects of the human conceptual organization of emotions. *Journal of Personality & Social Psychology, 45,* **1281-1288.**

cIvestigated whether certain elementary properties of the human conceptual system for categorizing emotions are pancultural or are specific to particular languages and cultures. From similarity judgments provided by 147 native speakers (mostly middle-aged and elderly) of 5 languages, multidimensional scalings of emotion-related words in Gujarati, Croatian, Japanese, Chinese, and English provided evidence of several pancultural properties. In all 5 languages, emotion-related words fell in roughly a circular order in a space definable by 2 dimensions: pleasure-displeasure and arousal-sleep. Similar results were obtained from unilingual and bilingual Ss.

422

Saito, H. (1981). [Use of graphemic and phonemic encoding in reading Kanji and Kana]. *Japanese Journal of Psychology, 52,* **266-273.** (In other language.)

Conducted 2 experiments with Japanese Ss to investigate whether phonological recoding is an obligatory stage of reading Japanese or whether the direct access to semantic representation is the general rule. Exp I used a word reading-out task and Exp II a sentence judgment task. In Exp I, Kana (Japanese characters) were read out faster than Kanji (Chinese characters), but in Exp II with the silent reading condition, Kanji were judged faster than Kana. Results suggest that Kana is superior to Kanji in access to the phonemic codes, but this does not imply that the meaning is comprehended more rapidly in Kana. In contrast, Kanji takes longer for reading out (decoding) than Kana but makes rapid access to semantic codes possible. In the silent reading of Kanji the direct processing from visual (graphemic) codes to meaning (semantic codes) is possible, whereas in Kana, the relation of graphemic codes to meaning is mediated by the phonemic system.

423

Shen, N. C. (1936). A note on the color preference of Chinese students. *Journal of Social Psychology, 7,* **69-81.**

424

Shen, N. C. (1937). The color preference of 1368 Chinese students, with special reference to the most preferred color. *Journal of Social Psychology, 8,* **185-204.**

The color preference of Chinese subjects was studied. The subjects were 1,368 Chinese senior middle school students (847 boys and 521 girls). They were given a test of color preference with six saturated Bradley colors and achromatic white. The method of paired comparisons was used. The results showed that the descending order of preference was: white, red, blue, green, yellow, orange, and violet. Judgments of preference were quite consistent. That the most preferred color is white is unusually significant, because in no other racial group studied so far has white been consistently the most preferred. It is suggested that the Chinese language is probably responsible for this result.

425

Shwedel, A. M. (1979). Information processing models of skilled reading: An examination of the relationship between Chinese orthography and coding tactics in primary memory. *Dissertation Abstracts International, 40,* **A1973.**

426

Smith, M. C., & Kirsner, K. (1982). Language and orthography as irrelevant features in colour-word and picture-word Stroop interference. *Quarterly Journal of Experimental Psychology: Human Experimental Psychology, 34A,* **153-170.**

Based on evidence that Chinese (C) yields more interference than English (E), I. Biederman and Y. Tsao suggest that the processes involved in reading C are more similar to those involved in color naming than those involved in reading E. In 3 experiments (with 52 C-E bilingual, 12 French (F)-E bilingual, and 20 E monolingual university students) conducted to evaluate the empirical foundation for this hypothesis, it was found that (1) C yielded less interference than E (and F) in between-S comparisons involving C-E bilinguals and E monolinguals or E-F bilinguals; (2) C print did not yield more interference than E print in within-S comparisons involving the orthogonal combination of print language (C or E) and naming language (C or E) among C-E bilinguals; and (3) compared with syntactic category, both language and orthography were relatively impotent variables in the object naming version of the Stroop task.

427

Su, H. Y. (1961). [Explanation of emotional age]. *Acta Psychologica Taiwanica,* **No. 3, 73-77.** (In Chinese.)

428

Sun, F. C., Morita, M., & Stark, L. W. (1985). Comparative patterns of reading eye movement in Chinese and English. *Perception & Psychophysics, 37,* **502-506.**

The authors examined eye-movement patterns among four skilled native Chinese readers, eight native Chinese whose recent reading experience had been primarily in English, and eight native English speakers. The subjects were university professors and graduate students. Skilled native readers of each language had similar eye-movement patterns when care was taken to compare identical reading tasks and material and also to consider the Chinese multicharacter word. The similarity implied that both printed languages have been optimized to fit visual and oculomotor physiology and also higher level cognitive processes. Eye-movement recordings taken while subjects read from horizontal Chinese text, now widespread, and classical vertical text indicated that subjects were more accustomed to horizontal text, suggesting that continued updating of reading skill is necessary.

429

Tada, H. (1975). Syllable effects on reaction and recognition times in reading letters in Japan. *Tohoku Psychologica Folia, 34,* **17-26.**

Conducted 3 experiments with 12 paramedical school females to examine the syllable dependent effects on reading pronunciation latency (Exps I and II), and the recognition-threshold (Exp III) for Japanese alphabets and Chinese characters. Results indicate that significant effects on latency were observed in Japanese alphabets, (i.e., words with a larger number of syllables required longer latency), but this was not necessarily true for Chinese characters. The recognition time was also affected by the number of syllables in 2-character words, but not in 1-character series. Findings are discussed in terms of the distinctive features between the "idiogram" such as Chinese characters and the phoneme-like Japanese syllabaries, and also with respect to the level of grapheme-phoneme correspondence.

430

Turnage, T. W., & McGinnies, E. (1973). A cross-cultural comparison of the effects of presentation mode and meaningfulness on short-term recall. *American Journal of Psychology, 86,* **369-381.**

Investigated the effects of language (Chinese or English), mode of stimulus presentation (visual or auditory), and noun frequency on short-term serial recall. Ss were 60 American students at the University of Maryland and 60 Chinese students at National Taiwan University. Visual input facilitated learning for Chinese Ss, but American Ss learned faster with auditory input. This finding is discussed in terms of qualitative differences in basic memory processes vs quantitative differences in common learning parameters across the 2 language groups. The major results are seen as compatible with past findings on persuasion, association, and unit-sequence interference in immediate memory.

431

Tzeng, O. J., Hung, D. L., & Wang, W. S. Y. (1977). Speech recoding in reading Chinese characters. *Journal of Experimental Psychology: Human Learning & Memory, 3,* **621-630.**

Two experiments, each with 20 Chinese graduate students, investigated whether phonemic similarity affected the visual information processing of Chinese characters. Exp I used a short-term retention paradigm and a sentence judgment task. In both experiments Ss' performance was found to be impaired by the introduction of phonemic similarity into the test materials. Results are discussed with respect to the issues of orthographical differences and of speech recoding in reading.

432

Tzeng, O. J. L., & Hung, D. L. (1978). [Reading Chinese characters: Some basic experimental studies]. *Acta Psychologica Taiwanica, 20,* **45-49.** (In Chinese.)

Reviewed recent developments in the experimental investigation of reading Chinese characters. Two major approaches are noted. The first concerns the problem of visual lateralization and the other focuses on the problem of phonemic recoding. Four experiments are described that attempted to clarify the above issues from an information processing perspective.

433

Tzeng, O. J. L., Hung, D. L., Cotton, B., & Wang, W. S. Y. (1979). Visual lateralisation effect in reading Chinese characters. *Nature, 282,* **499-501.**

Conducted 3 experiments on 20 Chinese graduate students to examine the visual lateralization effect in reading logographic symbols such as Chinese characters. Ss in Exp I were exposed to brief tachistoscopic presentation of a single character, and their task was to name the character as soon as possible. A left-visual-field-right-hemisphere superiority was found. In Exp II, the stimuli were 2 vertically arranged characters, and Ss were asked to name the stimulus terms as soon as possible. Exp III was the same as the 2nd except that the task was to decide whether these character-strings were correct semantic terms, using a manual response. A right-visual-field-left-hemisphere superiority effect was found in both Exp II and Exp III. These differential visual lateralization results reflect the function-specific property of the 2 hemispheres and cast doubt on the orthography-specific localization hypothesis proposed by earlier investigators.

434

Tzeng, O. J., & Wang, W. S. (1983). The first two r's. *American Scientist, 71,* **238-243.**

Discusses how, in evolutionary terms, speech emerged considerably earlier than writing. The terms used to describe units of all spoken language are described: feature, segment, syllable, morpheme, and word. A writing system may be categorized according to how these 5 types of units are represented in its symbols. The process of reading is then characterized by a correspondence between written script and spoken language. Research using the Stroop Color-Word Test is reviewed, which supports the contention that the relation between script and speech underlying all types of writing systems plays an important role in reading behavior. It was hypothesized that if the configuration is important in deciphering a logograph, then the reader has to pay attention to the position of every element it contains. It was consequently expected that the processing of logographs would involve more visual memory than the processing of alphabetic script. The memory performances of native English speakers and native Chinese speakers were compared to test this hypothesis. Nine items were presented to Ss either auditorily or visually. Results, together with previous research, highlight the influence of script on memory processes.

435

Wang, N. Y., & Cao, M. X. (1979). [Evaluated threshold of impairment for hearing of standard colloquial Chinese]. *Acta Psychologica Sinica, 11,* **313-318.** (In Chinese.)

Measured the thresholds of hearing for pure tones of more than 2,000 workers who had been exposed to various noise levels over a different number of years. Ss' ability to hear speech under everyday life conditions was also examined. Thresholds of impairment were evaluated by psychophysical statistical analysis. In comparison with the recommendation of 25 db of ISOR 1999, the result was about 5 db lower.

436

Ward, C. (1982). The psychological study of consciousness: Pitfalls and limitations. *Hong Kong Psychological Society Bulletin,* **No. 8, 37-45.**

Discusses the historical and cultural development of the theories of consciousness. The major shortcomings of current psychological research on consciousness are confinement to laboratory data, implementation of a unidimensional approach, and adaptation of a Western ethnocentric bias. Cross-cultural altered states of consciousnesss (ASC) data originate from 2 prime sources--ancient mystical traditions of established religions such as Buddhism and Hinduism, and assorted practices of folk religions. Trance and possession in Chinese society are briefly examined. They occur in 2 forms: ritual possession, usually voluntary, and possession by malevolent spirits. Mention is made of Chinese patients admitted to the hospital with possession syndrome who were later diagnosed as having hysteria, schizophrenia, or depression. In order to better study consciousness, a more holistic approach must be taken, examination of ACS in naturally occurring circumstances must be expanded, and there must be a dispersion of the ethnocentric view that equates "altered" with pathological.

437

Weist, R. M., & Crawford, C. (1972). Phonological and semantic representations of words, compartments of memory, and rehearsal. *Psychonomic Science*, *28*, **106-108.**

Presented a semi-free-recall task to 2 groups of 20 undergraduates: bilingual Ss from Hong Kong, fluent in Cantonese and English; and nonbilingual English-speaking Ss. The effect of inhibiting rehearsal on Ss' capacity to remember phonological and semantic representations was studied. The procedure used to retard rehearsal caused an overall decrement in the capacity of bilingual and nonbilingual Ss to remember words in both Cantonese and English. Inhibiting rehearsal did not cause a relatively greater decrement in the nonbilingual Ss' recall of foreign language words.

438

Wong, C. C. (1963). [The role of eye-movement in the development of perception and recognition in preschool children]. *Acta Psychologica Sinica*, **No. 1, 48-54.** (In Chinese.)

439

Wu, C. Y. (1962). The autistic effect of reward and punishment on directional perception. *Acta Psychologica Taiwanica*, **No. 4, 104-111.**

440

Wu, T. M. (1985). [A second experiment on the method on raising the level of children's intelligence]. *Acta Psychologica Sinica*, *17*, **38-45.** (In Chinese.)

The results obtained from two successive experiments support the author's viewpoint that intelligence can be enhanced through stimulating brain activity. This is a report on the second experiment, held in a middle school. A first-year class of 42 students and a fourth-year class of 44 students were used as experimental classes, and another first-year class of 43 students was used as the control class. The two experimental classes were asked to solve one problem within 10 minutes each morning in their own classrooms. During a whole semester, 64 such exercies were done. As a result, the mean IQs of the two experimental classes increased, but that of the control class remained the same.

441

Wu, Z. Y., & Li, D. M. (1986). [A comparative study of the characteristics of short-term memory in the morning and in the evening in adults of different ages]. *Information on Psychological Sciences*, **No. 3, 7-14.** (In Chinese.)

A comparative study was made of the short-term memory in the morning and in the evening in 70 subjects aged from 20 to 80. The purpose of the study was to explore the combined effect of the two factors, age and test time, on short-term memory. The Clinical Memory Scale was used to test short-term memory. The results showed: (1) The short-term memory of each age-group tended to be better in the morning than in the evening. (2) Each age-group had its own characteristic memory errors.

442

Xu, S. X. (1986). [A tentative study of the forgetting process of movement operation]. *Information on Psychological Sciences*, **No. 1, 11-15.** (In Chinese.)

443

Xu, Z. H., He, B. Y. et al. (1980). [A serial study on the relative spectral luminosity among Chinese people: Vol. 2. Scotopic relative spectral luminosity]. *Acta Psychologica Sinica*, *12*, **57-62.** (In Chinese.)

Determined scotopic efficiency functions through a brightness matching method using 14 points ranging in wavelength from 420 to 640nm. 24 Ss with normal vision were divided into groups of those aged more than or less than 30 yrs. The results indicate that (a) the Ss' average maximum spectral sensitivity equaled 515nm and (b) values in the short wave side of the spectrum decreased with increasing age.

444

Yang, B. M. (1986). [The influence of ways of training and predetermined criterion of the number of hits of shooting practice]. *Acta Psychologica Sinica*, *18*, **16-24.** (In Chinese.)

Two simulated experiments were performed to investigate some practical problems in marksmanship training. The main results were: (1) The score of those with a half-hour practice in two periods of 20 trials separated by a 14 to 18-minute rest interval was significantly higher than the score of those with 100 trials in succession, and virtually equalled the score of those with 100 trials with several rest intervals. (2) The important role of kinesthetic discrimination training in improving the method of shooting practice was manifested. (3) The score of those aiming at fulfilling a predetermined criterion of the number of hits was much higher than the score of those having no such criterion in mind. The significance of these results were discussed.

445

Yang, K. S., & Yang-Lee, P. H. (1973). The effects of anxiety and threat on the learning of balanced and unbalanced social structures. *Journal of Personality & Social Psychology, 26,* **201-207.**

Predicted that balance (a task variable) would interact with anxiety (a personality trait) and threat (a situational factor) in determining the rate at which a social structure was learned. Ss were high- and low-anxious female junior high students, (n = 40), as measured by the Chinese versions of the Manifest Anxiety Scale for Children and the Test Anxiety Scale for Children. The general prediction was confirmed by the following findings: (a) The balanced structure was learned more rapidly than the unbalanced one among high-anxious Ss while the 2 structures were learned at the same rate among low-anxious Ss. (b) Under nonthreat instructions, the balanced structure was learned faster than the unbalanced one at least on the last few trials, whereas under threat instructions, no significant difference was observed during the entire learning session. Data also reveal that high-anxious Ss performed better than low-anxious Ss in learning the balanced structure; the reverse was true when the unbalanced structure was learned.

446

Yang, Z. L. (1985). [An experiment on the process of concept formation: With a discussion about the negative effect of rote memory on concept formation]. *Information on Psychological Sciences,* **No. 5, 31-35.** (In Chinese.)

447

Yeh, J. S., & Liu, I. M. (1972). [Factors affecting recognition thresholds of Chinese characters]. *Acta Psychologica Taiwanica, 14,* **113-117.** (In Chinese.)

Obtained recognition thresholds for 72 Chinese characters varying in 4 factors (3 levels of meaningfulness, 2 levels of number of strokes, 2 levels of word formation, and 2 levels of word shape), combined factorially. The factor of meaningfulness was a between-S variable, and the other factors were within-S variables. As expected, the variables of meaningfulness and number of strokes were related to recognition threshold. The variables of word formation and word shape, which are peculiar to Chinese characters, had no effect on recognition threshold.

448

Yik, W. F. (1978). The effect of visual and acoustic similarity on short-term memory for Chinese words. *Quarterly Journal of Experimental Psychology, 30,* **487-494.**

Used 4 lists of Chinese words in a 2-by-2 factorial design of visual and acoustic similarity in a short-term memory experiment; Ss were 80 male armed forces personnel. In addition to a strong acoustic similarity effect, a highly significant visual similarity effect was also obtained. This was particularly pronounced in the absence of acoustic similarity in the words used. Results not only confirm acoustic encoding to be a basic process in short-term recall of verbal stimuli in a language other than English but also lend support to the growing evidence of visual encoding in short-term memory as the situation demands.

449

Yu, B. L. et al. (1985). STM capacity for Chinese and English language materials. *Memory & Cognition, 13,* **202-207.**

The authors reviewed the theoretical implications of a program of research on short-term memory (STM) using Chinese characters as stimuli and compared the findings with studies of STM that used English language materials. One major theoretical product of this research is an experimentally tested model that reconciles the chunking theory of STM capacity with the articulatory loop theory of A. D. Baddeley (1983), making good quantitative predictions of capacity compatible with both. Another result, obtained by using homophones as stimuli, is a demonstration that STM is mainly acoustically encoded, but that there are an additional 2 or 3 chunks of visually or semantically encoded STM available. Chunks are shown to play the same role in immediate recall and rote learning in both Chinese language and English language stimuli; and STM capacity, measured in chunks, is essentially the same for materials in both languages.

450

Yu, B. L. (1986). [Effects of code additivity of Chinese words and phrases]. *Acta Psychologica Sinica, 18,* **50-57.** (In Chinese.)

On the basis of Chinese double-phonetic compound words, code additivity was carried out according to morphological, phonetic, and semantic relationships of Chinese words. It was confirmed that Chinese words and phrases can be used as suitable verbal materials and can provide a new method for research of verbal memory. The effects of code additivity was not mainly reflected in the process of acquirement of verbal memory, but was reflected in spontaneous recovery and in transition from short-term memory to long-term memory. It could be considered that the effects of code additivity mainly influence long-term retention and retrieval of information, and not the acquirement of information. In addition, the number of encoded dimensions of words, as an independent variable, seemed unrelated to the serial-position curve under free recall.

451

Yu, B. L. (1986). [Relative efficiency of semantic and phonetic encoding in verbal memory]. ***Acta Psychologica Sinica*, *18*, 140-148.** (In Chinese.)

Two experiments were carried out, using control subjects to encode modes and loads of information. The purpose was to explore the relative efficiency of semantic and phonetic encoding in verbal memory. The results showed that performances of semantic encoding were better than those of phonetic encoding in either short-term or long-term memory, and this was also true in either one-trial recall task or multi-trial reconstructing-word-pairs tasks. Both semantic and phonetic information could be stored in either short-term or long-term storing system. It was concluded there is no inherent relation between the encoding of information and of memory in the two kinds of memory systems.

452

Yu, B. L., Brogan, J., Robertson, S., & Uttal, W. R. (1985). The detection of Chinese strokes and characters in visual noise. ***Perception & Psychophysics*, *38*, 23-29.**

The authors investigated the effects of experience, method, and stimulus form on the detectability of dotted approximations to Chinese strokes and characters when they are masked by random-dot visual noise. Subjects were three undergraduates with no previous exposure to Chinese pictographic calligraphy and three students who had been reading and writing Chinese pictographs throughout their lives. Results of two experiments showed that experience effects were limited. Even when small effects were present, they were in the direction opposite to that predicted. Similarly, method (static or dynamic) played only a minor role in determining performance. However, strong stimulus-form effects existed that were well predicted by a previously developed autocorrectional-type computational model of the dotted form detection process. This model is passive, automatic, and preattentive.

453

Yu, B. L., Jing, Q. C., & Sima H. (H. A. Simon). (1984). STM capacity for Chinese words and phrases under simultaneous presentation. In ***Issues in Cognition: Proceedings of a Joint Conference in Psychology*** **(pp. 317-329). Washington, DC: National Academy of Sciences and American Psychological Association. (Also** ***Acta Psychologica Sinica*, 1985 *17*, 361-368 in Chinese.)**

Using the standard immediate recall experimental design, the span of short-term memory (STM) for Chinese words and phrases was investigated. The data for single words, double-phonetic-compound words, and four-character idioms support the hypothesis that STM is capable of storing a fixed number of chunks, but with rather strong effects of familiarity and complexity on STM span. Furthermore, phonetic similarity caused a decrease in STM span. The morphological effects of the internal components of Chinese characters in forming chunks was also examined. Pseudocharacters and noncharacters from character components were made up. It was found that the component units, but not the full composite patterns, behaved as chunks. Finally, by comparing two different stimulus presentation procedures as to their effects on STM span, it was found that the strategy of controlling perception may increase STM span somewhat.

454

Yu, E. S. H. (1974). Achievement motive, familism, and hsiao: A replication of McClelland-Winterbottom studies. ***Dissertation Abstracts International*, *35*, A593.**

McClelland's procedures were replicated in a study of achievement motivation and its relations with filial piety and familism in Chinese teenagers. It was found that: (1) The teenagers upheld filial piety. (2) Verbal statements on achievement were uncorrelated with the need for achievement as measured by TAT stimuli. (3) The need for achievement was not significantly correlated with filial piety, the Familism scale, or with either the Extended Familism or the Nuclear Familism subscales. (4) Verbal statements on achievement were, however, significantly correlated with both filial piety and the Familism scale; the correlation was higher with the Extended Familism subscale than with the Nuclear Familism subscale, with or without any control variable. The findings suggested that Chinese achievement motivation is rooted more firmly in the collectivist than in the individualistic orientation.

455

Yu, G. F. (1986). [Reading of letter display in a picture and its subsequent memory effects]. ***Information on Psychological Sciences*, No. 1, 6-10.** (In Chinese.)

The reading of letter display in a picture and associated memory effects was discussed. It was concluded that: The reading route (site order) follows an order. It usually starts from the left, followed by the order of upper, middle, and lower sites, and terminates at the right. The upper-middle-lower site order amounts to 68.5% of the frequency. The memory route is basically similar to that of reading, although there are errors and omissions. Whether it is the reading route or the memory route, the upper-middle-lower site order is more frequent than other orders. The middle sites are particularly important to reading and memory.

456

Yu, H. S., Fang, L. L., & Zhang, J. T. (1980). [A measurement of the visual depth differential limen among Chinese male young people: Vol. 1]. *Acta Psychologica Sinica*, *12*, **298-302.** (In Chinese.)

Studied the distribution of the static-depth differential limen (DL) and its interrelation with stereoscopic vision in 1,293 Ss, aged 18-25 yrs. 51 Ss had abnormal stereoscopic vision, and 83 others demonstrated visual abnormalities on at least one of 7 ophthalmological tests. Results indicate a mean static-depth DL of 2.

457

Zajonc, R. (1970). Brainwash: Familiarity breeds comfort. *Psychology Today*, *3*, **32-35, 60-64.**

Various studies involving Turkish words, Chinese-like characters, and men's faces supported the hypothesis "that the mere repeated exposure of an unfamiliar stimulus is enough to increase one's attraction to that stimulus." Correlational evidence from word-frequency counts and experimental data from rats added further support. Possible explanations suggest that novel stimuli evoke uncertainty and conflict. The resulting stress is reduced and the stimulus becomes better liked when the individual develops a stable way of responding to the stimulus. Increased exposure encourages the development of such stable response patterns and, therefore, leads to increased attraction.

458

Zhang, G. J., & Simon, H. A. (1985). STM capacity for Chinese words and idioms: Chunking and acoustical loop hypotheses. *Memory & Cognition*, *13*, **193-201.**

The authors developed and tested a model that predicts short-term memory (STM) capacity, incorporating two factors: number of unfamiliar chunks and the average complexity of the chunks (number of syllables). Six experiments that used both Chinese and English language materials and included 38 Chinese scholars as subjects were conducted. One experiment, which used Chinese homophones, showed that STM had a nonacoustical (visual or semantic) component as well as an acoustical one. STM capacity for material encoded nonphonologically appeared to be no greater than three chunks, whereas acoustical STM had a capacity of up to seven chunks. This result was confirmed by an experiment using chunks (radicals) that did not possess highly familiar one-syllable names.

459

Zhang, M. L. (1986). [A preliminary study of relationship between structure of knowledge and cognition]. *Acta Psychologica Sinica*, *18*, **286-294.** (In Chinese.)

A preliminary study is presented on the relationship between knowledge and cognition, carried out on the basis of 4 years of teaching and clinical experimentation. The results showed that acquiring the structure of knowledge concerning the part-whole relationship in mathematics with the number 1 as the underlying basis was important. It permitted the child to form a better cognitive structure, which would contribute to the learning of new knowledge, the choice of strategies as well as the transfer of ability in learning mathematics.

460

Zhang, S. L., & Feng, B. L. (1985). [How field dependence affects concentrated and scattered character learning]. *Information on Psychological Sciences*, **No. 6, 14-19.** (In Chinese.)

The present experiment examined the effects of field dependence on concentrated and scattered learning of Chinese characters. The results showed that different cognitive styles suited different teaching methods. In concentrated character learning, field-independent pupils did better than field-dependent ones. Field-dependent pupils performed better in scattered character learning than in concentrated character learning. Therefore, cognitive style was an important factor which affected character learning achievement.

461

Zhang, T. Z., Sun, G., & Ma, J. H. (1986). [An experimental study of structural components of illusional figures]. *Acta Psychologica Sinica*, *18*, **174-184.** (In Chinese.)

462

Zhang, W. T., Peng, R. X., & Si, M. H. (1986). [STM capacity for Chinese characters and phrases]. *Acta Psychologica Sinica*, *18*, **133-139.** (In Chinese.)

The simplest information processing theory of short-term memory (STM) asserts that STM has a capacity for a fixed number of chunks. To gain a deeper understanding of STM capacity, it would be useful to compare the immediate recall span using Chinese characters and phrases with that using English words. Here, control experiments were conducted for comparison, using three kinds of Chinese materials: one-character words, two-character words and four-character phrases, each with two levels of familiarity, two manners of expression and two learning methods. The results showed that STM capacity approached more closely to constancy when measured in chunks than when measured in other units, but the STM span decreased slightly with increase in chunk complexity. Relative chunk constancy was also observed in the time required for rote learning of stimuli. The degree of familiarity of stimulus materials played only a moderate role in STM capacity. The visual STM span was larger than the auditory span. Analysis of the serial position of STM capacity showed that for the first half, STM through vision was better than that through audition. Some speculative explanations were offered.

463

Zhang, Z. H. (1985). [Size discrimination by sight and touch in school children, deaf-dumb children and adults]. *Information on Psychological Sciences*, **No. 3, 26-31.** (In Chinese.)

464

Zhang, Z. H., Lin, Z. X., & Mao, Y. Y. (1986). [Studies of color preference of Han and Korean children aged 4-6]. *Information on Psychological Sciences*, **No. 5, 6-14.** (In Chinese.)

This study investigated the color preference of preschool children. The subjects were 90 Han and 90 Korean children, aged 4 to 6 years. Various colored chips and clothes were used as stimuli. The results showed that, for Han children, the preference of color chips was, in a descending order: red, yellow, orange, purple, green, white, blue, and black; for Korean children: yellow, red, orange, green, purple, blue, white, and black. Regardless of whether the stimuli were chips or clothes, both groups of children preferred red, yellow, and orange the most, and purple and black the least.

465

Zheng, R. C., & Xiao, B. L. (1983). [A study of the creativity of high school students]. *Acta Psychologica Sinica*, *15*, **445-452.** (In Chinese.)

The Creative Thinking Exercises for High School Students (CTE) was administered to 812 high school students, whose creativity was evaluated by their teachers. The results indicated that: (1) The CTE is reliable and valid for evaluating high school students' creativity. Highly creative students displayed some common personality characteristics. (2) CTE scores were normally distributed. (3) The correlation between CTE scores and academic achievement was not very high. (4) Boys had significantly higher scores in flexibility than girls, but not in other aspects. (5) There were no significant differences between only-children and other children. (6) Among the students, cadres had higher CTE scores than others.

466

Zhou, Q., Wu, L. J., & Fang, P. (1986). [A study of experiments in the characteristics of teenagers' short-term memory development -- A tentative research into memory with the application of Signal Detection Theory]. *Information on Psychological Sciences*, **No. 3, 15-19.** (In Chinese.)

467

Zhu, Y. & Pang, K. Y. (1986). [The covariance decomposition of the mean probability score in decision theory and theory of signal detection]. *Acta Psychologica Sinica*, *18*, **35-42.** (In Chinese.)

The purposes of this paper were to introduce a covariance decomposition of the mean probability score in decision theory (CDMPS) and to explore the relation between the CDMPS and theory of signal detection (TSD). Two experiments were conducted according to the confidence rating method of TSD. The results indicated: (1) The CDMPS could discriminate a person's ability of judgment from his or her attitude when a decision was made. (2) The CDMPS had the same effect as the TSD in dealing with sensory events such as the sensation of weight.

The following references are also relevant to this chapter:

77, 88, 316, 479, 480, 484, 507, 516, 520, 529, 533, 535, 549, 578, 607, 615, 623, 624, 645, 646, 647, 668, 672, 686, 705, 725, 800, 928, 1023, 1033, 1051, 1099, 1219, 1979, 2363, 2593.

PHYSIOLOGICAL PSYCHOLOGY 5

Frequency data on citations in this chapter, in terms of content classification subcategories, are presented in Table 5.

Table 5: *Number of Citations by Content Classification, Language, and Geographical Area*

Content classification	Total	CL	EL	OL	PRC	T	HK	US
Physiological psychology	9	3	6	0	6	0	0	1
Neurology & electrophysiology	13	3	9	1	0	0	0	0
Physiological processes	1	1	0	0	0	0	0	0
Psychophysiology	7	6	1	0	5	0	0	0
Physiological intervention	5	1	4	0	1	0	0	0
Electrical stimulation	0	0	0	0	0	0	0	0
Lesions	0	0	0	0	0	0	0	0
Drug stimulation & psychopharmacology	6	0	6	0	1	0	0	0
Total		41	14	26	1	13	0	01

Note: CL = Chinese language; EL = English language; OL = other languages. PRC = People's Republic of China; T = Taiwan; HK = Hong Kong; US = United States (Chinese Americans--according to the frequency of the subject term Asian Americans).

There are only three subject terms used for indexing citations related to physiological psychology with a frequency of 10 or more: *Peoples Republic of China* (21), *Asia* (13), and *adults* (11).

A review of physiological psychology in the PRC over a 30-year period can be found in Chen, D. R. (1980). [Thirty years of physiological psychology in China: An historical retrospection and some basic problems]. *Acta Psychologica Sinica, 12(1)*, 22-29. (In Chinese.)

468

Barlow, J. B. (1971). *Contemporary brain research in China: Selected recent papers on electrophysiological topics.* **New York: Consultants Bureau.**

469

[Beijing Co-operative Research Group on Acupuncture Anaesthesia in Neurosurgery]. (1980). [The relationship between suggestibility and the effect of acupuncture on cerebral potentials evoked by painful stimulation]. *Acta Psychologica Sinica, 12,* **205-211.** (In Chinese.)

This study is further research on the relations between the suggestibility of cutaneous sensations (electric touch sensibility, electric pain) and the effect of acupuncture on cerebral potentials evoked by painful stimulation. The subjects were 30 normal adults. The role of acupuncture analgesia was observed through the inhibitory effect of acupuncture on cerebral potentials evoked by painful stimulation. The criterion used was the variation of amplitude P2 in the first somatosensory area. The method in the suggestibility experiment was the same as in the previous paper. The results were: (1) Acupuncture produced an inhibitory effect on pain. The majority of subjects (21/30) showed this effect. (2) Both electrical touch and pain thresholds increased under suggestion (by an average of 31.20% and 18.37% respectively). (3) There was no correlation between the degree of suggestibility and the inhibitory effect of acupuncture. It seemed that the faith of the subject in acupuncture analgesia bore no relation to the effect of acupuncture. Inductive suggestion played no important role in acupuncture analgesia.

470

Bell, C. C. (1981). Psychoneuroendocrinology, biorhythms, and Chinese medicine. *Journal of the National Medical Association, 73,* **31-35.**

471

Bennett, B., Fulker, D. W., & DeFries, J. C. (1985). Familial resemblance for general cognitive ability in the Hawaii Family Study of Cognition. *Behavior Genetics, 15,* **401-406.**

Maximum-likelihood estimates of familial correlations for general cognitive ability for three ethnic groups (Americans of European, Japanese, and Chinese ancestry) tested in the Hawaii Family Study of Cognition were similar to product-moment and intraclass correlations previously reported by the 3rd author and colleagues. Standard errors for the maximum-likelihood estimates were somewhat smaller. The estimation procedure used in the present study facilitated tests of alternative hypotheses; hypotheses of homogeneity of familial correlations among the 3 ethnic groups and of homogeneity among the various parent-offspring and sibling correlations were rejected.

472

Cai, T. W., Wu, R. L., Wang, J. H., Xu, G. H., & Chen, X. F. (1980). [Psychological aspects of components of pain: Vol. 2]. *Acta Psychologica Sinica, 12,* **424-431.** (In Chinese.)

Previous experiments found that strong pain consists of two different components: sensation and emotion. Electro-acupuncture exerts a certain influence on both of them. The results of this current experiment, performed on 25 subjects under normal conditions, showed that the main analgesic effect produced by electro-acupuncture is probably due to its influence on the emotional components of pain.

473

Chen, D. R. (1980). [Thirty years of physiological psychology in China: An historical retrospection and some basic problems]. *Acta Psychologica Sinica, 12,* **22-29. (English translation in** *Chinese Sociology and Anthropology,* **1980,** *12,* **78-96.)** (In Chinese.)

Emphasizes the importance of physiological psychology in basic and applied research for the modernization of psychology. Research is reviewed, and problems such as the viewpoint of naturalism in modern China are considered.

474

Courtney, A. J. (1984). A search task to assess visual lobe size. *Human Factors, 26,* **289-298.**

Using a sample of 18 Cantonese Chinese Ss (aged 15-52 yrs) that covered a wide range of acuity scores and age, very high correlations were obtained between time taken on a simple card-sorting task and visual lobe dimensions. With Ss younger than 30 yrs of age and having good acuity, similar but not so highly significant correlations were found. Only one card sorting session was required to produce useful data for between-S comparisons so that the card-sorting task may provide a simple, fast, and valid measure of a visual function of great importance to search performance. Also, a simple means of calculating visual lobe size from tachistoscopically presented stimulus material was tested and found to produce comparable results to those obtained using a more complex method of calculation involving data transformation.

475

Courtney, A. J., & Chan, H. S. (1985). Eight-axis visual-field mapping for targets embedded in a homogeneous competing background. *Perceptual & Motor Skills, 60,* **655-663.**

The authors investigated visual-field mapping on eight axes, using a careful definition of correct detection of a target (i.e., in terms of the size of the error made by subjects in estimating target positions). Six Chinese graduate engineering students attended four 1-hour sessions on separate days and were presented with four orientations. The subjects were shown 118 target locations four times over the four sessions. Immediately after presentation, the subject was required to give an estimate of the location of the target on a specimen card showing the possible target locations. Results showed that visual fields for subjects were irregular in shape, and there were differences among subjects. The eight-axis area correlated highly with area based on only the horizontal and vertical axes, but the latter area gave no indication of even gross irregularities in shape of the visual field.

476

DeFries, J. C. et al. (1979). Familial resemblance for specific cognitive abilities. *Behavior Genetics*, *9*, **23-43.**

Measures of familial resemblance (spouse correlations, regressions of offspring on midparent, single-parent/single-child correlations, and sibling correlations) are presented for members of the 2 largest ethnic groups tested in the Hawaii Family Study of Cognition. A battery of 15 individual tests of specific cognitive abilities (e.g., Primary Mental Abilities Vocabulary Test and Raven Progressive Matrices) was administered to 1,816 families consisting of both biological parents and children 13 yrs of age or older (6,581 individuals). Median spouse correlations (corrected for differences in test reliability) are 0.15 and 0.12 for Americans of European and of Japanese ancestry, respectively. With regard to the regressions of offspring on midparent value, corresponding median values are 0.50 and 0.35. Results of hierarchical multiple regression analyses, as well as the ordering of single-parent/single-child and sibling correlations, provide no evidence to support the hypothesis that spatial ability is influenced by a sex-linked, recessive gene.

477

DeFries, J. C. et al. (1982). Sex-by-generation and ethnic group-by-generation interactions in the Hawaii Family Study of Cognition. *Behavior Genetics*, *12*, **223-230.**

Subjected principal component scores for members of the 3 largest ethnic groups tested in the Hawaii Family Study of Cognition (J. R. Wilson et al, 1978) to an Ethnic Group * Sex * Generation ANOVA with unequal subclass numbers. The components spatial ability, verbal ability, perceptual speed, and visual memory, as well as general mental ability, were computed from the 15 cognitive tests for members of 369 American families of Japanese ancestry (AJAs), 93 families of Chinese ancestry, (ACAs), and 927 families of European ancestry (AEAs); total Ss, 4,677. Large and highly significant Sex-by-Generation and Ethnic Group-by-Generation interactions were found for measures of general and specific cognitive abilities. The Group-by-Generation interactions may be the result of the rate of development or decline of cultural factors. The influence of cultural factors is apparent in the high scores of daughters compared to their mothers.

478

Dixon, P. W., Roper, R. E., & Ahern, E. H. (1974). A preliminary study of the use of moxacautery for punishment and medical reasons as a discriminant of personality differences in Japanese nationals. *Psychologia: An International Journal of Psychology in the Orient*, *17*, **28-35.**

Discusses the use in Chinese and Japanese medicine of moxacautery, said to have curative qualities resulting from the stimulation of peripheral nerves and blood vessels. Moxacautery has also been used as a form of punishment for Japanese children. 25 Ss who had previously received moxacautery were tested with a version of the Edwards Personal Preference Scale. Females who had received moxacautery as punishment showed relatively poor socialization.

479

Guo, N. F., & Yin, W. G. (1986). [An experiment in the functional asymmetry of the two cerebral hemispheres in recognizing Chinese characters]. *Acta Psychologica Sinica*, *18*, **203-209.** (In Chinese.)

Past experiments showed that in correctly recognizing isolated Chinese characters, neither of the two hemispheres played a dominant role. In the present study, eight Chinese characters were set against four different background noises. The subjects were 10 male and 10 female college students. The time of appearance for the stimuli was 60 msec. The results of the experiment were: (1) Without noise interference, there was no marked difference between the left and right visual fields, nor was there any difference when the signal-to-noise ratio was 6.66. (2) It was only when the signal-to-noise ratio was 4 and the difficulty of recognition reached a fairly high level that the dominance of the right visual field became obvious. (3) Whatever the degree of difficulty, reaction time of the left visual field was shorter than that of the right, but in the correctness of recognition the right visual field displayed some dominance.

480

Hardyck, C., Tzeng, O. J. L., & Wang, W. S. (1978). Cerebral lateralization of function and bilingual decision processes: Is thinking lateralized? *Brain & Language*, *5*, **56-71.**

Reports 4 experiments utilizing tachistoscopic presentation of verbal and spatial stimuli to visual half-fields. 28 right-handed Chinese-English bilinguals served as Ss in Exps I and II, and 16 right-handed graduate students with no knowledge of Chinese served in Exps III and IV. Three experiments failed to find any cerebral lateralization effect of the type predicted from existing models of cerebral lateralization processes. One experiment found marked lateralization effects. Since the experiments differed only in the ratio of trials to experimental stimuli, it is argued that cerebral lateralization experiments detect only a memory process occurring after Ss have learned all the stimuli to be presented. When new stimuli are presented on each trial, no cerebral lateralization effects are found, suggesting that active ongoing cognitive processing is independent of lateralization.

481

Hoosain, R. (1984). Lateralization of bilingual digit span functions. *Perceptual & Motor Skills*, *58*, **21-22.**

36 right-handed Chinese-English bilingual undergraduates were tested on forward and backward digit spans in both Chinese and English in monaural listening tests. There was a significant right-ear advantage for forward digit span in Chinese but not in English, suggesting different hemispheric involvement.

482

Huang, Y. L., & Jones, B. (1980). Naming and discrimination of Chinese ideograms presented in the right and left visual fields. *Neuropsychologia*, *18*, **703-706.**

In a naming experiment, Chinese Ss showed no significant visual-field advantage for naming tachistoscopically presented Chinese characters. However, the 10 Chinese and 10 North American Ss tended to discriminate characters presented in the left visual field more accurately. Results are discussed in terms of the theories of hemispheric specialization.

483

Johnson, R. C. et al. (1984). Further investigation of racial/ethnic differences and of familial resemblances in flushing in response to alcohol. *Behavior Genetics*, *14*, **171-178.**

Data were presented in a previous paper by S. Y. Schwitters et al. on ethnic differences and family resemblances in the flushing response to alcohol. Using a sample of 1,288 subjects from 245 families, the present study used the same analyses as in the above study, as well as analyses pertaining to the extent and duration of flushing, association of flushing with other symptoms, and degree to which flushing influenced drinking behavior. Subjects belonged to one of the following ethnic groups: White, Chinese, Filipino, Hawaiian/part Hawaiian, Japanese, or other. A distinction was made between fast (one drink or less to evoke flushing) and slow (two drinks or more to evoke flushing) flushing. Substantial ethnic differences were found in flushing. Highly significant family resemblances in flushing were also found, but these did not conform to a single-locus genetic model. Extent of flushing was significantly related to flushing type, but duration of flushing and other symptoms resulting from alcohol use were not. The two flushing types appeared to have different amounts of influence on drinking behavior.

484

Kershner, J. R., & Jeng, A. G. (1972). Dual functional hemispheric asymmetry in visual perception: Effects of ocular dominance and postexposural processes. *Neuropsychologia*, *10*, **437-445.**

Investigated laterality differences in visual perception by assessing the effects of the directional postexposure scanning movements associated with reading habits, the visual half-field (VHF) in which stimuli were presented, and eye dominance on an immediate recall task. 40 Chinese bilingual graduate students (20 right-eye dominant and 20 left-eye dominant) were tested for their recall of forms, Chinese words, and English words. The stimuli were projected tachistoscopically in the left and/or right VHFs under conditions of simultaneous and successive presentation. Results demonstrate a right field superiority for verbal stimuli under both conditions and a left field superiority for nonverbal stimuli when presented successively. Right-eyed Ss were better in processing verbal materials and left-eyed Ss were better in the perception and recall of nonverbal materials. Findings support the validity of the psychophysiological model of asymmetrical cerebral functioning and demonstrate the importance of reading habits and eye dominance. Results are interpreted as preliminary support for Piaget's postulated relationship between perceptual and organic development

485

Kuang, P. Z., Luo, S. D., & Liu, S. X. (1980). [Thirty years of physiological psychology in China]. *Acta Psychologica Sinica*, *12*, **144-151. (Also in U.S. Publications Research Service (Trans.),** *China report: Science and technology* **(No. 53), 1980, August, Report No. 76,320, pp. 62-78.)** (In Chinese.)

Discusses the development of physiological psychology from the time when it was first characterized by Pavlov's learning theory and methods to present day achievements, experiences, problems, and prospects.

486

Kung, Y. H. (1958). [Typing of higher nervous activity of normal adults]. *Chinese Journal of Neurology and Psychiatry*, *4*, **362-367.** (In Chinese.)

487

Kupietz, S. S., Richardson, E., Gadow, K. D., & Winsberg, B. G. (1980). Effects of methylphenidate on learning a "beginning reading vocabulary" by normal adults. *Psychopharmacology*, *69*, **69-72.**

Required 9 21-37 yr old adults to learn a beginning vocabulary of 96 Chinese characters under placebo and 5 and 10 mg methylphenidate by 2 teaching methods that differed in the rate at which new items were introduced for practice. Using lists composed of 12 characters and their English equivalents, all items were presented prior to the start of practice trials (simultaneous method), or each item was introduced only as S practiced items previously presented (progressive method). Learning performance was analyzed in terms of total errors and errors made at 2 criterion stages in list acquisition. Overall performance was significantly facilitated by the low dose of methylphenidate, but only with the simultaneous method. Significant drug effects were also obtained at criterion stages that were associated with high error rates. It is concluded that drug effects are likely to be most pronounced in difficult learning situations and that dosage appears to be an important variable for further consideration.

488

Kusuma, A. (1980). The treatment of functional impotence by acupuncture. *American Journal of Acupuncture*, *8*, **39-45.**

The pathophysiology and therapy of functional impotence according to the Chinese Organ Phenomenon and the Five Element Theory are described. 42 cases of functional impotence, with ages between 23 and 47 yr and a duration of illness from 1 to 4 years, were treated. 33 cases showed good results (78.6%), 6 cases improved considerably (14.3%), while 3 (7.1%) cases failed to respond to acupuncture.

489

Leong, C. K., Wong, S., Wong, A., & Hiscock, M. (1985). Differential cerebral involvement in perceiving Chinese characters: Levels of processing approach. *Brain & Language*, *26*, **131-145.**

Three experiments with 24 right-handed Chinese undergraduates were designed to determine the accuracy and latency with which subjects recognized Chinese characters in the left and right visual half-fields (VHFs). Experiment I was a lexical decision task, in which the configuration of the stimulus (a real Chinese character or the mirror image of a real character) determined whether the grapheme was an actual character. Experiment II required phonological processing. Subjects had to decide whether a character (or a foil) matched the sound of an orally presented Chinese character. Experiment III required semantic processing, and subjects had to decide if a character (or a foil) belonged to a particular semantic category. In each experiment, single characters were presented unilaterally for 150 msec. There was a significant right VHF superiority for accuracy scores in Experiments II and III but not in Experiment I. None of the experiments yielded significant visual asymmetries in reaction time (RT). Findings do not support previous claims of orthography-specific laterality but instead show that laterality effects for morphemic stimuli vary with the orthographic, phonological, and semantic processing demands of the task.

490

Li, H. (1978). Hallucinogenic plants in Chinese herbals. *Journal of Psychedelic Drugs*, *10*, **17-26.**

Hallucinogenic plants from Chinese works are given in the order of their relative importance. The Chinese herbals and other related works cited here are given with the author's name first and arranged chronologically to give a historical perspective to this record. A bibliography to modern works is given at the end of the paper. It has to be noted that most of the earlier herbals have been lost and existed only as quotations in subsequent works. A number of these items have been reconstituted by later workers. The illustrations given here are from Chang Tsun-hui, the 1249 A.D. edition of Tang Shen-wei's Cheng-lei pen-tsao of 1108 A.D., which is one of the earliest illustrated pen-tsao extant.

491

Lin, C. S. (1982). [The perception and responses of college students with different GSR patterns to psychosocial stressors]. *Bulletin of Educational Psychology*, *15*, **85-96.** (In Chinese.)

Classified 42 Chinese undergraduates into a high-high amplitude group (H-H), a high-low amplitude group (H-L), and a low-low amplitude group (L-L), according to the change patterns of their galvanic skin response (GSR) waves. Ss were asked to recite Chinese poems and to complete subtests of the Raven Progressive Matrices. Lowest absolute skin resistance and subtest scores were recorded before and after their performance in front of classmates. Ss' perception of stressors was assessed by a rating scale of semantic differential type, with 16 school-life events as its concepts. Results show that (1) there were no differences in responses to psychosocial stressors among H-H, H-L, and L-L groups; (2) only half of the classifications were correct; and (3) there were no significant discriminant functions with which the H-H, H-L, and L-L groups could be classified. It is concluded that physiological indices, such as GSR waves, may not be used as a measure of personality.

492

Mendelson, J. H., & Mello, N. K. (1982). Hormones and psycho-sexual development in young men following chronic heroin use. *Neurobehavioral Toxicology & Teratology*, *4*, **441-445.**

Compared 16 former addicts who began heroin use during early puberty with 17 current heroin users and 10 drug-free controls with respect to psychosexual development and pituitary gonadal hormone levels. Ss were all males (aged 16-29 yrs) living in Hong Kong. Standardized interviews were conducted to assess sexual activity and desire. Plasma testosterone and luteinizing hormone (LH) levels did not differ between the former addicts and controls but were significantly suppressed in the current heroin users. Measures of sexual behavior and physical development did not differ significantly among the 3 groups.

Recurrent heroin use during early puberty did not significantly disrupt pubertal development. It is postulated that tolerance to opiate-induced suppression of pituitary gonadal hormones occurs in prepubescent as well as postpubescent males.

493

Nguy, T. V., Allard, F. A., & Bryden, M. P. (1980). Laterality effects for Chinese characters: Differences between pictorial and nonpictorial characters. *Canadian Journal of Psychology*, *34*, **270-273.**

20 Chinese undergraduates identified Chinese characters presented tachistoscopically to the left or right of fixation. The characters presented were of 3 types: pictorial--characters looking like the object they represent; single--nonpictorial characters; and combination--characters comprised of 2 other characters. The magnitude of the laterality effect observed was a function of the type of character viewed. The standard right visual field effect was found for single and combination characters, while no visual field difference was found for pictorial characters. Results suggest some right-hemispheric involvement in processing pictorial characters.

494

Schwitters, S. Y., Johnson, R. C., Johnson, S. B., & Ahern, F. M. (1982). Familial resemblances in flushing following alcohol use. *Behavior Genetics*, *12*, **349-352.**

47 sets of parents and 77 adult offspring from families of Caucasian, Chinese, or Japanese ancestry provided data regarding their use of alcohol and their flushing responses (FRs) following alcohol consumption. Results show substantial familial resemblances in FRs and suggest that the FR may be inherited as a genetic dominant.

495

Schwitters, S. Y., Johnson, R. C., McClearn, G. E., & Wilson, J. R. (1982). Alcohol use and the flushing response in different racial-ethnic groups. *Journal of Studies on Alcohol*, *43*, **1259-1262.**

2,338 men and 1,376 women of Caucasian, Chinese, Filipino, Hapa-Haole (half-Oriental, half-Caucasian) and Hawaiian or part-Hawaiian ancestries responded to a questionnaire on alcohol consumption and symptoms following consumption. A significant association between drinking behavior and flushing was found among males of Japanese ancestry, but not among subjects from the other ethnic groups.

496

Shi, R. H., & Yang, Z. L. (1980). [A comparison of effects of acupuncture and suggestion on the pain threshold]. *Acta Psychologica Sinica*, *12*, **341-347.** (In Chinese.)

497

Shimada, M., & Otsuka, A. (1981). [Functional hemisphere differences of kanji processing in Japanese]. *Japanese Psychological Review*, *24*, **472-489.** (In other language.)

Discusses some contradictions in research studies concerning functional hemisphere differences of kanji processing in Japanese. Kanji refers to a Japanese system of writing composed principally of Chinese characters. Some researchers claim that the right hemisphere is superior to the left one for kanji processing, but there are many inconsistencies in the research. Many clinical and experimental studies indicate that the left hemisphere is superior to the right one for the processing of written materials, regardless of the nature of the characters. However, these studies do not claim that the right hemisphere has a total lack of ability to process kanji. Rather, data are presented that indicate that the right hemisphere can process kanji words to some degree. A neuropsychological model of kanji processing is proposed, and it is suggested that the right hemisphere processes kanji words by the direct or lexical-semantic processing route.

498

Taylor, W. J. (1971). History and pharmacology of psychedelic drugs. *International Journal of Clinical Pharmacology, Therapy & Toxicology*, *5*, **51-57.**

Discusses various presently used psychedelic drugs. Cannabis or marijuana is an ancient compound used by the Chinese for scores of centuries. At present, there are estimated to be 8 million users in the United States. Many generations of American Indians have used mescaline in the form of peyote cactus buttons to alter consciousness. More recently, lysergic acid diethylamide (LSD), which was 1st synthesized in 1938, became a significant part of the psychedelic scene. Amphetamines or "pep pills" are also aggravating the current drug abuse problem. Organic solvents, anesthetics, and household spices can be used to produce psychotropic effects. "Glue sniffing" has great potential for serious damage to the liver, kidney, and central nervous system. Cocaine abuse is probably a much greater problem in this country than is generally realized. Alcohol, caffeine, and nicotine are socially acceptable pharmacological psychedelics which are causing physical dependence in millions of Americans. Little is known about the clinical pharmacology of most mood-altering chemicals and too little is being done to learn more. A drug "credibility gap" is being created between the generations, and physicians are contributing by making public statements before all the facts are known.

499

Tsao, Y. C., Wu, M. F., & Feustel, T. (1981). Stroop interference: Hemispheric difference in Chinese speakers. *Brain & Language*, *13*, **372-378.**

Hypothesized that more Stroop interference would occur in the nondominant hemisphere because the 2 processes involved in the Stroop effect (i.e., reading logographs and naming colors) are possibly localized in that hemisphere in Chinese-speaking Ss. 18 right-handed Chinese-English bilinguals were Ss. There were 3 conditions in each visual field: interference, reading, and naming. Each slide was presented for 150 msec preceded by a fixation dot. Ss were asked to verbally report as fast and as accurately as possible either the color words or the color names, depending upon the condition. RTs and error rates were analyzed. As expected, more Stroop interference was obtained when color words were presented in the left visual field.

500

Wang, J. S., Xin, D. G., Sun, C. H., & Lin, S. H. (1979). [The role played by the psychological factors in the clinical mechanism of acupuncture anaesthesia]. *Acta Psychologica Sinica, 11*, **88-97.** (In Chinese.)

Since 1965, several thousands of cases receiving acupuncture anaesthesia have been observed. The results show: (1) Psychological factors play an active role in reactions to needling, analgesia, regulation by acupuncture, and the efficacy of acupuncture anaesthesia. (2) Recognition, confidence, suggestion, individual experience of feeling pain, cooperation with medical members and, above all, emotional factors play an important role in acupuncture anaesthesia. (3) Both exaggeration and rejection of the effects of psychological factors on the acupuncture anaesthesia are unwarranted.

501

Wang, J. S., Xin, D. G., Sun, S. H., & Lin, S. H. (1980). [The effect of acupuncture anesthesia on 2-point discrimination sensation]. *Acta Psychologica Sinica, 12*, **438-444.** (In Chinese.)

This paper reviews the results of more than 10 years' study on the effect of acupuncture anesthesia on 2-point discrimination sensation. The results are : (1) Acupuncture heightens not only the pain but also the two-point discrimination sensation thresholds. (2) When the points of Hegu and Sanyinjiao are stimulated, durations of 25 minutes and 15 minutes are equally effective. The duration of 5 minutes is the least effective. (3) The factors influencing the heightening of two-point discrimination sensation by acupuncture have been determined. (4) There is a positive correlation between pain and two-point thresholds. The effect of needling on heightening the two-point threshold correlates closely with the effectiveness of acupuncture anesthesia.

502

Wu, W. P. (1973). *Chinese acupuncture* **(Trans. J. Lavier & Philip M. Chancellor). Elmsford, NY: British Book Centre.**

Presents an English translation of a French edition dealing with the history, the pathways, and techniques of the Chinese art of acupuncture and cauterization. Energic and symptomatic medicine are considered.

503

Xu, S. L., Tang, C. M., Song, W. Z., Sun, C. H., Xiang, M. J., Zhang, S. X., Liu, S. Q., Gong, X. L., Yu, Q. S., Liu, J. L., Feng, B. Y., Xu, M. Y., Men, X. W., & Zhang, C. L. (1979). [Patients' emotional state on entering the operation room, the effect of acupuncture anesthesia, and psychophysiological functions]. *Acta Psychologica Sinica, 11*, **77-87.** (In Chinese.)

The study was carried out during 1975-1976, and the Ss were 101 patients for lung resection under acupuncture anesthesia. The results showed: the emotional states before needle inserting, as assessed either by self-observation or by objective behavior observation, highly correlated with the effect of acupuncture anesthesia, this was especially the case with the latter assessment (P.001). The tensionals often had worse effect than the stables. Moreover, Pts who seemed stable at the beginning and then became tensional usually had bad effects. The emotional states were related to the following physiological and psychological functions: 1) Most of the emotional tensionals had greater fluctuations in respiration and pulse amplitude when lying quietly after entering the operation room (51Ss). 2) While inserting the acupuncture needle, the combined fluctuations of G.S.R., respiration and pulse amplitude were markedly larger for the tensionals than for the stables (P.001, 47Ss). 3) The pts with tensional or medial emotional states, the plasma 11-OHCS (as compared to that tested in the ward) increased more significantly than the stables (P.05, 47Ss). 4) All the stables completed the time estimating test more accurately on entering operation room than that performed in the ward, while the most of the tensionals showed worse performance than in the ward (P.01, 32Ss). 5) The pts that overconcerned about acupuncture anesthesia usually were the tensionals when entering the operation room (P.001, 99 Ss). 6) The results of the predicting test, based upon the combined responses of G.S.R., respiration and pulse amplitude during acupuncture in the laboratory before operation, were also highly correlated with the emotional states when entering the operation room (P.01, 101 Ss). 7) Oversensitive patients, evaluated through the compound cutaneous sensitivity tests of touch and pain before operation, usually were the emotionally tensionals when entering the operation room (P.01, 87 Ss). After the acupuncture induction, the catecholamines in blood of most of the tensionals increased while most of the stables had this blood substance decreased. However, the changes in catechoamines in blood were related with the effect of acupuncture anesthesia, pts. who have increased cathecholamine in blood often show bad effect.

504

Yan, G. C., & Zhu, Y. X. (1983). [Contribution of Liu Zhi's "Tian Fang Xing Li" to research on the human brain]. *Information on Psychological Sciences*, **No. 6, 21-23.** (In Chinese.)

505

Yang, L. N., Greenstadt, L., & Shapiro, D. (1985). [Effects of caffeine and stress on blood pressure: A cross-cultural comparison]. *Information on Psychological Sciences*, **No. 3, 39-44.** (In Chinese.)

506

Zhang, W. T., & Peng, R. X. (1983). The lateralization of hemispheric function in the recognition of Chinese characters. *Neuropsychologia*, *21*, **679-682.**

Conducted 2 experiments to investigate the lateralization of hemispheric functions. In Exp I, single Chinese characters, English words, and random dot forms were used as stimuli presented to the left or right visual field of 12 adults. In Exp II, 12 adults and 12 9-10 yr olds were asked to recognize single characters presented in one field and arabic numerals in the opposite field. Adults and children all showed left-hemisphere superiority in the recognition of characters. Some possible causes are given to explain why Chinese characters, being components of an ideographic language, show a superiority similar to that of phonetic languages.

507

Zhang, W. T., & Peng, R. X. (1984). [Cerebral laterality and the recognition of ideograms]. *Acta Psychologica Sinica*, *16*, **275-281.** (In Chinese.)

This is a study of the recognition of Chinese characters, words, and single Arabic numerals (ideograms) tachistoscopically exposed in the left and the right visual fields. Normal right-handed subjects were used. There was no difference between left and right visual fields for single Arabic numerals. A significant right-field (left hemisphere) superiority was shown for characters and words presented unilaterally and for characters presented bilaterally with Arabic numerals. A nonsignificant difference was obtained between left and right visual fields for words presented bilaterally with numerals and characters presented in center and lateral visual fields simultaneously. Still, the right visual field (left hemisphere) was dominant in the recognition of Chinese characters and words.

508

Zhao, Y. J., Xu, H. Z., Shen, J., & Liu, A. H. (1982). Biodetector experiments on human body radiation physics. *PSI Research*, *1*, **77-84.**

Discusses a method of detecting radiation associated with exceptional human functioning. Using nuclear emulsion and negative X-ray film, the authors observed multiple exposures produced by radiation emitted from Ss who were demonstrating exceptional capabilities. Among the exposures were images of written Chinese characters that were recognized by the gifted Ss. Imperfections in the method are delineated.

The following references are also relevant to this chapter:

3, 947, 948, 1010, 1041, 1388, 2635, 2641, 2642, 2644, 2757, 2784, 2965, 3189.

COMMUNICATION SYSTEMS 6

Frequency data on citations in this chapter, in terms of content classification subcategories, are presented in Table 6.

Table 6: *Number of Citations by Content Classification, Language, and Geographical Area*

Content classification	Total	CL	EL	OL	PRC	T	HK	US
Communication systems	26	4	20	2	2	1	0	1
Language and speech	133	66	61	6	40	1	10	2
Literaturre and art	12	1	11	0	3	18	0	0
Total		171	71	92	8	45	20	103

Note: CL = Chinese language; EL = English language; OL = other languages. PRC = People's Republic of China; T = Taiwan; HK = Hong Kong; US = United States (Chinese Americans--according to the frequency of the subject term Asian Americans).

Subject terms used for indexing citations related to communication systems are grouped according to geographical area, subject population, and topic. These are presented below, in a descending order of frequency. (The frequency of single-word subject terms includes those of compound terms in which the single word appears. Subjects terms used for indexing citations from other chapters may have been included. Terms with a frequency of less than 10 are not shown.)

Geographical area

59 Peoples Republic of China
52 Asia
23 Taiwan
13 Hong Kong

Subject population

40	children
24	school age children
23	students
15	college students
13	adults

Topic

120	language
56	Chinese characters
48	written language
33	development
31	reading
25	learning
22	perception
20	cross cultural differences
20	foreign languages
19	language development
15	word meaning
14	bilingualism
14	orthography
13	adulthood
13	literature
13	communication
12	cognitive processes
12	semantics
11	comprehension
11	word (phonetic units)
10	cognitive development
10	tachistoscopic presentation

Table 6 shows that the majority of citations belongs to the subcategory of language and speech (77.8%). As to geographical area, the PRC predominates. The subject terms *Chinese characters*, *written language* and, to a lesser extent, *orthography* appear with notably high frequencies, testifying that written Chinese has received special attention in research.

In recent years, considerable attention has been devoted to psychological and psycholinguistic studies of the Chinese language. Several edited books (Kao and Cheng 1982; Kao and Hoosain 1984; Kao and Hoosain 1986), an entire issue of *Acta Psychologica Taiwanica* (1978), and a bibliography (Ho 1979) on this topic have been published; another book (Kao 1986) focused on the psychology of Chinese calligraphy.

REFERENCES

Ho, D. Y. F. (1979). Chinese language and learning-learning behaviour: A bibliography of psychological and psycholinguistic studies. In R. Lord (Ed.), *Hong Kong language papers* (pp. 161- 184). Hong Kong: Hong Kong University Press.

Kao, H. S. R., & Hoosain, R. (Eds.). (1984). *Psychological studies of the Chinese language. Hong Kong:* The Chinese Language Society of Hong Kong.

Kao, H. S. R., & Hoosain, R. (Eds.). (1986). *Linguistics, psychology, and the Chinese language.* Hong Kong: Centre of Asian Studies, University of Hong Kong.

Kao, S. R. (1986). [*Psychology of Chinese calligraphy*]. Taipei: Great Eastern. (In Chinese.)

Kao, S. R., & Cheng, C. M. (Eds.). (1982). [*Psychological studies of the Chinese language*]. Taipei: Wen Ho. (In Chinese.)

509

Au, T. K. (1984). Counterfactuals: In reply to Alfred Bloom. *Cognition, 17,* **289-302.**

The author responded to A. Bloom's criticisms of the present author's (1983) study of Chinese and English counterfactual thoughts. Bloom's findings with respect to the Sapir-Whorf hypothesis were considered in detail.

510

Bain, B., & Yu, A. (1980). Raising children bilingually in the Alsace, Alberta and Hong Kong: "One parent, one language". *New Horizons,* **No. 21, 80-106.**

511

Bain, B., & Yu, A. (1982). [The cognitive styles of bilingual children under the condition of exposure to two languages]. *Acta Psychologica Sinica, 14,* **351-357.** (In Chinese.)

512

Bain, B., & Yu, A. (1983). Language, class and culture: Implications for first and second language acquisition in Hong Kong and Alberta. *New Horizons,* **No. 24, 63-82.**

513

Bloom, A. H. (1981). *The linguistic shaping of thought: A study in the impact of language on thinking in China and the West.* **Hillsdale, NJ: Erlbaum.**

514

Bloom, A. H. (1984). Caution--the words you use may affect what you say: A response to Au. *Cognition, 17,* **275-287.**

The author responded to T. K. Au's paper on Chinese and English counterfactual thoughts. Implications for the effects of linguistic labels on thought were discussed.

515

Chan, M. C., Chau, H. L., & Hoosain, R. (1983). Input/output switch in bilingual code switching. *Journal of Psycholinguistic Research, 12,* **407-416.**

21 Chinese-English bilingual undergraduates were asked to read a passage with spontaneous bilingual code switchings, compared with a unilingual Chinese translation of the passage, a unilingual English translation, a translation with random switchings, and a translation with only nouns switched into English (Exp I). There was no difference between the reading speed for the passage with natural switchings and the unilingual Chinese passage, thus questioning the need to postulate a bilingual input/output switch. The speed for reading passages with artificial switchings was slower. In a translation task, the naturally switched items required less time in Chinese-to-English translations compared with English-to-Chinese translations (Exp II with 20 Ss). This indicated that in natural code switchings, the English lexical items produced were more available, even though English is generally the weaker language.

516

Chang, H. W. (1984). The comprehension of complex Chinese sentences by children: Relative clause. *Chinese Journal of Psychology, 26,* **57-66.**

Forty-eight elementary school children equally divided into four age groups (grade 1, 2, 4 and 6) were tested for their comprehension of sentences containing a relative clause. Comprehension was assessed by asking children to act out with toys the meaning of test sentences. Depending on the grammatical function of the head noun in the main and relative clause, four types of constructions were possible: SS (head noun functions as subject in main and relative clause), SO, OS, and OO. Results indicated a clear difference in comprehension difficulty, with SS = SO OS = OO in an ascending order. The present finding together with previous results from English speaking children can best be accounted for by hypothesizing a combined disruptive effects on comprehension due to sentence interruption and rearrangement of the normal order of linguistic units.

517

Chao, T. (1986). Communicating through architecture: San Francisco Chinese restaurants as cultural intersections. *Dissertation Abstracts International, 46,* **A2467.**

518

Chau, A. W. L., Kao, H. S. R., & Shek, D. T. L. (1986). Writing time of double-character Chinese words: Effects of interrupting writing responses. In H. S. R. Kao, G. P. van Galen, & R. Hoosain (Eds.), *Graphonomics: Contemporary research in handwriting* **(pp. 273-288). Amsterdam, Netherlands: North-Holland.**

519

Chen, H. C. (1984). [Detecting radical component of Chinese characters in visual reading]. *Chinese Journal of Psychology, 26,* **29-34.** (In Chinese.)

In the present two experiments, subjects were asked to read a story that contained some misconstructed characters and to respond to each occurrence of a given radical component. The story was presented on paper in Experiment 1 and on a computer screen showing either 1 or 10 characters at a time in Experiment 2. In the paper and 10-character conditions, detection errors were significantly higher when the target was embedded in a correct character than when it was embedded in a misconstructed character. This difference, however, decreased dramatically in the 1-character condition. The results are discussed in terms of character perception and word recognition processes involved in the traditional tachistoscopic presentation and in conventional reading situations.

520

Chen, S. Y., & Wang, S. M. (1964). [The influence of related elements on reproduction of tachistoscopically presented series of words]. *Acta Psychologica Sinica*, **No. 2, 143-151.** (In Chinese.)

521

Chen, V., & Ryback, D. (1974). Language acquisition in Chinese children. *Acta Psychologica Taiwanica, 16,* **1-6.**

In this cross-sectional study, the speech patterns of five Chinese children were examined for types of errors and average length of utterance. Each child's speech was electronically taped during natural conversations with his or her parents. These tapes were then transcribed using the Yale system of romanization of Chinese. The youngest child, 14 months of age, provided too little speech for purposes of analysis. The remaining four children showed a remarkable absence of errors involving word order. Tonal errors appeared to decrease markedly with age. Sentence length appeared as a consistently increasing function of age. Mean length of utterance ranged from 2.5 morphemes for the 24-month old to 7.7 morphemes for the 32-month-old. These data were quite similar to those obtained from American children of similar ages.

522

Chen, Y. M., & Peng, R. X. (1985). [Preliminary study of semantic retrieval for Chinese language]. *Acta Psychologica Sinica, 17,* **162-169.** (In Chinese.)

Two experiments were conducted to investigate semantic retrieval in the Chinese language. In experiment 1, 23 two-character words selected from 13 sentences were used as stimuli in a free association test. The results indicated that semantic distance in terms of common sense relations between words was useful in predicting performance on the free association test. In experiment 2, true/false judgment reaction time was measured, using 38 (20 true and 18 false) sentences as stimuli. The findings agreed with the results obtained by Collins and Quillian. A difference in retrieval time between levels in which the sentences were stored was found. The results indicated that at the stage of information retrieval the morphology of Chinese characters is not an important factor.

523

Cheng, C. M. (1978). [A design of Chinese character input system with phonetic symbols as indexing keys]. *Acta Psychologica Taiwanica, 20,* **19-27.** (In Chinese.)

524

Cheng, C. M. (1981). [Perception of Chinese characters]. *Acta Psychologica Taiwanica, 23,* **137-153.** (In Chinese.)

Experiment 1 showed that a Chinese character was better perceived in tachistoscopic presentation when embedded in a word context than when embedded in a nonword context. Experiment 2 showed that a constituent of a Chinese character was better perceived in tachistoscopic presentation when embedded in a character context than when embedded in a pseudocharacter context, which was in turn better perceived than when the character was embedded in a noncharacter context. The advantage of pseudocharacter over noncharacter cannot be attributed to differential phonetic encoding in favor of pseudocharacter, because both are not readable. It also cannot be attributed to the existence of sequential redundancy among constituents in favor of pseudocharacter, because the two differ in positional redundancy of constituents rather than in sequential redundancy among constituents. The advantage of both character over pseudocharacter and word over nonword is interpreted to be a result of both character and word stimuli being coded semantically before the response is made. The findings of the two experiments indicated that both the word superiority effect and the character superiority effect were not sensitive to the complexity and frequency of usage of presented characters or words.

525

Cheng, C. M., & Sakurai, S. (1984). [The fuzziness of human concepts and its quantification]. *Chinese Journal of Psychology, 26,* **67-75.** (In Chinese.)

In the present study, the applicability of fuzzy set theory to Chinese verbal concepts was experimentally tested. The functions of some language operators, adverbs, negative markers, and adjectives, predicted by fuzzy set logic, were evaluated empirically. The subjects used a 5-point scale to judge the applicability of a set of phrases to squares of various sizes. The proportion of responses falling on the values of "most suitable" and "suitable" for each stimulus under each condition were determined. The results showed that fuzzy set theory described well the fuzziness of Chinese verbal concepts and that language operators could be considered as operators on the fuzzy set. However, for a complex term, the operational functions of a language operator could not be predicted precisely by fuzzy set logic. This latter result suggests that the analysis of semantic meaning is more suitable at the psycholinguistic than at the logical level.

526

Chu, C. P. (1969). An investigation of the development of language and vocabulary in elementary school children. *Acta Psychologica Taiwanica, 11,* **48-66.**

The main purpose of this study is to find out the developmental and sex differences in the use of language and vocabulary of elementary school children. The experiment used three specific TAT pictures, and controlled the manner of telling stories. The 60 subjects were from the average or above average socioeconomic status and school achievement levels. Comparison of the results with similar studies shows several common characteristics, such as increase of sentence length with increase of age; and higher percentage of good and complex sentence structures in the older group as well as comparable proportions of using the parts of speech in the younger group. Nevertheless, it was very difficult to combine or classify the various studies into a harmonious standard because of the different interests, and methodological and terminological bases of different investigators.

527

Chuang, S. C. (1974). A survey of Chinese bird and flower paintings. In J. L. M. Dawson & W. J. Lonner (Eds.), *Readings in cross-cultural psychology.* **Hong Kong: Hong Kong University Press.**

528

Connell, B. A., Hogan, J. T., & Rozsypal, A. J. (1983). Experimental evidence of interaction between tone and intonation in Mandarin Chinese. *Journal of Phonetics, 11,* **337-351.**

Determined in an experiment with 28 native Chinese speakers (aged 20-47 yrs) proficient in Mandarin how far the shape of a tone in Mandarin Chinese can be changed before it is consistently recognized as a different tone. Results show that perceptual changes in tone arose and that these changes corresponded generally with expectations based primarily on production data. The recognition of tone was stable over a wide range of pitch contour changes.

529

Covello, E. M. (1977). Symbolization of conscious states in the I Ching: A quantitative study. *Journal of Altered States of Consciousness, 3,* **111-129.**

The "I Ching" is an ancient Chinese text, initially used for divination, which consists of 64 separate aphorisms and their accompanying interpretations. The nature of each of these documents is purportedly decided by variations of a symbolic code. Each of a system of 64 symbols, or hexagrams, accompanies one document, the hexagram being the symbolic determinant. From this symbolic code, the "I Ching" can be viewed as a 64-fold division of conscious experience. One major question the present study addressed was whether the symbology accounts for the meaningful semantic dimensions of the text, or whether the 64 documents are a collection of arbitrary themes. Four different organizational schemas for the "I Ching" suggested by its authors and interpreters were tested to determine whether the texts follow an internal logic. Portions of R. Wilhelm's (1967) commentaries to each of the 64 hexagrams were content analyzed across a number of semantic categories. Results indicate that all 4 systems measure some meaningful aspect of the "I Ching". Thus the "I Ching" depicts a meaningful cosmology, organized into a system of symbols.

530

Crown, B. R. (1973). The People's Republic of China: A sampler of contemporary Chinese writing for the masses. *Social Education, 37,* **9-46.**

531

Devereux, G. (1979). The nursing of the aged in classical China: A study of the oral components of the Oedipus complex. *Journal of Psychological Anthropology, 2,* **1-10.**

An examination of a 2,100-yr-old Chinese text, Shih Chi, suggests the resurfacing of the Oedipus complex in senility, especially on an oral mode (i.e., breastfeeding). The discussion is based on a passage from the text in which an Imperial Chancellor is dismissed from his post in old age. While he required wet nurses (some of whom it is presumed were his concubines), he would only have intercourse with those women who had had no children. According to the author's interpretation of this and similar cases in the literature, intercourse with mother-surrogates becomes impossible, partly because of castration anxieties, and partly because of the unconscious fear that the "mother's" milk may turn into poison. Each step of the interpretation is illustrated with ethnographic examples of the mechanisms under consideration.

532

Eoyan, E. (1973). The solitary boat: Images of self in Chinese nature poetry. *Journal of Asian Studies, 32,* **593-622.**

533

Erickson, D. M., Mattingly, I. G., & Turvey, M. T. (1977). Phonetic activity in reading: An experiment with kanji. *Language & Speech, 20,* **384-403.**

Reading seems to require phonetic short-term storage even if the writing system is logographic. A short-term memory probe paradigm was used to test the ability of 12 undergraduates (10 Japanese, 1 Chinese, and 1 Korean) to recall kanji characters. When pairs of characters in a silently read list were homophonous, recall was significantly poorer than when the silently read list included no such pairs, presumably because of confusion in phonetic short-term storage. Since the kanji have no overt phonetic structure, it would seem that this kind of storage is involved in the reading of kanji not because of the particular structure of the writing system but because of the essentially linguistic nature of the task. Evidently the linguistic process cannot readily disperse with phonetic short-term storage. It is suggested, however, that the design of a writing system does not depend directly on linguistic process but rather on the partial and uneven awareness that users of the system have of certain aspects of this process.

534

Fang, S. P., Mei, K., Yang, C. M., Lin, F. W., Huang, J. H., Huang, Z. H., & Yang, S. Z. (1985). [A psychological model for evaluating Chinese graphemic input systems]. *Chinese Journal of Psychology*, *27*, **27-41.** (In Chinese.)

This study proposed an evaluation model for small-keyboard graphemic input systems for Chinese characters. Four input systems were analyzed and compared: HANG's three-corner coding, Multitech's Chinese-alphabet input, CDC's top-bottom coding, and the simplified indexing developed by Kiang. Five experiments were conducted to examine the relative efficiency of these systems at various stages. Experiment 1 measured the degree of congruency between the system-prescribed encoding and the user's intuition. Experiment 2 measured the degree of difficulty of graphemic decomposition. Experiment 3 measured the amount of training required to master the feature-code correspondence and the speed of code generation given the feature. Experiment 4 measured the amount of training required to master the encoding rules and the speed of character encoding. Experiment 5 measured the general efficiency of text handling. In general, three-corner coding and simplified indexing showed greater efficiency than the other two systems. A total of 10 measures were obtained and 3 of them were recommended to serve as predictors of the input speed of a given system.

535

Fang, S. P., Tzeng, O. J., & Alva, L. (1981). Intralanguage vs. interlanguage stroop effects in two types of writing systems. *Memory & Cognition*, *9*, **609-617.**

Three experiments investigated the relationship between word processing strategy and the orthographic structure of a written language; 30 Chinese-English, 30 Spanish-English, and 50 Japanese-English bilingual undergraduates served as Ss. Each S was asked to perform a modified Stroop color-naming task in which the stimulus and the response language were either the same or different. The magnitude of the Stroop effect was greater in the intralanguage than in the interlanguage condition. When the magnitude of reduction of Stroop interference from the intra- to the interlanguage condition was compared across all bilingual groups, an inverse relationship was found between the magnitude of reduction and the degree of similarity between the orthographic structures of the 2 written languages. It is concluded that reading logographic and phonetic symbols entails different processing mechanisms and that controversial issues in bilingual processing cannot be resolved without taking into account the effect of orthographic variations on the information-processing system.

536

Flege, J. E., & Davidian, R. D. (1984). Transfer and developmental processes in adult foreign language speech production. *Applied Psycholinguistics*, *5*, **323-347.**

The hypothesis that factors that shape children's production of their native language (L1) will also influence adults' pronunciation of sounds in a foreign language (L2) was tested. The final stops in consonant vowel consonant English words produced by 12 native speakers of English, Polish, Spanish, and Chinese were phonetically transcribed. The frequency with which these stops were devoiced, deleted, or fricativized was tabulated. The Spanish subjects showed the effect of a transfer process, producing word-final /b,d,g/ as fricatives. The subjects in all three nonnative groups resembled English-learning children in devoicing word-final /b,d,g/. Subjects whose L1 does not have word-final stops showed final stop deletion, which is commonly observed in English L1 acquisition. A number of language background variables were not significantly correlated with the accuracy of final stop production. These findings suggested that, in addition to transfer processes arising from L1/L2 phonetic and phonological differences, developmental processes similar to those affecting child L1 speech production also influence adult L2 speech production.

537

Fok, A., & Bellugi, U. (1986). The acquisition of visual spatial script. In H. S. R. Kao, G. P. van Galen, & R. Hoosain (Eds.), *Graphonomics: Contemporary research in handwriting* **(329-355). Amsterdam, Netherlands: North-Holland.**

538

Galtung, J., & Nishimura, F. (1983). Structure, culture and languages: An essay comparing the Indo-European, Chinese and Japanese languages. *Social Science Information*, *22*, **895-925.**

The present study examined the role of languages as carriers of structure and culture in European, Chinese, and Japanese societies. Language is considered to condition but not determine thought and to supplement other factors such as religion and technology in forming culture and structure, which in turn are reflected in language. Several differences were apparent among the languages examined. While the European languages endow space and time with relatively rigid and rather simple structures, there is considerable flexibility in these dimensions in Japanese. Chinese is more universal because it is more flexible in terms of space, time, and knowledge; and also in terms of relations to nature, to other human beings, and to the transpersonal. It stands out as the richest language family among the three compared.

539

Gleitman, L. R. (1985). Orthographic resources affect reading acquisition--if they are used. [Special Issue: Phonology and the problems of learning to read and write]. *RASE: Remedial and Special Education*, *6*, **24-36.**

Comments were given on an article by H. Stevenson, who interpreted his cross-linguistic studies as showing that differences in orthographies do not materially affect the reading-acquisition process or the prognosis for successful learning. Differences in the formatives and combinatorial principles of varying scripts, and differences in learning consequent on these, were analyzed. Stevenson's results were shown to derive from a faulty interpretation of comparisons among learning rates of Japanese, Chinese, and American learners.

540

Guo, K. J. (1984). [Information-processing and neural mechanics in the recognition of Chinese characters]. *Information on Psychological Sciences*, **No. 4, 31-36.** (In Chinese.)

541

Han, Y. H. (1964). [An experiment on learning Dot Patterns]. *Psychological Testing*, *11*, **24-28.** (In Chinese.)

542

Herrmann, D. J., & Raybeck, D. (1981). Similarities and differences in meaning in six cultures. *Journal of Cross-Cultural Psychology*, *12*, **194-206.**

Explored the use of multidimensional scaling in a cross-cultural investigation involving 6 cultures (Spain, Vietnam, Hong Kong, Haiti, Greece, US; N = 155, median age range 17-39 yrs) and 2 categories varying in abstractness (animals and emotions). Cross-cultural agreement in the scaling solutions was quite high but highest for the Emotions category. Additionally, the solutions of both categories across cultures revealed details that reflected culture-specific meaning. It is concluded that the multidimensional scaling procedure appears sensitive enough to cultural contexts to reveal meaningful intercultural differences and similarities in meaning.

543

Hightower, J. R. (1961). Individualism in Chinese literature. *JHI*, *22*, **159-168.**

544

Ho, D. Y. F. (1979). Chinese language and language-learning behavior: A bibliography of psychological and psycholinguistic studies. In R. Lord (Ed.), *Hong Kong language papers* **(pp. 161-184). Hong Kong: Hong Kong University Press.**

545

Hoosain, R. (1986). Language, orthography and cognitive processes: Chinese perspectives for the Sapir-Whorf hypothesis. *International Journal of Behavioral Development*, *9*, **507-525.**

546

Hu, C. Q., Zhu, Y. L., & Wu, W. Z. (1983). [The supporting effect of spoken language on written language--a neurolinguistic analysis of cases of brain damage]. *Acta Psychologica Sinica*, *15*, **349-354.** (In Chinese.)

This paper discusses four aspects of speech behavior--listening, speaking, reading, and writing--in three patients having brain damage in different locations. The usefulness of the so-called "supporting effect of spoken language on written language" was discussed.

547

Huang, J. T. (1982). [Perceptual separability and cohesive process in reading Chinese words]. *Acta Psychologica Taiwanica*, *24*, **49-58.** (In Chinese.)

The present study is an attempt to investigate the perceptual separability and cohesive process involved in reading Chinese characters composed of two constituents, each with an independent meaning. Perceptual separability, a perceptual break-down of the single Chinese word into two independent constituents, is expressed as a result of the bottom-up process. The cohesive process, a reintegration of the being-separated constituents, is solely affected by the top-down process. In two experiments subjects read Chinese characters embedded in semantic contexts differing in length and quality. Results from Experiment 1 suggested that perceptual separability accompanying a longer reading time of the experimental item occurred more often if the target word was embedded in a shorter semantic context. The findings might be due to the lack of semantic constraint on the target word. Experiment 2 demonstrated that perceptual separability could be shown if the target word and its surrounding context were severely degraded. Interactive models suggested by Neisser and by McClelland and Rumelhart are used to discuss the possible interaction between the bottom-up and the top-down processes in reading Chinese words.

548

Huang, Y. H., Pratoomraj, S., & Johnson, R. C. (1969). Universal magnitude symbolism. *Journal of Verbal Learning & Verbal Behavior*, *8*, **155-156.**

Magnitude symbolism appears to be conveyed by initial vowels, with the same vowels conveying the same symbolism in English, Chinese, and Thai. Data were obtained from 64 English, 276 Chinese, and 57 Thai Ss and support the position that universal phonetic symbolism exists.

549

Inoue, M. (1980). [Relations among the graphemic, phonemic, and semantic processings of Chinese characters (Kanji): A study by the graphemical matching task]. *Japanese Journal of Psychology, 51,* **136-144.** (In other language.)

20 college students completed a graphemical matching task in which they decided whether paired stimuli presented serially were graphemically identical. Three factors that could influence the RT in the matching task were manipulated: interstimulus interval (200 and 2,000 ms), word frequency (high and low), and type (5 conditions of the relations of a stimulus pair in the 3 processings). Results suggest that these 3 processings functioned in parallel and interactively, that they were carried out within 300 ms, and that the change of codes did not occur within 2,100 ms.

550

Jeng, C. I., Lai, M. W., & Liu, I. M. (1973). Category norms in Chinese and English from bilingual subjects. *Acta Psychologica Taiwanica, 15,* **81-153.**

Presents complete normative data (in Chinese and English translation) for responses to 54 verbal categories by Chinese college students. All but 2 categories from US studies by B. H. Cohen et al (1957) and by W. F. Battig and W. E. Montague (1969) were included. Data include all responses given by each S to each category name within 60 sec, and English-word responses within 30 sec to each of 56 categories of norms presented in English.

551

Kaiho, H., & Inukai, Y. (1982). [An analysis of Gestalt characteristics of 881 Japanese/Chinese Kanji]. *Japanese Journal of Psychology, 53,* **312-315.** (In other language.)

Rated the Gestalt characteristics of 881 Kanji on each of 10 scales. High reliability was found for all rating scales. Principal component analysis of the mean rating values of the Kanji for each scale showed 8 of the 10 scales to be appropriate for the measurement of complexity, compactness, elongation, openness, straightness, roundness, stability, and symmetry.

552

Kaiho, H., & Nomura, Y. (1983). [*The psychology of information processing of Kanji*]. **Tokyo: Kyoiku Shuppan.** (In other language.)

553

Kao, H. S. (1978). Phonetic motion variability: A preliminary study in the vocalization of Chinese sounds. *Acta Psychologica Taiwanica, 20,* **51-56.**

Investigated the nature of the intratask control motion and motion variability in the vocalization of 2 Chinese phonetic sounds, using 2 Mandarin-speaking Ss with training in the Chinese Phonetic System. Results show that the intratask motion pattern resembled a bell-shaped curve with a general acceleration-peak-deceleration trend for all 4 vocalization trials. The intratask motion variability curve also resembled a bell-shaped curve with peak variability in the middle of the task course.

554

Kao, H. S. R. (1986). [*Psychology of Chinese calligraphy*]. **Taipei: Great Eastern.** (In Chinese.)

555

Kao, H. S. R., & Hoosain, R. (Eds.). (1984). *Psychological studies of the Chinese language.* **Hong Kong: Chinese Language Society of Hong Kong.**

556

Kao, H. S. R., & Hoosain, R. (Eds.). (1986). *Linguistics, psychology, and the Chinese language.* **Hong Kong: University of Hong Kong, Centre of Asian Studies.**

557

Kao, S. R., & Cheng, C. M. (Eds.). (1982). [*Psychological studies of the Chinese language*]. **Taipei: Wen Ho.** (In Chinese.)

558

Kawai, Y. (1966). Physical complexity of the Chinese letter and learning to read it. *Japanese Journal of Educational Psychology, 14,* **1-10.**

It was hypothesized that the Chinese letter is basically composed by attaching the meanings to a special physical pattern. Paired-associate learning between a nonsense physical pattern composed randomly with lines and meaningful words was conducted. The stimuli were 12 physical patterns divided into 6 different complexity levels (c) and 2 irregularity (ir) levels. The responses were 12 2-syllabic meaningful words. Major results were: (1) Learning trials were statistically significant for the level of c, but not for the ir level, (2) there was a tendency for the more complex patterns to be easier to learn, and (3) the more complex letters were significantly more readable than less complex letters when the frequency of use was held constant. Results are discussed by making a distinction between the stimulus differentiation phase and the stimulus-response association phase in the learning of letters.

559

Klank, L. J., Huang, Y. H., & Johnson, R. C. (1971). Determinants of success in matching word pairs in tests of phonetic symbolism. *Journal of Verbal Learning & Verbal Behavior, 10,* **140-148.**

Exp. I with 240 undergraduates dealt with conditions under which Ss correctly match 1 member of a foreign word pair to its English equivalent. Ss matched antonym pairs, nonantonym pairs from opposite ends of the same semantic dimension, nonantonym pairs whose members are from different dimensions, nonantonym pairs from opposite ends of the same dimension and from different foreign languages, and pairs of antonyms not on the main dimensions of semantic space at above chance levels. Pairs from the same end of 1 of the 3 major dimensions of semantic space were not matched above chance expectancy. Exp. II with 47 undergraduates investigated sounds in English and Chinese words associated with semantic dimensions. Consistencies were found for words on dimensions of activity and potency but not evaluation.

560

Koriat, A., & Levy, I. (1979). Figural symbolism in Chinese ideographs. *Journal of Psycholinguistic Research, 8,* **353-365.**

Conducted 3 experiments with 120 15-35 yr old Hebrew-speaking Ss, who had no previous knowledge of Chinese. Ss were presented with 42 pairs of Chinese characters designating antonymic concepts and were required to match them with their corresponding Hebrew words. Examination of the character-referent relationships suggested that translation success was due to principles of figural symbolism rather than to pictographic representation of the attributes in question. The effects of figural symbolization on the invention and/or evolution of natural scripts are related to the manner in which the graphic medium has been fashioned to convey abstract concepts.

561

Koutstaal, C. W., Smith, O. W., & Knops, L. (1972). Intercorrelation of Greenberg and Jenkins' S scale and effort ratings of phonemic CCVCs by Ss from different groups of languages. *Perceptual & Motor Skills, 34,* **655-658.**

Obtained effort ratings for subvocalizing the 24 CCVCs of J. Greenberg and J. Jenkins's List 1 from native speakers of Bantu, Chinese, Dutch, English, Flemish, Spanish, and Swedish. It was predicted that the effort ratings would intercorrelate significantly as well as correlate significantly with S values of the CCVCs. Correlations ranged from .64-.89 with a median of .81. The predictions proved to be tenable on the basis of the data.

562

Kroger, R. O., Cheng, K., & Leong, I. (1979). Are the rules of address universal? A test of Chinese usage. *Journal of Cross-Cultural Psychology, 10,* **395-414.**

Questioned whether the alleged universality of R. Brown's (1965) invariant norm of address extends to Chinese usage and whether the alleged universal relationships between social power and intimacy and between inequality and equality hold for Chinese social structure. To answer these questions, 3 indices were developed to measure reciprocity, solidarity, and inequality in dyadic address exchanges. The indices permitted the precise comparison of empirical results with theoretical predictions and of address usage across languages. 70 18-76 yr old Chinese speakers reported actual address usage received from and sent to 27 interactants. Results reveal the structure of address usage among Chinese speakers and provide unequivocal support for Brown's prediction such that Chinese may be added to the series of languages that jointly support the claim for the universality of the invariant norm. The relationship between studies in the semantics of social structure and the emerging alternative social-psychological strategy of ethogeny is noted.

563

Kroger, R. O., Wood, L. A., & Kim, U. (1984). Are the rules of address universal? 3. Comparison of Chinese, Greek, and Korean usage. *Journal of Cross-Cultural Psychology, 15,* **273-284.**

The present study attempted to provide additional evidence for the invariant norm of address proposed by R. Brown (1965) and investigated the alleged universality of the invariant norm by comparing the nominal forms of address used by Korean speakers with those used by speakers of modern Greek and Chinese. Twenty-seven Korean speakers from Korea and 46 Korean speakers from Canada reported actual address usage in 34 dyadic relationships distributed over 6 categories based on the structure of Korean social relationships. Responses were coded in terms of three quantitative indices that assessed the degrees of reciprocity, solidarity, and inequality in dyadic address exchanges. Results supported Brown's description of address exchange and supported the universality of the rules of address. There were no significant differences in address usage between Korean speakers living in Korea and those living in Canada. A comparison of Korean, Greek, and Chinese usage revealed substantial cross-cultural consistency. The idea of subordination appears to be universal.

564

Kurcz, I. (1977). Cultural and linguistic determinants of phonetic symbolism. *International Journal of Psycholinguistics, 4*(7), **5-12.**

Conducted a study of phonetic symbolism based on "guessing" the meaning of words of a language unknown to the Ss (Polish high school and university students). Languages were Chinese, Japanese, Swahili, and Hungarian. Ss were differentiated for age (12 and 13 yrs, 16 and 17 yrs, and university students), sex, education, and perceptual ability: (a) auditory--music school students, (b) visual--students of painting, and (c) tactual-kinesthetic--students of sculpture. Words of a foreign language were presented in pairs, one element of which was to be judged as corresponding to a Polish word displayed simultaneously. Words were selected from abstract and sensory categories, the latter subcategorized as auditory, visual, tactual, and kinesthetic. Factors affecting the results were language type, word category, and experimental method used. Results demonstrate a general tendency to symbolize, but show the influences on this tendency of Ss' cultural and linguistic experience.

565

Kushner-Vogel, H. B. (1982). Word segmentation in the initial stages of second language learning. *Dissertation Abstracts International, 43,* **A586.**

566

Kvan, E. (1969). Problems of bilingual milieu in Hong Kong: Strain of the two-language system. In I. C. Jarvie (Ed.), *Hong Kong: A society in transition* **(pp. 327-343). London: Routledge & Kegan Paul.**

567

LaBarre, W. et al. (1972). Nonverbal aspects: Taking part in intercultural communication. In L. A. Samovar & R. E. Porter (Eds.), *Intercultural communication: A reader.* **Belmont, CA: Wadsworth.**

Examines cultural influences on nonverbal communicative behaviors. Topics include cultural differences in the use of body, limbs, and eyes; nonverbal behaviors of black Americans; comparison of Chinese and American emotional expression; postural habits of particular cultures; tactile experiences in different cultures; spatial relationships; interaction distances; and furniture arrangement patterns.

568

Leather, J. (1983). Speaker normalization in perception of lexical tone. *Journal of Phonetics, 11,* **373-382.**

Used 4 natives of Peking (aged 20-40 yrs) for whom Mandarin was the native language and 1 bilingual (Cantonese and Mandarin) phonetician to investigate speaker-normalization in the recovery of linguistically significant pitch information from voice fundamental frequency (FO). Ss listened to 2 sets of synthetic Mandarin speakers with different but overlapping voice ranges. Sets were presented in a lexical identification test. Individual Ss differed somewhat in the acoustic criteria by which they apparently decided lexical identity; all Ss significantly assigned ambiguous stimuli with identical absolute FO contours to different lexical categories depending on which speaker was heard to produce them. It is suggested that in the perceptual processing of FO, phonetic decisions are referenced to an inferred scaling of the source voice range.

569

Lee, K. S. (1981). [Logic and modern Chinese language]. *Yuwen Zazhi, 7,* **50-52.** (In Chinese.)

570

Lee, K. S. (1981). [A study on the symmetrical relation between concepts and words on modern Chinese language]. *Luoji Yu Yuyan Xuexi, 2,* **7-12.** (In Chinese.)

571

Lee, P. W. H., Luk, E. S. L., Yu, G. K. K., & Bacon-Shone, J. H. (1985). A developmental language screening scale for use in Hong Kong. *Hong Kong Journal of Paediatrics,* **No. 2, 152-165.**

572

Lee, Y. M. (1965). [An analysis of meanings of Chinese words]. *Acta Psychologica Taiwanica, 7,* **97-103.** (In Chinese.)

573

Lester, D. (1973). Phonetic and graphic symbolism. *Perceptual & Motor Skills, 37,* **592.**

Found evidence of phonetic symbolism for the Chinese language among English-speaking undergraduates, but no evidence of graphic symbolism.

574

Lester, D. (1974). Symbolism in the Chinese language. *International Journal of Symbology, 5,* **18-21.**

Determined whether evidence could be obtained for graphic and tonal symbolism in the Chinese language in addition to the evidence obtained in previous studies for phonetic symbolism. Data from 44 undergraduates show no evidence of graphic or tonal symbolism, indicating that the symbolic aspects of language may be limited to phonetic aspects.

575

Leung, J. (1985). Images of women in Chinese literature [Selected papers from the 1984 Annual Conference]. *Hong Kong Psychological Society Bulletin,* **No. 14, 71-77.**

Reviews classic and modern Chinese literature to assess how images of women evolved. From the 17th century onward, subtle changes in the role and status of women can be observed that foreshadow the 20th-century literature's emphasis on women's searches for identity and self-determination.

576

Li, J. Z., & Chen, Y. M. (1985). [An experiment in understanding ancient Chinese with the computer]. *Acta Psychologica Sinica, 17,* **235-242.** (In Chinese.)

The paper describes a computer system for understanding ancient Chinese (SUACH), using two stories written in ancient Chinese as the experimental material. The system can make syntactic and semantic analysis of every sentence contained in the two stories and translate them into modern Chinese. It also has the ability to answer questions about the syntactical function and meaning of certain words used in different contexts. Unlike Western languages, the Chinese language has no declensions. For instance, one cannot determine the case of a noun or the tense of a verb according to the morphology of Chinese characters. Neither does Chinese grammar contain adequate rules governing inflections. A tentative plan for the programming of ancient Chinese is presented and discussed, and is offered as an aid to learning ancient Chinese.

577

Li, J. Z., Guo, R. J., & Chen, Y. M. (1982). [A Chinese language understanding system--CLUS I]. *Acta Psychologica Sinica, 14,* **29-40.** (In Chinese.)

This is the first experiment on a Chinese language understanding system constructed on the principle of semantic network. It simulates a dialogue between a pupil and a teacher on knowledge about the characteristics and behavior of animals. A machine built on the basis of this system has limited reasoning abilities, including induction, and making inferences from partial information or indirect information; thus it is capable of answering questions which cannot be answered on the basis of only its own knowledge base. Because word order is important in Chinese, the system adopted "word order analysis" instead of the "case analysis" used by P. H. Lindsay, P. A. Norman, R. H. Simmons, and others. About 200 Chinese characters written in alphabetic form have been used for the input and output of the experiment; the program runs on a computer made in China.

578

Li, T. (1964). [A preliminary study on the perception of Chinese characters by six year children]. *Acta Psychologica Sinica,* **No. 2, 178-184.** (In Chinese.)

579

Lin, T. M. (1964). [A diagnostic test of Chinese phonetics]. *Psychological Testing, 11,* **101-111.** (In Chinese.)

580

Liu, I. (1978). [Methods of acquiring Chinese vocabulary]. *Bulletin of the Sun Yat-sen Cultural Foundation, 22,* **159-187.** (In Chinese.)

581

Liu, I. M. (1978). [Psychological studies of the Chinese language in Taiwan]. *Acta Psychologica Taiwanica, 20,* **1-4.** (In Chinese.)

582

Liu, I. M. (1983). [Cueing function of fragments of Chinese characters in reading]. *Acta Psychologica Taiwanica, 25,* **85-90.** (In Chinese.)

By using a FUJITSU MICRO 8 computer, it is possible to delete an upper left quarter, upper right quarter, lower left quarter, or lower right quarter of any Chinese character. The subject read stories and nonstories (all characters randomly arranged) of 120-character length with each character kept intact or one quarter deleted. Deleting an upper quarter of each character resulted in more reading errors than deleting a lower quarter. The effect of deleting a left quarter was not significantly different from the effect of deleting a right quarter. The obtained reading times can be fit by a mathematical equation that incorporates the conceptually-driven context factor and the data-driven cue factor in an interactive way.

583

Liu, I. M. (1984). [Production frequency of descriptive units for common verbs]. *Chinese Journal of Psychology, 26,* **95-100.** (In Chinese.)

Twenty commonly used verbs were selected on the basis of their frequency count. For each verb, the subject was allowed one minute to write down as many subject-object pairs as possible to complete sentences. Four to eight types of descriptive units were obtained for each verb by assigning subjects and objects to a small number of categories. The obtained classification of descriptive units for each verb defined not only the meanings of the verb but also its usages. It was concluded that the frequency analysis of descriptive units contributes to our understanding of the process of human thought as well as to efficient language learning.

584

Liu, I. M., & Chen, C. L. (1980). [Reading efficiencies for Chinese logography and phonographic simulation]. *Acta Psychologica Taiwanica, 22,* **23-28.** (In Chinese.)

Exp I investigated the effects on reading efficiency of attaching the phonetic alphabet to Chinese words. When the degrees of comprehension were approximately equal, the phonetic alphabet alone (phonographic simulation) was found to be inferior to conditions of Chinese words alone and of Chinese words accompanied by the phonetic alphabet; the latter 2 conditions were equally efficient. In Exp II, placing the phonetic alphabet to the left of Chinese words was found to cause inferior reading efficiency compared to placing the phonetic alphabet to the right and compared to reading Chinese words alone. This result rules out an explanation based on inattention for the results of Exp I. Findings are compatible with the notion of cerebral lateralization and have implications for the best way to print Chinese words accompanied by the phonetic alphabet in order to increase reading efficiency.

585

Liu, I. M., & Chuang, C. J. (1970). [Scaling 1,200 Chinese characters for meaningfulness]. *Acta Psychologica Taiwanica, 12,* **33-52.** (In Chinese.)

Divided 1200 Chinese characters into 4 equal sets. Ss were 2000 undergraduates, divided into 4 equal groups who wrote down the 1st associate and, at the same time, rated the association value by means of a 5-point scale. For each character, Ss were to respond within 10 sec. Data, based on 1/2 of the Ss, were analyzed according to scale value, popular response, 2nd popular response, percentage of responses, and number of distinct responses to each character.

586

Liu, I. M., & Chuang, C. J. (1971). [Scaling 1,200 Chinese characters for meaningfulness (continued)]. *Acta Psychologica Taiwanica, 13,* **75-190.** (In Chinese.)

Lists the word associations elicited by 1,200 Chinese characters in the order of frequency. The associations for each character were collected from 250 freshmen by asking them to write down the 1st associate.

587

Liu, I. M., Chuang, C. J., & Wang, S. C. (1975). *[Frequency count of 40,000 Chinese words]*. **Taipei: Luck Books Company.** (In Chinese.)

588

Liu, I. M., Yeh, J. S., Wang, L. H., & Chang, Y. K. (1974). [Effects of arranging Chinese words as units on reading efficiency]. *Acta Psychologica Taiwanica, 16,* **25-31.** (In Chinese.)

Experiment I investigated: (1) the effect of aggregating Chinese characters constituting a word (while providing a space between words) on the recognition threshold of sentences; and (2) the effect of varying the number of words within a sentence (with the number of characters kept constant) on the recognition threshold of sentences. In Experiment II the effect of manipulating the space between words and the effects of the variables used in Experiment I on the recognition threshold of sentences were studied, while the span of each sentence was kept the same. The two variables used in Experiment I were studied in Experiment III by controlling the size of Chinese characters and by minimizing artifacts inherent in the general limit method as a threshold measuring technique. It was found that, contrary to expectation, the effect of arranging Chinese words as units within a sentence was to raise the recognition threshold. Whether this finding reflects a memory process affecting recognition threshold or subject's established habit of reading awaits further experimentation.

589

Liu, I. M., & Yeh, Y. Y. (1977). [Studies of Chinese anagrams: Vol. 1. Anagrams of one-character words]. *Psychological Testing, 24,* **24-31.** (In Chinese.)

In the present study, one-character words were split into three parts. Anagrams were then constructed by a random arrangement of the three parts constituting a word. According to the results of Experiment I, the order of the three parts in the anagrams affected the solution time. The solution time also depended on the frequency of the solution words. However, the frequency of the three parts in the anagrams did not affect the solution time. In Experiment II, the effect of similarity between the structure of Chinese characters and that of anagrams on the solution time was studied. It was found that the effect of this similarity was more predominant than the effect of frequency of the structures of characters, indicating that a perceptual factor overshadows a learning factor in solving Chinese anagrams.

590

Liu, Y. T. (1965). [Experimental studies on the effects of pictorial material and writing in learning characters]. *Acta Psychologica Sinica,* **No. 3, 198-205.** (In Chinese.)

The principal contradiction in learning characters in first grade primary school children was the connection of sound, form and meaning. The principal aspect of the contradiction was the form of characters. The more effective method for solving the contradiction was the method by which the children learn writing in connection with reading and explanation of the meaning of characters.

591

Liu, Z. J. (1985). [On the psychological approach in literature as reflected in Liu Xie's Wen Xin Diao Long]. *Acta Psychologica Sinica, 17,* **115-122.** (In Chinese.)

Liu Xie (465-532 A.D.), a Chinese literary critic, was the author of Wen Xin Diao Long, a comprehensive work on literary theory. The article is an attempt to study some of his thoughts contained in this classical work from a psychological point of view.

592

Loehr, M. (1961). The question of individualism in Chinese art. *JHI, 22,* **147-158.**

593

Lohr, J. M., & Staats, A. W. (1973). Attitude conditioning in Sino-Tibetan languages. *Journal of Personality and Social Psychology, 26,* **196-200.**

594

London, I. D. (1975). Interviewing in sinology: Observations on methods and fundamental concepts. *Psychological Reports, 36,* **683-691.**

Offers experientially and analytically based observations to maximize the contribution that the interview, as a research instrument, can make to sinology. 4 major aspects of the interview as communication-in-depth are discussed: the linguistic, perceptual, attitudinal, and assumptive.

595

Lu, C. H., & Ma, L. Y. (1959). [Studies on certain rules of abbreviations and variations in the project of romanizing Chinese spelling system]. *Acta Psychologica Sinica,* **No. 2, 117-126.** (In Chinese.)

The present study is an investigation into the project of romanizing Chinese. The authors conducted research in a farmers' spelling class of Ting Hsien and discovered mistakes were made on certain of the spelling rules by 70% to 90% of the class and two-thirds of the teachers. An analysis of examination papers of 548 grade-school teachers, night-school teachers and members of the spelling class for training illiteracy-eliminating cadres, also revealed that about 30% of this group made mistakes on these same rules. The authors proposed that these rules be revised as follows: (1) To cancel the abbreviated forms iu, ui, and un of multiple vowels iou, uei, uen. (2) To retain the umlaut "..", on the top of u that follows j, q, and x. (3) To remove the rule of changing i into y and u into w. Instead, the use of a sound-separator "," is sufficient.

596

Lundbaek, K. (1982). China in transcultural communication research. *Social Science Information, 21,* **887-899.**

Discusses 4 basic questions that arise during any kind of transcultural communication research: (1) Is the transmission a direct or an indirect one? (2) Is it intentional? (3) What is the code? (4) Is there a 2-way or only a 1-way traffic on the communication channel? Four types of transcultural communication research are discussed with reference to China: studies of influence, similarities, accuracy of transmission, and reception.

597

Lust, B., & Chien, Y. C. (1984). The structure of coordination in first language acquisition of Mandarin Chinese: Evidence for a universal. *Cognition, 17,* **49-83.**

Data obtained from a standardized elicited imitation test of 68 Chinese children in Taiwan, showed that subjects who were acquiring Mandarin Chinese (a left-branching language) as their first language, systematically preferred VO sentences with a backward reduction pattern ((V + V)) over those with a forward reduction pattern (V(O + O)). The subjects' responses to SV coordinate sentences differed systematically from their VO responses. The authors explained this apparent paradox in terms of an interaction in early language acquisition between children's sensitivity to a predominant Chinese topic-comment structure (in SV) and their sensitivity to the abstract, specifically grammatical concept of principal branching direction.

598

Lyczak, R., Fu, G. S., & Ho, A. (1976). Attitudes of Hong Kong bilinguals toward English and Chinese speakers. *Journal of Cross-Cultural Psychology, 7,* **425-438.**

210 bilingual Hong Kong Chinese university students evaluated the taped voices of Chinese and English speakers on 13 traits (e.g., honesty, competence, intelligence, and occupational status). Ss were unaware that speakers were actually bilinguals speaking once in each language. Chinese "guises" of the speakers were rated more favorably on 7 traits (kind, trustworthy, considerate, serious of purpose, humble, honest and friendly) and English guises on 4 traits (good looking, intelligent, well-off, and competent). Factor analysis of ratings revealed 2 major factors, one consisting of traits related to character, and the other of traits related to success. Chinese guises were favored on the former and English guises on the latter.

599

McCoy, M. K. (1973). Adverbs of frequency in Chinese and English. *Psychologia: An International Journal of Psychology in the Orient, 16,* **164-173.**

Attempted to show that certain frequency-indicating adverbs in both Chinese and English have imprecise meanings and that it is not a sound practice to use such words to discriminate frequency in questionnaires and self-report inventories. All Ss were bilingual college students. It was established that despite a lack of agreement as to absolute frequency referred to by a particular word, individuals operate with a frequency construct which enables words to be rank ordered in a relatively stable way from person to person.

600

McGinnies, E., & Turnage, T. W. (1968). Verbal association by Chinese and American students as a function of word frequency and mode of presentation. *Psychological Reports, 23,* **1051-1060.**

Obtained associations from 40 Ss each at National Taiwan University and the University of Maryland to words presented either vocally or in writing. The words varied in frequency of occurrence for both languages. American Ss produced more associations than the Taiwanese Ss under all conditions. In both samples number of associations increased with frequency of the stimulus words. Printed Chinese, however, enjoyed a significant advantage over spoken Chinese in evoking associations to infrequent words. This finding, which was not obtained for the English words, was attributed to (1) more frequent exposure of Taiwanese to low frequency words in print than in speech and (2) increased identifiability of infrequent Chinese words when printed. Implications for more effective communication between the 2 language communities were discussed.

601

Miao, X. C. (1982). [Strategies for Chinese sentence comprehension]. *Information on Psychological Sciences*, **No. 6, 9-15.** (In Chinese.)

The present study is an attempt to reveal what role word order and semantics play and how these two factors interrelate when one interprets Chinese utterances. Comparisons were made between the comprehension strategies used by native Chinese speakers and native English speakers who could speak Chinese. The results showed that Chinese subjects relied more heavily on a semantic factor--lexical meaning--than on word order in interpreting Chinese utterances, whereas the native English speaking subjects relied both on word order and the lexical meaning. However, they used word order strategy more frequently. The author proposes that two factors account for the difference between the responses of two groups of subjects.

602

Miao, X. C. et al. (1984). [An re-examination of the roles of word order and lexical meaning in Chinese sentence comprehension]. *Information on Psychological Sciences*, **No. 6, 1-7.** (In Chinese.)

This study tested the extent of Chinese reliance on lexical meaning in comprehending utterances, and explored the differences in comprehension between adults and children. One hundred and twenty subjects were divided into six age groups from 4 years to adult. The results were: (1) Subjects of all ages relied both on word order and lexical meaning in comprehending simple Chinese utterances. (2) Lexical meaning was more important in adult's comprehension. (3) Comprehension, to a great extent, depended on the strategies employed by the listener and the subjects preconstructed sentence models.

603

Miller, J. (1972). Plays and players. In R. A. Hinde (Ed.), *Non-verbal communication*. **Cambridge, England: Cambridge University Press.**

Discusses the nonverbal behavior of dramatic artists which give meaning to the verbal core of the material and to the silences between utterances. Various uses of vocal, facial, postural, and manual components are described. Differences in nonverbal expression in various dramatic art forms and in the Western naturalistic and Chinese stylistic theater are considered.

604

Minford, J. (1985). Translation as treason [Special issue: Psychology in political contexts]. *Hong Kong Psychological Society Bulletin*, **No. 15, 43-50.**

Presents a history of translation and translation studies in China, arguing that the Chinese language functions as a psychological wall surrounding Chinese culture. In the 1st half of the 19th century, translators were considered as breakers of the wall of language and therefore traitors in their betrayal of a whole culture. It is contended that this theme of translation as treason runs throughout subsequent Chinese history; the gradual evolution of a humanistic, liberal tradition of translation during the 1920's and 1930's was disrupted by the Sino-Japanese War in 1937 and by the coming to power of the Chinese Communist Party in 1949. The importance of cultural understanding to translation and the collaboration of cross-cultural psychologists with translators are discussed.

605

National Institute for Compilation and Translation. (1967). *A study on the high frequency words used in Chinese elementary school reading materials*. **Taipei, Taiwan: Chung Hwa.** (In Chinese.)

606

Ng, B. (1967). An analysis of the compositions of bilingual children in the fifth grade. *Dissertation Abstracts International*, *27*, **A3632-3633.**

607

Nomura, Y. (1978). [The information processing of Chinese characters (Kanji): Chinese reading, Japanese reading and the attachment of meaning]. *Japanese Journal of Psychology*, *49*, **190-197.** (In other language.)

To investigate the hypothesis that the Japanese people attach the meaning to Kanji or Chinese characters at the first glance, not by Ondoku (Chinese reading) but by Kundoku (Japanese reading), a series of Kanji were presented to Ss using the incidental learning paradigm in such a way that the effects of 3 variables on the information processing of Kanji could be adequately analyzed. The 3 variables were the probability of relative appearance of Ondoku, the type of presentation, and the type of reading. The results support the above hypothesis and suggest the possibility that Ss translated Kundoku to Ondoku when they were required to pronounce in Ondoku.

608

Nomura, Y. (1979). [Information processing of Chinese characters (kanji): Retrieval processes in Chinese-style reading (on) and Japanese-style reading (kun)]. *Japanese Journal of Psychology, 50,* **101-105.** (In other language.)

In a factorial design, a series of kanji were presented to Japanese Ss without furigana (phonetic signs) or with on- or kun-furigana; Ss were instructed to read each kanji in either on or kun. Results support the hypothesis that the presence of appropriate phonetic furigana would shorten the search time required for reading a kanji in on or kun. Results also support the theory that Japanese Ss attach meaning to a Chinese character by reading it in Japanese style at first sight of the character.

609

Oetomo, D. (1985). The Chinese of Pasuruan: A study of language and identity in a minority community in transition. *Dissertation Abstracts International, 45,* **A2860.**

610

Oller, J. W., Hudson, A. J. & Liu, P. F. (1977). Attitudes and attained proficiency in ESL: A sociolinguistic study of native speakers of Chinese in the United States. *Language Learning, 27,* **1-27.**

611

Olney, R. L., & Scholnick, E. K. (1976). Adult judgments of age and linguistic differences in infant vocalization. *Journal of Child Language, 3,* **145-155.**

59 college students judged the relative ages of pairs of vocalizations sampled either from a Chinese infant at 0.6, 1.0, and 1.6 yrs or from an American infant at the same ages. The judgments were 88% accurate, with the easiest judgments contrasting the 0.6 and 1.6 samples (96% accurate). With 1 exception, age contrasts for the Chinese infant were as easy to judge as those for the American infant. However, a 2nd sample of 85 college students was unable to judge the linguistic community of the vocalizer when age was held constant, whether the data were drawn from infant samples of 0.6, 1.0, or 1.6 or from adults babbling to babies. These data led to speculations on the kinds of cues speakers of different languages use to discriminate infant vocalizations, and whether these cues are age-specific or language-specific. The data presently suggest the former, but the present study has methodological limitations, and generalizations are limited to 1 specific language contrast, English and Chinese.

612

O'Mahony, M., & Tsang, T. (1980). A preliminary comparison of Cantonese and American-English as taste languages. *British Journal of Psychology, 71,* **221-226.**

Compared 15 monolingual American-English-speaking Americans of Chinese descent (21-22 yrs old) with 10 Cantonese/American-English bilingual Chinese (20-24 yrs old) living in America to examine their taste descriptions for a set of aqueous solutions. Cantonese, unlike other languages, did not appear to differ greatly from American-English in its general taste descriptive strategy and depth of vocabulary, although Cantonese speakers had a tendency to use "glutamic" as a descriptive term for monosodium glutamate.

613

Osaka, R. (1976). Functional classification of visual behavior by Chinese characters. *Psychologia: An International Journal of Psychology in the Orient, 19,* **234-238.**

Chinese language is the only ideographic language still used. Its elements number more than 50,000 characters. Consulting a voluminous Chinese-Japanese dictionary, it was found that there are approximately 350 characters which relate to vision or use of visual apparatus. After redundant ones were omitted, 250 characters were classified into morphology, physiology, pathology, psychology, and miscellany sections. The psychology section was further divided into 5 modes of vision (i.e., unintentional, intentional, mental/spiritual, emotional, and social). Oriental thinking was revealed in the varieties of the character classification.

614

Osgood, C. E. (1975). *Atlas of affective meanings.* **Urbana, Il: University of Illinois, Institute for Communications Research.**

615

Osgood, C. E. (1979). From Yang and Yin to and or but in cross cultural perspective. *International Journal of Psychology, 14,* **1-35.**

Studied 8 postulates, derived from ancient Chinese metaphysics, governing the dynamics of interactions among cognitions, utilizing both linguistic and psychological evidence. The postulates were used to predict the performance of native speakers of 12 languages (American English, Belgian Flemish, Swedish, Finnish, Hungarian, Serbo-Croatian, Dutch, Iranian Farsi, Hindi, Malaysian, Thai, and Japanese) on a simple cognitive task: the insertion of the equivalents of "and" or "but" in the conjunction of pairs of familiar adjectives. The comparably measured affective meanings of the pairs of adjectives were found to predict the differential usage of "and" and "but" equivalents with high precision, and results displayed high consistency across all 12 languages. The universality of bipolar organization of human cognizing is suggested.

616

Osgood, C. E., May, W. H., & Miron, M. S. (1975). *Cross-cultural universals of affective meaning.* **Urbana, Il: University of Illinois Press.**

617

Pedersen, P. (1983). Learning about the Chinese culture through the Chinese language. *Communication & Cognition, 16,* **403-412.**

Discusses the importance of implicit metaphors within the pictographic characters of written Chinese, and the manner in which studying the Chinese language reveals attributes of the Chinese culture, based on the author's experience in using and translating the Church Youth Research Inventory from English into Chinese. It is suggested that language defines the boundaries of culturally appropriate behavior. Problems of achieving equivalence in translation and in accurate communication between English- and Chinese-speaking persons are discussed. Examples are provided of implicit metaphorical meaning within the written Chinese language as it relates to the words and concepts frequently used in counseling.

618

Peng, D. L., Guo, D. J., & Zhang, S. L. (1985). [The retrieval of information about Chinese characters in making similarity judgments under recognition conditions]. *Acta Psychologica Sinica, 17,* **227-234.** (In Chinese.)

Using the procedures provided by S. M. Condry and A. Levy, 30 fifth-grade and 30 college students were asked to judge the graphic, phonetic, or semantic similarities of Chinese characters under different distracting conditions. The differences in reaction time (RT) for similarity judgments between the college students and the schoolchildren were significant. Within the same age group, the RT for graphic similarity was the shortest; characters similar in sound required a longer RT, and synonyms the longest. The RT difference between the second and third catagories was not significant. The results also showed that the distractive effect of graphic similarity was greater than that of phonetic similarity on synonym judgments. On the basis of these results, the authors hold that coding sound may not be a necessary step in processing the meaning of characters. In addition to the graphic-phonetic-semantic channel in information processing of Chinese characters, the graphic-semantic channel must also be available.

619

Peng, R. X. (1982). [A preliminary report on a statistical analysis of the structure of Chinese characters]. *Acta Psychologica Sinica, 14,* **385-390.** (In Chinese.)

The structures of 3000 printed Chinese characters selected from Chinese textbooks for elementary schools were statistically analysed. Each character was divided into four quadrants: upper-left (UL), upper-right (UR), bottom-left (BL), and bottom-right (BR). On the basis of strokes in the UL and the BR quadrants, same or similar shapes were grouped together and were called subpatterns. The results showed that UL subpatterns have a stronger effect than BR subpatterns in the formation of characters. However, UL subpatterns are more complex, in that there are always strokes in addition to those composing the radical of the subpattern; BR subpatterns are simpler, without strokes extra to the subpattern itself. It appears more advantageous to rely on BR subpatterns for initial classifications in the design of an automatic multistage system for Chinese character recognition.

620

Riegel, K. F. (1968). Comparison of restricted associations among six languages. *Journal Of Social Psychology, 75,* **67-78.**

Tested native speakers of English, German, French, Spanish, Japanese, and Chinese. There were 12 males and 12 females in each group and the same 7 types of restricted associations to the same 35 stimulus nouns were obtained in all languages. There were large interlingual differences in response variability and response differentiation, i.e., in the repetition of responses to the same stimuli under different types of restrictions. The method also proved useful for quantification of the similarity in meaning or substitutability of alternate translated stimuli.

621

Ritsema, R. (1984). Analyzing: A study of the 40th hexagram in the I Ching. *Spring,* **77-104.**

Chinese texts were translated in a word-to-word manner to show the images and terms that occur. In part 2, an analysis of the trigrams and counter hexagram includes the name, image, family, action, word explanations, and paraphrasing explanations of the text of the 40th hexagram of the I Ching.

622

Rouam, F., & Duche, D. J. (1982). La main dans la symbolique du corps [The hand in the body symbols system]. *Psychologie Medicale, 14,* **1341-1346.** (In other language.)

Drawing on examples from Chinese and Hebrew culture, the authors explore the use of the hand in picture and ritual to symbolize the passing on of knowledge and tradition from one person or generation to another. They also speculate on the possibility of a nonlinguistic symbol system that uses the body instead of spoken language for communication.

623

Saito, H., Inoue, M., & Nomura, Y. (1979). Information processing of Kanji (Chinese characters) and Kana (Japanese characters): The close relationship among graphemic, phonemic, and semantic aspects. *Psychologia: An International Journal of Psychology in the Orient, 22,* **195-206.**

Discusses the origin and formation of Kanji and Kana in both linguistic and information-processing terms, focusing on the interrelationship between information extraction and the graphemic, phonemic, and semantic aspects of Kanji. Both theoretical and experimental work on the 2 systems are considered. Findings support the idea that both phonemic processing and semantic processing of Kanji are carried out simultaneously since the characters are arranged in 2 dimensions--information can be extracted from Kanji first by minimal core encoding, with graphemic, phonemic, and semantic processing following in a parallel manner.

624

Sasaki, M., & Watanabe, A. (1984). [Cultural origin of "kusho" behavior]. *Japanese Journal of Educational Psychology, 32,* **182-190.** (In other language.)

The present paper explored the origin of spontaneous writinglike finger movements, "kusho," demonstrated by the Japanese and investigated whether kusho behavior (KB) was based on Kanji learning experience. In Experiment I, 21 Chinese undergraduates were observed while completing a Kanji grapheme test. Findings revealed that all subjects used KB to facilitate the integration of Kanji graphemes. In Experiment II, 83 Japanese, 21 Chinese, and 23 non-Kanji culture undergraduates were observed while performing three English work tasks (forward spell reading, backward spell reading, and work completion). Results showed that 60-80% of the Japanese subjects exhibited KB in each task, while non-Kanji subjects displayed no KB. Analysis of the functional role of KB in the English word completion task indicated that KB augmented the performance of the Japanese subjects as it had in the Kanji grapheme test; however, for the non-Kanji culture subjects, it had a disturbing effect. The cultural background of kusho behavior and its specificity for the Japanese were discussed.

625

Sasanuma, S., Itoh, M., Mori, K., & Kobayashi, Y. (1977). Tachistoscopic recognition of Kana and Kanji words. *Neuropsychologia, 15,* **547-553.**

626

Seidenberg, M. S. (1985). The time course of phonological code activation in two writing systems. *Cognition, 19,* **1-30.**

The author conducted two studies of word recognition in two writing systems, English and Chinese, that are structured along different principles (alphabetic and logographic, respectively). In Experiment 1, 22 native speakers of Cantonese were presented with two sets of stimuli containing four types of characters, a result of crossing the factors type (phonogram, nonphonogram) and frequency (high, low). The phonograms are compound characters containing phonetics that provide information relevant to pronunciation. In Experiment 2, 48 undergraduate native speakers of English were also presented with two sets of stimuli but consisting of words with regular and irregular sound-spelling correspondences of high and low frequency. The results indicated that in each writing system, a large pool of higher frequency words is recognized on a visual basis, without phonological mediation. Phonology only enters into the processing of lower frequency words. Findings are consistent with a parallel interactive model of word recognition in which orthographic and phonological information are activated at different latencies.

627

Shen, B. (1927). An analysis of eye movements in the reading of Chinese. *Journal of Experimental Psychology, 10,* **158-183.**

628

Shen, Y., & Wang, S. X. (1983). [The compilation of materials on speech measurement]. *Acta Psychologica Sinica, 15,* **316-328.** (In Chinese.)

629

Shen, Y., & Wang, S. X. (1983). [Experimental study on multiple-choice in speech discrimination]. *Acta Psychologica Sinica, 15,* **402-409.** (In Chinese.)

630

Shih, C. P. (1964). [Preliminary report on a Punctuation Yest]. *Psychological Testing, 11,* **96-100.** (In Chinese.)

631

Shu, J. I. (1979). The portrayal of Chinese on network television as observed by Chinese and White raters. *Dissertation Abstracts International, 40,* **B2825-2826.**

632

Steinberg, D. D. (1972). Semantic universals: Investigations in Japanese, Chinese, Slovenian, Finnish, and English. *Working Papers in Linguistics* **(University of Hawaii),** ***4,*** **67-83.**

633

Steinberg, D. D. (1975). Semantic universals in sentence processing and interpretation: A study of Chinese, Finnish, Japanese, and Slovenian speakers. *Journal of Psycholinguistic Research, 4,* **169-193.**

The universality of certain aspects of sentence interpretation was investigated with native speakers of a variety of language families; Ss were 66 Mandarin-, 63 Finnish-, 70 Japanese-, and 61 Slovenian-speaking undergraduates. Ss were given, in their own language, the same 156 affirmative and 156 corresponding negative sentences to sort into categories solely on the basis of sentence samples. The categories represented semantic sentence interpretations based on information value and nonsensicality. Ss generally sorted the same sentences (translation equivalents) into the same categories (e.g., Informative, The person is a man; Redundant, The man is a person; Contradictory, The chair is a spouse; Amphigorously Redundant, The chair is not a spouse). A semantic feature analysis indicated that Ss based their interpretations on particular interactions of features. Sets of rules and operations utilizing such feature combinations were formulated and attributed to the Ss. Such knowledge is postulated to be universal to speakers of all languages.

634

Stevenson, H. W. (1981). [Culture, orthography and reading lessons in Chinese and English]. *Information on Psychological Sciences,* **No. 3, 28-35.** (In Chinese.)

635

Sun, J. T. (1923). [Symbolism in the Chinese written language]. *Psychoanalytic Review, 10,* **183-189.** (In Chinese.)

636

Takata, G. (1975). An examination of cultural differences in the use of English mood words: A multidimensional scaling analysis. *Dissertation Abstracts International, 35,* **B5094.**

637

Tang, H. C. (1933). [The psychology of calligraphy in primary schools]. *Chung Hwa Educational Review, 21; 21,* **59-64;** *21,* **63-68;** *21,* **75-78.** (In Chinese.)

638

Tang, T. C. (1964). [A study on the relation between written and spoken language in lower grade school children]. *Acta Psychologica Sinica,* **No. 2, 185-193.** (In Chinese.)

Three experiments were carried out to investigate the development of written and spoken language in primary school children of the second grade. The results were: (1) In the second grade, the quantity and other characteristics of the children's vocabulary in written and spoken language did not differ. The children could use written language to express their ideas mastered orally. (2) Training oral expressions of children through group discussion helped to raise the quality and quantity of written language. (3) Children of the second grade were not capable of correcting their written language, but this ability began to develop at this age. Based on these results, the author proposed some suggestions to improve the quality of children's composition.

639

Tang, T. C., Chow, S. Y., & Chen, J. Y. (1965). [Methods in teaching orthography and their effects on memory]. *Acta Psychologica Sinica,* **No. 4, 299-306.** (In Chinese.)

Children's memory of correctly written characters is related to the teaching methods of orthography. One of the best methods to overcome wrongly written characters is to let the children analyse the structure of the characters and to practice writing the characters together with other related characters. Since memory effects do not increase proportionally with the amount of practice, an optimal practice schedule should be adopted.

640

The Co-operative Research Group for Studying Concept Acquisition in Bilingual Children. (1983). [Concept acquisition in bilingual children]. *Acta Psychologica Sinica, 15,* **162-168.** (In Chinese.)

This study aimed to determine whether logical concepts acquired in one language could be transferred to another language, following earlier studies with bilingual children in Australia and Malaysia. The subjects were a group of children 4-7 years of age who were bilingual in Chinese (the language of the Han nationality) and the language of the Uygur nationality, and a group of 5 year-old children who were bilingual in the Shanghai dialect and the Beijing dialect. After being pretested in both languages or dialects respectively, they were trained in one language or dialect in the conservation of weight, post-tested in their other language or dialect, and were tested again one month later in both languages or dialects. The results showed that the concept acquired in one of their languages or dialects was immediately available in the other. This tends to support Piaget's view that thinking is independent from language. However, it seemed that the children would do slightly better in concept acquisition if trained in their native language.

641

The National Language Research Institute. (1976). [A study of the use of Chinese characters in modern newspapers]. *The National Language Research Institute Report, 56,* **Tokyo, Japan.** (In other language.)

642

Tong, J. S. (1971). Chinese writing as a mentalist symbolic system. *International Journal of Symbology, 2,* **21-28.**

With regard to Chinese writing, a "symbol" is defined here as "a concrete sign or character that represents either a figurative object or an abstract idea by reason of relationship, association, convention, or pictorial aptness". An attempt was made to explore the special symbolic value in the Chinese writing system. Ideographic writing is here demonstrated to be a symbolization par excellence of language, because the ideograms represent not only overt speech sounds, but more importantly, the internal linguistic processes producing and ordering them. The 4 basic principles of symbolization in Chinese writing are explained and illustrated with characteristic examples. It is also demonstrated that Chinese writing as a mentalist symbolic system can represent the most abstract ideas through a crystallization of concretism.

643

Tong, L. Q., & Li, W. F. et al. (1979). [The influences of the number of strokes and the parts of speech on remembering Chinese characters by young children]. *Acta Psychologica Sinica, 11,* **202-206.** (In Chinese.)

644

Tsai, L. S., & Abernethy, E. (1928). The psychology of Chinese characters: Vol. 1. Complexity of character and difficulty of learning. *Journal of Experimental Psychology, 11,* **430-442.**

645

Tsao, C. Y., & Shen, Y. (1963). [The recognition of Chinese characters by primary school children under tachistoscopic conditions: Vol. 2. The effect of the structure of characters]. *Acta Psychologica Sinica,* **No. 4, 271-279.** (In Chinese.)

The purpose of this study was to analyze the effect of the structure of characters on recognition. Three experiments were conducted. The results indicated: (1) Degree of similarity between the structure of characters influenced the recognition. (2) Characters with the same contour but different in content were more difficult to identify than the characters with the same content but different in contour. (3) Familiar radicals played an important role in the reproduction of unfamiliar radicals. Children tended to replace the new radical with familiar ones.

646

Tsao, C. Y., & Shen, Y. (1963). [The recognition of Chinese characters by primary school children under tachistoscopic conditions: Vol. 3. The central effects on recognition]. *Acta Psychologica Sinica,* **No. 4, 280-286.** (In Chinese.)

Using familiar and unfamiliar phrases as materials, this study was an investigation of the central effects on recognition. Results indicated that no visual duration threshold (VDT) difference was found between familiar phrases of 2-6 words, but the VDT difference was significant when the word order of these same phrases was changed. For the unfamiliar phrases no such difference was found under the same condition. On the other hand, the VDT for the familiar phrases with word order changed was significantly higher than the unfamiliar phrases. It is suggested that central effects may affect recognition in two ways; facilitating and interfering. Problems of the storage systems of language in human brain were discussed.

647

Tsao, C. Y., & Shen, Y. (1963). [The recognition of Chinese characters under tachistoscopic condition in primary school children: I. Preliminary experiments on method]. *Acta Psychologica Sinica,* **No. 3, 203-213.** (In Chinese.)

Three experiments were conducted to investigate: (1) the relationship between visual duration threshold (VDT) and the size and brightness of stimulus; (2) VDT of words, phrases and disconnected word-groups; (3) VDT of familiar and unfamiliar words under different procedures. The results were: (1) under brief exposures (below 20 ms.), size x brightness x VDT approximated a constant; (2) the VDT difference was significant between single word and disconnected word groups (2-4 words) but not significant between single words and phrases (2-4 words); (3) VDT for familiar words were all about 10 ms. under different procedures (re-cognition or reproduction); (4) VDT difference between familiar and unfamiliar words was highly significant.

648

Tsao, C. Y., & Shen, Y. (1965). [Developmental studies on the recognition and generalization of Chinese characters in primary school children: Vol. 2. Development of generalization and its relation to recognition]. *Acta Psychologica Sinica,* **No. 2, 121-134.** (In Chinese.)

Hull's and Smoke's methods for the study of concept formation were adopted which included 4 tests: recognition, generalization, identification and reproduction. It was found that there were 3 types of developmental curves: (1) recognition and generalization--negatively accelerated; (2) identification--positively accelerated; (3) concepts of figures--simple accelerated curve. Correlations between different indices on generalization and recognition of different Chinese characters were significant. The results support the hypothesis that the ability of generalization is one of the basic factors which promotes the recognition of Chinese characters.

649

Tsao, C. Y., & Shen, Y. (1965). [Developmental studies of the recognition and generalization of Chinese characters in primary school children: Vol. 3. Development of the discrimination of detail]. *Acta Psychologica Sinica*, **No. 2, 135-140.** (In Chinese.)

An experiment designed to study the development of visual discrimination of Chinese characters was applied to primary school children of the 1st, 2nd and 5th grades. The discrimination task required subjects to match a standard character with an identical one, the latter being grouped in a list of characters varying according to different principles. The results were: (1) Significant difference was found between 2nd and 5th grades. (2) Changes in character structure caused more errors in 2nd and 5th grades than in the 1st grade. This suggested that central storage plays a part in the recognition process.

650

Tsao, C. Y., & Shen, Y. (1965). [Developmental studies on the recognition and generalization of Chinese characters in primary school children: I. Development of recognition under tachistoscopic condition]. *Acta Psychologica Sinica*, **No. 1, 1-9.** (In Chinese.)

In this experiment, the development of recognition of letters, familiar and unfamiliar Chinese characters, and Korean characters was studied. Three types of developmental curves were found: (1) negative accelerated curve for familiar Chinese characters; (2) positive accelerated curve for unfamiliar Chinese characters; (3) simple accelerated curve for Korean characters. It was suggested that there were two important developmental changes in the process of mastering Chinese characters by primary school children: one was found immediately after the first month of learning Chinese characters and the other was between the 1st and 2nd grade. Under different teaching conditions, the occurrence of the second change might be found in different stages of the 1st grade.

651

Tseng, H. C., Chang, L. H., & Chen, C. K. (1965). [The relative frequencies of the various stroke-types of the Chinese ideograms]. *Acta Psychologica Sinica*, **No. 3, 212-214.** (In Chinese.)

652

Tseng, S. C., Chang, L. H., & Wang, C. C. (1965). [An informational analysis of the Chinese language: I. The reconstruction of the removed strokes of the ideograms in printed sentence texts]. *Acta Psychologica Sinica*, *4*, **281-290.** (In Chinese.)

The strokes of the Chinese ideograms in printed sentences selected from recent newspapers were removed at various percentages in three different ways: (1) omitting the anterior strokes of the ideograms; (2) omitting the posterior strokes; and (3) omitting strokes which would not seriously change the configuration of the ideograms. College students were asked to reconstruct the removed strokes. The results indicated that the remaining strokes of the anterior part of the ideograms left by the second type of omission were easier to reconstruct than those of the posterior part left by the first type of omission, while those left by the third type of omission produced the best reconstruction. The average subject, given limited time to work, was able to reconstruct the mutilated ideograms with 55% of the strokes omitted, while superior subjects, given unlimited time, were able to restore as much as 75% of the omitted strokes. From these results the lower bound on redundancy in terms of strokes adopting all the simplified ideograms is estimated to be about 78%. Implications of the findings for further simplification of the Chinese ideograms and for the design of more efficient and more simplified typewriters and printers are suggested.

653

Tsien-Lee, M. (1969). Sound and meaning in Chinese language: A study of phonetic symbolism. *Psychologica Belgica*, *9*, **47-58.**

Investigated the existence of phonetic symbolism in Chinese language. Test material consisted of 8 3-dimensional objects enabling all possible combinations of the big-small, heavy-light, and pointed-round qualities and the Chinese phonetic auxiliary symbols. Ss were 650 Chinese children and 792 adults. They were asked to devise a name for the nonsense objects either by means of freely chosen sounds fitting to the qualities of the objects, or by choosing the suitable sounds from the list of the Chinese phonetic auxiliary symbols. The analysis focused on the relation between the qualities of the objects (weight, size, form) and the sounds devised or chosen by the Ss. The results support the hypothesis of universal phonetic symbolism.

654

Tzeng, O. J. L., Garro, L., & Hung, D. L. (1977). Research in Chinese characters: A call for interdisciplinary endeavor. *Journal of Chinese Linguistics*, *5*, **349-354.**

655

Tzeng, O. J. L., Hung, D. L., & Garro, L. (1978). Reading the Chinese characters: An information processing view. *Journal of Chinese Linguistics, 6,* **270-288.**

656

Van Bezooijen, R., Otto, S. A., & Heenan, T. A. (1983). Recognition of vocal expressions of emotion: Three-nation study to identify universal characteristics. *Journal of Cross-Cultural Psychology, 14,* **387-406.**

Results of 3 experiments show that 48 18-28 yr old Dutch, 40 21-28 yr old Taiwanese, and 41 16-17 yr old Japanese students were able to identify Dutch vocal expressions of emotion beyond chance expectancy. Inspection of the confusion data revealed that, in addition to symmetrical confusions, there were quite a few confusions that were asymmetrical. The outcomes of a multidimensional scaling suggest that confusions were a function of similarity in levels of activity of the emotions concerned rather than, for example, similarity in evaluative meaning. It is concluded that there are universally recognizable characteristics of vocal patterns of emotion and that these characteristics are primarily related to the activity dimension of emotional meaning.

657

Wang, X. (1986). Mirror writing and the development of Chinese written language. In H. S. R. Kao, G. P. van Galen, & R. Hoosain (Eds.), *Graphonomics: Contemporary research in handwriting* **(pp. 321-328). Amsterdam, Netherlands: North-Holland.**

658

Warner, R. (1976). The relationship between language and disease concepts. *International Journal of Psychiatry in Medicine, 7,* **57-68.**

The Sapir-Whorf hypothesis, well-known in anthropological linguistics, postulates that language may not only describe the world we inhabit but also mold the way we experience it; similarly, an individual's language may determine his/her conception of disease. Possible relationships between linguistic features and disease concepts are cited for the Eskimo, the Navaho, and the Chinese, and it is suggested that, in European languages, the extensive use of spatial metaphors to express abstract concepts may encourage a more rigid categorization of disease and inhibit the ability to conceive of multiple factors in disease causation. The use of nouns rather than verbs to express the idea of illness could lead to a static view of disease, and tends to separate illnesses as distinct entities rather than defining them as aspects of bodily functioning. The bipolar structure of Indo-European languages, setting subject against predicate and noun against verb, may play a part in the persistence of the mind-body dichotomy and restrict the holistic perception of man with nature. These linguistic features, in leading to a conception of disease as a rigidly defined, unchanging, unicausal thing, may encourage an overuse of surgery to remove that which is intruding upon the patient and lead to difficulty in perceiving social and psychological factors in disease.

659

Weakland, J. H. (1956). Lusin's "Ah Q": A rejected image of Chinese character. *The Pacific Spectator, 10,* **137-146.**

660

Wingeier, D. E. (1980). Generative words in six cultures. *Religious Education, 75,* **563-576.**

Identified the words "most weighted with existential meaning", following P. Friere's concept of generative words. Ss were 88 young people in 3 US groups (from a Methodist church in Georgia, a Congregational church in Illinois, and a Protestant seminary in the Midwest) and 3 foreign groups (Protestant teacher trainees in Haiti, university students in Shanghai, and young Japanese). Each S was asked to specify 3 words describing the realities of life as currently experienced and 3 words describing their hope for the future in their country. Group discussion clarified the subjective meanings of the words, and comparisons were made among the 6 groups. Implications for religious education are drawn primarily from Friere's concepts and secondarily from the current research data.

661

Wong, P. K., & Lau, S. (1983). [A study of the relative efficiency in learning pronunciation by using National Phonetic Symbols and Hanyu Pinyin]. *Acta Psychologica Taiwanica, 25,* **109-120.** (In Chinese.)

The National Phonetic Symbols and Hanyu Pinyin are popular Mandarin phonetic systems used in learning Mandarin in Hong Kong. The present research was an attempt to determine which system is easier for middle school students. An experimental investigation was held in a middle school. Subjects were divided into two groups. One group learned National Phonetic Symbols (NPS) and the other learned Hanyu Pinyin (HP). Each group consisted of 20 Grade 7 students and 20 Grade 10 students. The results showed that there was a significant difference between the pronunciation performance of the two groups, with better pronunciation performance in the HP group than the NPS group. This result was attributed to the positive transfer from the familiar English alphabets to the HP system. In the analysis of the incorrect responses, it was found that the difficulties encountered by the NPS group were the close similarities among symbols and the different phonetic representations of "yin" "ying", etc. The difficulties in the HP group were syllable boundaries, the letters separating syllables, and "u" "e" each representing two phonemes respectively. The common difficulty of the two systems was the confusion of the retroflex with the alveolar and blade-alveolar.

662

Wu, J. T., & Liu, I. M. (1978). [On the process of sentence production]. *Acta Psychologica Taiwanica, 20,* **65-81.** (In Chinese.)

663

Yamadori, A., Nagashima, T., & Tamaki, N. (1983). Ideogram writing in a disconnection syndrome. *Brain and Language, 19,* **346-356.**

664

Yang, J. B. (1979). [A study on the number index system of Chinese characters in accordance with the characteristics of their structures]. *Acta Psychologica Sinica, 11,* **293-303.** (In Chinese.)

The results of a study on the number-index system of Chinese characters based on their structure are presented. The suggested system may be used in dictionary or catalogue compilations. Through further improvement, it may also be used in information retrieval, file searching, and so on.

665

Yang, K. S., & Cheng, C. M. (1974). [Pattern of Chinese-character arrangement and character-searching efficiency]. *Acta Psychologica Taiwanica, 16,* **73-86.** (In Chinese.)

The present experiment was designed to investigate the differences in search efficiency among 9 arrangement patterns, varying in size and dimension of the character block, of Chinese characters. The subjects were 135 university women. Each subject was instructed to search the display screen for one predetermined character on each trial. The time interval between the display of the characters on the screen and the pressing of keys to indicate the correct location of the chosen character was recorded as the main measure of search efficiency. It was found that, among the 9 patterns used, the efficiency was highest for the 6 x 0 arrangement (6 characters in a row in each block), and lowest for the 2 x 2 arrangement, The proposed reasons for the efficiency of the 6 x 0 arrangement are: (1) The number of characters per block is similar to the average human span of attention or comprehension; and (2) the characters in each block are arranged in a one-dimensional format, which requires less scanning tt only 2 significant differences for the normal group. The finding was interpreted as indicating that the author's psychotherapy is effective and, furthermore, that it is only e

666

Yang, K. S., & Tzuo, H. Y. (1961). The functional relationship between the pleasantness value and the character-number of the Chinese classical poem. *Acta Psychologica Taiwanica,* **No. 3, 125-131.**

This experiment was an investigation of the relative pleasantness values of different character-numbers of a Chinese classical poem. Twenty-four fourth-grade pupils whose ages ranged from 9 years and 2 months to 10 years and 2 months were individually asked to compare the pleasantness values of the nine kinds of character-numbers, using the method of paired comparisons. The results obtained substantiate the following conclusions: (1) There was a functional relationship between the pleasantness value and the character-numbers of the Chinese classical poem. (2) Among the nine kinds of character-numbers, the one with 5 had the greatest pleasantness value, followed by those with 4, 3, 7 and 6; the group with 9, 8, and 10 had the least value. The character-number of 2 was a special case which is not significantly different from any of the others.

667

Yang, K. S., & Yang-Lee, P. H. (1971). [Desirability, meaningfulness, and familiarity ratings of 557 Chinese personality-trait adjectives]. *Acta Psychologica Taiwanica, 13,* **36-57.** (In Chinese.)

Presented 557 Chinese personality-trait adjectives to 3 samples of about 150 college students for rating on desirability, meaningfulness, or familiarity. Normative rating data in the form of means and standard deviations were tabulated, with the 557 adjectives arranged and numbered in order of increasing desirability. While the mean ratings on desirability of the adjectives were bimodally distributed, those on the other 2 variables had a negatively skewed distribution. Correlations of the 3 variables with 1 another for different adjectives were: (a) desirability-meaningfulness, r = .28 (p .001); (b) desirability-familiarity, r = .30 (p .001); and (c) meaningfulness-familiarity, r = .82 (p .001). The adjective list with normative values is evaluated in terms of its uses in personality and social-psychological research, and some general remarks about its limitations are made.

668

Yin, W. G. (1984). [A study of tachistoscopic recognition of Chinese characters and nonsense shapes]. *Acta Psychologica Sinica, 16,* **282-288.** (In Chinese.)

Sixty Chinese university students were requested to recognize Chinese characters and nonsense shapes presented tachistoscopically. The results showed that most subjects, both right-handed and left-handed, manifested the bilateral effect of the two hemispheres in their responses. The percentage of subjects who showed no visual field difference in reading Chinese characters was 60%; in the case of nonsense shapes, 56.66%. This experiment is different from those which test European-American subjects with syllabic words as stimuli. It indicates that Chinese character recognition seems to follow a special process.

669

You, H. S. (1964). [Preliminary studies on the forgetting of auxiliaries and of substantives in first grade junior middle school pupils]. *Acta Psychologica Sinica*, **No. 4, 377-380.** (In Chinese.)

Pupils were required to memorize 4 paragraphs of text materials (3 paragraphs of classical prose and 2 paragraphs of modern prose). By means of recall made at various intervals after memorization, the retention of substantive and auxiliary words was examined, which gave the following results: (1) The forgetting ratio was greater for auxiliary words. (2) There were two kinds of manifestations in forgetting: omission and error. This might be due to generalization and inhibition that took place in the higher nervous activity. 3) Pupils' knowledge and experience affected the understanding of the text; idiomatic expressions also influenced the reproduction.

670

Young, B. M. (1971). Psycholinguistics in a cross-cultural context. *Psychologia*, *14*, **106-111.**

671

Yu, B. C., & Liu, I. M. (1982). [Applicability of the model of Chinese sentence comprehension to English sentences]. *Acta Psychologica Taiwanica*, *24*, **59-63.** (In Chinese.)

This study investigated the applicability of a model of Chinese sentence comprehension to English sentences and to Western subjects. The results indicated: (1) For two-proposition sentences, the right-incremented (RI) sentences were comprehended faster than the left-incremented (LI) sentences; (2) the two-proposition sentences were comprehended faster than the compound sentences; and (3) an atypical pattern of sentence-picture verification latencies was obtained, consistent with the results of Liu (1980). In summary, these results support the generality of the model of sentence comprehension established for Chinese sentences and Chinese subjects.

672

Yu, B. L. (1985). [Effects of encoding modes of word lists on recall]. *Information on Psychological Sciences*, **No. 5, 12-17.** (In Chinese.)

673

Zee, E. (1980). Tone and vowel quality. *Journal of Phonetics*, *8*, **247-258.**

Speakers of a tone language, Taiwanese, were instructed to produce vowels with 2 contrasting tones--high and low. Results show that vowel quality was affected by tonal difference, although not systematically for different vowels and for different speakers.

674

Zhang, J. L., Qi, S. Q., & Lu, S. N. (1981). [A preliminary study of the perceptual configurations of Chinese consonants]. *Acta Psychologica Sinica*, *13*, **76-85.** (In Chinese.)

Chinese consonant confusion matrices were obtained with articulation tests for natural syllables in several transmission conditions. It was found that analogical and numerical transmission conditions were very similar such that the configurations that were deduced from the confusion matrices reflected the perceptual features of Chinese consonants. Exceedingly important perceptual features of Chinese consonants were voicing, aspiration, frication, and place.

675

Zhang, W. T., Peng, R. X., & Sima, H. (H. A. Simon). (1984). STM capacity for Chinese words and idioms with visual and auditory presentations. In *Issues in Cognition: Proceedings of a Joint Conference in Psychology* **(pp. 331-344). Washington, DC: National Academy of Sciences and American Psychological Association.**

676

Zheng, D. C. (1983). [Recognition of Chinese synonyms and homonyms in the light of the theory of signal detectability]. *Information on Psychological Sciences*, **No. 6, 37-40.** (In Chinese.)

In light of the theory of signal detectability, research was carried out to investigate students' recognition of Chinese vocabulary and the problem of the transformation of recalled Chinese vocabulary. The results indicated that synonyms were more confusing than homonyms in terms of recognition, and that students in junior or senior middle schools were evidently superior to students in primary schools in recognition ability.

677

Zhu, M. S., & Wu, J. Z. (1981). [Factors affecting the comprehension of sentences by children]. *Information on Psychological Sciences*, **No. 1, 23-27.** (In Chinese.)

678

Zhu, Y., & Li, M. D. (1985). [The keyword method and English word acquisition]. *Acta Psychologica Sinica*, *17*, **170-176.** (In Chinese.)

This experiment was designed to test the Keyword Method of building vocabulary as it is used in English-speaking countries. The results showed that the Keyword Method is not nearly as successful for Chinese students as it is for native speakers of English. But a new Keyword Method designed by the investigators has proved helpful to Chinese students in translating Chinese into English.

679

Zhu, Z. R. (1966). [Comparison of three criteria of character recognition by primary school children]. *Acta Psychologica Sinica*, **No. 2, 118-123.** (In Chinese.)

The following references are also relevant to this chapter:

58, 75, 241, 266, 337, 357, 368, 379, 399, 408, 419, 433, 434, 452, 460, 685, 688, 700, 704, 766, 842, 855, 927, 1036, 1038, 1060, 1069, 1093, 1144, 1539, 1742, 1834, 1911, 1950, 2010, 2014, 2103, 2210, 2398, 2399, 2450, 2633, 2713, 3015, 3369.

DEVELOPMENTAL PSYCHOLOGY 7

Frequency data on citations in this chapter, in terms of content classification subcategories, are presented in Table 7.

Table 7: *Number of Citations by Content Classification, Language, and Geographical Area*

Content classification	Total	CL	EL	OL	PRC	T	HK	US
Developmental psychology	106	29	75	2	31	18	10	3
Cognitive & perceptual development	203	150	52	1	121	27	13	0
Psychosocial and personality development	166	68	98	0	28	57	33	5
Total	475	247	225	3	180	102	56	8

Note: CL = Chinese language; EL = English language; OL = other languages. PRC = People's Republic of China; T = Taiwan; HK = Hong Kong; US = United States (Chinese Americans--according to the frequency of the subject term Asian Americans).

Subject terms used for indexing citations related to developmental psychology are grouped according to geographical area, subject population, and topic. These are presented below, in a descending order of frequency. (The frequency of single-word subject terms includes those of compound terms in which the single word appears. Subjects terms used for indexing citations from other chapters may have been included. Terms with a frequency of less than 10 are not shown.)

Geographical area

197 Peoples Republic of China
172 Asia
114 Taiwan
58 Hong Kong
18 United States

Subject population

330	children
151	school age children
103	adolescents
82	preschool age children
28	infants
28	students
24	Asians
14	adults
12	aged
11	gifted
11	human females

Topic

224	development
100	cognitive development
79	age differences
73	cross cultural differences
61	sex
49	cognitive processes
48	perception
44	language
39	socialization
37	attitudes
37	learning
36	personality
33	childrearing practices
33	intelligence
33	language development
30	adolescence
28	family
27	ability
26	human sex differences
24	psychology
24	thinking
22	ethnic groups
22	behavior
19	achievement
19	development psychology
19	education
18	concept learning
18	parent child relations
18	concept formation
17	parental attitudes
16	curriculum
15	mathematics
14	curriculum development
13	adulthood
13	concepts
13	longitudinal studies
13	teaching
12	academic achievement
12	intellectual development
12	moral development
12	sociocultural factors
11	adjustment
11	numbers
11	psychosocial development
10	childhood development
10	comprehension
10	concepts

10	motivation
10	personality development
10	racial and ethnic differences
10	socioeconomic status
10	status

Table 7 shows that: (a) Citations in cognitive and perceptual development (42.7%) exceed those in psychosocial and personality development (35.0%), (b) Chinese-language citations exceed English- language ones, and (c) citations pertaining to the PRC are more numerous than those pertaining to Taiwan. However, content classification subcategory interacts with both language and geographical area. In cognitive and perceptual development, Chinese- language citations are almost three times as numerous as those in English; citations pertaining to the PRC predominate, being more than four times as numerous as those pertaining to Taiwan. But in psychosocial and personality development, English-language citations exceed Chinese-language ones; citations pertaining to Taiwan are more than twice as numerous as those pertaining to the PRC. It appears that psychologists in the PRC have devoted more attention to cognitive and perceptual development, whereas psychologists in Taiwan have devoted more attention to psychosocial and personality development.

An inspection of terms indexing subject populations reveals a clear imbalance. Children and, to a lesser extent, adolescents have received most of the attention in research; infants have received much less; adults and the aged have been neglected. It appears that the notion of life-span development has yet to be taken seriously by researchers. Also, the low frequency of the term *moral development* suggests that this important topic has been neglected.

A book on behavioral development in Chinese children was edited by Yang and Chang (1974); a review of the empirical literature on socialization may be found in Ho (1986).

REFERENCES

Ho, D. Y. F. (1986). Chinese patterns of socialization: A critical review. In M. H. Bond (Ed.), *The psychology of the Chinese people* (pp. 1-37). Hong Kong: Oxford University Press.

Yang, K. S., & Chang, C. H. (Eds.). (1974). *[Behavioral development of Chinese children].* Taipei: Huan Yu. (In Chinese.)

680

Abbott, K. (1980). The first three years of child development: A theoretical consideration of change in Chinese societies. *Hong Kong Psychological Society Bulletin*, **No. 4, 19-32.**

Describes the mutual interaction of 3 factors in a social system: cultural values, childrearing practices, and personality development. Each factor in this triad is also influenced by other variables, such as technological change and urbanization. Two important studies of developmental patterns during the 1st 3 yrs of life are reported in detail: (1) M. Mahler's 5-yr study, begun in 1963, of middle-class European and American mothers and their children from 6 mo to 3 yrs old, which produced extensive empirical data and theoretical formulations; and (2) the 5-yr study, begun in 1967, by C. E. Field and F. M. Bader of almost 600 children in Hong Kong, from birth onwards. Comparison of childrearing practices and child development patterns in the 2 samples reveals significant differences; overall, the Chinese pattern emphasizes the group and the interdependence of its members on each other, while the Western pattern fosters individualism. However, both systems are in the process of change, since neither excessive independence nor excessive interdependence are consistent with a highly technological society.

681

Aboud, F. E. (1977). Interest in ethnic information: A cross-cultural developmental study. *Canadian Journal of Behavioural Science*, ***9*, 134-146.**

A total of 159 White, Indian, and Chinese Canadian kindergartners and 1st graders were introduced to 3 picture book characters from each of 5 ethnic groups: Indian, Black, White, Chinese, and Eskimo. These books were then used as stimulus materials for measuring the children's self-identification, information seeking, role taking, and social perception. The information-seeking measures were found to be related in a very minor way to attitude. However, it is proposed that the stage of development of self-identification influenced the child's selection of ethnic information.

682

Abu-Saad, H. (1984). Cultural components of pain: The Asian-American child. *Children's Health Care*, ***13*, 11-14.**

The investigator interviewed 13 female and 11 male first-generation children of Asian born parents to determine how subjects perceived, described, and responded to painful experiences. Information was elicited regarding causative factors and word descriptors of pain, feelings, and coping strategies when in pain. The subjects could identify sources of pain, use words to describe their pain, and respond to painful experiences in accordance with known cultural indicators. Results showed that girls identified more frequently than boys psychological causes of pain, a finding that reflects the cultural expectation that girls are more sensitive and emotional about behavioral expressions than boys. The finding that older girls described more psychological causes of pain than the younger group suggested the delineation of children's cognitive stages in the development of health and illness concepts. Girls more often chose affective and evaluative words to describe pain while boys chose sensory descriptors.

683

Abu-Saad, H. (1984). Cultural group indicators of pain in children. *Maternal-Child Nursing Journal*, ***13*** **187-196.**

The investigator examined how 24 Arab-American (ARA), 24 Asian-American (ASA), and 24 Latin-American (LA) children perceived, described, and responded to painful experiences. The subjects were interviewed over a 6-month period at home, in school, or at a recreational facility; the interview schedule was adapted from a pain questionnaire developed by M. Savedra et al. Findings showed that the range of physical and psychological causes of pain did not differ widely among the 3 groups, suggesting that causative factors of pain in children are likely to be universal. ARA and LA subjects were more likely to use sensory words to describe pain, while ASA subjects tended to use more affective and evaluative words. The range and type of description of subjects' feelings varied by group, as did coping strategies. Implications for managing and assessing children's pain coping strategies by health professionals were discussed.

684

Adkins, M. K. (1978). Children's drawing in the People's Republic of China. *Theory into Practice*, ***17*, 401-409.**

Love of labor, class struggle and class consciousness, patriotism, physical culture, serving the people, furthering the political movement, and worship of Mao and the Communist Party are the themes of Chinese children's drawings, books, and cartoons. These themes are consistent with the Chinese use of art to exert political influence on the masses. Drawing skills are developed by copying model pictures that contain these themes. 10 pictures by 6-yr-olds are included.

685

Au, T. K. (1983). Chinese and English counterfactuals: The Sapir-Whorf hypothesis revisited. *Cognition*, ***15*, 155-187.**

This is a report on a series of five studies with 989 subjects, 8 to 21 years old, designed to replicate a study by A. H. Bloom (1981) that provided evidence supporting a weak version of the hypothesis of linguistic relativity and determinism proposed by E. Sapir (1949) and B. L. Whorf (1956). Using both Chinese and English versions of a new counterfactual story as well as one used by Bloom, findings were obtained that suggest that the mastery of the English subjunctive is probably tangential to counterfactual reasoning in Chinese.

686

Ayabe, H. I., & Santo, S. (1972). Conceptual tempo and the Oriental American. *Journal of Psychology, 81*, **121-123.**

15 male and 15 female 2nd graders of Japanese or Chinese extraction and 15 male and 15 female of Filipino, Hawaiian, Samoan, or Portuguese extractions were randomly assigned to 1 of 3 Matching Familiar Figures (Kagan's Instrument for reflection-impulsivity) testing conditions, fast, slow, and control. It was hypothesized that the Japanese and Chinese traditional values of perseverance and reservedness would manifest itself in the production of few errors and extended latencies. When Ss were asked to "go as fast as you can", Japanese and Chinese American children produced significantly fewer errors than the other racial group. No other significant differences were found.

687

Baber, F. M. (1973). Problems of preschool children in Hong Kong. *Hong Kong Journal of Mental Health, 2*, **8-10.**

688

Bain, B., & Yu, A. (1980). Cognitive consequences of raising children bilingually: One parent, one language. *Canadian Journal of Psychology, 34*, **304-313.**

Used A. R. Luria's (1961) language and cognition paradigm in a longitudinal study of 88 mother-father-child triads of which 30 were from France, 31 from Canada, and 27 from Hong Kong. At first testing, children were 22-24 mo of age and at later testing 46-48 mo old. There was 1 bilingual and 2 unilingual groups (10 Ss/group) at each of the 3 locations. Parents of the bilingual groups were instructed on how to raise their children according to J. Ronjat's (1913) "1 parent, 1 language" principle. No significant differences in performance between the younger groups were found. At the older age level, all bilingual groups obtained significantly higher scores compared to all unilingual groups. Results held regardless of language combinations or cultural milieu.

689

Beck, S. S. (1981). A study of patterns of mental ability and language development of Chinese-American children in a two-language environment. *Dissertation Abstracts International, 42*, **A1518.**

690

Borke, H. (1973). The development of empathy in Chinese and American children between three and six years of age: A cross-cultural study. *Developmental Psychology, 9*, **102-108.**

Administered a series of social interaction situations representing the 4 emotions of happy, afraid, sad, and angry to 288 American children and 288 Chinese children. 24 girls and 24 boys, 1/2 from middle-class families and 1/2 from disadvantaged families, were tested at 6-mo intervals between 3 and 6 yrs of age. Children from both cultural groups exhibited similar overall trends in their ability to recognize other people's emotional responses. By 3 yrs of age, the majority of American and Chinese children could differentiate between happy and unhappy reactions in other people. Perception of afraid, sad, and angry feelings developed somewhat later and appeared to be influenced by social learning. Results of a previous investigation that very young children are capable of empathic responses are confirmed. The awareness of other people's feelings by young children from very different cultural backgrounds suggests that empathy may be a basic human characteristic related to social adaptation.

691

Breiner, S. J. (1980). Early child development in China. *Child Psychiatry & Human Development, 11*, **87-95.**

A psychiatrist compares his direct observations of child rearing in China with reports from other Western professionals. The discrepancy between psychiatric knowledge in the cities and absence of it among teachers in the provinces is stressed. Differences between contented children and conforming children are pointed out. It is concluded that the Chinese emphasis on conforming and on discipline and the failure to acknowledge emotional factors result in psychopathology going undetected or being misdiagnosed in the children.

692

Bronson, G. W. (1972). Infants' reactions to unfamiliar persons and novel objects. *Monographs of the Society for Research in Child Development, 37*, **Serial No. 148.**

693

Cao, Z. F., Zhao, S. W., Sun, C. S., Lu, J., Liu, J. H., & Liu, F. (1983). [Development of the concept of intersection set in children and adolescents in the five regions in China]. *Information on Psychological Sciences*, **No. 5, 1-8.** (In Chinese.)

694

Chan, J. (1978). Parent-child interaction and personality. *New Horizons*, **No. 19, 44-52.**

695

Chan, J. (1979). Effects of parent-child interaction on verbal and other intellectual abilities: An empirical study. *New Horizons*, **No. 20, 19-30.**

696

Chan, J. (1981). Correlates of parent-child interaction and certain psychological variables among adolescents in Hong Kong. In J. L. M. Binnie-Dawson, G. H. Blowers & R. Hoosain (Eds.), *Perspectives in Asian cross-cultural psychology* **(pp. 112-131). Lisse, Netherlands: Swets & Zeitlinger.**

This is a study on parental treatment, teaching, and discipline from the child's point of view, based on a stratified sample of 1,408 secondary school students from 14 schools in Hong Kong. Using the Parent Image Differential, three favorable factors, Concerned, Democratic, and Rational, and three unfavorable factors, Restrictive, Demanding, and Autocratic, were identified for both fathers and mothers. The results clearly showed that generally mothers were viewed more favorably than fathers. Boys experienced stronger restrictive treatment and demanding teaching by the father, as well as stronger autocratic discipline by both parents, than did girls. It was felt that most findings were in accord with those of previous investigations.

697

Chan, J., Eysenck, H. J., & Gotz, K. O. (1980). A new Visual Aesthetic Sensitivity Test: III. Crosscultural comparison between Hong Kong children and adults, and English and Japanese samples. *Perceptual & Motor Skills*, *50*, **1325-1326.**

Applied the Visual Aesthetic Sensitivity Test to 539 Hong Kong children of Chinese extraction (aged 7 yrs and over) and to 202 adults. Their responses were compared with those of 1,115 English and Japanese children and adults. Somewhat lower scores were recorded for the Hong Kong children and adults. 200 11-18 yr old female Germans were also tested. Their difficulty levels for the items were not dissimilar to those observed in England and Japan.

698

Chang, C. H. (1985). Achievement motivation in five groups of first graders in South Taiwan. *Dissertation Abstracts International*, *45*, **A2036.**

699

Chang, C. K., & Chu, W. B. (1964). [An experimental study in the formation of children's sense of duty in school work]. *Acta Psychologica Sinica*, **No. 2, 194-202.** (In Chinese.)

The authors studied the following problems: (1) The relationship between children's sense of duty in school work and their achievement scores. (2) The relationship between motivation and habitual behavior in the psychological structure of the sense of duty in school work. (3) The role of explanation, demonstration, supervision and children's self-evaluation in the formation of the sense of duty in school work. (4) The transference of the sense of duty in school work to other activities and the development of moral traits in the sense of duty in general among children.

700

Chang, H. W. (1985). [Semantic relations of single-word utterances by young children acquiring Mandarin Chinese]. *Chinese Journal of Psychology*, *27*, **1-11.** (In Chinese.)

This report presents a part of the data from a longitudinal study of the initial stages of Chinese children's acquisition of Mandarin. The subjects were four children whose mean age was 14 1/2 months at the beginning of the study. Over a period of one year, 10 recordings of utterances were made for each child with a 3 to 4 weeks interval between consecutive recordings. The analysis was based on the framework by Greenfield and Smith who classified early semantic relations into 13 basic categories. The data indicated that the order of acquisition of semantic relations was fairly constant when the 13 relations were grouped into four basic classes: performative, volition, and performative objects; action, or state of agent and state of object; words relating an object with location or another object; and words dealing with the modification of events. This order of appearance agrees with that found for English in general. In addition, the data indicated that Chinese children at this stage had an initial comprehension of the Chinese interrogative form "V-not-V" (somewhat analogous to English yes/no questions).

701

Chang, K. S. F., Lee, M. M. C., Low, W. D., Chui, S., & Chow, M. (1965). Standards of height and weight of southern Chinese children. *Far Eastern Medical Development Journal*, *1*, **101.**

702

Chang, K. S. F., Ng, P. H., Lee, M. M. M. C., Chan, S. J. (1966). Sexual maturation of Chinese boys in Hong Kong. *Pediatrics*, *37*, **804-811.**

703

Chang, P. H. (1979). Children's literature and political socialization. In G. C. Chu & F. L. K. Hsu (Eds.), *Moving a mountain: Cultural change in China*. **Honolulu, HI: University Press of Hawaii.**

704

Chang, S. T., Chan, L. T., & Shen, T. L. (1957). [The effects of words in children's generalized cognitions]. *Acta Psychologica Sinica*, *1*, **134-142.** (In Chinese.)

Eight school children took part in an experiment on the interaction of the first and the second signal systems. Ivanov-Smolensky's method was used. The results showed that there was more transfer from the first to second signal system than from the second to the first. The amount of transfer from the second to the first system has no correlation with age and grade, and a rather negative correlation with school scores and records. The results were discussed with reference to the aim and method of teaching in elementary schools.

705

Chang, T. C., & Hwang, H. T. (1963). [An experimental study on the time perception in 6-7 years old children]. *Acta Psychologica Sinica*, No. 3, 214-221. (In Chinese.)

706

Chang, W. H. (1964). [The Draw-A-Man Test and intelligence]. *Psychological Testing, 11*, 60-78. (In Chinese.)

707

Chang, W. J. (1974). [An analysis of interpersonal relationships of gifted children]. *Psychological Testing, 21*, 53-57. (In Chinese.)

708

Chang, Y. H. (Ed.) (1968). [*Children's language and thinking*] (2nd ed.). Taipei: Chung-hua. (In Chinese.)

709

Chao, C. S. (1979). [*Chinese adolescents' moral judgment and cognitive development*]. Unpublished master's thesis, National Taiwan University, Taipei. (In Chinese.)

710

Chen, C. M. (1977). [Effects of birth order, socioeconomic status, and childrearing practices on children's creativity]. *Research in Education & Psychology, 1*, 228-229. (In Chinese.)

711

Chen, H. C. (1984). [The child's moral cognitive development: A perspective on recent research]. *Acta Psychologica Sinica, 16*, 466-474. (In Chinese.)

The author reviewed the research on moral cognitive development of the child, which has been conducted since the 1960s by several successors to Piaget and L. Kohlberg. The present author supported some of the theories of these 2 psychologists and raised points of discussion or criticism regarding others. It was suggested that although Western methodology should be approached critically, Chinese psychologists should benefit from its use to advance research on the moral development of children and adolescents in China.

712

Chen, H. C., & Ho, C. (1986). Development of Stroop interference in Chinese-English bilinguals. *Journal of Experimental Psychology: Learning, Memory & Cognition, 12*, 397-401.

One hundred and twenty Chinese-English bilingual students in Grades 2, 4, and 8, and 10 students in college, used both Chinese and English to name the colors of patches and Chinese and English words that consisted of incongruent color names. Subjects of all levels showed greater within- than between-language interference when responding in their primary language, Chinese. When English was the response language, however, a developmental shift from greater between-language interference to greater within-language interference was observed. These results argue against E. Magiste's language proficiency hypothesis and suggest that the pattern of the between- and within-language interference in bilinguals is determined by both language similarity and language proficiency. Further implications of the obtained results for language processing of bilinguals and for the traditional horse race model of the Stroop effect were also discussed.

713

Chen, H. C., & Li, B. S. (1982). [A study of moral judgment of children about the public and private property damage]. *Acta Psychologica Sinica, 14*, 318-325. (In Chinese.)

714

Chen, H. C., & Wang, L. W. (1983). [An experimental study of the influence of interesting game activity on intelligence development in kindergarten children]. *Acta Psychologica Sinica, 15*, 169-177. (In Chinese.)

This study explored the relationship between playing games and intellectual development in kindergarten children. The subjects were 30 boys and girls 4 years and 8 months of age. They were given 7 months of educational training, twice per week. The results indicated that playing games according to the children's interests under adult instruction markedly enhanced intellectual development in children.

715

Chen, H. N., & Su, C. W. (1977). [The perception of parent-child relationships and its relation to adjustment of adolescents]. *Bulletin of Educational Psychology* (Taiwan Normal University), *10*, 91-106. (In Chinese.)

Relationships between childrearing practices and the personal and social adjustments of adolescents in Taiwan were explored. The subjects were 321 sophomores from six different junior high schools in Taipei. The Parent-child Relation Questionnaire and the California Test of Personality were administered. The results were: (1) Parents from the upper class tended to be more loving, protecting, and used more psychological rewards than lower-class parents. Parents from the lower class were more rejecting, neglecting, and used more punishment than upper-class parents. (2) Generally speaking, girls from the upper class had better personal and social adjustments than girls from the lower class. However, this trend was not found for boys. (3) Being loving, protecting, and casual, and using psychological and physical rewards had positive effects on the personal and social adjustments of adolescents. Parental demanding, neglecting, rejecting attitudes, and using psychological and physical punishments had negative effects. (4) Girls were more readily influenced by the childrearing behaviors of their parents than boys. (5) Childrearing practices appeared to have deeper influences on the personal adjustment of adolescents than on their social adjustment. (6) The subjects' intelligence was not related to their adjustment or to their perceived parental childrearing behaviors.

716

Chen, I. H. (1978). [The development of moral judgment among Taiwan adolescents]. *Bulletin of Kaoshung Teachers' College of Education*, *6*, **93-159.** (In Chinese.)

717

Chen, I. Y. (1978). [*A study on political socialization in Chinese students in Taiwan*]. **Taipei: Chia-Hsin Cultural Foundation.** (In Chinese.)

718

Chen, K. W. (1985). [A preliminary study on the affiliation of the only child]. *Acta Psychologica Sinica*, *17*, **264-270.** (In Chinese.)

This study compares the sociability of only and nononly children between 3 to 12 years of age. The subjects were 482 only children and paired nononly children in 4 kindergartens and 14 primary schools in urban and suburban Beijing. Questionnaires were used, supplemented by observation, interviews, case studies, and peer evaluations. The results showed that there was no significant difference in sociability between only and nononly children in urban Beijing; in suburban Beijing, a significant difference in favor of nononly children was found for boys, but not for girls.

719

Chen, L. C. (1982). [A comparative study of the cognitive development of gifted and normal students]. *Bulletin of Educational Psychology*, *15*, **215-225.** (In Chinese.)

Conducted 2 experiments to (1) explore cognitive abilities in normal and gifted children and (2) assess the possibility of acceleration in the gifted. In Exp I, 112 normal and 112 gifted children in Grades 3-6 were selected from 3 elementary schools in Taipei. Each S was tested with 10 questions presented in the order of symbolic item, pictoral item, and then manually operational real materials. In Exp II, 192 gifted children in Grades 3-6 were randomly assigned to 3 groups, and each group was presented an enactment or an iconic or symbolic representation of materials. It was found that (1) the cognitive abilities of the gifted were superior to those of the normal Ss; (2) the cognitive developmental ability of enactment was the highest ability in all grade levels of gifted and normal Ss, followed by the iconic representation and the symbolic representation; and furthermore, the gifted used more symbolic representation than did normal Ss; (3) it was possible to accelerate the cognitive ability of the gifted children by using more enactment.

720

Chen, L. C. (1983). [The study of the college graduates' identity status development]. *Bulletin of Educational Psychology*, *16*, **89-98.** (In Chinese.)

Two hundred and fifty-one college graduates (158 males and 93 females) in Taiwan responded to a number of scales measuring identity status development (diffusion, foreclosure, moratorium, and identity-achievement status), self-certainty, occupational decision, satisfaction of learning scale, and perceived parental socialization styles. The results revealed that: (1) Most of the female graduates were in the moratorium group; male graduates were more likely to be identity achievers. (2) Graduates who had higher self-certainty tended to be identity achievers. (3) The evidence revealed that perceived parental socialization styles significantly differentiated the identity status groups from one another.

721

Chen, L. C. (1985). [The application of Bruner's theory in cognitive development of the elementary and junior high school students]. *Bulletin of Educational Psychology*, *18*, **191-228.** (In Chinese.)

This study tested J. S. Bruner's theory of representation and explored its applicability to instruction. Five experimental observations were made. The results were: (1) There was a significant difference between boys and girls in cognitive development; enactive representational ability was the highest at all grade levels, with iconic representation the next, and symbolic representation the lowest. Cognitive representational ability increased with grade levels. (2) Gifted children used more symbolic representation than normal and mentally retarded children did. (3) The group taught by the proper sequence, from enactive to iconic and then to symbolic, was superior to the group taught by symbolic representation directly. (4)

Evidence from comparing fourth grade children who were taught mathematical concepts supposedly difficult for them with a control group showed that the acceleration of cognitive development was feasible.

722

Chen, L. C. (1986). [A study of junior high students' cognitive developmental ability and creativity]. *Bulletin of Educational Psychology*, *19*, **85-104.** (In Chinese.)

This study tested the applicability of Bruner's theory of representation and explored the relationship between cognitive developmental ability and creativity. A battery of instruments including the Test of Cognitive Representation, the Torrance Tests of Creative Thinking, Figural Form A, and Verbal Form B were given to 160 junior high school students. The main findings were: (1) There were significant differences among grades, sexes, and ability groups in symbolic representational and iconic representational ability. (2) There were no significant differences in grades, and sex on the creativity scales. Nevertheless, the students in the first section ability grouping were superior to the students in the second section ability grouping. (3) There was a relationship between cognitive developmental ability and creativity. However, there was no significant influence of cognitive ability on creativity.

723

Chen, L., & Wang, A. S. (1965). [A developmental study of color and form abstraction in children]. *Acta Psychologica Sinica*, **No. 2, 154-162.** (In Chinese.)

This was an experimental study of color and form abstraction in 267 children, ranging from 2-8 years in age. Three definite stages of development were established: (1) pure form abstraction before the age of 3 years; (2) a stage of color dominance, with a peak at about 4 1/2 years; (3) the dominance of identity-abstraction after the age of 6 years. Subjective factors, such as color and form preferences, sex differences and intelligence, were ruled out as playing significant roles in the differences of abstraction. Various hypotheses were discussed and a hierarchy in the cognitive process was supported.

724

Chen, L., & Wang, A. S. (1965). [A follow-up study of color and form abstraction in children of different ages]. *Acta Psychologica Sinica*, **No. 2, 163-164.** (In Chinese.)

Fifty-one children (who previously participated in the same study) in the age groups of 2-3 years, 3-4 years and 5-6 years were again examined after an interval of one year to observe if they did follow the trend of the 3-stage development as suggested. The results confirmed former conclusions that repetition did not make children adopt the methods of their respective old solutions but helped them achieve a solution appropriate to a more advanced stage. This finding argues for the role of exercise in mental development.

725

Chen, L., & Wang, A. S. (1965). [Color and form preferences]. *Acta Psychologica Sinica*, **No. 3, 265-269.** (In Chinese.)

A total of 537 pre-school children and university students were studied. No developmental trend was observed among the various age groups of children in either color or form preferences. Pre-school children were, as a rule, more uniform in their rankings of color preferences, than were university students. The judgments of children with regard to different forms were less uniform than those of the students. Nevertheless, the circle was preferred by all age groups, and there was a tendency for adults to prefer a rectangle of the so-called golden section, while children preferred squares. No sex difference was observed among children for either color or form preferences, though adults did show some sex difference in color preferences. Children formed more concrete images with different forms, while there was no such tendency with regard to colors. It was suggested that adults might form different associations for particular colors.

726

Chen, M. J. (1981). Directional scanning of visual displays: A study with Chinese subjects. *Journal of Cross-Cultural Psychology*, *12*, **252-271.**

60 Chinese 8th graders and university students were tested on a naming task using 6 types of material. Results show no difference between the 2 groups in their preference for direction of scan; the scanning patterns were highly systematic and unaffected by stimulus materials. In spite of the fact that Chinese readers are accustomed to reading Chinese either from top to bottom, right to left, or left to right, Ss chose to scan predominantly from top to bottom and from left to right when presented with patterned arrays of familiar stimulus materials. Further analysis of Ss' scanning patterns suggest that a general top-to-bottom and left-to-right scanning tendency prevails in the Chinese Ss' performance.

727

Chen, S. M. (1973). [A study on the relationship between socio-economic levels and preschool children's ability to imitate and to comprehend speech]. *Bulletin of Educational Psychology*, *6*, **113-120.** (In Chinese.)

The main purpose of this study is to investigate the relationship between socioeconomic level and children's ability to imitate and comprehend speech. The subjects were 32 kindergarten children, equally divided by sex; 16 were drawn from a low socioeconomic level and 16 from a high socioeconomic level. Speech imitation and speech comprehension tasks were designed to test the subjects' abilities to control 10 syntactic structures. The results indicated that: (1) The performance of children from the high socioeconomic level was significantly superior to that of children from the low socioeconomic level. (2) There were no significant differences between boys and girls. (3) Significant interrelationships were obtained among the variablies of intelligence, abilities of speech comprehension, and abilities of speech imitation.

728

Chen, S. M. (1976). [A study on the behavior of categorization in primary school children]. *Bulletin of Educational Psychology, 9,* **57-72.** (In Chinese.)

The main purpose of this study was to examine children's categorization behavior in relation to socioeconomic level and age. The subjects were 120 first-, third-, and fifth-grade children. The instruments were 32 color pictures. Each child was asked to choose the pictures which were alike in some way, and to state the basis on which they were chosen. Two scoring methods were used: (1) content analysis--responses were classified according to four attributes, global-descriptive, analytic-descriptive, relational, and inferential; and (2) structure analysis--responses were classified into three grouping structures, superordinate, complexity, and thematic. The results were: (1) Inferential and analytic-descriptive attributes used in grouping showed an increasing tendency with age, whereas relational and global-descriptive attributes showed a decreasing tendency; superordinate grouping structure showed an increasing tendency with age, whereas complexity showed a decreasing tendency. (2) As compared with those of children of a low socioeconomic level, responses of children of a high socioeconomic level reflected more superordinate, but less complexity, grouping structure; they also reflected relying more on inferential and analytic-descriptive, but less on global-descriptive and relational, attributes as the basis of grouping.

729

Chen, S. M. (1981). [A study of the parent-child relationship of Chinese school children]. *Bulletin of Educational Psychology, 14,* **173-187.** (In Chinese.)

Studied 2,112 children's perceptions of changes in their parents' childrearing practices. Ss in Grades 1-9 were administered the Parent-Child Relations Questionnaire; Ss in 1st, 4th, and 7th grades were administered the Tennessee Self-Concept Scale, Children's Locus of Control Scale, and the Emotional Maturity Scale. Children perceived that parental demands decreased with age. Males perceived more parental demand and punishment than females. There were significant correlations between perceived childrearing practices and internality, self-concept, emotional maturity, and behavioral problems of children.

730

Chen, S. M. (1984). [Parent-child relationship of Chinese gifted children]. *Bulletin of Educational Psychology, 17,* **131-150.** (In Chinese.)

731

Chen, Y. F. et al. (1981). [Investigations into the aspirations and learning interests of primary school pupils]. *Information on Psychological Sciences,* **No. 4, 26-31.** (In Chinese.)

Preliminary investigations were conducted on the personal aspirations and learning interests of higher-grade pupils in a primary school. On the whole, the pupils' school consciousness appeared to be developing satisfactorily, in that they were able to consider the requirements of duty and responsibility when thinking about their personal aspirations. Achievements were better in the main academic subjects, such as Chinese language, arithmetic, and English. They also showed greater interest and confidence in these subjects. Some problems pertaining to their personal aspirations and learning interests were also revealed.

732

Cheng, L. (1979). The role of play in early childhood: Some personal observations of Hong Kong preschool children. *Hong Kong Psychological Society Bulletin,* **No. 2, 27-32.**

Observed the play of 10 preschool children who participated in a playgroup at a university in Hong Kong as well as their neighborhood. In addition, extensive information was obtained from conversations with their parents. The importance of play in child development is discussed in terms of the contrasting views of Piaget and Freud. Characteristics (curiosity and high mobility) of children's play, limitations of play in Hong Kong, and some solutions to these limitations are included in the discussion.

733

Cheng, T. H., & Lee, M. K. (1960). [An investigation into the scope of the conception of numbers among 6-7 years old children]. *Acta Psychologica Sinica,* **No. 1, 28-35.** (In Chinese.)

This study attempted to discover the scope of 6 to 7 year old children's grasp of the conception of numbers, in order to make suggestions for the compilation of 1st year primary school arithmetic textbooks. Eighty-four 1st year primary school and top class infant school children took part. It was found that in grasping the conception of numbers less than 100, the children recognized the cardinal numbers, the ordinal numbers, understood their real significance and did calculations. These four aspects varied in the course of development. The grasp of the first aspect far exceeded that of the other three. Children's estimates of the quantity of objects were greatly influenced by the spatial arrangement of the given objects.

734

Chern, Y. H. (1978). [Moral judgment development in Chinese adolescents]. *Journal of Education* **(Kaoshung Normal College), 98-159.** (In Chinese.)

735

Cheung, F. M. C. (1979). Self-perception, cultural norm and development: Case studies of 36 Chinese women.

736

Cheung, F. M. C., Chau, B. T. W., & Lam, M. C. (1986). *Caretaking forms and styles in urban Hong Kong: A pilot study on three-year-old children* **(Occasional Papers 14). Hong Kong: Chinese University of Hong Kong, Centre for Hong Kong Studies.**

737

Cheung, K. N., Salili, F., & Lee, H. W. (1986). Adolescents' attitude toward sex education in Hong Kong. *New Horizons* **(The Journal of Education, Hong Kong Teachers' Association), No. 27, 78-90.**

738

Cheung, T. S. & Tam, S. Y. (1984). *An analysis of the self-esteem of adolescents in Hong Kong: Configurations and determinants^ (Occasional Report No. 5). Hong Kong: Chinese University of Hong Kong, Centre of Hong Kong Studies.*

739

Chi, C. (1986). Locus of control, sex of dyad and cooperative/competitive behavior in Chinese and American children. Dissertation Abstracts International, 46, *A2230-2231.*

740

Chi, G. Y. (1969). [How Chinese college students spend their leisure time]. National Chengchi University Journal *(Taiwan),* **19,** *167-202. (In Chinese.)*

741

Chi, W. H. (1977). [A study of youth's intelligence development in the Ami tribe in Taiwan]. Research in Education & Psychology, 1, *83-96. (In Chinese.)*

The population of the Ami tribe is about 90,000, being 38.3% of the total mountain people. They are distributed along the seashore region of the Taitung and Hwa-lian plains. Little research has been done on the education of the mountain people. This study investigated the intellectual development of young people among the Ami tribe. The Culture Fair Intelligence Test (scale 2) was administered to 574 students from Grades 1 to 3 and 1,675 students from Grades 3 to 6. The results were: (1) The intelligence scores increased with age. (2) Males scored higher than females. (3) Students in nonmountainous areas scored significantly higher than students from mountainous areas.

742

Chiang, J. S., & Costello, J. R. (1983). The acquisition of syntax in first and second language learning. IRAL: International Review of Applied Linguistics in Language Teaching, 21, *19-33.*

Presents data indicating that the language-learning capability of adolescents and adults acquiring a 2nd language differs from that of children acquiring their 1st language. 475 junior and senior high school students in Taiwan who were native speakers of Chinese but were studying English as a 2nd language completed a test that required them to translate sentences from English to Chinese. The sentences required Ss to distinguish the subject of each verb in simple and embedded sentences and to determine to whom a pronoun referred. This test was structurally identical to that administered by C. Chomsky (1969) to 40 children (aged 5-10 yrs) learning their 1st language. Ss in the current investigation were graded on whether the difficulty associated with a particular structure was translated correctly. Comparisons between the test results of the 2 populations indicate that those learning a 2nd language mastered sentence structures in a different sequence than did native speakers. Results are discussed in terms of neurolinguistics and implications for language teachers.

743

Chiang, Y. (1940). A Chinese childhood. *London: Methuen. (Republished New York: John Day, 1952; New York: Norton, 1963).*

744

Chien, M. F. (1978). [Impact of parental attitudes on adjustment of elementary school children]. Bulletin of Educational Psychology, 11, *63-86. (In Chinese.)*

Used the Parental Childrearing Behavior Questionnaire, the Chinese Revision of the California Test of Personality, and the Test of Parental Attitudes Toward Childrearing Practices to study the effects of parents' attitudes on 217 5th graders. The "loving" dimension of childrearing behavior had more influence than the "demanding" dimension on the Ss' adjustment. Children of warm-restrictive and warm-permissive parents were better adjusted, both personally and socially, than children of hostile-authoritarian and hostile-neglectful parents. Girls were more readily influenced than boys by parental attitudes. Parents' attitudes had a greater effect on children's personal adjustment than on their social adjustment.

745

Chien, M. F. (1980). [Intellectual development of Chinese children and adolescents]. Bulletin of Educational Psychology, 13, *95-117. (In Chinese.)*

A 2nd-yr report on a 3-yr longitudinal study analyzed the mental development of 688 elementary and junior high school students using the Progressive Matrices (PM), the WISC-R, Cognitive Abilities Test, and the Matching Familiar Figures Test. The mean scores of 2nd-, 5th-, and 8th graders on the PM and WISC-R were significantly higher than scores 1 yr before. Score improvements decreased significantly with increasing grade levels. There were significant correlations between intelligence and verbal, mathematical, and global academic achievements of the 5th- and 8th graders.

746

Chien, M. F. (1981). [The growth of intelligence in Chinese school children]. Bulletin of Educational Psychology, 14, *125-147. (In Chinese.)*

This is the third-year report on a study of the intellectual development of Chinese children and adolescents. The subjects were 2,115 students for the cross-sectional approach and 654 students for the longitudinal approach. They were drawn by stratified sampling from two elementary schools and two junior high schools in Taipei. The Progressive Matrices and the Chinese revision of Wechsler Intelligence Scale for Children were administered. The main results were: (1) The growth of intelligence of Chinese school children was most rapid in the primary grades, and thereafter growth occurred at a progressively decreasing rate. (2) Verbal intelligence correlated much more highly than nonverbal intelligence with academic achievement in various academic subjects.

747

Chien, M. F. (1982). [Creative thinking abilities of gifted children in Taiwan, Republic of China]. Bulletin of Educational Psychology, 15, *97-110. (In Chinese.)*

Investigated creative thinking in 420 gifted and 458 average children selected from 4 elementary and 3 junior high schools in the Taipei area. Ss completed the General Classification Test, Chinese versions of the Stanford-Binet Intelligence Scale and WISC-R, and the Torrance Tests of Creative Thinking. Data were subjected to ANOVA, trend analysis, and multiple regression analysis. Findings indicate that (1) in the fluency, flexibility, and originality aspects of creative thinking, gifted 4th, 6th, and 8th graders were significantly superior to their classmates of average intelligence; (2) the creative thinking abilities of gifted Ss increased with age; and (3) there were significant correlations between creativity and intelligence, physical fitness, and self-concept characteristics, as well as parent-child relationships in Ss.

748

Chien, M. F. (1983). [Factors related to peer interaction among school children]. Bulletin of Educational Psychology, 16, *71-88. (In Chinese.)*

The purposes of this study were to investigate peer relationships of school children and to find out factors influencing peer interaction among them. Subjects were 76 fourth graders, 74 fifth graders, and 78 sixth graders from one elementary school in Taipei city. A sociometric test, the Chinese Revision of the California Test of Personality, and the Test of Parental Attitudes toward Childrearing Practices were administered to the subjects in regular classroom settings. The data were statistically treated by the stepwise multiple regression technique. The main findings of the study were as follows: (1) Academic achievement of school children was the most important factor influencing peer interaction among them. (2) All measures of the factors could account for 44% to 55% of the variation in sociometric scores of the fourth, fifth, and sixth graders.

749

Chien, Y. C., & Lust, B. (1985). The concepts of topic and subject in first language acquisition in Mandarin Chinese. Child Development, 56, *1359-1375.*

The authors tested 95 children who were acquiring Mandarin Chinese as their 1st-language in Taiwan, using an elicited imitation task on a set of coordinate sentences and on a set of sentences related to equi-construction. It was hypothesized that if young children are sensitive to the presence of a grammatical subject they should distinguish topic and subject in equi-constructions. Findings provided evidence that young children acquiring Mandarin Chinese differentiate the concept of subject from the concept of topic, even though Chinese is topic-prominent. Results were discussed in terms of the implication that even for highly topic-oriented languages like Chinese, it is necessary to attribute to young children some sensitivity to formal grammatical concepts as well as semantic or pragmatic ones in 1st-language acquisition.

750

Child psychiatry in Shanghai. (1974). International Child Welfare Review, *No. 22-23, 16-20.*

751

Chiu, L. H. (1971). Manifested anxiety in Chinese and American children. Journal of Psychology, 79, *273-284.*

Administered the children's manifest anxiety scale to 381 American 4th and 5th grade children from 2 geographical areas of Indiana. A Chinese translation of the same test was administered to 613 Chinese children at the same grade levels and from 2 different geographical locations in Taiwan. Results show that (a) for both grade levels, the Chinese Ss obtained significantly higher scores than the American Ss on both the Anxiety and Lie scales; and (b) within each cultural group, girls were found to be more anxious than boys, and Ss from 1 geographical area to be more anxious than Ss from the other area. It is concluded that for sampling to be adequate the geographical location of samples should be given serious consideration in cross-cultural studies.

752

Chiu, L. H. (1972). Manifest anxiety in children with analytic and nonanalytic cognitive style. Perceptual & Motor Skills, 35, *406.*

Administered the Sigel Cognitive Style Test and the Children's Manifest Anxiety scale to 310 American and 220 Taiwanese 4th and 5th graders. Cognitive style scores identified 2 groups of 71 American and 2 groups of 48 Taiwanese analytic and nonanalytic Ss. No significant differences were found in anxiety scores between the 2 American subsamples. However, nonanalytic Taiwanese obtained significantly higher anxiety scores than analytic Taiwanese, supporting previous findings with Americans.

753

Chiu, W. C. (1982). [A study on the physique and physical fitness of Chinese gifted children]. Bulletin of Educational Psychology, 15, *19-29. (In Chinese.)*

Investigated differences in physique and physical fitness between 421 gifted children and 457 average children in Grades 4, 6, and 8 selected from 4 elementary schools and 3 junior high schools. Findings show that gifted Ss were greater than average Ss in (1) body height, sitting height, and length of lower limbs; (2) muscular power; (3) agility, flexibility, speed, and endurance; and (4) throwing ability for 4th-grade boys and 4th- and 6th-grade girls. Average Ss excelled at muscular strength and throwing ability for 6th- and 9th-grade boys and for 9th-grade girls.

754

Chiu, W. C., Su, C. W., & Hwang, C. H. (1967). [Physical and psychological development in relation to menarcheal age in school girls in Taipei area]. Psychology and Education, 1, *1-19. (In Chinese.)*

The main objective of this study was to determine the age of the first menstruation of Chinese girls and to investigate their psychological condition at that period. Based on data collected on 2,246 girls in Taipei, the mean age of reaching sexual maturity was found to be 13.4 years--very similar to findings reported in Western countries. There were very large individual differences in physical development among the girls. Some had their first period at the age of 11, whereas others had not reached maturity until 17. Girls at puberty differed from younger ones in attitudes toward the opposite sex, and in interests in movies, games, and leisure reading. They became more self-conscious than younger girls and tended to feel that their parents did not understand them. Also, many girls at puberty had little knowledge of their own physical development; as a consequence, anxiety and tension were very common.

755

Chiu, W. C., Su, C. W., & Hwang, C. H. (1968). [Physical and psychological development in relation to menarcheal age in school girls in Taiwan]. Psychology and Education, 2, *1-22. (In Chinese.)*

This study is a continuation of the authors' research into physical and psychological development in relation to menarcheal age in school girls in Taipei. The subjects were 8,790 school girls in Taichung, Tainan, Kaohsiung, and Hualien in Taiwan. Both rural and urban populations were represented. The data were combined with those collected in Taipei. The size of the entire sample was 11,036. It was found that the mean age of sexual maturation of school girls in Taiwan was 13.37 years. This was nearly identical to that for Taipei alone and was very similar to findings reported in Western countries. The whole range of the age of onset of puberty was, however, rather great. Those who were urban and of high socioeconomic status, and whose parents had better education, tended to reach maturity at an earlier age. After puberty, girls tended to become more self-conscious, to have a greater need for independence and increasing feelings that they were not understood by their parents. Generally, they showed a negative attitude toward their menstration, which apparently caused a great deal of anxiety due mainly to lack of information.

756

Chu, C. H. (1960). [The theory of child mental development in the light of Marxism]. Acta Psychologica Sinica, *No. 2, 115-127. (In Chinese.)*

The present paper dwells on the theory of child mental development from the Marxian point of view. Six problems are discussed: (1) two contradictory points of view concerning mental development; (2) heredity as the biological premise of mental development; (3) the determining significance of environment and education; (4) intrinsic cause (intrinsic contradiction) as the motivating force; (5) interrelations between education and mental development; and (6) age-dependent stages of development.

757

Chu, C. H., Chen, K. M., & Wu, F. K. (1964). [An experimental study on children's conceptions of left and right]. Acta Psychologica Sinica, *No. 3, 229-236. (In Chinese.)*

The present study was a systematic replication of experiments performed by Piaget and Elkind. The findings of this study were fundamentally the same as the two previous experiments. There was no more than a year's discrepancy in the results of the age levels at which the tests were passed, and the stages of development were similar. Despite such similarities, the authors provided alternative interpretation of the results.

758

Chu, C. P. (1970). A study of the effects of maternal employment for the preschool children in Taiwan. Acta Psychologica Taiwanica, 12, *80-100.*

Compared 20 mothers who were employed with 20 who were not employed, each with a child in kindergarten. All Ss were of average or above average socioeconomic status and were interviewed, using a modified form of the Mother's Interview Schedule of R. R. Sears and Y. M. Wang. Data indicate that working mothers (a) give less time and personal care to their children and are less responsive to the child's crying; (b) are less strict toward the child's general behavior, but more strict toward eating and toilet training processes; (c) give more praise for obedience but may punish for dependency; (d) have higher self-esteem as individuals; and (e) delegate more housework and child care to their husbands. It is noted that the children of working mothers appear to demand more attention and need more love than children of nonworking mothers. A reproduction of the Mother's Interview Schedule is included.

759

Chu, C. P. (1971). Children's problem solving on the discovery of a principle. Acta Psychologica Taiwanica, 13, *25-35.*

This paper presents a modification and extension of Heibreder's study on children's problem-solving behavior. Fifty subjects were chosen for studies on developmental and experimentally manipulated effects. The results showed that there were many items reflecting age differences. Age groups beyond 5 1/2 years old showed marked superiority in problem solving behavior. The group aged from 7 1/2 to 8 1/2 years could even compete with adults in some aspects, such as giving many various kinds of reasons, and using generalization to solve problems. The presentation order of problems affected the children's ability to give reasons for their choice of answers. Cultural differences also had effects on later development.

760

Chu, C. P. (1974). Parental attitudes in relation to young children's creativity: Cross-cultural comparison. Acta Psychologica Taiwanica, 16, *53-72.*

This is a cross-cultural study of parental attitudes and creativity in American and Chinese children. The subjects were 72 preschool children, divided into four groups: American-middle class, American-lower class, Chinese-middle class, and Chinese-lower class. Tests of creativity included the Uses Test, the Picture Construction Test, and the Freedom Test. Parental attitudes were measured with the Parental Attitudes Research Instrument. The results showed that: (1) Chinese children scored higher on fluency, and American children scored higher on originality. (2) Chinese parents used more authoritarian control, but they also had closer relationships with their children. (3) Sex and socioeconomic differences (favoring middle-class children) were present in both American and Chinese groups.

761

Chu, C. P. (1975). The development of differential cognitive abilities in relation to children's perceptions of their parents. Acta Psychologica Taiwanica, 17, *47-62.*

Parent-child relations and the cognitive abilities of children in Taiwan were studied. The subjects, 301 4th, 5th, and 6th graders, were given the California Test of Mental Maturity (Short Form), the Torrance Tests of Creative Thinking, and modified forms of the Parent-Child Relation Questionnaire (father and mother). The results showed that for girls, but not for boys, significant positive correlations, with a few exceptions, were obtained between perceived positive parental attitudes (protecting, loving, rewarding, and being casual) and both verbal and nonverbal aspects of convergent and divergent abilities. Significant negative correlations were obtained between perceived negative parental attitudes (rejecting, demanding, neglecting, and punitive) and these abilities; these negative correlations were more often found between opposite-sex parents and children than between same-sex parents and children.

762

Chu, L. (1979). The sensitivity of Chinese and American children to social influences. Journal of Social Psychology, 109, *175-186.*

320 Chinese (C) and American (A) 2nd graders were exposed to experimental treatments (e.g., material reinforcement and model status/competence manipulations), and their imitation of the choices of 40 models in a paired setting was analyzed. As compared to a single, continuous measurement of imitation, a 2-dimensional conformity/anticonformity/independence framework was more discriminative and was able to show the following cultural differences: (a) more Cs were either conformers or anticonformers, and more As were independent of the model's choice; (b) Cs were more sensitive, whereas As were more indifferent to the status/competence treatments of the model; and (c) C girls conformed more than C boys, whereas no difference was found between A girls and boys. The

material reinforcement used failed to significantly influence either group. F. L. Hsu's (1970) hypothesis that Cs are socialized earlier in life and are more responsive to environmental influences than As was partly supported.

763

Chuang, C. J. (1973). [The factors of grade and school achievement in concept formation of children]. Acta Psychologica Taiwanica, 15, *54-58. (In Chinese.)*

The purposes of this experiment were to clarify how conceptual ability develops and the relationship between conceptual ability and school achievement. Based on their school grades, subjects were divided into five groups. The concepts of direction, number, and movement were tested. The development of conceptual ability for students in grades 1 to 5 was continuous, and was significantly related to school achievement.

764

Chung, S. K., & Hwang, K. Y. (1984). [Leisure activities of the elderly]. Journal of Education & Psychology, 7, *119-143. (In Chinese.)*

This study investigated how the elderly in Taipei City participate in leisure activities. Subjects were 781 elderly with an age above 65 years old. Subjects were interviewed and given a Questionnaire on Leisure Activities of Aging. The results were: (1) Ten of the most frequent leisure activities that the elderly participated in were watching television, walking, reading, house keeping, visiting, taking care of grandchildren, listening to the radio, gardening, religious activities, and climbing. (2) The participation time was early morning, evening, or unfixed time, and the places were their home and neighborhood. (3) The purposes of their participation were mostly to kill time and to provide physical exercise for health. (4) Five of the least frequent but most favorite activities were traveling, climbing, visiting, seeing a movie, and gardening; these activities were limited because of their physical and financial problems.

765

Chung, Y. J. & Jamie, B. (1967). Studies in adolescent behavior and culture patterns in Hong Kong. *Unpublished master's thesis, University of Hong Kong.*

766

Clumeck, H. (1979). A parallel between child and adult language: A study in the phonetic explanation of sound patterns. Journal of Child Language, 6, *593-598.*

Documents a sound substitution used by a Mandarin-speaking girl (studied from the age of 1 yr 10 mo to 2 yrs 10 mo), demonstrates how this substitution is paralleled in adult language by sound correspondences across a variety of Chinese dialects, and proposes a phonetic explanation for the facts from both child and adult language.

767

Cohen, T. B. (1977). Observations on school children in the People's Republic of China. Journal of the American Academic Child Psychiatry, 16, *165-173.*

During a 3 weeks' visit to the People's Republic of China, the author made behavioral observations and found no evidence to contradict Chinese claims of marked improvement in physical and mental health of children in the 25 years since the revolution. Prostitution, child abuse, delinquency, and drug addiction have been sharply curtailed by severe control, employing shaming and guilt induction. Birth control is widely practiced, and children's needs have priority. However, disapproval of individualism seems to inhibit a true "hatching" of personalities. Decreased creativity and curiosity are likely casualties of the strict containment of drives.

768

Cohen, T. B. (1981). Preventive implications of the effect of varying cultures on drive organization: Focus on People's Republic of China. Journal of Preventive Psychiatry, 1, *29-36.*

Prevention of mental illness in children requires an understanding of the interaction of nature and nurture. Vulnerability (nature/genetic) interacts with risk (nurture/environment) to establish mental health or illness. This article discusses the child who is a victim of his/her environment acting against the developmental process itself. Sociologists' view of personality development is described. The psychoanalytic theory of object relations and identification can be translated into the language of role and social structure. Children absorb their culture through diverse exposures and communications, their impulses are harnessed and channeled, and they receive training for social participation. Observational data on the People's Republic of China is used to examine claims that drug and alcohol addiction, child abuse, venereal disease, teenage pregnancy, and juvenile delinquency were eliminated in one generation. How the Chinese control sexual and aggressive drives is described, and their efforts to foster early secondary narcissism are examined. Speculation is made about the effects of severe drive control on the inhibition of creativity and a lack of curiosity.

769

Condon, W. S., & Sander, L. W. (1974). Synchrony demonstrated between movements of the neonate and adult speech. Child Development, 45, *456-462.*

Explored the possibility that there is a correspondence between sound segments of adult speech and points of change in neonate movement. One-hour observations of 16 normal neonates in awake-active states were videotaped or sound-filmed and analyzed frame-by-frame. Frames were judged as a "hit" or a "miss" (discrepancy) in terms of the correspondence between the analysis of speech segments (within phone, phone boundary, and word boundary) and that of body movement (process units for heel, elbows, shoulders, hips, and feet). A comparison between the speech and body movement in 1 2-day-old S is detailed. Results show a correspondence between adult speech and infant movement in all 16 Ss (14 of which were 2 hrs-2 days of age). Evidence of sustained movement synchrony over speech segments appeared regardless of whether (a) the speaker was present and addressing the infant or a tape-recording was used, (b) Chinese or American-English was spoken, or (c) infants were supine or helped. Findings reveal a complex interactional system which suggests that infant motor organization is entrained by the pattern of adult speech over many months from birth; this system may underlie later developmental implanting of speech.

770

Cook, H., & Chi, C. (1984). Cooperative behavior and locus of control among American and Chinese-American boys. Journal of Psychology, 118, *169-177.*

Cooperative behavior and the effect of locus of control were investigated in American (n = 64) and Chinese-American (n = 75) boys aged 8-10 years. The subjects from two ethnically homogeneous, lower middle-class, urban Catholic schools were administered the Nowicki-Strickland Locus of Control Scale for Children. Nineteen external and 12 internal American subjects and 15 external and 15 internal Chinese-American subjects were randomly paired into groups of internal, external, and mixed locus-of-control dyads, yielding a 2 * 3 between-subjects design. Each pair played a cooperative board game, with latency to achieve a goal the major dependent measure. Results indicated that: (a) overall, Chinese-Americans were significantly more external than Americans and, when matched on locus of control, were significantly more cooperative than Americans; (b) external dyads were significantly more cooperative than internal or mixed dyads; and (c) in mixed dyads, Chinese-Americans took significantly less time, indicating they were more cooperative than Americans. Findings suggested the importance of the role that cultural context plays in the socialization process.

771

Davis-Friedman, D. (1979). Field research report: The urban elderly in China. China Exchange Newsletter, 7, *2-4.*

772

Dawson, J. L., Young, B. M., & Choi, P. P. (1973). Developmental influences on geometric illusion susceptibility among Hong Kong Chinese children. Journal of Cross-Cultural Psychology, 4, *49-74.*

Hong Kong Chinese developmental results are presented to test cross-cultural developmental theories relating to changes in illusion susceptibility with age. The Muller-Lyer (M-L) and Sander-Parallelogram (S-P) illusion data confirm the expected decrease in 3-12 yr. olds and the later increase in 21 yr. olds due to exposure to a more sophisticated environment. Data also supported the hypotheses regarding contiguous and noncontiguous versions of the Horizontal-Vertical (H-V) illusions. The U.S., Hong Kong, and Arunta cross-cultural comparisons also support the "carpentered world hypothesis", while H-V illusion susceptibility was also related to ecologically valid desert/urban differences in habits of perceptual inference. However, intersample differences in retinal pigmentation and the cross-sectional nature of the study may have influenced the results.

773

Dawson, J. L., Young, B. M., & Choi, P. P. C. (1974). Developmental influences in pictorial depth perception among Hong Kong Chinese children. Journal of Cross-Cultural Psychology, 5, *3-22.*

Presents a developmental model of expected age trends and sex differences in the acquisition of 3-dimensional picture perception (3DPP). 212 Chinese males and 240 females from nursery, elementary, and secondary schools completed a battery of psychological tests, including the Chinese 3DPP Test, measures of photographic depth perception, the Chinese Socialization Scale, and the Rod and Frame Test. Data support the expected increase in 3DPP in Ss aged 3-17 and the expected superiority of males in 3DPP after age 8; these differences are thought to stem from increased testosterone output after that age, which stimulates the development of cholinergic inhibitory perceptual processes, and interacts with the appropriate cultural-educational stimuli to result in better 3DPP skills in male Ss. Lower socioeconomic levels, field dependence, "harsher" socialization, and more traditional attitudes were associated with lower 3DPP scores, while data from J. W. Berry's study of Eskimo Ss suggest that Eskimos had higher 3DPP scores than the Hong Kong Chinese.

774

de Boysson-Bardies, B., Sagart, L., & Durand, C. (1984). Discernible differences in the babbling of infants according to target language. Journal of Child Language, 11, *1-15.*

Presented, in 2 experiments, samples of babbling productions of 6-, 8-, and 10-mo-old infants from different language backgrounds (French, Arabic, and Chinese) to a total of 88 adult native speakers of

French whose task was to identify the infants from their own linguistic community. Results show that certain language-specific metaphonological cues render this identification possible when the samples exhibit long and coherent intonation patterns. At 8 mo, identification scores in Exp I were clearly positive and stable across judges. Probability of correct identification was found to be closely related to certain dimensions of speech. In Exp I, samples from 8-10 mo olds were characterized by long productions involving patterns of pitch and intensity. In Exp II, samples from 10-mo-olds were extracted from highly articulated productions of reduplicated babbling that were poorer in prosodic cues. The segmental indications that were present in the fully syllabic productions of canonical babbling did not allow the judges to identify the infants correctly from their own linguistic community. These results seem to support the hypothesis of an early influence on babbling of the metaphonological characteristics of the target language.

775

Dennis, W. (1966). Group values through children's drawings. *New York: Wiley.*

776

Department of Education, Shanxi Normal University (1979). [Psychological analysis of a mathematics competition in primary shcool children]. Acta Psychologica Sinica, 11, *287-292. (In Chinese.)*

777

Devoy, J. (1969). Personality development in three cultures: A comparative analysis of middle class White Americans, lower class Negro Americans in the urban north and southern working class Chinese. International Social Work, 12, *38-47.*

778

Dien, D. S. (1982). A Chinese perspective on Kohlberg's theory of moral development. Developmental Review, 2, *331-341.*

Discusses contextual problems of L. Kohlberg's (1969) theory of moral development using the Chinese culture as an example and to point to a new direction for cross-cultural research. The Western view of humans as autonomous beings who make free and rational choices as moral agents is clearly reflected in Kohlberg's stages of moral development as well as in his methodology. The Confucian view of humans as integral parts of an orderly universe with an innate moral sense to maintain harmony is quite different. The preferred mode of resolving human conflict in China is reconciliation and collective decision making rather than individual choice, commitment, and responsibility, as in the West. In light of these fundamental differences in the 2 cultural traditions, an alternative to Kohlberg's theory is suggested, based on J. Youniss's interpretation of Piaget's conception of moral development, with attention paid to cultural variation in the definition of moral maturity and to the developmental process.

779

Dien, D. S. (1984). A Chinese perspective on Kohlberg's theory of moral development. Annual Progress in Child Psychiatry & Child Development, *85-97.*

Discusses contextual problems of L. Kohlberg's (1969) theory of moral development using the Chinese culture as an example and to point to a new direction for cross-cultural research. The Western view of humans as autonomous beings who make free and rational choices as moral agents is clearly reflected in Kohlberg's stages of moral development as well as in his methodology. The Confucian view of humans as integral parts of an orderly universe with an innate moral sense to maintain harmony is quite different. The preferred mode of resolving human conflict in China is reconciliation and collective decision making rather than individual choice, commitment, and responsibility, as in the West. In light of these fundamental differences in the 2 cultural traditions, an alternative to Kohlberg's theory is suggested, based on J. Youniss's interpretation of Piaget's conception of moral development, with attention paid to cultural variation in the definition of moral maturity and to the developmental process.

780

Ding, Z. Y. (1984). [The development of thought process of elementary schoolchildren]. Acta Psychologica Sinica, 16, *139-146. (In Chinese.)*

781

Ding, Z. Y., & Ha, Y. M. (1983). [Development of children's ability in color discrimination]. Information on Psychological Sciences, *No. 2, 14-17. (In Chinese.)*

782

Dixon, J. (1981). The welfare of urban youth in China 1949-79. Journal of Adolescence, 4, *1-12.*

Outlines the range of policies and programs that have emerged in China since 1949 to promote the welfare of young people in the city. Factors include the encouragement and decline of out-of-school activities for adolescents, delays in assigning them jobs, and their experience with compulsory and permanent transfer to the countryside. There is evidence of weakening family discipline and a confusion about youth's role in Chinese society. It is concluded that responses to these factors have not been effective.

783

Donohue, N., & Colletta, N. J. (1977). The child and his surroundings: The ecology of child development on a Malaysian rubber plantation. International Child Welfare Review, *No. 32, 24-46.*

Presents findings from a study of child development in Malay, Chinese, and Indian laborer families on a rubber plantation in West Malaysia. Three factors affecting development were emphasized: socioeconomic conditions, child-rearing/family interaction patterns, and nutritional/health variables. Interviews and observations of the families were conducted, and data related to cultural group membership, the nature of the production process and its management by European authority, geographic isolation, illiteracy and immobility, male and female role structure, attitudes toward education, and socialization patterns are presented. It is concluded that although there are differences in cultural interactions as expressed in child-rearing patterns, the similarities in socioeconomic and health conditions make the environment homogeneous for the children.

784

Douglas, J. D., & Wong, A. C. (1977). Formal operations: Age and sex differences in Chinese and American children. Child Development, 48, *689-692.*

60 Hong Kong Chinese and 60 American adolescents were given 3 Piagetian tasks of formal operations in order to assess cultural, age, and sex differences. Significant effects were demonstrated: American Ss performed at a more advanced level than Chinese Ss; 15-yr-olds were more advanced than 13-yr-olds; and males performed better than females. Chinese females demonstrated the lowest scores on each of the tasks. Results support previous findings in emphasizing the importance of the milieu and are discussed in terms of the need to consider sex differences, particularly on tasks of formal operations.

785

Eicher, C. E., & Wood, R. W. (1977). An investigation of elementary children's perceptions of selected countries of the world. Education, 98, *82-90.*

Used an open-ended questionnaire employing the words The World, China, India, and Nigeria to examine 300 1st-6th graders' perceptions of those concepts. Results show that (a) younger Ss described the words mostly in reference to their immediate environment, (b) TV played an important role in perception, (c) there appeared to be a movement toward objective understanding with increased age, and (d) all Ss exhibited stereotypes and lack of understanding of the words.

786

Ekblad, S. (1982). Kinas nya barn: Barnuppfostran, livsvillkor, familje politik *[China's new children: Childrearing, conditions for growth, and family policy]. Stockholm, Sweden: Natur & Kultur. (In other language.)*

787

Ekblad, S. (1984). Children's thoughts and attitudes in China and Sweden: Impacts of a restrictive versus a permissive environment. Acta Psychiatrica Scandinavica, 70, *578-590.*

With a restrictive-permissive frame of reference, this study explores how children in Sweden and China come to behave in accordance with cultural values and the price they have to pay for doing so. The subjects were 273 school children (about 11-12 years old) from six cities, and 49 preschool children (aged 6-7 years old) from 10 cities in China; the Swedish children (329 and 48) were drawn from a single community. Despite acknowledged limitations, the overall findings confirmed two hypotheses: (1) Chinese children learn to control their emotions to a greater extent than Swedish children, and (2) Chinese children learn to orient towards collective norms, as opposed to Swedish children who are more individualistically oriented.

788

Eysenck, S. B., & Chan, J. (1982). A comparative study of personality in adults and children: Hong Kong vs England. Personality & Individual Differences, 3, *153-160.*

The 90-item adult version of the Eysenck Personality Questionnaire (EPQ) was translated into Chinese and administered to 270 male (mean age 22.34 yrs) and 462 female (mean age 22.68 yrs) in Hong Kong. In a 2nd study the 81-item version of the Junior EPQ was translated into Chinese and given to 698 boys and 629 girls (aged 7-15 yrs). Reasonably valid scales for use in Hong Kong are suggested for both adult and junior forms of the questionnaire. In a direct comparison of British and Chinese (Hong Kong) groups, using reduced scales comprising only items both scoring keys had in common, Hong Kong adults scored higher on Psychoticism and Social Desirability and lower on Extraversion than the British. Children from Hong Kong scored lower on Extraversion and Neuroticism but higher on Social Desirability than their British counterparts. Indexes of factor comparison were universally high, indicating that the major dimensions of personality were very similar in Hong Kong Chinese as in British Ss.

789

Fan, C. R., & Zhou, Z. F. (1983). [On the developmental pattern of intelligence in children from birth to six years]. Acta Psychologica Sinica, 15, *429-444. (In Chinese.)*

790

Fang, F. X. (1983). [A preliminary study of 4-6 year-old children's representation of moving objects]. Acta Psychologica Sinica, 15, *70-79. (In Chinese.)*

Children 4-6 years of age were asked to represent the motion of horizontally moving, down-tilting, and falling objects. It was found that the ability to represent the motion of these objects had already developed. Preschoolers not only paid attention to the static status of the objects, but also began to gradually understand the processes of motional transformation. Training could accelerate the development of motional representation, and the effect of training increased with age.

791

Fang, F. X. (1985). [Preschoolers' ability to tell animate from inanimate objects]. Acta Psychologica Sinica, 17, *62-70. (In Chinese.)*

This is a study of childrens' ability to differentiate animate from inanimate objects. Preschool children were asked four types of questions concerning actions, parts, mental states, and reciprocal ability concerning objects. The results showed: (1) Preschoolers, even at 3 years of age, were able to distinguished a person from not only a rock but also a doll. They did not attribute the characteristics of animate objects (e.g., a person) to inanimate objects (e.g., a rock or a doll). (2) The children's identification of a person, a rock, or a doll was based not only on the movement or stillness of the object, but also on the parts or materials of which it is made, its origin, properties, and functions. The 3-year-olds were able to distinguish a person from a doll according to endogenous movements or movements produced by an external agent. (3) The children's understanding of the distinction between animate and inanimate objects proceeded from external to internal characteristics, from analysis to integration, and from appearance to reality. Their ability to make distinctions is directly related to the understanding of causality, the cause of movement, and the basic knowledge about objects.

792

Fang, F. X. (1985). [An experiment on the use of classifiers by 4 to 6 years old]. Acta Psychologica Sinica, 17, *384-392. (In Chinese.)*

In the present study, 4 to 6-year-old children speaking Mandarin or Cantonese and bilingual overseas Chinese children in the same age group were tested for their ability to use some of the common classifiers with the objects shown to them through pictures. This was followed by another test for their ability to generalize four classifiers among a number of novel objects called by pseudo names. The results showed that the 4-year-olds' ability to use classifiers was poor, but their ability improved quickly with age. The usage of basic common classifiers was learned by the end of the preschool period. Dialect and foreign language were both important variables which had strong effects on the children's ability. The development of such ability was also found to be closely related to the cognitive development of abstract thinking and the power of generalization.

793

Fang, F. X., & Fang, G. (1986). [A preliminary experiment on preschooler's ability of classification]. Acta Psychologica Sinica, 18, *157-165. (In Chinese.)*

A modified Piagetian's class inclusion task and a simplified classification task were presented to preschoolers. The results indicated: (1) The ability to solving class inclusion problem was facilitated by three factors: endowing general class with the common attributions of perception; highlighting the common attributions in instruction; and comparing sub-class with general-class by counting performance. (2) Several stages were involved in solving the class inclusion problem. (3) The hierarchical structure of class was shown in the child 3 to 4 years old when familiar stimuli were manipulated in a simplified task of classification.

794

Fang, G., Ekblad, S., Li, W. F., Wu, N. Y., & Liu, F. (1982). [A study of the interrelation between direct and indirect cognitive components in the cognitive development of children aged 4-6 years]. Acta Psychologica Sinica, 14, *326-334. (In Chinese.)*

The purpose of this experiment was to analyze the influence of three different conditions (using concrete objects, photos or pictures, and verbal instructions) on children's counting, manual operation, and comparing, so as to explore the role played by the relationship between direct and indirect cognitive components in these cognitive processes. The subjects were 89 children aged 4 to 6 years. The results showed: (1) Manual operation based on photos differed significantly from that based on verbal instructions. (2) Counting using concrete objects differed significantly from counting using photos in the 5-year-old group. (3) No significant difference was found between using pictures and using photos. It appeared that children's cognitive processes resulted from the interaction between direct and indirect cognitive components.

795

Fang, G., Fang, F. X., & Liu, F. (1984). [A study of the development of children's cognition of time sequence (I)]. Acta Psychologica Sinica, 16, *165-173. (In Chinese.)*

The purpose of this study is to explore the development of children's cognition of time sequence within a day (morning, afternoon, evening) and its extension (yesterday evening, tomorrow morning), as well as the relativity of time sequence itself. The results indicated that children of 5 to 6 years of age correctly understand time sequence within a day, but 4-year-olds cannot. The 7-year-olds know well the relativity of time sequence. Children's comprehension of time sequence is related to their own experiences. The development of temporal words and the cognition of temporal relations facilitate each other.

796

Fang, G., Fang, F. X., & Liu, F. (1984). [The development of children's cognition of the sequence of time (II)]. Acta Psychologica Sinica, 16, *250-258. (In Chinese.)*

The purpose of this study was to explore children's cognition of time sequence within longer time periods, such as weeks and seasons. It was found that preschool children are able to understand time sequence within a week, but have great difficulty with time sequence within a year. In conjunction with those of a previous study, the present results show that the length of the time period is one important factor in the cognition of time sequence; and that this cognition proceeds from close to far and from short to long periods.

797

Fang, G., & Liu, F. (1981). [The development of children's cognition of velocity of moving objects (I)]. Acta Psychologica Sinica, 13, *21-29. (In Chinese.)*

This study explored children's cognition of velocity at different ages. The subjects were 140 children from 4 to 10 years old. Individual tests were used. The subjects were asked to make a comparison of the velocities of two toy cars moving simultaneously and uniformly at the same speed, under four experimental conditions. After the child had made each judgment, the experimenter asked him to give a reason for his answer, regardless of whether the answer was correct or not. The results indicated that children's abilities in judging velocity were fairly intercorrelated, and that there was a definite consistency in reactions of the same child to different test items.

798

Fang, G., & Liu, F. (1981). [The development of children's cognition of the velocity of moving objects (II)]. Acta Psychologica Sinica, 13, *273-279. (In Chinese.)*

The full results of this research on children's cognition of velocity are: (1) In comparing velocities, children develop from relying on beginning and ending points in space and time to relying on integrating the time-space process. Children's cognition of velocity develops from part to whole. (2) The effect of the relative positions of moving objects is earlier and stronger than that of their distance. (3) The space factor has a stronger effect than the time factor. The effect of the beginning and ending time of moving objects is much stronger than that of the duration of movement. (4) The development of cognition of velocity accelerates when children are about 7-8 years old. (5) Cognition of velocity develops through recognizing and resolving contradictions in the perception and conception of motion. (6) Children develop the basic internal conditions for forming the concept of velocity by the age of 10.

799

Fang, G., & Liu, F. (1983). [The development of children's cognition of velocity of two moving light-spots]. Acta Psychologica Sinica, 15, *59-69. (In Chinese.)*

This study explored further the development of children's cognition of velocity. The subjects were 205 children from 5 to 11 years old, divided by age into seven groups of 28 or 30. Individual tests were adopted. Two light-spots moving simultaneously and uniformly at the same speed under three experimental conditions were presented. The subjects were asked to make a comparison of the velocities of the two moving light spots. After each trial the subject was asked to give the reason for his answer. The results indicated: (1) The characteristics of the development of children's cognition of velocity were the same as those obtained in a former experiment using moving toy cars. (2) There were differences in results between the present and the former experiment: Beginning from age 8, the frequency of judging velocities according to the distance between the two light spots increased with age; the superior effect of the spatial factor decreased when the children could not integrate both spatial and temporal factors. (3) Some older children actively used various strategies to solve problems presented by the experimenter.

800

Feldman, D. H. (1969). The fixed sequence hypothesis ethnic differences in the development of spatial reasoning. Dissertation Abstracts International, 30, *B1884.*

801

Feldman, D. H., & Markwalder, W. (1971). Systematic scoring of ranked distractors for the assessment of Piagetian reasoning levels. Educational & Psychological Measurement, 31, *347-362.*

Attempted to determine if a map reading test could be used to assess both a child's map reading skill and his level of reasoning ability according to Piaget's theory of cognitive development. The latter would be assessed by the analysis of the child's choice of distractors. A new instrument for measuring spatial reasoning was designed and validated based on conceptual analysis of a geographic map. All 25 items were designed to induce responses indicative of the 4 reasoning levels suggested by Piaget. The sample included 270 5th, 7th, and 9th graders evenly distributed across 3 different ethnic groups (black, white, and Chinese). The results tend to indicate that the instrument devised may be capable of measuring reasoning stage levels as well as map achievement. Results also show that children of different ethnic backgrounds tend to go through the same set of developmental stages and that children of specific developmental levels tend to select distractor indications of that level.

802

Feng, S. J., Song, J., & Tong, L. Q. (1980). [An experimental study on children's ability to generalize terms in sentence groups]. Acta Psychologica Sinica, 12, *226-234. (In Chinese.)*

This study explored the development of children's ability to generalize terms. Nine groups of sentences were used as test materials, consisting of one, two or three terms ("factors"). Subjects were required to generalize them. The subjects were 150 children aged from 8.5 to 12 years, divided into groups of 30 by age. The results indicated that the development of children's ability to generalize terms was not completely correlated with the increase of age, and was different in speed and grade. Between the age group of 8.5-9 and the age group of 11-12, the differences were significant. In other age groups, the development of ability was slow.

803

Feng, Z. L., Zhang, X. Y., & Wang, X. P. (1984). [Experimental research on controlled mastery of concepts]. Acta Psychologica Sinica, 16, *147-154. (In Chinese.)*

This is an experimental research on the efficiency of controlled mastery of concepts in class teaching. The results suggested that controlled mastery could improve the students' ability to master concepts. The effect seemed stable. The correct action cultivated could be transferred to learning new concepts in different areas. Teaching with this method affected positively all students; it was particularly helpful to low- and medium-level performers. The researchers hold that the advantage of this method comes from integrating concepts with actions.

804

Field, C. E., & Baber, F. M. (1973). Growing up in Hong Kong. *Hong Kong: Hong Kong University Press.*

805

Flavell, J. H. et al. (1983). A comparison between the development of the appearance-reality distinction in the People's Republic of China and the United States. Cognitive Psychology, 15, *459-466.*

The 1st author et al reported 3 experiments on the development of the appearance-reality (AR) distinction in American 3-5 yr olds. The experiments assessed the children's ability to distinguish between and correctly identify real vs apparent object properties (color, size, and shape); object identities; object presence-absence; and action identities. The present study replicated Exp 2 with Chinese preschoolers. The American sample consisted of 24 31/2-4 yr olds and 24 41/2-5 yr olds; the Chinese sample was identical to the American sample. Stimuli were 4 highly realistic-looking imitation objects. Findings show that the error patterns, age changes, and absolute levels of performance were similar in the 2 samples. The most noteworthy cross-national similarities were that (1) younger Ss in both samples seemed to show at least some beginning ability to make the AR distinction and (2) older Ss performed significantly better than younger ones, suggesting that the ability may undergo considerable development during this particular year of early childhood in both cultures.

806

Fong, S. L. M. (1968). Identity conflicts of Chinese adolescents in San Francisco. In E. B. Brody (Ed.), Minority group adolescents in the United States. *Baltimore: Williams & Wilkins.*

807

Fowler, W., & Swenson, A. (1979). The influence of early language stimulation on development: Four studies. Genetic Psychology Monographs, 100, *73-109.*

In a series of 4 studies, 15 infants were stimulated for a mean of 7 mo (between the mean ages of 5.4 and 12.3 mo) in language processes mediated through tutoring parents. The program consisted of language labeling in 6 common caregiving and play activities. Development was assessed through the Griffiths Mental Development Scale for Testing Babies from Birth to Two Years and the Receptive Expressive Emergent Language Scale, parent records, and tape recordings. Mean Griffiths language gains for both sexes, infants from parents with high and low education levels, and English, Italian, and Chinese speaking homes all exceeded 32 points, compared to maximum nonlanguage scale gains of 19.4 points. At 18 mo, follow-up mean language and nonlanguage scores on 10 Ss remained stable. Through 42 mo, Ss in Study 2 were superior in language and counting skills and high average on other abilities. Process measures indicated a constant acquisition order for basic language dimensions, but rate and content were highly influenced by experience.

808

Freedman, D. G. (1971). An evolutionary approach to research on the life cycle. Human Development, 14, *87-99.*

The evolutionist sees the influence of phylogeny at all points of the life cycle; and evolutionary theory is both a fruitful source of ideas and a powerful explanatory tool in the study of human behavior. This paper reports various empirical studies that illustrate these points. For example, in pairs of fraternal and identical twins observed over the first year of life identicals were substantially more alike than fraternals in smiling, vocalizing and attending to mother. Newborns of various ethnic groups were demonstrably different on measures of temperament. Differences in the biologically adaptive role of the sexes appear in humans (e.g., females in infancy and in adolescence show more affiliative behavior than males; boys show more preoccupation with dominance hierarchies than girls; men react differentially to pictures in which secondary sex characteristics, beards and breasts, are present or absent).

809

Freedman, D. G. (1974). Human infancy: An evolutionary perspective. *Hillsdale, NJ: Erlbaum.*

810

Freedman, D. G., & DeBoer, M. M. (1979). Biological and cultural differences in early child development. Annual Review of Anthropology, 8, *579-600.*

Part 1 presents an overview of studies showing ethnic differences in newborn behavior; Part 2 includes a more selective review of the sex-difference literature, focusing on cross-cultural findings in social behavior. Cross-cultural differences in infant behavior are reviewed in studies of Chinese, Caucasian, and Japanese; Navajo and Hopi; sub-Saharan Africans, Jamaicans, and Afro-Americans; Balinese; Australian Aboriginals; and Puerto Ricans, Guatemalans, and Mexicans. The sex-difference literature suggests that prepubertal boys and girls differ with respect to aggression, dominance, nurturance, and movement in space. Directions are suggested for research on these phenomena.

811

Freedman, D. G., & Freedman, N. C. (1969). Behavioural differences between Chinese-American and European-American newborns. Nature, 224, *1227.*

812

Fuchs, E. (1976). Youth in a changing world: Cross-cultural perspectives on adolescence. *Hague, Netherlands: Mouton.*

Presents a series of 20 papers on the cultural context of, and growth and health care in, adolescence. Topics include development patterns in New Guinean and West African communities, psychotherapy in adolescents, aspects of mental illness among Puerto Rican adolescents in New York, parental authority and family size in China, and psychological correlates of family socialization in the US and Korea.

813

Gabrenya, W. K., Wang, Y. E., & Latane, B. (1985). Social loafing on an optimizing task: Cross-cultural differences among Chinese and Americans. Journal of Cross-Cultural Psychology, 16, *223-242.*

The authors examined whether members of group-oriented cultures such as the Chinese would be less likely than members of individualistic cultures to exhibit "social loafing"--a phenomenon in which people exert greater effort when they work individually than when they do so in a group that obscures identifiability of members' individual inputs. Eighty Chinese and 72 U.S. schoolchildren in the sixth and ninth grades performed an auditory tracking task that required counting tone patterns alone and in pairs. Americans evidenced social loafing on this task, whereas Chinese exhibited the opposite pattern ("social striving"), performing better in pairs than alone. Alternate sources of this cultural difference in social loafing within the global group-orientedness variable were proposed.

814

Gallin, B. (1967). Emerging individualism in changing rural Taiwan. Journal of China Society *(Taipei),* **5,** *3-8.*

815

Gao, Z. F. (1980). [Psychological analysis of the selfish behavior of preschool age only children]. Xinli Kexue Wenzhai^ [Psychological Science Digest], *1,* **21-24.** (In Chinese.)

This is a study on the behavior of only children aged 4 to 6 years conducted by the staff of the Shanghai School for Teachers of Young Children. The results showed higher percentages of only than nononly children who pick their food, throw temper tantrums frequently, and are unfriendly toward their peers.

816

Gardiner, H. W., & Suttipan, C. S. (1976). Parental tolerance of aggression: A study of preadolescents in Thailand. *Adolescence, 11,* **573-578.**

817

Gilliom, M. E. (1978). Citizenship education in the People's Republic of China. *Theory into Practice, 17,* **389-395.**

Chinese children as young as 56 days old may enter a nursery that is attached to a factory where the mother is employed. By 2 years of age they are surrounded by political posters and are taught songs, dances, and plays celebrating workers, peasants, and productive labor. For children aged 3 to 5 years, kindergartens focus on early academic skills, but the content of the material is political. This indoctrination continues into the primary school, which lasts from 7 to 12 years. Primary schools have a pupil-operated workshop, which may be run in cooperation with a local industry. Middle schools typically offer politics, Chinese language, mathematics, physics, chemistry, English, history, geography, practical knowledge of agriculture and industry, and physical training. Specific examples of the 10-year emphasis on politics are given.

818

Goodnow, J. J. (1962). A test of milieu effects with some Piaget's tasks. *Psychological Monographs: General and Applied, 76,* **1-22 (Whole No. 555). (Also in Air Force Contract, 1963, AF 49 (638)-682.)**

819

Goodnow, J. J., & Bethon, G. (1966). Piaget's tasks: The effects of schooling and intelligence. *Child Development, 37.* **573-582.**

820

Goodnow, J. J., Young, B. M., & Kvan, E. (1976). Orientation errors in copying by children in Hong Kong. *Journal of Cross-Cultural Psychology, 7,* **101-110.**

Asked 39 3-4 yr olds and 42 5-7 yr olds from Hong Kong to copy a number of geometric shapes. Orientation errors corresponded with 2 types of error observed in US samples: inversions of shapes regarded by children as having "right-side-up" and "wrong-side up" positions, when presented for copying in a "wrong-side-up" orientation; and left-right reversal of a shape inconsistent with the usual sequence of strokes in young children's copying. Results suggest the presence of common features in the way perception of a visual pattern is translated into a copied form.

821

Goodnow, R. E. (1961). *Measurement of personality traits resulting from the interaction of abilities and environment: Vol. 3. Analysis of differential abilities in the Chinese.* **New York: Human Ecology Fund, 8-12.**

822

Gordon, I. E., Zukas, M., & Chan, J. (1982). Responses to schematic faces: A cross-cultural study. *Perceptual & Motor Skills, 54,* **201-202.**

32 Brunswik schematic faces--formed from combinations of features associated with responses of Good, Bad, Happy, and Sad--were rated on Good-Bad and Happy-Sad scales by 30 British undergraduates and 114 school children (aged 12-13 yrs) from Britain, Hong Kong, and Zambia. All groups responded in similar ways to the faces. Omitting pupils from the faces shifted ratings toward the Bad and the Sad ends of the scales.

823

Green, N. (1969). *An exploratory study of aggressive behavior in two preschool nurseries.* **Unpublished master's thesis, University of Chicago, Committee on Human Development, Chicago.**

824

Grimley, L. K. (1974). A cross-cultural study of moral development. *Dissertation Abstracts International, 34,* **A3990.**

825

Harris, P. L., Guz, G. R., Lipian, M. S., & Zhu, M. S. (1985). Insight into the time course of emotion among Western and Chinese children. *Child Development, 56,* **972-988.**

In four experiments, 48 children 4-6 years old from China and 96 children 4-6 years old from the U.K. were assessed for their insight into the time course of emotion. The subjects were asked about happy and sad episodes and about experiences from their own lives and story episodes. Results showed that Western and Chinese 6-year-olds exhibited a highly consistent pattern: they judged that an initially intense emotional reaction, positive or negative, would wane gradually over time. They made the same claim regarding their emotional reaction to experiences that they recalled from their own lives. Four-year-olds were less consistent. In two experiments, they failed to show the gradual waning pattern that characterized the judgments of 6-year-olds. However, when stringent precautions were taken to ensure that 4-year-olds fully understood the rating scale, they too judged that emotion wanes gradually over time. Implications for current accounts of children's insight into emotion were discussed.

826

He, C. K., & Chen, C. H. (1963). [An experimental study of the development of causality thinking in pre-school children: Vol. 2]. *Acta Psychologica Sinica,* **No. 4, 296-303.** (In Chinese.)

The experimental study showed: (1) Causality thinking in pre-school children. (2) Children's active attitude (or mental set) and eagerness to find out the solution of the problem were essential conditions for the development of causality thinking; (3) There were several stages in the transformation of actions into thoughts, and their characteristics varied with different age levels; (4) Reversibility in thinking was revealed in the discovery of the conservation of quantity of liquid in 6-7 year old children but not in 3-4 year old children.

827

He, C. K., Chou, L. C., Hsu, H. C. (1962). [An experimental study of the development of causality thinking in pre-school children: Vol. 1]. *Acta Psychologica Sinica,* **No. 2, 136-150.** (In Chinese.)

The results of the present experimental study showed that: (1) Pre-school children are able to realize the causality in simple physical phenomena; (2) The process of the development of causal thinking is the process from the external practical action of reflecting the causal relations between objects to the formation of image of causality, and finally, to an internal causality thinking; (3) The causal thinking of preschool children does not grow spontaneously but develops gradually under social and educational influences.

828

He, J. Q. (1982). [An investigation in cognitive development of the relation between part and whole in children--on solving problems of inclusive division not by the division method in children of 6-7 years of age]. *Acta Psychologica Sinica*, *14*, **41-49.** (In Chinese.)

222 children aged 6-7 years were asked to solve problems of inclusive division of various forms. These children did not know multiplication and division methods. The results indicated that: (1) The children showed some ability in dealing with the part-whole relationship concerning numbers, but only to a certain level. They used three different methods in solving problems of inclusive division: a non-arithmetical method, successive addition or subtraction of equal numbers, and composition and decomposition of equal numbers. (2) The mastering of the part-whole relationship in inclusive division depends on the children's understanding of the relations among the total number, the number of sets into which the total number is divided, and the number of the elements in each set.

829

He, J. Q., Liu, J. H. et al. (1983). [The cognitive development of part-whole relationship concerning geometrical figures in 5-11 years old children]. *Acta Psychologica Sinica*, *15*, **80-87.** (In Chinese.)

830

Hickrod, L. J. H., & Hickrod, G. A. (1965). Communist Chinese and the American adolescent subcultures. *China Quarterly*, **No. 22, 171-180.**

831

Ho, D. Y. F. (1974). Early socialization in contemporary China [Abstract]. In *Proceedings of the Twentieth International Congress of Psychology*, **1972, (pp. 442). Tokyo: University of Tokyo Press.**

A 4-week visit to Mainland China in 1971 enabled the author to obtain some first-hand information on the early socialization of Chinese children. It was found that a great number of children are placed in nurseries and kindergartens, where peer group relations play a decisive role in influencing behavior. Social-environmental, rather than hereditary, factors in development are emphasized. "Education through persuasion" is fully endorsed, whereas punishment and the use of coercion are rejected as inferior techniques of training. Great emphasis is placed on the cultivation of independence, self-government, and the willingness to take initiatives. It is suggested that personality development in future generations may be radically different from that of their forefathers.

832

Ho, D. Y. F. (1975). Traditional Chinese approaches to socialization. In J. W. Berry & W. J. Lonner (Eds.), *Applied cross-cultural psychology* **(pp. 309-314). Amsterdam, Netherlands: Swets & Zeitlinger.**

833

Ho, D. Y. F. (1979). Parental education is not correlated with verbal intelligence or academic performance in Hong Kong pupils. *Genetic Psychology Monographs*, *100*, **3-19.**

Investigated the relationship between parental education and children's academic ability. Ss were 1,945 Chinese pupils in Grades 4 and above from 9 primary and secondary schools in Hong Kong. Two Chinese tests constructed by the investigator, the Idioms Test and the Proverbs Test, served as measures of verbal intelligence. Examination marks and behavioral ratings were also obtained. Results show that parental education was not related to verbal intelligence or to academic performance, even when age, sex, family size, and interschool variation were controlled. This lack of relationship was also evident when the effects of father's and mother's education were considered jointly in a series of ANOVAs. Results illustrate the danger of generalizing findings on one group to another with widely differing sociocultural characteristics and throw doubt on the importance of parental education as a factor in intellectual academic ability.

834

Ho, D. Y. F. (1979). Sibship variables as determinants of intellectual-academic ability in Hong Kong pupils. *Genetic Psychology Monographs*, *100*, **21-39.**

To study the need for investigating birth order in conjunction with other variables and the relevance of such an investigation in Chinese society, a scheme for sibship classification was devised, taking into consideration sex of siblings and birth order in the total sibship or in the same-sex sibship simultaneously. Data were obtained on verbal intelligence and academic performance from 1,945 Hong Kong school pupils. Two main findings emerged: (a) a quadratic relationship between sibship size and intellectual-academic measures, and (b) the inferiority of last-borns in verbal intelligence. Results are discussed with special reference to the conclusions of L. Belmont and F. A. Marolla and to the confluence model of R. B. Zajonc and G. B. Markus.

835

Ho, D. Y. F. (1981). Traditional patterns of socialization in Chinese society. *Acta Psychologica Taiwanica, 23,* **81-95.**

Salient features which characterize Chinese traditional patterns of socialization were described: overriding emphasis on the development of moral character through education and providing the child with a wholesome environment; placing primary responsibility for socialization in the home; using shaming and punishment, including the physical, as common techniques of training; leniency toward infants and young children, in contrast to the imposition of strict discipline on older children; clear differentiation of sex roles and of parental roles. Above all else, filial piety was the prime guiding principle for socializing children.

836

Ho, D. Y. F. (1986). Chinese patterns of socialization: A critical review. In M. H. Bond (Ed.), *The psychology of the Chinese people^ (pp. 1-37). Hong Kong: Oxford University Press.*

837

Ho, D. Y. F., & Kang, T. K. (1984). Intergenerational comparisons of child-rearing attitudes and practices in Hong Kong. Developmental Psychology, 20, *1004-1016.*

The present research comprises two studies, one focusing on maternal child-rearing attitudes and practices and the other on paternal roles and attitudes in Hong Kong. Intergenerational comparisons are made possible by having 17 pairs of grandmothers and mothers and 20 pairs of grandfathers and fathers from the same families serve as informants. An interview schedule was used in the first study, and a questionnaire and two attitude scales were used in the second study. Results show that the fathers depart more from the traditional orientation concerning child training and filial piety and tend to be more involved in child care than the grandfathers. On the other hand, intergenerational comparisons of maternal care are mostly nonsignificant (at the .05 level). Despite important changes that have taken place, continuity with the past remains strong, such as in the control of sex and aggression. A high degree of intergenerational commonality remains in attitudes and conceptions concerning human nature, the importance of social-environmental influences in character formation, and the desired characteristics expected of children when they grow up.

838

Hofmann, R. J., & Trepanier, M. L. (1982). A cross-cultural influence on some basic graphic representations of young Chinese and American children. Journal of Genetic Psychology, 141, *167-175.*

Euclidean and topological scores as determined from graphic representations of 11 models were obtained from 53 Chinese and 98 American children aged 4-6 yrs. As hypothesized by Piagetian theory, topological scores showed a primacy over Euclidean scores in both cultures at all age levels. Chinese Ss appeared to perform better than American Ss in a systematic fashion, suggesting cultural effects on the development of representational space.

839

Hong, D. H. (1984). [Some characteristics of memory development in children aged 3 to 14 years]. Information on Psychological Sciences, *No. 2, 18-20. (In Chinese.)*

Memory tests were administered to 3,511 children aged 3-14 years. The results indicated that children in 3-6 and 7-9 age groups showed rapid memory development. The rate of memory development between 3 to 14 years tended to decline as a function of age. Short-term memory developed rapidly before 9 years, and came to a standstill at about 11; long-term memory continued to develop as age increased.

840

Hong, D. H., & Wang, H. Y. (1983). [Comparison of memory activity of backward and excellent pupils in junior middle school]. Acta Psychologica Sinica, 15, *185-191. (In Chinese.)*

841

Honigmann, J. J. (1948). Review of F. L. K. Hsu's Under the ancestors' shadow: Chinese culture and personality. Psychiatry, 11, *321.*

842

Hoosain, R. (1979). Forward and backward digit span in the languages of the bilingual. Journal of Genetic Psychology, 135, *263-268.*

50 7th-grade and undergraduate Chinese bilinguals (Chinese and English) in Hong Kong were tested for forward and backward digit span in the respective languages. Despite years of instruction in English, the difference between forward digit span in Chinese and in English was significant. The difference between backward digit span in the 2 languages was much smaller. Forward and backward digit span appeared to reflect different cognitive processes. Some developmental differences were noted, and a bilingual auditory storage index is suggested as one indication of bilingual development.

843

Hoosain, R. (1983). Memorization of classical Chinese. Psychologia: An International Journal of Psychology in the Orient, 26, *193-197.*

Examined whether there were cognitive reasons for the use of memorization in classical Chinese studies. 114 Hong Kong 12th graders who were asked to learn passages in literary- or colloquial-style Chinese that were relatively more difficult or easy, with rote learning or meaningful learning instructions. It was found that those with a rote learning set were superior in verbatim reproduction and equally good in understanding, compared to those with a meaningful learning set. The significance of difficulty and learning set is discussed, particularly with reference to the habit of memorization in learning classical Chinese. It is suggested that a pedagogic reason for memorization of literary-style Chinese is that it provides better overall results.

844

Hrboticky, N., & Krondl, M. (1984). Acculturation to Canadian foods by Chinese immigrant boys: Changes in the perceived flavor, health value and prestige of foods. Appetite, 5, *117-126.*

The authors examined changes in the perceived flavor, health value, and prestige in 36 first-generation and 18 second-generation 14-16 year old Chinese males to investigate their acculturation to Canadian foods. The subjects' food perceptions were then correlated with an acculturation index measuring ethnic language use and compared to the food perception ratings of 44 age- and sex-matched Canadian Anglophones. Results indicated that, for Chinese subjects, the type and degree of change in perceived flavor, health value, and prestige ratings varied for individual foods. The second-generation subjects and subjects with more accultured patterns of language use gave higher hedonic flavor and prestige ratings to dessert, snack, and fast foods. These subjects also exhibited better discrimination between foods rich and poor in nutrients as assessed by changes in perception of health value. Food perceptions of the second-generation Chinese were also found to approach those of the Canadian Anglophones. The results suggested that diet westernization may have nutritionally undesirable effects for immigrants.

845

Hsiang, W. C., & Soong, S. C. (1941). The growth rate of Chinese. American Journal of Physical Anthropology, 28, *357-373.*

846

Hsieh, C. C. (1964). [Studies on the ability of moral judgment in adolescents]. Acta Psychologica Sinica, *No. 3, 258-265. (In Chinese.)*

This study was an attempt to test the assumption that the ability of moral judgment of adolescents is closely related to their intellectual levels. The subjects were required to make judgments of the moral behavior of characters described in a written text. Considerable number of adolescents showed the ability to make judgments based on the nature of the moral deed, to analyze concrete situations and to discriminate between matters of primary importance and matters of secondary importance. Marked individual differences in moral judgment were also noticed.

847

Hsieh, S. N. (1976). [The development of role-taking ability in Chinese elementary school children]. Bulletin of Research Institute of Education *(Taiwan Normal University),* **18,** *25-82. (In Chinese.)*

848

Hsu, C. C. et al. (1982). The temperamental characteristics of Chinese babies. Annual Progress in Child Psychiatry & Child Development, *323-329.*

Administered the revision of the Infant Temperament Questionnaire to the mothers of 349 4-8 mo old infants in Taiwan. The face validity of the questionnaire was supported within the different context: The distribution of scores was normal, and the mothers had no trouble in answering the questions. While the general pattern of results was similar to those found in W. B. Carey and S. C. McDevitt's (1978) American sample, differences were found that may be interpreted in terms of response biases, racial differences, or a combination of these. Data are analyzed for possible effects of sex and socioeconomic status, and these findings are in turn compared to previous results. Observational studies are considered necessary to understand the nature of cultural differences in temperament.

849

Hsu, C. C., See, R., Lin, C. C., & Yang, S. K. (1976). Sex and intellectual development as measured by Raven's Progressive Matrices: A six-year longitudinal study. Psychiatria et Neurologia Paediatrica Japonica, 18, *81-88.*

850

Hsu, C. C., Soong, W., Stigler, J., Hong, C., & Laing, C. (1981). The temperamental characteristics of Chinese babies. Child Development, 52, *1337-1340. (Republished in* **Annual Progress in Child Psychiatry & Child Development,** *1982, 323-329.)*

Administered the revision of the Infant Temperament Questionnaire to the mothers of 349 4-8 mo old infants in Taiwan. The face validity of the questionnaire was supported within the different context: The distribution of scores was normal, and the mothers had no trouble in answering the questions. While the general pattern of results was similar to those found in W. B. Carey and S. C. McDevitt's (1978) American sample, differences were found that may be interpreted in terms of response biases, racial differences, or a combination of these. Data are analyzed for possible effects of sex and socioeconomic status, and these findings are in turn compared to previous results. Observational studies are considered necessary to understand the nature of cultural differences in temperament.

851

Hsu, E. H. (1946). On the application of Vienese Infant Scale to Peiping babies. Journal of Genetic Psychology, 69, *217-220.*

852

Hsu, F. L. K., Watrous, B. G., & Lord, E. M. (1961). Culture pattern and adolescent behavior: A comparison of Hawaii Chinese and Chicago White adolescents. International Journal of Social Psychiatry, 7, *33-53.*

It is argued that, in contrast to Americans, Chinese parents do not seem to assume the existence of a children's world qualitatively different from that of adults. Chinese children are regarded as little adults who will become adults after adult models. They are not excluded from the adult world, except in the area of sex; they participate in familial, social, and ceremonial functions in the presence of adults, as a matter of course. Thus the child entering into the adult world has few surprises awaiting him; he has long been initiated into, and prepared for, his adult roles in society.

853

Hsu, M. R. (1978). [The relationships between determinants of sub-culture and childrearing attitudes]. Bulletin of Research Institute of Education, 20, *411-486. (In Chinese.)*

854

Hsu, M. S. (1979). Father absence, son's masculinity, and behavioral adjustment: New evidence from modern Taiwan. Bulletin of the Institute of Ethnology *(Academia Sinica), No. 48, 79-88.*

The present paper examines the effect of long-term father absence on sons' masculinity and adjustment difficulties. The subjects were 82 eighth-grade students in northern Taiwan, 40 of whom were from fishermen's homes. Mean durations of father absence, over a period of the past 2 years, were 11.5 months for the fishermen and 6.3 months for the non-fishermen. The results indicated that, for boys but not for girls, duration of father absence was significantly and positively correlated with measures of masculinity and maladjustment.

855

Hu, H. C. (1950). Chinese folk literature and the Chinese child. *Unpublished document, Columbia University Research in Contemporary Cultures, New York.*

856

Huang, W. S. (1978). On longevity. Bulletin of the Institute of Ethnology *(Academia Sinica), No. 46, 139-151.*

In this paper, the author develops the problem of longevity as seen in the China, India, and the West (represented by the US and the Soviet Union). Based on the author's theory of the integral culture of the West and the East, a program for the prolongation of life for modern men and women is proposed. Also discussed were Indian theories of yoga concerning how to live to one hundred years or more, and the Chinese emphasis on the Tao of Longevity as seen by the Taoists.

857

Huang, W. Y. (1976). [A research on the relation between parental discipline and personality traits of public junior high school students]. Thought and Word, 14, *54-65;* **14,** *41-60. (In Chinese.)*

This is a study of academic and social adjustment in relation to parental attitudes among public junior high school students in Taiwan. It was found that, for both boys and girls, rejecting and inconsistent parental attitudes tended to be associated with low achievement motivation and poor learning attitudes; placing expectations on children tended to enhance their achievement motivation; and occupational interests were mostly uncorrelated with parental attitudes. There was no clear-cut contrast between boys and girls in the pattern of correlations between parental attitudes (both father's and mother's) and measures of personal and social adjustment, learning attitudes, achievement motivation, and occupational interests.

858

Huang, X. T., & Zhang, Z. J. (1979). [An experimental study of time perception of children aged 5-8 years]. Acta Psychologica Sinica, 11, *166-174. (In Chinese.)*

This experimental study showed that: (1) The time perception of children in 5-year old group is not very accurate and steady because they cannot use the standard measure of time. (2) Children in the 6-year old group generally cannot use the standard measure of time and their reproductions of long time intervals are not accurate and steady, a result similar to that of children in the 5-year old group; but their reproductions of short time intervals are more accurate and steady. (3) Children in the 7-year old group are able to use the objective standard measure of time; but there are only few who can use the subjective standard measure of time. (4) Children in the 8-year old group can actively use the standard measure of time. The accuracy and steadiness of their time perception tend to approach the level of adults.

859

Huang, Y. F. et al. (1985). [A study of the development of the ability for logical inference in Chinese school pupils and students]. Information on Psychological Sciences, *No. 6, 34-39. (In Chinese.)*

860

Hung, B. K. M., Ling, L., & Ong, S. G. (1985). Sources of influence on infant feeding practices in Hong Kong. Social Science & Medicine, 20, *1143-1150.*

Among 714 Hong Kong mothers with infants aged 4 weeks to 6 months, bottlefeeding subjects were influenced more by the medical professionals who did not support breastfeeding and by the mass media, particularly TV advertisements on infant formulas. Successful breastfeeding subjects were influenced more by their social networks through which they were told of the dangers of bottlefeeding. Failed breastfeeding subjects experienced a lack of support from friends and relatives, and were more sheltered from the influence of the mass media and social networks. Several recommendations to promote breastfeeding were made.

861

Hwang, C. H. (1979). [A study of internal-external locus of control of Chinese school pupils]. Bulletin of Educational Psychology, 12, *1-14. (In Chinese.)*

Studied the locus of control of Chinese school pupils using the Nowicki-Strickland Locus of Control Scale for Children for 4th-12th grade students, and its simplified form for 1st-3rd grade students. Internality was found to increase with age. Internality also showed a significant positive correlation with self-acceptance, emotional maturity, and perceived child-rearing practices of the parents. Neuroticism was negatively correlated with internality.

862

Hwang, C. H., & Lan, M. H. (1980). [Social schemata of Chinese school children]. Bulletin of Educational Psychology, 13, *13-26. (In Chinese.)*

Studied social schemata in 253 3rd-, 6th-, and 9th graders, using a free placement of felt figures technique and analysis of voluntary verbal responses of Ss. Results indicate placements of figures reflect a "social schemata" that may be common to different cultures. There seem to be some indications that, with increasing age, awareness of how people relate to one another also increases.

863

Ikels, C. (1975). Old age in Hong Kong. Gerontologist, 15, *230-235.*

Interviews with 78 residents of homes for the aged in Hong Kong suggest that, while traditional roles in this urban community have been undermined, the traditional ethic of filial piety has not been abandoned. Changes in attitudes toward 3-generation households are noted.

864

Inn, K. (1983). Assessment of self-concept: Bilingual Asian-American children. In M. Chu-Chang (Ed.), Asian and Pacific-American perspectives in bilingual education: Comparative research *(pp. 172-193). New York: Columbia University Teachers College Press.*

865

Iwanaga, M. (1973). Development of interpersonal play structure in three, four, and five year-old children. Journal of Research & Development in Education, 6, *71-82.*

Examined interpersonal play structure by naturalistic observation of 30 children (10 each of ages 3, 4, and 5 yrs) attending an all-Chinese urban nursery school. A typology of 4 categories was defined from a cognitive role-taking perspective, key factors being the ways in which Ss assigned roles to themselves and peers and the ways in which these roles were enacted. Results are based on behaviors of each of 20 children recorded for each minute of a 15-min interval in terms of the types and the amount of time spent in various interpersonal structures. Findings suggest that the 4 types of structure appear in a sequential progression with a strong relationship between CA and highest level of interpersonal structure attained (p .001). Sex differences were found with respect to the amount of time spent in various types of interpersonal structure at each age.

866

Jahoda, G. (1958). Child animism: Vol. 1. A critical survey of cross-cultural research. Journal of Social Psychology, 47, *197-212.*

867

Jamias, M. F., Pablo, R. Y., & Taylor, D. M. (1971). Ethnic awareness in Filipino children. Journal of Social Psychology, 83, *157-164.*

Investigated Filipino children's self-perception in terms of ethnic identity and assessed how accurately they recognized sketches of persons representing 2 important out-groups, i.e., Americans and Chinese. Each of the 90 Tagalog male Ss (6, 8, and 10 yr. old) was administered a picture identification test designed to assess Ss' ethnic affiliation. Results demonstrate that the frequency of identifying with an ethnic group increased with age and that children identified more often with their regional group than with the national group. Ss were more accurate in recognizing Chinese pictures than those representing Americans, implying that accuracy of ethnic perception is related to the frequency of contact with the group.

868

Jaquish, G. A., & Ripple, R. E. (1984). Adolescent divergent thinking: A cross-cultural perspective. Journal of Cross-Cultural Psychology, 15, *95-104.*

Assessed divergent thinking in 119 9-17 yr old Cantonese-speaking Chinese residents of Hong Kong. Ss responded in writing to a divergent-thinking assessor based on auditory stimuli. Scores were obtained for fluency, flexibility, and originality of thought. Adolescents scored significantly higher than preadolescents on all 3 divergent-thinking measures. MANOVA indicated an overall absence of main effects for sex and Sex * Age interactions. Results are compared to a study conducted by the present authors with American adolescents.

869

Jiao, S. L., Ji, G. P., & Jing, Q. C. (1986). Comparative study of behavioral qualities of only children and sibling children. Child Development, 57, *357-361.*

The authors investigated the socialization of only and nononly children in Chinese society. The subjects were 993 rural and urban kindergarten and primary school children, aged 4-6 and 9-10 years; 180 pairs of only and nononly children were matched by age, sex, socioeconomic status, and family structure and size. Peer ratings were made on seven behavioral qualities: independent thinking, persistence, behavior control, frustration proneness, cooperation, peer prestige, and egocentrism. Results based on the 180 matched pairs showed no significant difference in independent thinking for rural children; for the urban, only children were rated higher than nononly children among the younger group, but lower than nononly children among the older group. In both rural and urban areas, only children were consistently rated higher on egocentrism, but lower on cooperation, persistence, and peer prestige than nononly children.

870

Jin, S. Y. (1948). Physical growth of Chinese infants. Journal of Pediatrics, 32, *273-277.*

871

Jin, Y. (1980). [Attach importance to research on psychological phenomena of only children]. Xinli Kexue Wenzhai *[Psychological Science Digest],* **1,** *46-47. (In Chinese.)*

872

Johnson, R. C. (1983). Age and cohort effects on personality factor scores across sexes and racial/ethnic groups. Personality & Individual Differences, 4, *709-713.*

Analysis of Adjective Check List data on 2,576 Ss from White, Chinese, and Japanese ancestry from the Hawaiian Family Study of Cognition (J. R. Wilson et al., 1979) showed that substantial differences existed across ethnic groups and sexes in generational changes in status among groups residing in Hawaii. Age differences in personality were remarkably consistent across the sexes and ethnic groups. It is concluded that generational differences in personality factor scores in these populations result from age rather than cohort effects.

873

Kagan, J., Kearsley, R. B., & Zelazo, P. R. (1977). The effects of infant day care on psychological development. Evaluation Quarterly, 1, *109-142.*

A longitudinal investigation was conducted to assess the psychological effects of an experimental day care program on children aged 3.5-29 months. The subjects were 45 Chinese and 63 Caucasian children from working- and middle-class families who were cared for at a special group care center 5 days per week; the major control groups consisted of children reared totally at home and matched with the experimental subjects in terms of ethnicity, social class, and sex. The subjects' cognitive development was assessed on the Bayley Scales of Infant Development and four other measures; their attachment to mother, play and social behavior, and behavior on a visit to an unfamiliar day care center were also evaluated. Data gathered during the last two assessments, at ages 20 and 29 months, revealed little difference between the day care and home control subjects with respect to cognitive functioning, language, attachment, separation protest, and play tempo; the only simple effect of rearing involved behavior with unfamiliar peers. There was an interaction among ethnicity, social class, and rearing: Among working-class Chinese subjects, the day care experience facilitated cognitive development and reduced apprehension in unfamiliar situations; this effect did not occur among Caucasians.

874

Kagan, J., Kearsley, R. B., & Zelazo, P. R. (1978). Infancy: Its place in human development. *Cambridge, MA: Harvard University Press.*

The development of 116 infants (53 Chinese and 63 Caucasions) from working- and middle-class families in the Boston area was studied for a period of 2 years. Of these infants, 67 were cared for at home, 33 attended day-care centres, and 16 had mixed care experiences. The results showed that ethnic differences, mostly in situations involving excitability and temperament, were the least equivocal and the most coherent. The Chinese infants, both those from the day-care center and those brought up at home, were less vocal, less active, less likely to smile to many (but not all) of the laboratory episodes, and more apprehensive in social and separation situations; they were quieter, stayed closer to the mother, played less when they were with unfamiliar children or adults, and cried more often following maternal departure; finally, they showed consistently more stable heart rates during laboratory episodes. This cluster of qualities imply a disposition toward inhibition.

875

Kail, R. V. (1974). Familiarity and attraction to stimuli: Developmental change or methodological artifact? Journal of Experimental Child Psychology, 18, *504-511.*

113 7-, 9-, and 11-yr-old children viewed a series of stimuli, consisting of Chinese characters exposed a different number of times. Following exposure to the stimuli, Ss ranked the stimuli according to liking. 7 and 9 yr olds preferred the more familiar characters to those seen less frequently, but the oldest children preferred novel stimuli. In rankings taken 3 wks after original exposure a subsample of 11 yr olds preferred the more familiar characters. Results suggest that discrepancies obtained in previous research on the affective consequences of mere exposure are of methodological rather than developmental origin. Possible critical differences in procedure are discussed.

876

Keats, D. M., Keats, J. A., & Wan-Rafaei, A. R. (1976). Concept acquisition in Malaysian bilingual children. Journal of Cross-Cultural Psychology, 7, *87-99.*

143 Malaysian 5-yr-olds who were bilingual in English and Malay and English and Chinese were pretested in both languages, then trained in one language on the conservation of weight, post-tested immediately on their other language, and post-tested again from 1 to 2 mo later in both languages. Immediate improvements were obtained after training, but other untrained control groups also showed improvement on the delayed post-test. It is concluded that language plays a minor part in the acquisition of cognitive concepts and that young children will perform at a slightly higher level on these tasks if tested in their native language.

877

Keats, D. M., Keats, J. A., & Wan-Rafaei, A. R. (1977). Performance of Malay and Chinese children on vocabulary and operational tasks in two languages. Australian Psychologist, 12, *63-68.*

Investigated the role of language in the acquisition of conservation concepts by 143 urban Malaysian 5-6 yr olds. Almost all Ss were receiving some form of education. 75 were bilingual in Malay and English (M-E), and 68 were bilingual in Chinese and English (C-E). Scores for both languages were obtained from each S on the Peabody Picture Vocabulary Test (PPVT). A standard procedure for testing operational thinking was given once in each of S's languages. Results show that M-E Ss scored significantly higher in operational thinking on the Malay version than on the English, but scores of the C-E Ss on Chinese and English versions did not differ significantly. Scores of both M-E and C-E Ss were significantly higher on the English version of the PPVT than on Malay/Chinese versions. Significant correlations of .63 and .59 between scores on the English version of the operational thinking test and scores on the Malay/Chinese versions were obtained for M-E and C-S Ss, respectively, whereas correlations between scores on the English version of the PPVT and scores on the Malay/Chinese versions were not significant. Overall order of difficulty of the operational tasks was number, the easiest; followed by volume, weight, and quantity; and then class inclusion, the most difficult. It is concluded that disturbing effects of language on operational thinking are relatively unimportant.

878

Keats, J. A. et al. (1983). Parents, friends, siblings, and adults: Unfolding referent other importance data for adolescents. International Journal of Psychology, 18, *239-262.*

Notes that few studies have examined the importance of referent others. One reason may be ignorance of appropriate methods for analyzing the data. This paper reports 2 comparative studies of referent others for adolescents. (One study compared Ss in 4 Western countries--96 Australian, 84 French, 100 Norwegian, and 149 American 12-, 15-, and 18-yr-olds--and the other compared 120 Australian and 120 Malay, 120 Chinese, and 120 Indian (the 3 latter groups were from Malaysia) 12-, 15-, and 18-yr-olds. Data were analyzed by the "unfolding" method. Adolescents ranked parents first in importance, followed by friends, adults, and then siblings. Parents were perceived as less similar to friends than they were to siblings or adults. Rankings of referent others varied more by question content than by nationality.

879

Keislar, E. R., Hsieh, H., & Bhasin, C. (1972). An intercultural study: Discrimination and informal experience. Reading Teacher, 26, *171-179.*

Tested a total of 153 4-5 yr. olds in Taipei, Formosa; Delhi, India; and Los Angeles. The test consisted of 45 items, 15 in each of the respective languages used: Chinese, Hindi, and English. The performance of children from 4-51/2 yr. old in 3 different countries demonstrated that it is not until 5 yr. old that children begin to discriminate the writing elements in their native language relatively better than they do those of other languages. The general growth of all children with all languages is viewed as the result of maturation and growth. Competence in dealing with written language is perhaps enhanced by home interest and parents who take an interest in their child's language development.

880

Kessen, W. (Ed.). (1975). Childhood in China. *New Haven, CT: Yale University Press.*

This report is based on a visit to the People's Republic of China in 1973 by the 13 members of the American Delegation on Early Childhood Development. It covers the Chinese family, nurseries, kindergartens and primary schools, language development, health and nutritional factors.

881

Keyes, S. (1979). The development of spatial ability in Hong Kong Chinese adolescents: Sex-role stereotypes and patterns of cognitive ability. Hong Kong Psychological Society Bulletin, *No. 2, 21-26.*

Examined spatial ability in 150 10-, 13-, and 16-yr-olds using performance and nonverbal tests. Because previous research has shown that males, on the average, perform better on spatial tests than females, the author attempted to control for sex-role stereotyping by developing a 104-item rating scale of school subjects and activities the students deemed important for a boy and a girl to be good at, and qualities of character a boy and a girl should possess. 13- and 16-yr-olds rated themselves according to how well each term described them and how frequently they engaged in each activity. The relationship between conformity to a stereotype and performance on spatial tests was then examined. Results show that although there were distinct male and female stereotypes for each sex, there was a variation in the degree of sex-appropriate conformity. This variation, however, appeared to be independent of test performance. On every test (both spatial and verbal), there were no differences between the sexes on test performance. Differences in the behavior of Ss in the testing situation are discussed.

882

Keyes, S. (1980). Sex differences in cognitive abilities and sex-role stereotypes in Hong Kong Chinese adolescents: A developmental study. (Doctoral dissertation, Harvard University, Mass., 1982). Dissertation Abstracts International, 41, *B709.*

883

Keyes, S. (1983). Sex differences in cognitive abilities and sex-role stereotypes in Hong Kong Chinese adolescents. Sex Roles, 9, *853-870.*

Administered a battery of cognitive tests, including the Block Design subtest of the WISC, to 96 13- and 16-yr-old Hong Kong Chinese students to assess spatial, fluency, and verbal abilities. Ss also completed the Chinese Sex Role Inventory. Sex differences were discovered in patterns of performance, with males performing better on tests of spatial ability and females performing better on tests of fluent production. Sex differences in sex-role identification were also discovered. There were, however, no significant relationships between sex-role identification and patterns of ability. Biological sex was found to be the best predictor of a male or female pattern of performance. Results indicate that a reformulation of a sex-role identification hypothesis is warranted. Suggestions for further research on the relationships among sex-role identification, cultural values, and personal adjustment are presented.

884

Ko, R. (1959). Developmental tasks of adolescents in Hong Kong. Journal of Education *(University of Hong Kong),* **17,** *54-57.*

885

Koo, L. C., Wong-Tam, V. C. W., & Ho, C. Y. (1986). Factors affecting breast-feeding among Hong Kong Chinese. Asia-Oceania Journal of Obstetrics and Gynaecology, 12, *469-477.*

886

Kou, T. (1982). Self-esteem of immigrant monolingual Chinese and bilingual Chinese-English speaking children. Dissertation Abstracts International, 43, *A1863.*

887

Kuan, S. W., Wang, H. T., Liu, S. C., & Cheng, T. H. (1961). [An experimental study of the relation between the understanding of causality and the mastery of causality conjunctions and the development of language in pre-school children]. Acta Psychologica Sinica, *No. 1, 51-56. (In Chinese.)*

The present investigation is an attempt to study the relation between the understanding of causality, the mastery of causality conjunctions and the development of language in pre-school children. The results were: (1) The understanding of causality and the mastery of causality conjunctions varied with age. (2) The trend of the understanding of causality by pre-school children is: a) from the reflection of external causes to the discrimination of latent internal ones; b) from a global reflection of causal relations to a more differentiated and exact understanding; c) from references to the concrete cause of the particular phenomenon to the reflection of a more general law. (3) The mastery of the causality conjunctions (because .. therefore) depends upon the understanding of cause and effect relation. It is essential, therefore, for children to understand such relations for the development of language in pre-school children.

888

Kuang, P. T. (1962). [The age aspect in the dynamics of delayed inhibition in children]. Acta Psychologica Sinica, *No. 1, 18-27. (In Chinese.)*

This is a study of the dynamics of delayed inhibition in children of different ages (9, 12 and 15 year-olds). The experimental results indicated: (1) The younger the child, the longer the pre-reaction phase and the more difficult the development of delayed inhibition; (2) The younger the child, the stronger the after-effect inhibition and the longer the duration of after-effect inhibition; (3) The functional role of the second signal system in the formation of delayed conditioned reflex increases with the age.

889

Kuo, E. C. Y. (1974). The family and bilingual socialization: A sociolinguistic study of a sample of Chinese children in the United States. Journal of Social Psychology, 92, *181-191.*

Explored the relationships between the family and bilingual socialization of the child among 47 2-6 yr old preschool Chinese children in a US city. Measures included ratings of the child's oral bilingual balance, parental interviews, and child's scores on the Peabody Picture Vocabulary Test. It was found that, besides the general language orientation of the family, parental attitudes and behaviors regarding the 2 languages involved were significant variables related to the relative bilingual proficiency of the child. Findings support the general belief that the family is an important socializing agent for the language learning of the preschool child, although its influence seems to decrease with the increase of the age of the child.

890

Kuo, H. H. (1937). A study of the language development of Chinese children. Chinese Journal of Psychology, 1, *334-364.*

891

Kuo, S. L. (1984). [The difference of socioeconomic status and parental attitudes between gifted children and average children in elementary school]. Journal of Education & Psychology, 7, *197. (In Chinese.)*

892

Kuo, S. Y. (1975). [The effect of tremendous discrepancy between parents' expectations and children's actual intelligence on children's achievement motivation]. Bulletin of Educational Psychology, 8, *61-79. (In Chinese.)*

The purpose of this study was to investigate the effect of discrepancies between parents' expectations and children's actual intelligence on children's tendency to achieve success and to avoid failure. The subjects were 681 eighth graders randomly selected from public junior schools in Taipei. All the subjects were given both an intelligence test and a Questionnaire of Parents' Expectations. The main findings were: (1) Boys in the moderate-expectation group had a stronger tendency to achieve success than boys in the high- or the low-expectation groups. (2) Boys in the high-expectation group had a stronger tendency to achieve success than boys in the low-expectation group. (3) Girls in the moderate-expectation group had a stronger tendency to achieve success than girls in the low-expectation group. (4) Boys in the high-expectation group had a stronger tendency to avoid failure than boys in the low-expectation group. The data seemed to support the conclusion that a large discrepancy between parents' expectations and children's intelligence had a bad effect on the tendency to achieve success, especially in the case of boys.

893

Kuo, Z. Y. (1964 - 1965). Notes on some behavior characteristics of Chinese children from Mainland China. Journal of Education ^ (University of Hong Kong), ***22,*** **39-43.**

894

Lau, S., Cheung, K. F., & Chau, S. F. (1982). Reactions to inequities by internal and external control adolescents. *Journal of Social Psychology, 118,* **243-247.**

From a pretest of 136 Chinese 9th- and 10th-grade students, a total of 88 internal and external control students were chosen as Ss on the basis of their scores on the Nowicki-Strickland Locus of Control Scale for Children. Ss read an overreward or underreward story and were asked to imagine how they would react in those situations. As predicted, internal locus of control had a positive effect on imagined performance and external control a negative effect. Overreward also had a positive effect on imagined performance and affect. Overreward and underreward created differential effects only on the internals and not on the externals. Specifically, internals indicated that they would perform faster and felt more positive when overpaid than when underpaid, whereas the performance and feelings of externals remained unchanged in the overreward and underreward conditions.

895

Layman, E. M. (1969). Developmental psychology in East Asia: A preliminary report. *Psychological Record, 19,* **273-294.**

Reviews briefly the history of psychology in East Asia and describes the present status of developmental psychology in Japan, Nationalist China (Taiwan), and Mainland China. In Japan psychology is mostly experimental, and developmental studies cover a broad spectrum. In Taiwan the functionalist-behaviorist tradition continues, and developmental psychology stresses studies of personality, social development, and mental testing. Psychology in Mainland China is similar to that in the USSR, and developmental psychology deals mostly with concept formation, conditioning, classroom learning, and perception.

896

Lee, M. M. C., Chang, K. S. F., & Chan, M. M. C. (1963). Sexual maturation of Chinese girls in Hong Kong. *Pediatrics, 32,* **389-398.**

897

Lee, R. H. (1949). [Review of *Under the ancestor's shadow* **by F. L. K. Hsu].** *American Journal of Sociology, 54,* **554-555.**

898

Lee, T., Miao, H. C., & Wu, C. C. (1962). [The development of the understanding of fable and metaphor in school children]. *Acta Psychologica Sinica,* **No. 2, 125-135.** (In Chinese.)

A study of the development of understanding fables and metaphors in school children of four different ages indicated: (1) The level of understanding the figurative meaning of fable and metaphor by school children increases with age; from understanding the specific details and giving the superficial explanation of the phrases to understanding the figurative meaning in specific detail, and finally, revealing the general implication and the abstract principles without regard to detail. (2) The level of understanding the different natures and degrees of fable and metaphor showed some characteristics of thinking.

899

Lee, Y. P. (1887). *When I was a boy in China.* **Boston: Lothrop, Lee & Shepard.**

900

Leifer, A. (1972). Ethnic patterns in cognitive tasks. *Proceedings of the Annual Convention of the American Psychological Association,* **7, 73-74.**

Assessed culturally reinforced cognitive abilities in economically disadvantaged preliterate children. Capabilities of 80 disadvantaged preschoolers (20 each from Chinese, Italian, Negro, and Puerto Rican backgrounds) were assessed in a constructional task, body understanding, copying geometric forms, and in verbal ideational fluency. Chinese Ss significantly exceeded all other groups in constructional ability and in body understanding. Italian, Negro, and Puerto Rican Ss significantly exceeded the Chinese group in verbal ideational fluency. There were no differences in the ability to copy geometric shapes. Using these strengths for further cognitive growth was the primary application of the findings.

901

Leiter, R. G. (1938). *A comparative study of the general intelligence of Caucasian, Chinese, and Japanese children as measured by the Leiter International Performance Scale.* **Unpublished doctoral dissertation, University of Southern California.**

902

Leong, C. K., Cheng, S. C., & Das, J. P. (1985). Simultaneous-successive syntheses and planning in Chinese readers. *International Journal of Psychology, 20,* **19-31.**

Simultaneous-successive syntheses and planning as cognitive processing constructs were investigated. The subjects were Chinese children, 66 fourth graders and 63 sixth graders. Measures of simultaneous-successive processing and planning included the Colored Progressive Matrices, the Memory-For-Designs test, an auditory serial recall task, the Illinois Test of Psycholinguistic Abilities Sequential Memory subtest, a sentence repetition task, a visual search task, and the Trail-Making Tests A and B. Principal factor and promax analyses provided evidence of the independent factors. Simultaneous and successive components contributed to composite reading with varying degrees of variance at each grade level. A. R. Luria's dichotomous processing paradigm provides a useful framework for research into patterns of reading.

903

Leung, L. (1979). Sex-role adoption in free play among Hong Kong kindergarten children. *Hong Kong Psychological Society Bulletin,* **No. 2, 33-35.**

Investigated whether (1) children adopt sex-appropriate roles regardless of the sex of their playmates, (2) children who play sex-appropriate roles are spontaneously aware of complementary roles, and (3) children spontaneously select sex-related toys. 19 girls and 14 boys were divided into 4-41/2 and 51/2-6 yr old groups and were videotaped in pairs in a richly furnished room of their own. Age-matched Ss were paired with a member of the same and then a member of the opposite sex. Data were quantitatively scored according to sex-role play, pretend play, awareness of complementary roles, and the selection of sex-related toys. Results show that sex-role adoption began with role preparation; the reciprocal interaction of sex-role play, apart from the awareness of complementary roles, involved sharing and cooperation; and there was an abstraction of rules during role play in that Ss decided on themes, changes, and rules of play.

904

Leung, M. W., Ray, J. J., & Lew, W. J. (1983). The comparative measurement of motivation towards educational and occupational achievement among Hong Kong Chinese. *Journal of Social Psychology, 120,* **143-145.**

Administered occupational motivation (J. J. Ray, 1979) and academic motivation (E. J. Furst, 1966) scales to 81 male Chinese students (modal age 15 yrs). Findings suggest that although different types of motivation do generalize to some extent, the generalizable aspect may not necessarily be the aspect responsible for variations in actual achievement.

905

Lew, C. K. (1986). Personality: Elderly versus other age groups. *Dissertation Abstracts International, 46,* **B3600.**

906

Li, A. K. (1973). A parental attitude scale in Chinese. *Psychologia: An International Journal of Psychology in the Orient, 16,* **174-176.**

Describes a research instrument to measure parent attitudes relating to personality development of the child. The initial statements were composed of items taken from the Parent Attitude Research Instrument, the Parent Attitude Survey, and items written by the investigator. A principal component analysis was performed on the computed Pearson product-moment correlations among the 20 items of the scale and the factors rotated by Varimax rotation. Three principal component factors were isolated. The appendix presents the Parent Attitude Scale, written in Chinese.

907

Li, A. K. F. (1974). Parental attitudes, test anxiety, and achievement motivation: A Hong Kong study. *Journal of Social Psychology, 93,* **3-11.**

Obtained data on parental childrearing patterns and attitudes from the parents of 61 male and 72 female 5th and 6th graders shortly after they took the Secondary Schools Entrance Examination in Hong Kong. The children also were administered Sarason's Text Anxiety Scale for Children and the Thematic Apperception Test as a measure of need achievement (nAch). Hypotheses about parental attitudes of dominance, fostering of dependency, and favoring of communication were confirmed for boys but not for girls. Data suggest cultural as well as sex differences in parent-child relationships. The finding that girls had significantly higher mean nAch scores than boys supports the idea that girls may react to a comparative lack of parental attention by finding other sources of recognition and satisfaction (e.g., intellectual achievement).

908

Li, B. S., Cen, G. Z., Ye, H. Z., Lu, J. M., & Shao, W. M. (1985). [Development of collective ideas in primary school children]. *Information on Psychological Sciences,* **No. 1, 11-15.** (In Chinese.)

Nine paired stories involving judgment of the intentions and consequences of behavior were designed to study the development of collective ideas. Ninety primary school children aged 7, 9, or 11 were interviewed to examine the developmental processes of dedicating themselves to collective responsibility, honor, and interest. The result showed that collective ideas occurred at about 7 years of age, and the major changes in judgment occurred at the age of 9.

909

Li, B. S., Lu, J. M., Cheng, X. C., Zhang, C. F. (1984). [A study of children's punishments as seen by themselves]. *Information on Psychological Sciences,* **No. 5, 1-5.** (In Chinese.)

More than 3,000 children aged 7 to 13 from 15 districts in China were interviewed to examine their responses to various types of punishments involved in two hypothetical stories. The experiment included three parts: (1) choosing the alternatives between expiatory and retributive punishments; (2) giving suggestive punishments; and (3) choosing alternatives among expiatory, retributive and reproaching punishments. The results revealed a developmental pattern of punitive values; choice of retributive punishment decreased with age, choice of reproaching punishment increased with age, and expiatory punishment was not dominant at any age.

910

Li, D., Zhang, F. J., & Jin, Y. (1985). [Characteristics of children's deductive reasoning for hypothetical judgment]. *Information on Psychological Sciences,* **No. 1, 4-10.** (In Chinese.)

This study explored the development of children's deductive reasoning in hypothetical judgments, and compared the developmental characteristics with the age levels of syllogism of categorical judgment. Two hypothetical judgments in formal logic, the sufficient conditional and the necessary conditional, were used as propositions to construct four patterns of reasoning problems. The results indicated: (1) The accuracy rate of hypothetical reasoning increased with age, with an acceleration phase between the 6th grade of primary school and the 1st grade of junior middle school. (2) Primary school children's ability to master the reasoning pattern for "non affirmative" judgments was approximately one year later than their mastery of categorical deductive reasoning. (3) The age levels of hypothetical reasoning varied with the degree of involvement with test material.

911

Li, F. L. (1970). [A case study of child training and education in rural Taiwan]. *Bulletin of The Institute of Ethnology* **(Academia Sinica), No. 29, 151-198.** (In Chinese.)

912

Li, H. (1986). [A study of children's cartoon cognition development]. *Information on Psychological Sciences,* **No. 5, 15-20.** (In Chinese.)

913

Li, H. T. et al. (1982). [An investigation of the development of intelligence of children less than three years of age]. *Information on Psychological Sciences,* **No. 1, 27-39.** (In Chinese.)

914

Li, H. Z., & Hu, R. X. (1983). [Direct inference ability on the judgement of full names in young children]. *Acta Psychologica Sinica, 15,* **453-460.** (In Chinese.)

915

Li, M. C., Cheung, S. F., & Kau, S. M. (1979). [Competitive and cooperative behavior of Chinese children in Taiwan and Hong Kong]. *Acta Psychologica Taiwanica, 21,* **27-33.** (In Chinese.)

72 Chinese children in Hong Kong (ages 4-12 yrs) and 144 Chinese elementary school students in Taiwan participated in 2 experiments to identify competitive vs cooperative reward structure. Ss were divided into 4 groups, and each group played the Madsen Cooperative Board under either competitive or cooperative conditions. Results from both experiments suggest that (1) older children were more cooperative, (2) Ss continued to cooperate even when the reward structure changed from cooperative to competitive, and (3) male Ss tended to be more cooperative than females.

916

Li, M. G., Li, X. T., Ge, H. K., & Wei, X. Q. (1984). [A study of hand preference in children]. *Information on Psychological Sciences,* **No. 2, 1-7.** (In Chinese.)

An experiment involving catching objects with the right or the left hand was designed to study hand preference. The subjects were 700 children of 1-7 years of age. The results showed that hand preference appeared mostly between 1 to 3 years; the critical age was 2 years. There was a slight difference between boys and girls. Alternations between right- and left-handedness occurred in some of the children. There was a positive correlation between the handedness of parents and that of their children.

917

Li, P. S., & Chou, K. S. (1964). [Motivational characteristics of moral behavior in children]. *Acta Psychologica Sinica,* **No. 1, 25-32.** (In Chinese.)

Questionnaires were distributed to 297 pupils of 9-16 years, to investigate their moral motivation under hypothetical and real situations. The results were: (1) Primary school children of 3rd and 4th grades were aware of the social implications of their behavior, but their behavior was rarely motivated self-consciously. Middle school pupils could comprehend, in a more systematic and generalized way, the moral significance of their behavior; the self-conscious character of their moral motivation was of a higher level. (2) Motivational struggle between moral and immoral behavior was a reflection of children's moral consciousness in actual life situations. (3) Moral motivation of primary school children was mainly determined by contradictions of environmental and inner factors, whereas motivation of middle school pupils was mainly determined by contradictions of environmental factors reflected in their consciousness.

918

Li, S. H. (1974). [The development of classificatory ability in Chinese children]. In K. S. Yang & C. H. Chang (Eds.), *[Behavioral development of Chinese children].* **Taipei: Huan-yu Publishing Co.** (In Chinese.)

919

Li, W. F., & Liu, F. (1982). [An experimental study of the development of childrens's cognition of two spatial relationships]. *Acta Psychologica Sinica, 14,* **174-183.** (In Chinese.)

This is a study of the cognitive development concerning two spatial relationships, equality of areas and verticality, in children 5-11 years of age. Mastery of the principle "equals minus equals will be equals" was investigated through studying children's judgments about the equality of areas. The result indicated that children's judgment of equality of areas may be divided into two types, one based on direct perception and one on reasoning, with a transitional stage between the two. In dealing with verticality, a medial phase developed gradually, from perpendicularity to the slope to perpendicularity to the level. Both of these results showed cognitive development with increasing age: a period of rapid development at 6-7 years when the children's achievements differed significantly, and a relatively stable period at 7-9 years when their achievements showed little or no increment. In the latter period the children's cognition was liable to be influenced by experimental conditions, and their achievements were more changeable than those of other age groups. This might be characteristics of the medial, transitional phase of development.

920

Li, W. F., & Liu, F. (1983). [Research on the development of cognition of space in 5-13 years old children]. *Acta Psychologica Sinica, 15,* **88-97.** (In Chinese.)

This was a continuation of experimental research on the development of cognition of two kinds of space relation. The inner occupied area was changed into a circular form. The results indicated that in the discrimination of children there was a transition from intuitional judgment to inferential judgment. In the same discrimination the intuitional and inferential activities are interlocked, thus the parts of occupied area conforms into a whole, but discrimination of the leftover areas is bound by intuition. Children could understand that equal amount subtract equal amount the remainder is equal, but they were not able to use this to solve the four types of problems. So to pass these transitions, the children must be able to solve three connected problems, this again proves through discrimination of areas there exists this kind of development of cognition of space in children.

921

Li, X. T., Li, M. G., Ge, H. K., & Jin, K. H. (1984). [An experimental study of grasping with the left or the right hand by children 6 months to 3 years of age]. *Acta Psychologica Sinica*, *16*, **214-222.** (In Chinese.)

A study of object grasping with the right or the left hand was designed to determine hand preference in 300 children from 6 months to 3 years of age. The results showed that the frequency of using the right or the left hand was around 50% within the first year. The percentage of right-handed children increased with age, reaching 69.4% at 1 to 1-1/2 years, 71.3% at 1-1/2 to 2 years, 76.9% at 2 to 2-1/2 years, and 81.5% at 2-1/2 to 3 years. The frequency of boys' right-handedness increased faster than that of girls. There were cases of object grasping with both hands, but the incidence decreased rapidly after 1-1/2 years of age. The percentage of left-handedness was higher in children with one or two left-handed parents than in children with two right-handed parents.

922

Li, Y. (1959). [An analysis of the psychological characteristics of primary school 5-6th grade students participating in agricultural work]. *Acta Psychologica Sinica*, **No. 5, 293-302.** (In Chinese.)

In this study, the author analyzed the characteristics manifested by primary school students in agricultural labor, in the understanding of discipline to be observed during work, and in the evaluation of their own and others' work. The students' understanding of discipline was mainly reflected in the following three aspects: the students' behavior when working individually; their obedience to the discipline; and their spirit of collectivism. These three aspects corresponded respectively to the three different levels (from the lower to the higher levels) of development of a child's mentality. Both the children's manifestation during the work and their evaluation of their own and others' labor were closely related to these three levels of understanding of the discipline. The author attempted to reveal the major psychological factors affecting the difference in the moral quality of the students.

923

Lin, C. D. (1981). [A study of the development of number concepts and operational ability in schoolchildren]. *Acta Psychologica Sinica*, *13*, **289-298.** (In Chinese.)

This study investigated the critical period and the unity of stability and variability of age characteristics in the development of number concepts and operational thinking in schoolchildren. The author believes that the structure of thinking is a system which has direction and form under the control of principles. The development of the structure of thinking in schoolchildren was also studied.

924

Lin, C. D. (1983). [Study on the development of thinking flexibility of operation in schoolchildren]. *Acta Psychologica Sinica*, *15*, **419-428.** (In Chinese.)

This was an experimental study of thinking flexibility or divergent thinking in mathematical operations by schoolchildren. The results showed: (1) No critical period was found in the development of thinking flexibility in schoolchildren. (2) Learning experiences played an important role in the development of thinking flexibility. It was argued that divergent thinking is a generalization process. Divergent thinking and convergent thinking are both aspects of the dialectical unity of thinking. Convergent thinking is a basis for divergent thinking; divergent thinking is the further development of convergent thinking. Both are important in teaching.

925

Lin, C. S. (1967). [A study on language development of preschool children]. *Bulletin of Institute of Educational Research* **(Taiwan Normal University),** *9*, **138-296.** (In Chinese.)

926

Lin, C. S. (1967). [A comparison of the mean length of sentences between orphanage children and ordinary children]. *Psychological Testing*, *14*, **403-408.** (In Chinese.)

927

Lin, C. S. (1968). [A comparison of variables of language development between preschool boys and girls]. *Psychology and Education*, *2*, **121-137.** (In Chinese.)

The subjects in this study were 36 preschool children, equally divided by sex. Their language responses were observed under two different situations: (a) the child-child situation in which the subject played with toys with another child; and (b) the adult-child situation in which the subject discussed the content of pictures with the experimenter. Fifty consecutive verbal responses were recorded in each situation for every child. Data were obtained on the total number of words and the total number of different words; the mean length, kinds, and complexity of sentences; the type-token ratio; and percentages of the different parts of speech. It was found that there were no significant sex differences, except that girls seemed to have a greater tendency than boys to use complex sentences. There were significant differences between the language spoken in the child-child situation and that in the adult-child situation.

928

Lin, C. S. (1972). An experimental study of the visual eidetic imagery of Chinese school children. *Dissertation Abstracts International, 33,* **A1025. (Also** *Psychology & Education,* **1971,** *5,* **49-119.)**

929

Lin, H. T., & Hwang, C. J. (1967). [A study of intelligence of Southern Taiwan primary school children by the draw-a-person test]. *Acta Psychologica Taiwanica, 9,* **74-80.** (In Chinese.)

930

Lin, J. S. (1981). [Experimental study on the development of children's cognition of the relations between parts and whole (II) - Combination and decomposition of numbers in children of 4-7 years old]. *Acta Psychologica Sinica, 13,* **159-167.** (In Chinese.)

931

Lin, L. Y., & Chang, H. W. (1984). [Preschoolers' number skills: Counting and numerical magnitude comparison]. *Chinese Journal of Psychology, 26,* **3-17.** (In Chinese.)

The present study investigated Chinese preschoolers' ability in counting and comparing number magnitudes. The subjects were 48 children between 3 1/2 and 5 1/2 years of age. In Experiment I, they were asked to count from 1 to as far as they could; Experiment II involved comparing pairs of numbers ranging from 1 to 9. Results from Experiment I indicated that if a child could count beyond 10, he would show definite knowledge of the underlying pattern of the Chinese number system. Furthermore, frequency of counting errors such as skipping, turning back, and the use of nonstandard counting words all decreased with age. In magnitude comparisons, when a child was uncertain about the numbers, he tended to choose the second number of the pair to be compared as the answer. Also, performance was better when the probing question used the word "more" rather than "less."

932

Lin, P. C. (1980). [A study of Piagetian cognitive development and psychometric IQ in junior and senior high school students]. *Acta Psychologica Taiwanica, 22,* **33-49.** (In Chinese.)

The present study used 1915 junior and senior high school students as subjects to investigate the relationship between Piagetian cognitive development and psychometric IQ. The main findings of the study were: (1) The reliabilities and validities of Longeot's and Lawson's revised group Piagetian tests are rather good. (2) Formal reasoning increases with age, but concrete reasoning does not. (3) Piagetian cognitive development correlates moderately with some IQ measures such as numerical reasoning and verbal comprehension. (4) Many students in junior and senior high school haven't entered the formal operation period.

933

Lin, S. C. (1971). Phonetic development of Chinese infants. *Acta Psychologica Taiwanica, 13,* **191-195.**

Tape-recorded the sounds emitted by 6 Chinese infants. The appearance of sequences of consonants and vowels are listed. Mispronounced consonants are indicated and discussed. Aspirated /p, t, k, ts/ were difficult for the Ss to produce; they were pronounced as unaspirated.

934

Lin, S. H. (1984). [The relationship of age to cognitive development and language ability in grade school children]. *Journal of Education & Psychology, 7,* **198.** (In Chinese.)

935

Ling, L., Hung, B. K. M., & Ong, S. G. (1985). A study of infant feeding practices in Hong Kong. *Journal of the Hong Kong Society of Community Medicine, 15,* **15-24.**

936

Liou, S. C. (1974). [Conception of conservation in Chinese children]. *Bulletin of Research Institute of Education* **(Taiwan Normal University),** *16,* **97-160.** (In Chinese.)

937

Liu, C. B. (1981). Vegetable consumption patterns, dietary intake and nutritional status of preschoolers in Taiwan. *Dissertation Abstracts International, 41,* **B2973.**

938

Liu, C. H. (1950). The influence of cultural background on the moral judgment of children (Doctoral dissertation, Columbia University, 1950). *Dissertation Abstracts, 10,* **319-321. (University Microfilms No. 1869, 104p.)**

939

Liu, C. H., Wang, H. T., Fan, T. J., & Chang, M. L. (1963). [An investigation in the development of concepts in children of 4-9 years: Vol. 1. Experimental studies on classification and generic naming]. *Acta Psychologica Sinica,* **No. 4, 287-295.** (In Chinese.)

This study was an investigation of the classification of various objects. Seventy-two children (4-9 years old) were given objects (depicted on cards) which could be divided according to different categories of varying levels. Each child was asked: (1) to sort according to his own ideas of classification; (2) to pick up the cards according to specified classifications; and (3) to give the generic name to previously sorted cards. The results showed that: (1) The percentage of correct responses increased with age. (2) In general, the children were more successful in the second task than in the first; and better in the first task than in the third. (3) Variations in successful performance were shown in different age groups. Differences were also found in the classification of different objects in the same level.

940

Liu, F. (1981). [The current developmental psychology in China with particular reference to the development of number-concepts of 3-12 year old Chinese children]. *Acta Psychologica Sinica, 13,* **117-123.** (In Chinese.)

Reports on a lecture delivered at the 22nd International Congress of Psychology held in Leipzig, East Germany, July 6-12, 1980. The current status of developmental psychology in China is discussed, including a cooperative study on the development of number concepts and arithmetic operational abilities in 3-12 yr old children.

941

Liu, F. (1981). [On some of the peculiarities of developmental and educational psychology in our country]. *Information on Psychological Sciences,* **No. 1, 7-9.** (In Chinese.)

942

Liu, F. (1982). Developmental psychology in China. *International Journal of Behavioral Development, 5,* **391-411. (Republished in** *Acta Psychologica Sinica,* **1982,** *14,* **1-10.)**

Discusses the ancient and modern history of Chinese developmental psychology as well as current emphases in this field. Developmental psychological concepts had already been formulated within ancient Chinese philosophy by such philosophers as Confucius and Xunzi. However, modern Chinese developmental psychology was strongly inspired by European and American psychology. Research in developmental psychology has been promoted since 1977, with particular reference to children's cognitive development and educational reform. Current research projects concern the following areas: cognitive development (development of the number concept and operational abilities), language development, the relation of thinking and language, personality and moral development, supernormal children and mental retardation.

943

Liu, F., Lu, J., Shen, J. X., Lai, C. G., Zhang, Z. J., Liu, J. X., Ding, S. N., Xu, X. C., Cao, Z. F., & Wang, P. F. (1981). [A study on the development of number concepts and operational abilities of 7-12 year olds in 10 districts in China]. *Acta Psychologica Sinica, 13,* **135-149.** (In Chinese.)

Reports on studies of 959 7-12 yr olds from 10 districts in China. The development of number recognition (including transfer between figure and number), ordinals and sets of series, composition/decomposition of numbers, and number operations and applications were explored. In addition, the authors discuss the relationships between learning and the development of arithmetic concepts, the process of this development, the environmental effects, and the stages of learning development.

944

Liu, F., & Zhao, S. W. (1983). [A study on the development of 8-15 year-old's concept of intersection set and their ability in resolving intersection problem - Studies on the development of children's cognitive structure (I)]. *Acta Psychologica Sinica, 15,* **156-161.** (In Chinese.)

This study explored children's development of the concept of intersection set, and the process of solving intersection problems. The subjects were 151 children 8-15 years of age. They were tested on three intersection problems of different degrees of difficulty, presented through words, pictures, and physical objects. The results suggest that primary school pupils have the mental facility for mastering problems involving simple intersection sets. The cognition of intersection involves interactions between concepts, images, and sensorimotor manipulations. The process of solving intersection problems is an active one: The children ponder actively, formulate strategies, and form related concepts with the help of pictures and manual manipulations.

945

Liu, J. H., Wang, X. T., & Zhang, M. L. (1982). [The development of children's cognition of the part-whole relationship concerning number and arithmetic]. *Acta Psychologica Sinica, 14,* **263-271.** (In Chinese.)

This is a comprehensive report of 9 experiments. From the first 4 experiments, 12 criteria were proposed for the comprehension of part-whole relationships. These 12 criteria were then used in 3 experiments (using integers, geometrical figures, and fractions) designed to investigate the reaction of children to part-whole relationships; finally, 2 teaching experiments were carried out. On the basis of the results obtained, the authors discussed how understanding the intrinsic nature of number and arithmetical concepts facilitates cognitive processes, the age characteristics, developmental levels, and periods of accelerated growth in the comprehension of part-whole relationships. That children's cognition of part-whole relationships may be effectively applied to learning arithmetic was also discussed.

946

Liu, S. C., Chao, C. C., Li, S. C., Kuo, C. Y., Tai, C. L., & Muo, H. H. (1964). [A preliminary study on the characteristics of memory for pictorial and verbal materials in primary school children]. *Acta Psychologica Sinica*, **No. 2, 170-177.** (In Chinese.)

The subjects of this experiment consisted of three groups of school children (aged 7-8, 9-10 and 11-12 years). The children's memory for pictorial and verbal materials showed: (1) For both pictorial and verbal materials, the quantity and accuracy of retention improved with age. (2) Memory for pictorial materials was superior to that for verbal materials. The lower the age, the more striking was this difference. (3) Scores for memorizing concrete verbal materials were higher than for memorizing abstract verbal materials, this difference decreasing with age. (4) Only a small portion of the 7-8 year olds could make use of "attempt to recall" as a method for memorization, while some of the 9-10 year old children used associations and classifications as methods for memorization. The oldest group were capable of consciously employing all the above-mentioned methods in memorizing the test materials.

947

Liu, S. Y., & Wu, C. E. (1962). [A developmental electroencephalographic study of children and youths aged 8 to 20 years]. *Acta Psychologica Sinica*, **No. 3, 173-185.** (In Chinese.)

Investigations of spontaneous and "evoked" potentials were carried out on 910 normal children and youths aged 8 to 20 years. Stimulation of subjects with "threshold" single and repetitive flashes of light, produced the following results: (1) The occipital rhythmic activity increased in frequency but decreased in amplitude with age. (2) Theta waves disappeared first from the occipital region, then from the temporal region and finally from the parietal region. (3) There were positive correlations between the phenomenon of "dicrotic" and "multicrotic" and the development and maturation of the cerebral cortex of children and youths. Display of the phenomenon of "dicrotic" and "multicrotic" decreased with age. (4) The percentage of "blocking" responses elicited by "threshold" single flashes increased with age. (5) "Driving" responses elicited by "threshold" repetitive flashes showed that neurons of the cerebral cortex of children and youths have high plasticity. (6) There is a period of acceleration of the brain's development at about 13-14 years of age.

948

Liu, S. Y., Wu, C. E., & Sun, W. L. (1962). [The electroencephalogram of pre-school children from 4 to 7 years]. *Acta Psychologica Sinica*, **No. 3, 186-196.** (In Chinese.)

Electroencephalographic (EEG) investigations of spontaneous and "evoked" potentials were performed on 758 normal preschool children. "Evoked" potentials were produced by "threshold" single and repetitive flashes of light. The results were: (1) EEGs in children aged 4-7 years showed both alpha and theta waves. (2) From 4-7 years the occipital rhythmic activity increased in frequency but amplitude remained high with age. (3) The vast majority of children aged 4-7 years showed the phenomena of "dicrotic" and "multicrotic". (4) "Blocking" responses elicited by "threshold" single flashes on preschool children were typically infrequent and of short duration. (5) "Driving" responses elicited by "threshold" repetitive flashes on preschool children were occasionally shown, although there was a narrow range of "driving" frequency and absence of afterdischarge. (6) The results suggest that there is a period of acceleration of brain's development between 5-6 years of age.

949

Liu, T. L. (1983). [The effects of multimodal behavior group and life skills group experiences on college students' anxiety levels and developmental task achievement]. *Journal of Education & Psychology*, **6, 99-144.** (In Chinese.)

The effects of group settings of life-skills training and multimodal behavior on college students' development task achievement were examined. 48 students were randomly assigned to a life-skills group (LSG), a multimodal behavior therapy group (MBG), and a control group. The LSG and MBG groups received eight treatment sessions within seven weeks, but the control group received no treatment. The descriptive posttest data gave evidence of postive therapeutic outcomes for both the LSG and the MBG interventions on the achievement of three developmental tasks and five developmental subtasks, viz Developing Autonomy, Developing Purpose, Developing Mature Interpersonal Relationship, Developing Emotional Autonomy, Developing Life-style Plan, Developing Intimate Relationships with Opposite Sex, Developing Mature Relationships with Peers, and Developing Tolerance. Interactions between sex and treatment were found on two developmental tasks (Developing Autonomy and Developing Purpose) and three developmental subtasks (Instrumental Autonomy, Mature Life-style Plans, and Mature Career Plans). The data showed that the LSG intervention was better than MBG intervention on the achievement of Intimate Relationships with Opposite Sex, but the intervention was better than the LSG's on the achievement of Emotional Autonomy and Tolerance. Because these two kinds of intervention were adopted in the Chinese society for the first time, some variables were not well controlled, such as experience of leaders; therefore further research is recommended.

950

Lo, H. Y., & Hwang, K. K. (1980). The parental child-rearing practices as perceived by Chinese teenagers and their social and personal adjustment. *Proceedings of the First Asian-Pacific Conference on Juvenile Delinquency*. **Taipei: Pacific Cultural Foundation.**

951

Lu, C. M. (1979). [Self concept characteristics of Chinese children and adolescents]. *Bulletin of Educational Psychology, 12,* **123-132.** (In Chinese.)

This study investigated developmental trends of the self-concept of Chinese children and adolescents. The subjects were 1,033 male students and 1,059 female students in Grades 1 to 9 from two elementary and two junior high schools. The self-concept scale (following the Tennessee Self Concept Scale) was administered in regular class settings. The scores of self-concept scale were treated as criteria, and grade levels as predictors. A trend analysis showed that: (1) The mean scores of the self-concept scale were high, which indicated that the self-concept characteristics of Chinese children and adolescents were sound and positive. (2) The linear regression lines (descending), but not the nonlinear regression lines, were a good fit to the self-concept scores predicted by grade levels.

952

Lu, C. M. (1980). [A study on the self concept development of Chinese school pupils]. *Bulletin of Educational Psychology, 13,* **75-84.** (In Chinese.)

This is a part of a 3-year longitudinal study on the physical and psychological development of Chinese school pupils. A total of 687 youngsters (335 males and 352 females) were sampled from two elementary schools and two junior high schools in Taipei. The self-concept scale, following the Tennessee Self Concept Scale, was administered to the subjects twice in the regular class settings, with a 1-year interval. Changes of scores of the self-concept scale were treated as dependent variables, and sex and grade level were independent variables. Statistical analyses revealed that: (1) The self-concept characteristics of elementary school boys and girls, and junior high school male students did not change with age; but some of the self-concept characteristics of junior high school female students decreased with age. (2) Sex differences in changes in self-concept characteristics were not significant for elementary schoolchildren; the same was found for junior high schoolchildren, except for family self. (3) For both sexes, the effects of grade level on changes in self-concept characteristics were not significant.

953

Lu, C. M. (1981). [A three year follow-up of the self concept of Chinese children and adolescents]. *Bulletin of Educational Psychology, 14,* **115-124.** (In Chinese.)

309 male and 339 female elementary and junior high school students were administered the Tennessee Self-Concept Scale 3 times in regular class settings. Findings indicate that Ss had positive self-concepts, and with the exception of identity they did not change with age.

954

Lu, C. M. (1982). [The self concept characteristics of Chinese gifted students]. *Bulletin of Educational Psychology, 15,* **111-126.** (In Chinese.)

Investigated self-concept characteristics of 420 gifted and 464 average students from 4 elementary and 3 junior high schools. A revised Tennessee Self-Concept Scale was administered to Ss in their classes. It was found that (1) the self-concept characteristics of gifted Ss were less positive than those of the average Ss; (2) the self-concept characteristics of the female gifted Ss were more positive than those of male gifted Ss; and (3) the straight regression lines were a good fit to the scores of ethical self and personal self as predicated by the grade levels of gifted Ss.

955

Lu, C. Y. (1968). [Revision of the California Test of mental maturity]. *Acta Psychologica Taiwanica, 10,* **22-39.** (In Chinese.)

956

Lu, C. Y. (1981). [A study on the development of interests in Chinese school pupils]. *Bulletin of Educational Psychology, 14,* **15-30.** (In Chinese.)

This is a short report on a 3-year study of the interest development of Chinese school pupils, using both cross-sectional and logitudinal approaches. The subjects were 2,111 youngsters (1,063 males and 1,048 females) sampled from two elementary schools and two junior high schools in Taipei. A questionnaire consisting of 17 sets of items concerning school-related interests, recreational preferences, and personal and social interests was administered once a year. The major findings were: (1) Interest in basic academic subjects, such as Chinese, did not change with age, but interest in mathematics steadily declined as the children grew older. (2) Interest in extracurricular activities and technical subjects changed considerably during childhood and adolescence. To a greater extent than was anticipated, similarities were found in the interest patterns of both sexes throughout the period of junior high school. Differences between grade groups were not significant.

957

Lu, C. Y. (1982). [A study on the development of interests in Chinese school gifted pupils]. *Bulletin of Educational Psychology*, *15*, **1-17.** (In Chinese.)

Conducted a 3-yr longitudinal study on the physical and psychological development of 424 gifted and 468 normal children from 4 elementary schools and 3 middle schools in the Taipei area. Ss completed a questionnaire consisting of 10 sets of items in 3 fields: school-related interests, recreational preferences, and personal and social interests. Results indicate clear differences between the gifted group and normal group. A majority of gifted Ss were highly interested in Chinese and elementary science. However, Ss' interests varied according to their intellectual and maturational levels.

958

Lu, J. (1981). [Research on the logical reasoning ability of 4-9 year old children--verifications of some of Piaget's experiments]. *Acta Psychologica Sinica*, *13*, **30-34.** (In Chinese.)

This paper seeks to verify Piaget's claims concerning the acquisition of conservation in children. The preliminary results demonstrated the development of logical thinking in the acquisition of conservation of children aged 4 to 9 years. They also showed that the developmental levels of conservation of substance, weight, and volume of these children were almost similar, whereas in Piaget's experiments they were different.

959

Lu, J. (1984). [An experimental study of the concrete-abstract transformation by children aged 4-7 years]. *Acta Psychologica Sinica*, *16*, **8-14.** (In Chinese.)

The study is to analyze the cognitive process of transformation form concrete to abstract and abstract to concrete.

960

Lu, J. (1984). [The development of number concepts in young children]. *Information on Psychological Sciences*, **No. 3, 1-7.** (In Chinese.)

The question of whether the child's notion of numbers is acquired from perception or from counting remains controversial. An experiment with children 2-5 years old supported the view that the notion of numbers was acquired in the order of discrimination, perception, and counting. Children younger than 3.5 years of age were better in recognizing than in counting numbers; the reverse was found for children older than 3.5 years. It might be concluded that the age of 3.5 years was a transition from recognizing to counting numbers.

961

Lu, J., & Lu, W. J. (1981). [A preliminary study of class inclusion in children from 3 to 7 years old]. *Acta Psychologica Sinica*, *13*, **266-272.** (In Chinese.)

This is an experimental study of the concept of class inclusion in preschool children. According to Piaget, preschool children cannot understand this concept. In this investigation, different methods were designed from the method used by Piaget, and the preschool children showed better results in understanding the concept of class inclusion.

962

Lu, J., Zhang, Z. J., & Chen, A. F. (1985). [Development of the concept of equally divided areas in children aged 5 - 11]. *Information on Psychological Sciences*, **No. 4, 8-14.** (In Chinese.)

963

Lu, S. J., & Li, H. Y. (1985). [A study on the stability of the concept of length among Zang (Tibetan) and Han children between the ages of 5 and 11 years]. *Acta Psychologica Sinica*, *17*, **71-79.** (In Chinese.)

This is a study of the stability of the concept of length among Zang (Tibetan) and Han children on the Qinghai Plateau between 5 to 11 years of age. The children were asked to compare the lengths of two or three objects. The results indicated that the stability of their concept of length increased with age. Significant differences between Zang and Han children were found only in the 11-year-old group. The development of the stability of the concept of length underwent four stages, corresponding roughly to increases of age, but there was no clear-cut transition from one stage to another. Differences in cultural and educational backgrounds clearly influenced this development.

964

Ma, H. K. (1985). Cross-cultural study of altruism. *Psychological Reports*, *57*, **337-338.**

Completion of an altruism scale by 78 Chinese (mean age 17.1 years) and 213 English (mean age 15.1 years) subjects revealed that they were more altruistic toward persons who were more closely related and that, apart from the stranger variable, the mean ratings in the two cultural samples were very close.

965

Ma, H. K. (1985). A cross-cultural study of sex differences in human relationships. *Psychological Reports*, *56*, **799-802.**

The validity of an altruistic hierarchy of human relationships was tested in a cross-cultural study involving 259 male and 260 female Chinese and 215 male and 185 female English high school students and adults. Subjects were presented with 2 hypothetical dilemmas and asked to what degree they would be willing to sacrifice themselves for another individual's survival. It was hypothesized that the probability for a subject to perform an altruistic act would depend on the relationship with the other individual, with probability decreasing in the following order of relationships: close relatives; best friends; strangers who are weak, young, or elite; common strangers; and enemies. Results generally supported the proposed hierarchy of human relationships; however, female subjects in both samples were more altruistic than the male subjects, and Chinese subjects were generally slightly more altruistic than English subjects.

966

Mao, Y. Y. (1984). [A comparative study of the adaptative behavior between the only-child and the non-only child]. *Acta Psychologica Sinica, 16,* **240-249.** (In Chinese.)

The adaptive behaviors of only and nononly children in nurseries were compared. The subjects were 48 pairs of only and nononly children aged 3 to 4 1/2 years. Observations were made and questionnaires were administered. The results showed no significant differences in adaptative behavior between only and nononly children, or between boys and girls, during their first month in kindergarten. Factors which influence adaptative behavior, indications of suitability for admission, and effective teaching methods for decreasing children's separation anxiety when entering nurseries were discussed.

967

Mao, Y. Y., Fan, C. R., & Over, R. (1983). Lateral symmetry in duration of grasp by infants. *Australian Journal of Psychology, 35,* **81-84.**

Tested 34 Chinese infants aged 63-135 days to determine how long each S maintained grasp of a rattle. The mean duration of grasping did not differ consistently for the left hand and the right hand. This result contrasts with the asymmetry in grasp favoring the right hand found by P. J. Caplan and M. Kinsbourne (1976) with American infants of similar ages using the same procedures.

968

Mao, Y. Y., & Zhou, Z. F. (1986). [A longitudinal study of the mental development of children from birth to 36 months]. *Acta Psychologica Sinica, 18,* **113-122.** (In Chinese.)

Using a tentative mental scale, the authors administered the mental tests to 29 children each month from birth to 36 months. At the same time they recorded and analyzed the mothers' detailed reports. The purposes were: (1) to collect the children's normative data in five areas (gross motor, fine motor, language, adaptive behavior and personal-social behavior) in their first three years; and (2) to study the factors which affected the mental development of children under three years of age. The patterns of the developmental process, mental activity levels of performing cognitive tasks, influences of personality upon mental development of children and the main indicators of mental abilities were discussed.

969

Mardell-Czudnowski, C., Hwang, C. H., & Wang, T. M. (1986). Cross-cultural adaptation of a developmental test (DIAL-R) for young children in Taiwan. *Journal of Cross-cultural Psychology, 17,* **475-492.**

Developmental Indicators for the Assessment of Learning-Revised (DIAL-R), a developmental test for children 2 to 6 years old, was modified minimally and translated for use in Taiwan. After it was normed on a stratified sample of 322 children in Taipei, analyses of internal consistency, construct validity, test-retest reliability, and concurrent validity all indicated that the test meets the standards of a technically adequate screening test for that culture, giving it criterion-referenced meaning. Whereas the normative data suggest that most skills develop at comparable ages in the two cultures, there are some notable exceptions, some of which develop earlier in American children, others of which develop earlier in Chinese children. These differences were discussed in context with environmental and cultural components, giving the test construct-referenced meaning.

970

Marks, S. C. (1985). A study of the intellectual development of Chinese children. *Dissertation Abstracts International, 46,* **A931.**

971

Martin, R. (1975). The socialization of children in China and in Taiwan: An analysis of elementary school textbooks. *The China Quarterly,* **No. 62, 242-262.**

972

Masangkay, Z. S. et al. (1972). The development of ethnic group perception. *Journal of Genetic Psychology, 121,* **263-270.**

Attempted to trace the development of children's impressions of ethnic groups and to determine the role of their mothers' perceptions on this process. Each of 52 Phillipine mothers and their 10- and 15-yr-old children were assessed in terms of their attitudes and specific stereotypes of Tagalog (in-group) and Chinese (out-group) people. Results demonstrate that children develop ethnic attitudes at an early age but that the attribution of specific traits to different ethnic groups occurs later in the socialization process. The relationship between mothers' impressions of specific groups and those of their children was relatively low, suggesting that other agents are significant in the development of children's ethnic perception.

973

Mead, M., & Wolfenstein, M. (Eds.). (1955). *Childhood in contemporary cultures.* **Chicago, IL: University of Chicago Press.**

974

Meng, H. W., Song, H. Y., Dong, Q., & Wang, X. P. (1982). [A study of the development of part-whole picture perception at 4-8 years of age]. *Acta Psychologica Sinica, 14,* **184-189.** (In Chinese.)

Children's picture perception of parts and wholes was investigated. The subjects were 98 children 4-8 years of age. The pictures used were those in which both the parts and the wholes had independent meaning. The results showed: (1) The ability to perceive both the parts and the wholes increased with age; the parts were perceived at an earlier age than the wholes. These results were similar to those reported by Western investigators. (2) By age 8, part-whole integration was achieved by the majority (83%) of the children.

975

Meng, Z. L., & Campos, J. J. (1984). [The influence of different emotions on mental performance in infancy]. *Acta Psychologica Sinica, 16,* **231-239.** (In Chinese.)

The influence of happiness and distress on mental task performance in infancy was studied. The subjects were infants from Denver aged 16 months and and from Beijing aged 16-18 months. The two samples showed no significant difference. The results indicated: (1) The performance of the "happiness" group was better than that of the "distress" group. (2) Intensity of happiness had a curvilinear relation with performance, with the middle level being optimal. Intensity of distress was linearly and inversely related with performance.

976

Meng, Z. L., Yan, J., & Meng, X. D. (1985). [A preliminary study of the facial expression patterns of infants]. *Acta Psychologica Sinica, 17,* **55-61.** (In Chinese.)

This study used pictures of one-year-old Chinese babies showing their facial expressions of six emotions, happiness, surprise, sadness, anger, disgust, and fear. It also included discriminative and labeling tests. The patterns shown are basically the same as those of non-Chinese babies described by Izard in "Max." The results support the contention that there are basic patterns of facial emotional expression in human infancy which are invariant across cultures.

977

Miao, X. C. (1986). [Young children's understanding of interrogatives - The developmental peculiarities of answering WH questions in young children]. *Information on Psychological Sciences,* **No. 5, 1-5.** (In Chinese.)

The main purpose of this investigation was to explore how young Chinese children comprehend interrogatives in terms of their answers. The subjects, 160 children aged 3-7 years, were asked to answer questions concerning who, what, where, when, how, and why. The results indicated that most 3-year-olds were able to answer who, what, and where questions; most 4-year-olds were able to answer when and how questions; and it was not until the age of 5 that children could appropriately answer why questions. These findings were compared with those in other countries.

978

Moran, L. J. (1981). Evidence for the universal structure of the child's cognitive dictionary. *Journal of General Psychology, 105,* **149-154.**

Administered the same free-word association list, in English, Mandarin Chinese, and Japanese, respectively, to children and adults in the US, Taiwan, and Japan. Most of the children, but almost none of the adults, evidenced a primary response mode involving actions (rip-shirt, chair-sit). Results provide evidence for the probable endogenous construction of a universal child's cognitive dictionary, with a structure derived from sensorimotor action schemes as proposed by Piaget (1980).

979

Moran, L. J., & Huang, I. N. (1974). Note on cognitive dictionary structure of Chinese children. *Psychological Reports, 34,* **154.**

Obtained free-word associations from 74 4-6 yr old Chinese children to a list of 66 stimulus words previously used with Japanese and North American children. For the Chinese groups as for the others, the most frequent response was the enactive, or "action upon referent", indicating this as a cross-cultural organizing principle of cognitive dictionary structure.

980

Morland, J. K., & Hwang, C. H. (1981). Racial/ethnic identity of preschool children: Comparing Taiwan, Hong Kong, and the United States. *Journal of Cross-Cultural Psychology, 12,* **409-424.**

Compared more than 200 preschool children (4-6 yrs old) from 4 racial/ethnic groupings in 3 sociocultural settings on racial/ethnic identity, using a picture interview. One of the settings, Taiwan, was relatively homogeneous in racial/ethnic makeup; the 2nd, Hong Kong, was nonstratified; the 3rd, the US, was stratified. In Taiwan and Hong Kong, Ss were Chinese; in the US they were Afro- and Euro-

American. The major hypothesis was supported, because Taiwan and Hong Kong Ss differed from Afro- and Euro-American Ss on racial/ethnic preference, self-preference, and self-perception; from Euro-American Ss on classification ability; and from Afro-American Ss on self-classification. It is concluded that a crucial factor in the development of racial/ethnic identity was not so much whether the society was multiracial/ethnic or homogeneous, but whether racial/ethnic groupings in the multiracial/ethnic society were stratified.

981

Nan, B. H. B. (1973). *The development of the concept of space as observed in children's drawings: A cross-national/cross-cultural study.* **Doctoral Dissertation, University of California, Berkeley.**

982

Nationwide Research Group on Adolescent Mental Development. (1985). [A study of the thinking development of adolescent students from 23 provinces and cities in China]. *Acta Psychologica Sinica, 17,* **286-295.** (In Chinese.)

This study was an attempt to investigate the thinking development of first and third year students of junior high schools and second year students of senior high schools. The results were: (1) The stages of development of thinking are: (a) formal logical thinking, which begins to prevail in the first year of junior high and matures by the second year of senior high; and (b) dialectical logical thinking, which emerges in its initial form in the first year of junior high and begins to take hold in the second year of senior high. (2) The overall level of the development of thinking is about the same in boys and girls, though both have their own characteristics. (3) There are differences in the development levels of student thinking between different types of high schools.

983

Ng, P. P. T. (1984). *Socio-demographic patterns of leisure behaviour of adolescents in Hong Kong* **(Occasional Paper No. 4). Hong Kong: Chinese University of Hong Kong, Centre for Hong Kong Studies.**

984

Ng, S. H. (1983). Children's ideas about the bank and shop profit: Developmental stages and the influence of cognitive contrasts and conflict. *Journal of Economic Psychology, 4,* **209-221.**

Administered a questionnaire dealing with the operation of bank and shop transactions to 96 Hong Kong boys (aged 6-13 yrs). The developmental progression in the understanding of the bank, though more complex in the Hong Kong sample, was found to be essentially similar to that of a Scottish sample reported by G. Jahoda. It was found that a full understanding of the bank emerged at 10 yrs of age while that of shop profit emerged at age 6, both showing a precocity over the Scottish sample. The present author also considered the roles of cognitive differentiation and conflict and experimentally tested for any new understanding that might result from the experience of cognitive contrasts and conflict. The experience produced a significant improvement in the understanding of the bank among 10-13 yr old boys and of shop profit among 8-10 yr old boys.

985

Ng, S. H. (1985). Children's ideas about the bank: A New Zealand replication. *European Journal of Social Psychology, 15,* **121-123.**

The author investigated what children in New Zealand know about the bank, using data from interviews with 140 first to fourth graders, aged 7 to 12 years. A Hong Kong study by the present author showed that the development of the understanding of bank interest and profit was essentially similar to that of a Scottish sample reported by G. Jahoda. It also uncovered two minor stages in addition to Jahoda's 6 stages. The present study confirmed the presence of these two stages as well as the others; and, like the Scottish sample, it showed a New Zealand "lag" behind Hong Kong. The results showed that the maturity of ideas about bank activity and income was clearly related to age. However, this relationship was asymmetrical; advancing age was not always correlated with mature ideas.

986

Ni, L. (1962). [Study of the causes of maladjustment of adolescents through the use of projective test]. *Acta Psychologica Taiwanica,* **No. 4, 32-52.** (In Chinese.)

987

Niem, T. I. C., & Collard, R. R. (1972). Parental discipline of aggressive behaviors in four-year-old Chinese and American children. *Proceedings of the 80th Annual Convention of the American Psychological Association, 7,* **95-96.**

This study attempted to discover if there were cultural differences between a group of Chinese and American children in kind and amount of aggressive behavior and in parental discipline of aggression. The subjects were 17 Taiwanese and 17 American 4-year-old children. Results were based on daily records kept by the mothers for 30 days describing aggressive incidents of the children and discipline methods used. Chinese subjects were found to show significantly less physical aggression and more tantrums and more verbal aggression than American subjects. Chinese parents used significantly more love-oriented and less non-love-oriented techniques of discipline than did American parents.

988

Niu, J., & Zhang, S. F. (1983). [Survey on learning ability of 1400 students of Han, Bai and Dai nationality in Kunming, Dehong and Dali City in Yunnan province]. *Acta Psychologica Sinica, 15,* **395-401.** (In Chinese.)

989

Olsen, N. J. (1971). Sex differences in child training antecedents of achievement motivation among Chinese children. *Journal of Social Psychology, 83,* **303-304.**

The author administered a verbal measure of achievement motivation to 36 children 6 to 10 years old in a Taiwanese village. Their mothers responded to the Six Cultures Mother Interview, from which four items concerning independence training were selected. Two of the items, low reward for dependent overtures and early training in self-reliance (feeding and dressing), were found to be significantly related to achievement motivation in boys, as was a summary score based on all four items. Independence training was unrelated to achievement motivation in girls.

990

Olsen, N. J. (1975). Social class and rural-urban patterning of socialization in Taiwan. *Journal of Asian Studies, 34,* **659-674.**

Data were gathered on social class, determined on the basis of the occupation of the family's main wage earner, and rural urban patterning of socialization in Taiwan. A structured interview schedule was given to 107 mothers. The results showed that high-status urban mothers placed more emphasis on self-reliance, and less emphasis on conformity to authority and control of aggression, than low-status urbanites. They were also more affectionate and rewarding with their children, and were more inclined to use love-oriented than power-assertive modes of discipline. Rural mothers were at the opposite extreme on all these dimensions. Maternal educational level was found to be more important than social class as a determinant of affection, the use of love-oriented discipline, conformity, and values of self-reliance. In contrast, social class had a greater impact on aggression control and power-assertive discipline. This social class and rural-urban patterning of socialization appeared to be very similar to that observed in other countries.

991

Olsen, N. J. (1976). The role of grandmothers in Taiwanese family socialization. *Journal of Marriage & the Family, 38,* **363-372.**

Interviews were conducted with mothers and grandmothers in 49 carefully selected three-generation Taiwanese families. The following tentative conclusions are favored. As compared to their daughters-in-law, Taiwanese grandmothers are more concerned with aggression control and behavioral conformity, but are less punitive and less demanding of obedience and self-reliance. There is little difference in the socialization attitudes and practices of grandmothers according to whether their husband is also present in the family or not, but the correlation of mother and grandmother scores is consistently higher when both grandparents are present. Grandmothers are not likely to play a dominant role in the rearing of school age children. In almost half of the sample families, mothers exceed grandmothers in providing both nurturance and discipline. However, the likelihood that a grandmother will act as a source of nurturance is higher if she is widowed. Finally, there tends to be a "fit" between caretaking responsibilities and socialization attitudes. Both grandmothers and mothers are most punitive when they have responsibility for discipline, and are most affectionate in their attitudes when they are in charge of providing nurturance. Self-reliance training is least emphasized when mother and grandmother share responsibility for child care. Of particular significance is that widowed grandmothers participate more in the nurturing aspects of child care, but that nonwidowed grandmothers have more influence on the childrearing attitudes of their daughters-in-law. Taiwan is typical of many of the world's societies in that succession to family decision making responsibility ordinarily passes from father to eldest son. Upon the death of her husband, an older woman is no longer a member of the generation in which power resides. She still retains formal authority for the domestic side of family life, but her actual power declines.

992

Ong, E. N. (1985). The coping styles of Oriental youth. *Dissertation Abstracts International, 45,* **A3588.**

993

Ou, G. (1969). Youth in Hong Kong. In J. H. Masserman (Ed.), *Youth: A transcultural psychiatric approach.* **New York: Grune & Stratton.**

994

Ozawa, A., & Nomura, Y. (1981). [The effects of discrimination and decoding process on the reading of Kanji and Kana script in young children]. *Japanese Journal of Educational Psychology, 29,* **199-206.** (In other language.)

In Exp I, 32 kindergarten Ss read either 4 Kanji or ideographic scripts; the latency of correct reading was recorded. Results show that Ss reading the ideographic script read more quickly although there was no difference in the latency condition between the 2 groups. Results suggest that similarities between ideographic scripts and real things facilitated the decoding process. In Exp II (32 Ss), results support the hypothesis that meaningfulness facilitated the decoding processes and that this decoding was more effective in 4-letter than 2-letter conditions. In Exp III, 32 Ss learned the reading of 4 Kanji scripts; their latency responses were recorded. Kun (Japanese-style reading) was learned more quickly than On (Chinese-style reading), and simple scripts more quickly than complex ones. Latency of reading increased trial by trial. Results indicate that discrimination and decoding processes affected reading processes and that these processes were independent of one another.

995

Pedersen, P. (1983). The effect of group differences among church-related youth in Indonesia, Malaysia, and Singapore. *Counseling & Values, 27,* **130-141.**

Explored the extent to which "church-relatedness", as one among many group differences along with ethnicity, nationality, language, and belief, is reflected in self-described priorities and concerns of youth in Malaysia, Singapore, and Indonesia. Results indicate that traditional values seem to be important for church-related youth with different backgrounds. Chinese youth concerns were more self-centered, while Indonesian concerns emphasized sociopolitical responsibilities. Chinese-speaking youth emphasized priorities of family and national welfare, while English-speaking youth were more concerned about achievement and successful interpersonal relationships. Sumatran youth were more achievement-oriented and individualistic, and the Javanese youth emphasized social and political concerns. Church-related youth were not homogeneous in their concerns, with differences of language, nationality, ethnicity, and belief clearly dividing the church-related affiliations depending on the situational context described by each item.

996

Petzold, M. (1983). *Entwicklungspsychologie in der VR China: Wissenschaftsgeschichtliche Analyse, Entwicklungspsychologische Forschung und ihre Anwendung* **[Developmental psychology in the People's Republic of China: Science policy analysis, research in developmental psychology and its application]. Saarbrucken, Germany: Breitenbach.** (In other language.)

997

Poon, B. (1981). Infantile sexuality of Hong Kong Chinese: Oedipus, Hsueh, or else? *Hong Kong Psychological Society Bulletin,* **No. 6, 32-47.**

Topics discussed are Freud's (1933, 1936, 1962, 1973) account of the Oedipus conflict and B. Malinowski's (1960) proposal on infantile sexuality. A theory of Chinese infantile sexuality is proposed.

998

Poston, D. L., & Yu, M. Y. (1985). Quality of life, intellectual development and behavioral characteristics of single children in China: Evidence from a 1980 survey in Changsha, Hunan province. *Journal of Biosocial Science, 17,* **127-136.**

Data were collected on 1,069 children in Changsha in the Hunan Province of China to compare single-child families with multiple-child families regarding the quality of life, intellectual development, and behavior. The results on comparing these two types of families were generally similar to those obtained in the US and other Western countries. Single children had a better quality of life and performed better intellectually than children with siblings. With regard to behavior, they were similar to children with siblings, but were generally more cooperative and less hostile.

999

Prior, M., Kyrios, M., & Oberklaid, F. (1986). Temperament in Australian, American, Chinese, and Greek infants: Some issues and directions for future research. *Journal of Cross-Cultural Psychology, 17,* **455-474.**

Ratings of temperament in 4- to 8- month-old infants were compared across four cultural groups (American, Chinese, Australian, and Greek-Australian) using the revised Infant Temperament Questionnaire. Significant differences were found on all dimensions, with American and Australian infants being most alike and Greek and Chinese being very different from these two groups. Generally, positive or "easy" temperament profiles characterized American and Australian infants while a "difficult" profile emerged for Greek-Australian infants. Biological and cultural explanations were considered in interpretations of the obtained differences. It was concluded that there are important cultural effects on temperament ratings but that such effects are complex and require more careful investigation.

1000

Research Group in the Study on Ideals, Motives and Interests of Adolescents (1982). [The study in ideal, motive and interest of adolescents in school in ten provinces and cities]. *Acta Psychologica Sinica, 14,* **199-210.** (In Chinese.)

Research results show that most Chinese adolescents possess strong ideals and that these ideals provide the basis of their outlook on life. It is argued that education must arouse the students' motives, foster their interests, and deal with the relation between these factors and ideals.

1001

Ripple, R. E., Jaquish, G. A., Lee, H. W., & Spinks, J. A. (1983). Intergenerational differences in descriptions of life-span stages among Hong Kong Chinese. *International Journal of Intercultural Relations, 7,* **425-437.**

Investigated intergenerational differences in descriptions of life-span stages using 248 9-63 yr old Hong Kong Chinese (128 males, 79 females). Ss generated 3 words that, in their opinions, described each of 8 age stages, 0-9 through 70-79 yrs. Response protocols were scored positive, neutral, or negative, and the easiest and hardest age decades to describe were identified. Results indicate that younger age groups were easiest to describe; older age groups and Ss' own age group were hardest to describe. Females were significantly more positive than males in their descriptions. There was a tendency for older age groups to be more positive in their descriptions than younger Ss. Younger age decades were described more positively than older ones. The traditional concepts of Chinese socialization practices, the Confucian concept of filial piety, and other cross-cultural research are discussed.

1002

Ryback, D. (1974). Child-rearing and child care among the Sino-Thai population of Bangkok. *Journal of Social Psychology, 92,* **307-308.**

1003

Salili, F., & Hoosain, R. (1981). Acquisition of bitransitive sentences in Persian and Chinese: Differences between comprehension and production tests. *Perceptual & Motor Skills, 53,* **475-482.**

48 Iranian and 48 Chinese children, aged 3-5 yrs, were tested for their comprehension and production of 2 forms of bitransitive sentences in their respective languages. There was evidence that sentential forms in which the transfer object was mentioned next to the transfer action were acquired better by the Ss than those in which the 2 were separated by the recipient of the transfer object. Sentences that were closer in structural or semantic aspects to extralinguistic experiences were handled better. Some differences were obtained between sentence comprehension and sentence production, apparently due to psychomotor factors in language-related behaviors.

1004

Scofield, R. W., & Sun, C. W. (1960). A comparative study of the differential effect upon personality of Chinese and American child training practices. *Journal of Social Psychology, 52,* **221-224.**

1005

Shen, D. L., Liu, J. Q., & Lin, J. Q. (1983). [An experimental study of the development of motor skills in middle school students]. *Information on Psychological Sciences,* **No. 5, 26-30.** (In Chinese.)

1006

Shen, J. X., Liu, F. et al. (1984). [Research on the development of "Volume" concept of 5-17 years old children and youth]. *Acta Psychologica Sinica, 16,* **155-164.** (In Chinese.)

1007

Shiang, J. (1986). "Heart" and self in old age: A Chinese model. In M. I. White & S. Pollak (Eds.), *The cultural transition: Human experience and social transformation in the Third World and Japan^ (pp. 211-239). Boston: Routledge & Kegan Paul.*

1008

Shiao, K. S. (1975). [The analysis of the values of children]. Thought and Word, 13, *46-53. (In Chinese.)*

1009

Shu, T. Y., Mon, C. L., & Chang, P. Y. (1960). [Contradictions and social influence in child mental development]. Acta Psychologica Sinica, *No. 3, 154-161. (In Chinese.)*

1010

Silverberg, R., Obler, L. K., & Gordon, H. W. (1979). Handedness in Israel. Neuropsychologia, 17, *83-87.*

Found that the handedness scores of 1,171 Israeli high school students were independent of ethnic origin, socioeconomic class, and reading direction. The distribution was significantly different from Taiwanese and British populations reported in the literature. Cultural and genetic factors giving rise to the differences in the distribution are discussed.

1011

Sollenberger, R. T. (1968). Chinese-American childrearing practices and juvenile delinquency. Journal Of Social Psychology, 74, *13-23. (Also* **Child & Family,** *1969,* **8,** *279-288.)*

From intensive interviews of 69 Chinese-American mothers on childrearing practices and personal observations over a period of 7 wk., it is concluded that the low delinquincy rate in Chinatown, New York City, is probably due to the following: (1) The integrated family and indulgence of the child for the 1st 6 yr. reduce frustrations to a minimum, (2) physical aggression and competitive behavior is strongly discouraged, (3) within the family and the community, the child is continuously in contact with good models of behavior, and

(4) parents accept complete responsibility for the proper social behavior of the child.

1012

Steward, D., & Steward, M. (1974). Early learning in the family: A report of research in progress. Character Potential, 6, *171-176.*

Studied teacher-learner dyads for 3 different ethnic groups: Chinese, Anglo, and Mexican-American. Mothers were videotaped teaching 3-yr-old boys (their own and others') 2 games, 1 a sorting task, the other a motor task. Coders with 10 hrs training coded "parent-interaction" codes for teaching learning loops with reliability in excess of .85. Teaching strategies and child responses differed by ethnic group and by mother teaching own or another's son. Implications for education, particularly religious education, are discussed.

1013

Steward, M., & Steward, D. (1973). The observation of Anglo-, Mexican-, and Chinese-American mothers teaching their young sons. Child Development, 44, *329-337.*

Observed parents teaching preschool-age children a sorting and a motor-skill game. 6 mothers and their own 3-yr-old sons from 7 ethnic groups participated: middle-class Anglo-American, lower-class Anglo-American, English-speaking Mexican-American, bilingual Mexican-American, Spanish-speaking Mexican-American, English-speaking Chinese-American, and Chinese-speaking Chinese-American. Interaction was videotaped. Coders were selected from each ethnic group. Data were coded using a parent interaction code which analyzed programmatic variables: total time, input, and pacing; and teaching-loop variables: alert, format, child response, and feedback. The single best predictor of maternal teaching, or child response, was ethnicity. Children in this study experienced different learning environments which may result in different skills and expectations brought by them into the classroom.

1014

Stigler, J. W. (1983). Abacus skill in Chinese children: Imagery in mental calculation. Dissertation Abstracts International, 43, *B3387.*

1015

Stigler, J. W., Smith, S., & Mao, L. W. (1985). The self-perception of competence by Chinese children. Child Development, 56, *1259-1270.*

Cultural differences in self-perceptions of competence between Chinese and American elementary schoolchildren were investigated. A Chinese translation of the Perceived Competence Scale for Children was administered to 714 children in Grade 5 in Taiwan, and results were compared with four American samples studies by S. Harter that employed the same scale. The results showed a nearly perfect replication of the factorial validity of the four subscales (Cognitive Competence, Social Competence, Physical Competence, and General Self-Worth) in the Chinese sample. Also similar across the two groups was a high correlation between perceived cognitive competence and actual achievement in school. However, cultural differences were also found. Chinese subjects tended to underrate their competence compared to American subjects, except in the social domain, where higher ratings were judged to reflect a difference in social reality. Judging oneself as important to one's peers loaded on the Cognitive subscale for the Chinese and the Social subscale for the Americans. Chinese subjects also differentiated satisfaction with oneself from the desire to change for the better.

1016

Su, C. S. (1972). [A study of Chinese children's moral judgment]. Bulletin of Research Institute of Education *(National Taiwan Normal University),* **14,** *271-363. (In Chinese.)*

1017

Su, C. W. (1968). A developmental study of the child's concept of life. Psychological Testing, 15, *522-529.*

1018

Su, C. W. (1969). [A study of aggressive behavior in preschool children]. Psychology and Education *(Taiwan Normal University),* **3,** *11-28. (In Chinese.)*

Time samples of aggressive behavior were obtained from preschool children of 3 to 5 years of age in Taiwan during free play and during doll-play sessions. The main findings were: (1) The frequency of aggressive responses, particularly for girls during doll play, increased with age. (2) Boys showed more aggressive responses than girls during free play, but there was no significant difference during doll play. (3) During free play, boys showed more physical than verbal aggressive responses, but girls showed a nearly equal number of physical and verbal aggressive responses. (4) During free play, there was not a single aggressive response directed against the teachers, although there were some directed against other adults. (5) There was no correlation between the frequencies of aggression during free play and during doll-playing sessions. The children were quite inhibited in the doll-play situation, with which they were unfamiliar. (6) A clear majority of the mothers responded in interviews that they would "absolutely not tolerate" aggressive behavior directed against parents; the percentages were much lower if the behavior was directed against siblings or against children in the neighborhood.

1019

Su, C. W. (1973). [Children's discovery of the conservation of number, mass, weight, and volume]. Psychological Testing, 20, *1115-1129. (In Chinese.)*

1020

Su, C. W. (1975). [Maternal child rearing attitudes and practices in relation to aggressive behavior of school children]. Bulletin of Educational Psychology *(Taiwan Normal University),* **8,** *25-44. (In Chinese.)*

The aggressive behavior of 111 children, 50 boys and 61 girls, from three third grade classes was rated by their classmates. Concurrently, the mothers of all subjects were interviewed individually to obtain information about their child-rearing attitudes and practices. The results were: (1) Maternal punishment for aggression at home increased the children's aggressive behavior both in school and at home. (2) Maternal rejection and shaming seemed to instigate aggressive behavior both in school and at home. No significant correlations were found between the child's aggressiveness and the variables of maternal restrictiveness, lack of nurturance, and parental disharmony. (3) The mother's own aggressive behavior was not significantly related to the child's aggressive behavior in school or at home or to the child's sex-role identification. Internalization of parental standards did not seem to be an important factor for suppressing aggressive behavior. (4) Children of higher socioeconomic status showed less aggressive behavior than children of lower socioeconomic status. (5) Maternal child rearing attitudes and practices had stronger effects on the aggressive behavior of girls than on that of boys. (6) Maternal authoritarian attitudes toward children were unrelated with the child's aggressive behavior. However, girls of mothers with democratic attitudes showed less aggressiveness in school; but this relationship did not hold for boys. Children of mothers who had more marital conflicts and refused to assume their home-making roles were more aggressive at home.

1021

Su, C. W. (1975). [Parental childrearing practices as related to moral behavior in adolescence]. Acta Psychologica Taiwanica, 17, *109-124. (In Chinese.)*

This is a study of parental child-training practices and moral development. The subjects were seventh-grade children in Taiwan. They were assessed on several dimensions of moral behavior, such as guilt intensity, resistance to temptation, moral judgment orientation, honesty, and consideration for others by means of story completion tests and peer nomination. Parental discipline and child-rearing practices were measured by the Parent-Child Relations Questionnaire. The children reported that both fathers and mothers relied more on induction (explaining why the unwanted behavior is wrong and what consequences it would have) than on love withdrawal or power assertion. There was a tendency for both parents to rely more on induction when disciplining daughters than when disciplining sons, and more on power assertion and love withdrawal when discipling sons than when disciplining daughters.

1022

Su, C. W. (1978). [Similarity of attitudes between adolescents and their parents as related to their adjustment]. Bulletin of Educational Psychology, 11, *25-36. (In Chinese.)*

This study aimed to understand the attitudes held by adolescents and their parents regarding four family concepts ("my family," "my father," "my mother," and "my child") and to explore the relationship between the similarity of attitudes between adolescents and their parents and adolescents' adjustment. Subjects were 194 sophomores from four different junior high schools in Taipei and their parents. Semantic differential technique was used to measure the attitudes of adolescents and their parents. California test of personality was given to subjects to measure their personal and social adjustment. The following results were found: (1) There was a high degree of similarity of attitudes between adolescents and their parents regarding to "my family", "my father" and "my mother". However, there was significant difference of attitude between adolescents and their parents on "my child". Parents' ratings about their children were generally better than the adolescents self ratings. (2) The degree of similarity of attitudes between adolescents and their parents regarding the four family concepts had nothing to do with the adjustment of adolescents. (3) The degree of similarity between adolescents and their parents' self-rating was significantly related to the personal and social adjustment of adolescents.

1023

Su, C. W. (1979). [Basic emotional development of children and adolescents]. Bulletin of Educational Psychology, 12, *99-114. (In Chinese.)*

A sample of 1,436 schoolchildren from grade 4 to grade 9 were studied as to their self-expressed happiness, anger, sadness, fears and worries, and their reactions to these emotions. Generally speaking, the children and adolescents tended to regard school success and personal achievement as the happiest experiences; the percentage increased with age. This was followed by holidays or festivals, and recreational activities; the percentages decreased with age. The most frequently mentioned incidences of anger by the children were behaviors of other people, frustration from school work, and personal restrictions. Mentioning belongings broken or lost, behaviors of other people, and being punished increased with age, more so by boys than by girls. The most frequently mentioned fears were natural disasters, being left alone in the dark, accidents, injuries, and threats to personal safety. For the adolescents, the above mentioned fears decreased with age; instead, fears of school life and the future increased. Sad experiences centered around sickness and death of family members; the percentage decreased with age. The most frequently mentioned worries of the subjects were school work, being punished, family life, peer relationships, and personal weakness. The major patterns of responses were almost the same for both children and adolescents.

1024

Su, C. W. (1980). [A developmental study on the manifest anxiety of children and adolescents and its related factors]. Bulletin of Educational Psychology, 13, *85-94. (In Chinese.)*

This study investigated anxiety manifested by children and adolescents and its correlates. The subjects were 242 children in the fifth grade and 254 adolescents in the eighth grade from two elementary and two junior high schools. They were given the Children's Manifest Anxiety Scale, Tennessee Self-Concept Scale, Children's Internal-External Control Scale, Emotional Maturity Scale, Eysenck's Juvenile Personality Inventory, Parent-Child Relation Questionnaire, and Raven's Standard Progressive Matrices. The results indicated that adolescents had higher anxiety scores than elementary school children. Girls had higher anxiety scores than boys. The manifest anxiety scores were not consistently related to intelligence test scores and school achievement. They were significantly and negatively related to some personality factors, such as self-concept, internality, and emotional maturity. A multiple regression was made, using scores of the parent-child relation questionnaire as predictors and children's manifest anxiety score as the criterion. The regression coefficients were significant only for adolescents. The predictors accounted only for 11-24% of the variance of the criterion.

1025

Su, C. W. (1981). [A longitudinal study on the development of basic emotions of school children and adolescents]. Bulletin of Educational Psychology, 14, *79-102. (In Chinese.)*

This is a longitudinal study of the development of basic emotions of school children and adolescents. The subjects were 212 third grade children, 216 sixth grade children, and 231 ninth grade adolescents. A questionnaire on self-expressed happiness, anger, sadness, fears and worries, and reactions to these emotions was administered twice, with a 2-year interval. The results indicated that developmental trends were more evident for the emotions of happiness, anger, and fear than sadness and worry. They also varied according to the sex of the subject.

1026

Su, C. W. (1982). [A study on the development of basic emotions of gifted children and adolescents]. Bulletin of Educational Psychology, 15, *67-84. (In Chinese.)*

Studied the development of emotions in 141 gifted and 163 average 4th graders, 293 gifted and 327 average 6th graders, and 131 gifted and 142 average 8th graders. Ss were from 4 elementary and 3 secondary schools in the Taipei area. Results indicate that there were no differences between gifted and ordinary Ss on their scores of emotional stability or their responses to happy or frightening situations. However, there were differences in their responses to situations provoking anger and sadness. Gifted and ordinary Ss dealt with their emotions in similar manners.

1027

Su, C. W., Chu, C. P., & Liu, H. H. (1971). [A study on motor development from four- through fourteen-year old children]. Bulletin of Educational Psychology, 5, *121-145. (In Chinese.)*

The main purposes of this study were to evaluate motor ability of children between 14 to 16 years old and to adapt the Lincoln Oseretsky Motor Developmental Scale for use with Chinese children. The scale was administered to 570 children in this age range, half males and half females. Analysis of the results showed that: (1) The odd-even split-half reliability coefficient for all subjects was .95. The split-half reliability coefficients at each age level ranged from .33 to .81 for male children, and from .58 to .81 for female children. (2) The correlations of total score with age for male and female children were .94 and .83 respectively. Item analysis indicated that every one of the 36 items was capable of discriminating between the performance of children from the age range 6 through 14. For the youngest group, 21 of the 36 items had the capacity to discriminate between the children's performances. (3) There were no sex differences in the performances of children younger than the age of 12. Above that age, girls performed significantly better than boys. No differences were found among children from families of different socioeconomic statuses. (4) Iranian children performed best, followed respectively by Chinese and American children.

1028

Su, C. W., Chu, C. P., & Liu, H. H. (1974). [The development of motor skill in Chinese children]. In K. S. Yang & C. H. Chang (Eds.), [Behavioral development of Chinese children*]. Taipei: Huan-yu Publishing Co. (In Chinese.)*

1029

Su, C. W., Hwang, C. H., Lu, C. M., & Chen, S. M. (1979). [Parent-child relationship and personality development of Chinese school children]. Bulletin of Educational Psychology *(Taiwan Normal University),* **12,** *195-212. (In Chinese.)*

Studied the relationship between parental childrearing practices and personality development in 2,084 students in Grades 1-9. Ss were administered the Parent-Child Relation Questionnaire, Tennessee Self-Concept Scale, Children's Locus of Control Scale, Emotional Maturity Test (Grades 4-9) and Junior Eysenck Personality Inventory (Grades 7-9). Teachers also rated problem behaviors for 1st-, 4th-, and 9th-grade Ss. Multiple regression analysis indicated that most personality variables could be significantly predicted by parental childrearing practices. This influence was greater for students in upper grades than for those in lower grades. Self-concept, internality, and emotional maturity were more susceptible to parental influence than neurotic and problem behaviors.

1030

Su, C. W., & Jong, J. T. (1984). [A longitudinal study on motor development of infants from birth to one year old]. Bulletin of Educational Psychology, 17, *73-98. (In Chinese.)*

This is a longitudinal study of the motor development of infants from birth to one year of age. The subjects were 28 infants. Each subject was observed in his or her home monthly. It was found that age, but not sex, was a very important predictor of motor development. The data obtained were similar to those of a cross-sectional study reported by Su et al. earlier. All of the infants' motor development was orderly. It was also found that early stimulation and good nutrition had a great influence on the development of infants.

1031

Su, C. W., & Jong, J. T. (1985). [A study about how mothers take care of their infants]. Bulletin of Educational Psychology, 18, *117-148. (In Chinese.)*

This study examined how mothers take care of their infants. Using questionnaires we interviewed 504 Chinese mothers whose infants ranged from birth to one year old. The items selected for discussion were the infants' sleeping patterns, diet, health, crying behavior, toilet training, and maternal feelings. The results showed that mothers' attitudes toward taking care of their male and female infants were similar. However, mothers liked boys more than girls. The socioeconomic level of the family was a very important factor in determining methods of infant care.

1032

Su, H. Y. (1962). [An investigation of the emotional development of the problem youth through the use of Pressey's Attitude-Interest Test]. Acta Psychologica Taiwanica, *No. 4, 53-64. (In Chinese.)*

1033

Sun, S. L. (1964). [Age differences in Muller-Lyer illusion]. Acta Psychologica Sinica, *No. 3, 223-228. (In Chinese.)*

Measurements in Muller-Lyer illusion were taken for children ranging from 6 to 18 years of age and adults. The results were: (1) The illusion showed no sex difference, but changed with different age levels, decreasing from 6-16 years of age; (2) Involvement of thought processes decreasde the illusion; (3) Adults with different professional experiences showed some differences in the illusion.

1034

Sung, B. L. (1985). Bicultural conflicts in Chinese immigrant children. Special Issue: Family, kinship and ethnic identity among the Overseas Chinese. Journal of Comparative Family Studies, 16, *255-269.*

The author examined bicultural conflict resulting from the clash between the customs of a newly adopted country and the values, customs, traditions, and heritage of the country from which an individual has emigrated. This problem was examined in relation to the difficulties (e.g., confusion, anxiety) it poses to Chinese immigrant children. Cultural differences were examined with regard to aggressive behavior, sexuality, thrift, affection, dependency, individualism, sports, tattling, education, respect for authority, and heroes and heroines. It was suggested that, faced with situations where courses of action are diametrically opposed or radically different, the immigrant child is often immobilized, not having the maturity to evaluate or modify choices or to adjust his/her values. It was concluded that both teachers and parents should be aware of these potential conflicts, avoid exacerbating the differences, and encourage in the immigrant child a healthy respect for cultural differences.

1035

Tan, H. K., & Stacey, B. G. (1981). The understanding of socio-economic concepts in Malaysian Chinese school children. Child Study Journal, 11, *33-49.*

120 Malaysian Chinese school children, aged 6-15 yrs, were interviewed to determine their understanding of socioeconomic concepts. The interview was based on a series of questions dealing with money, buying/selling, savings, banks, gambling, and a simple picture arrangement task. Results show significant age and sex effects and a positive relationship between age and understanding of socioeconomic concepts.

1036

Tan, T. Y. (1977). [Sex, psychosocial environment, and linguistic behavior in primary school children]. Research in Education & Psychology, 1, *224-225. (In Chinese.)*

1037

Tang, G. W. (1982). Abortion in single girls in Hong Kong. Journal of Adolescent Health Care, 2, *213-216.*

Examined the psychosocial factors and sexual behavior in 100 15-25 yr old women requesting an abortion. Ss were interviewed before their abortion regarding demographic and reproductive information. Six weeks after the abortion they were interviewed about their feelings about the operation. 70% were educated to Form III level (Grade 10 US equivalent), and these did not come from broken or disturbed homes. The adequacy of their prepregnancy use of contraception was significantly and positively related to their level of formal education. Ss all became pregnant by their boyfriends. 60% had engaged in sex because of romantic love. Ss did not show serious or prolonged sequelae at a follow-up conducted 8-10 wks after the abortion.

1038

Tang, J. (1984). [A study of the comparison of children's ability to transform active and passive forms in Chinese sentence structure]. Acta Psychologica Sinica, 16, *182-192. (In Chinese.)*

This study investigated the development of children's ability to transform active into passive sentence forms and vice versa in the Chinese language. The subjects were 208 children, including deaf, retarded, and normal pupils aged 9 to 13 years, and 21 deaf and mute children aged 14 to 18 years. Ten groups of sentences were used as test materials, each of which was composed of one active sentence and one passive sentence. All active and passive sentence forms in Chinese were represented. The results indicated that as a group normal children performed better than deaf children, who in turn performed better than retarded children. For normal children, the significant period in developing the ability to transform sentences fell between 10 to 11 years; for the retarded, between 12 to 13; and for the deaf, shortly after 12-13. These three groups showed identical trends in all kinds of transformations. No regular relationship was found between transformational ability and studies in language or arithmetic.

1039

Tao, G. T., Qiu, J. H., Yu, L., Tseng, W. S., Hsu, J. (1986). [Family background and behavior patterns of only and non-only children]. Chinese Journal of Neurology and Psychiatry, 19, *321-324. (In Chinese.)*

To investigate the family backgrounds and behaviorial patterns of children in urban and suburban areas, home visits were made and a questionnaire was administered to 587 preschool children. The survey revealed that behaviorial problems in both only and nononly children were related to the sex of the child, parental education and occupation, and urban-rural differences. In urban areas, only children were less likely than nononly children to be physically aggressive and get into fights, destructive of their possessions, unfriendly toward and ill-treat others; however, in rural areas, they were more likely to be overly tied to or dependent on adults, complain about being lonely, and have bad eating habits. Rural children were more likely than urban children to be aggressive, both physically and verbally, and less likely to feel embarrassed about their bad behavior. Urban children were more likely to have poor eating habits, and be destructive of their possessions, jealous, shy or timid, lacking in concentration and attention span.

1040

Teng, E. L., Lee, P. H., Yang, K. S., & Chang, P. C. (1976). Handedness in a Chinese population: Biological, social, and pathological factors. Science, 193, *1148-1150.*

Conducted a questionnaire survey of 4,143 Chinese, about half in elementary schools and half in colleges. Social pressure for right-handed writing and for eating was effective but showed little indirect influence on hand use in other activities. Neither primiparous birth nor birth to older mothers affected handedness. Twinning, however, seemed to be associated with both decreased right-handedness and lower intelligence.

1041

Teng, E. L., Lee, P. H., Yang, K. S., & Chang, P. C. (1979). Lateral preferences for hand, foot and eye, and their lack of association with scholastic achievement, in 4143 Chinese. Neuropsychologia, 17, *41-48.*

Conducted a hand preference questionnaire survey using Chinese students--2,102 4th and 5th graders and 2,041 undergraduates. Social pressure for right-handed writing and eating was effective, but showed limited transfer influence on other activities. The general features of the distribution showed the same characteristics found in Caucasian samples. Distributions of lateral preferences in foot and eye uses and the intercorrelations among hand, foot, and eye preferences, were also comparable with Western results. No difference was obtained between the grade-school sample and the university sample, indicating a lack of association between lateral preferences and intelligence in the nonclinical population.

1042

The Collaborative Group for Research on the Acquisition of the Concept of Conservation. (1985). [A study of the acquisition of the concept of conservation]. Information on Psychological Sciences, *No. 6, 20-33. (In Chinese.)*

The study examined whether children's learning experience or underlying structure of thinking played a more important role in the acquisition of the concept of conservation. Subjects were three groups of 4 1/2 to 6 1/2 year old children with different cultural backgrounds from two different regions. None of the children were able to conserve weight. Age was an important factor in training the acquisition of the concept of weight. Cultural background had no effect on ability to conserve weight. The training procedure greatly benefited those subjects who had developed a certain logical structure of thinking. Without training being given at an appropriate time, progress would be retarded.

1043

The Cooperation Study Group of Oral Speech of Preschool Children. (1981). [Investigations into the development of speech of preschool children]. Information on Psychological Sciences, *No. 5, 30-37. (In Chinese.)*

This is a general summary of the results of six studies conducted under the same research program by five colleges and one middle school in different parts of China. Three hundred and eighty children aged from 2-6 years were tested. This paper consists of three parts: (a) The development of syntactic structures, (b) the length of sentences, and (c) the use of words of different parts of speech and comprehension of function words.

1044

The Co-operative Research Group on Children's Cognitive Development. (1982). [A study of 4-11 year old children's development of the stability of concepts in mathematics]. Acta Psychologica Sinica, 14, *272-284. (In Chinese.)*

Four sets of 3 or 5 test items were used to examine the stability of children's concepts in mathematics. In each of 13 districts in China, children between 3 to 11 years of age were examined individually with the "clinical method." No ethnic or sex differences were found. The stability of concepts seemed to develop in the following order: number, length, area, and volume.

1045

The Co-operative Research Group on Child's Conception of Numbers (1979). [The development of conception of number in children 3-7 years old in nine districts throughout China, and their ability to perform arithmetical operations: A general report]. Acta Psychologica Sinica, 11, *108-117. (In Chinese.)*

Conducted 9 experiments with similar procedures that tested 780 3-7 yr old children's conception of cardinal and ordinal numbers and their ability in addition-subtraction operations in 9 districts throughout China. Results are discussed in terms of S's development of counting ability, conception of group and addition-subtraction operations, conception of serialization and the relationship between cardinal and ordinal numbers, the conservation of number, mathematical reasoning, and the part different cognitive processes play in the conception of numbers.

1046

The Study Group on Children's Cognitive Development. (1984). [Development of the concept of length in children age 5 to 12 years in the five regions in China]. Information on Psychological Sciences, *No. 2, 8-12. (In Chinese.)*

1047

The Study Group on Moral Development. (1983). [An investigation of children's concepts of justice: A comparison with Piaget's data]. Information on Psychological Sciences, *No. 1, 15-21. (In Chinese.)*

Following Piaget's procedure, an attempt was made to study children's conceptions of justice. Responses were collected to questions about four stories which depicted possible violations of one's rights and personal integrity. The subjects were 1,585 primary and junior high school students. The results appeared to substantiate Piaget's proposal concerning the child's increasing acceptance of reciprocity as a principle with age.

1048

The Study Group on Moral Judgment of Children. (1982). [An investigation of the development of moral judgment in children]. Information on Psychological Sciences, *No. 1, 22-26. (In Chinese.)*

The studies of J. Piaget and D. Elkind were replicated. Four paired stories were given to 2,788 children in 18 districts of China to investigate their moral judgments. The results indicated that: (1) The critical period from objective to subjective responsibility was 6-7 years of age. (2) The critical period for making moral judgments that are independent of sanctions was 8-9 years. (3) With intentionality held constant, most children at all age levels judged personal injury as more culpable than property damage. Under unintentional conditions, responses to two kinds of damages were independent of the age; whereas under intentional conditions, they were not completely independent, and the variation appeared between 7 to 9 years.

1049

Tien, J. L. (1982). A descriptive cross-cultural study on factors associated with self-perceptions of aging among Anglo-Americans, Chinese-Americans, and Chinese in Taiwan. Dissertation Abstracts International, 43, *B1798.*

1050

Ting, T. Y. (1964). [The development of children's ability of picture observation]. Acta Psychologica Sinica, *No. 2, 161-169. (In Chinese.)*

This study is an experimental study of 120 children observing 3 pictures of different contents. The results showed: (1) The level of the children's ability to observe pictures was influenced by contents of the picture and the instruction. The results do not confirm Binet's contention that it is solely determined by the innate intelligence or "age". (2) The development of the children's ability to observe pictures could be considered as consisting of four stages: recognition of "individual objects"; recognition of "spatial relations"; recognition of "causal relations"; and recognition of "content as a whole".

1051

Ting, T. Y., Pan, C., Luo, M., & Sun, Y. M. (1964). [Memory of disconnected words, digits and pictures in school children]. Acta Psychologica Sinica, *No. 1, 33-40. (In Chinese.)*

Elementary school children served as subjects memorizing lists of words, digits and series of pictures. The results were: (1) The efficiency of memory was different, for different materials memorized. Concrete and lively pictorial materials were easily learned and better remembered than abstract materials. (2) Memory of "related" materials was better than "unrelated" materials, especially with concrete lively pictorial materials and delayed reproductions. (3) Children of the first grade realized that "related" materials were easier to commit to memory. They tried also to construct meaningful connections to facilitate memory. (4) The efficiency of memory increases with grade levels. The increase was more striking with "related" materials and in immediate reproductions.

1052

Tobin, J. J., & Friedman, J. (1984). Intercultural and developmental stresses confronting Southeast Asian refugee adolescents. Journal of Operational Psychiatry, 15, *39-45.*

Explored how critical issues of adolescence (separation, identity, and sexuality) interact with critical issues of being a refugee (loss and grief, survivor guilt, trauma reactions, and cultural discontinuity) among adolescent refugees from Southeast Asia. Refugees came from Vietnam, Laos, and Cambodia; between one-third and one-half were ethnically Chinese. In the Southeast Asian view of the life cycle, age serves as an important social and individual organizing principle. Subjects were conscious of being outside the normal ages in marrying, finishing education, getting a job, and having children. Case illustrations of how oedipal issues have been complicated by trauma reactions, survivor stress, and cultural discontinuity were given. It was suggested that cohorts of refugee children will be at risk until they reach stability in adulthood.

1053

Torrance, E. P., Gowan, J. C., Wu, J. J., & Aliotti, N. C. (1970). Creative functioning of monolingual and bilingual children in Singapore. Journal of Educational Psychology, 61, *72-75.*

Gave 1063 mono- and bilingual Chinese and Malayan 3rd, 4th, and 5th graders Figural Form A of the Torrance Test of Creative Thinking. The test booklets were translated and all instructions given in the native languages of the Ss. Fluency, flexibility, and elaboration were scored according to the standard guides of the test. A guide for scoring originality was based upon data from the Singapore culture, and was developed on the same principles as the United States version of the test. Results show that the monolinguals scored higher than the bilinguals on fluency and flexibility (p .01), but that the direction of the trend is reversed for originality and elaboration. The overall difference for elaboration is significant at about the .05 level but is not significant for originality. If corrections are made for number of responses, the trend toward the superiority of the bilinguals over the monolinguals on originality and elaboration becomes stronger.

1054

Treiman, R. (1984). Individual differences among children in spelling and reading styles. Journal of Experimental Child Psychology, 37, *463-477.*

Previous studies have found differences among children in their relative reliance on spelling-sound rules and word-specific associations in reading words. Children at one end of the continuum ("Phoenicians") rely heavily on spelling-sound rules; children at the other end ("Chinese") are more likely to use specific associations. This study found evidence for a Phoenician-Chinese continuum in spelling as well as in reading. 22 4th graders and 24 3rd graders completed a spelling test, a reading test, and a rapid reading test. Ability to spell nonsense words (e.g., prunt) correlated more highly with ability to spell regular words (e.g., grunt) than with ability to spell exception words (e.g., front). Ss who were skilled at rules tended to overgeneralize them to exception words. In addition, a measure of rule use in spelling correlated with measures of rule use in reading. Implications for the study of reading-disabled individuals are discussed.

1055

Treiman, R., & Baron, J. (1983). Individual differences in spelling: The Phoenician-Chinese distinction. Topics in Learning & Learning Disabilities, 3, *33-40.*

Discusses the processes that children and adults use to spell and read single words, concentrating on differences between those who use "Phoenician" and those who use "Chinese" rules. Phoenician refers to a reliance on spelling-sound rules; Chinese refers to a reliance on word-specific associations. Evidence suggests that Phoenicians are better able to read and spell than Chinese. This finding implies that learning the rules of reading and spelling are mandatory for ease in these competencies. Also, special attention may be needed for children who speak nonstandard dialects.

1056

Tsai, S. L. (1985). [A study of socioeconomic status, child-rearing attitudes, school environments, and junior high students' assertiveness and adjustment]. Bulletin of Educational Psychology, 18, *239-264. (In Chinese.)*

Assertiveness and adjustment of 941 junior high students were investigated. The dependent variables were parental child-rearing attitudes, myths of nonassertion, assertiveness (self-respect and self-expression), self-confidence, social anxiety, anxiety, and interpersonal relationships. The independent variables were sex, nature of school and class, experience of being a class cadre, participation in noncurricular activities in the school, and ability grouping. The results were: (1) Assertiveness was significantly correlated with socioeconomic status, child-rearing attitudes, experience of being a class cadre, participation in noncurricular activities, nature of school, ability grouping, myths of nonassertion, self-confidence, social anxiety, and interpersonal relationships. (2) There were interactions among ability grouping, sex, and nature of the school with regard to self-respect and assertiveness; similarly, there were interactions among ability grouping, sex, and nature of class with respect to self-expression.

1057

Tse, J. K. (1978). Tone acquisition in Cantonese: A longitudinal case study. Journal of Child Language, 5, *191-204.*

There have been relatively few studies on tone acquisition, as compared to studies on the acquisition of segmentals, morphology, and syntax. Still fewer are the studies on Chinese language acquisition. The present paper reports on a longitudinal case study of a Cantonese-speaking child aged 2 yrs 8 mo and considers the implications of tone acquisition for tone studies in general, and Cantonese tonology in particular.

1058

Tse, S. M. (1980). Acquisition of the Chinese language by young children: An overview. Acta Psychologica Taiwanica, 22, *41-50.*

Traces major studies of acquisition of Chinese that were done in China and in North America from 1759 to 1979. Emphasis is placed on the early period of a child's linguistic development (up to 3 yrs of age).

1059

Tsung, L. T. (1954). [An analysis of the results of general motor ability tests for elementary school children]. Psychological Testing, 2, *116-121. (In Chinese.)*

1060

Van, Y. Y., & Zian, C. T. (1962). [Special aspects in memorizing Chinese characters by elementary school children]. Acta Psychologica Sinica, *No. 3, 219-230. (In Chinese.)*

The learning of Chinese characters by 160 Grade 1 pupils from two elementary schools in Shanghai was systematically studied. Relations among the phonetic sound, the meaning, and different parts that form the characters had to be learned. Beginners often neglected details in these relations. Three factors are important in learning Chinese characters: the child's level of physical and mental development, the method of instruction, and learning rules governing the formation of Chinese characters.

1061

Wan, C. W., Fan, C. R., & Lin, G. B. (1984). [A comparative study of certain differences in individuality and sex-based differences between 5 to 7 year-old onlies and non-onlies]. Acta Psychologica Sinica, 16, *383-391. (In Chinese.)*

A comparison was made on behavioral differences between only children and nononly children aged 5 to 7 years in six day-care centers in Beijing. The subjects were 138 only and 127 nononly children (120 boys and 145 girls). Five categories of 16 behavioral items, dependency, independence, helpfulness, friendliness, and aggressiveness were observed. The only significant difference found between only and nononly children was in dependency among the 5-year-olds. It was also found that girls were significantly more friendly and less aggressive than boys.

1062

Wang, C. C. (1965). [A developmental study of eye movement in pre-school children]. Acta Psychologica Sinica, *No. 3, 259-264. (In Chinese.)*

1063

Wang, C. C. (1965). [Movement of the eye and development of visual object-perception in children of pre-school age]. Acta Psychologica Sinica, 32, *259-264. (In Chinese.)*

1064

Wang, H. T., Liu, C. H., & Fan, T. J. (1964). [An investigation into the development of concepts in children of 4-9 years: Vol. 2. Generalization development as reflected in children's ability to classify]. Acta Psychologica Sinica, *No. 4, 352-360. (In Chinese.)*

This is the second report on an investigation into development of concepts in children of 4-9 years of age. This study comprised two parts: investigation of the developmental trends reflected in children's ability to classify, and investigation of the age at which classification can be seen as a turning point in conceptual thinking. One hundred and eight children of 4-9 years were each asked to sort objects depicted on cards, according to his or her own ideas of classification. Another 72 children in the age groups of 5, 5-6, and 6 performed the second part of the experiment. The results were: (1) Children under 4 failed to carry out classification. (2) Children of 5-6 years showed a rudimentary ability to classify but their classification was mainly on the perceptual level. (3) Beyond 6-7 years, the children showed a conceptual ability in classification. Their conceptual thinking seemed to reach a new level. (4) In children from 4-9 years old, the turning point from perceptual to conceptual thinking as reflected in ability to classify seemed to fall between the age of 5-6.

1065

Wang, P. Y. (1963). [Growth of grip strength of Zhejiang children]. Acta Psychologica Sinica, *No. 3, 237-246. (In Chinese.)*

1066

Wang, P. Y. (1963). [Physical development of Zhejiang children]. Acta Psychologica Sinica, *No. 4, 336-346. (In Chinese.)*

1067

Wang, X. T., & Zhang, M. L. (1985). [On children's memory and cognition: Vol. 1. A study on the memory of serial configuration by children between 4 - 6 years of age]. Acta Psychologica Sinica, 17, *393-400. (In Chinese.)*

1068

Wang, X. Y. (1985). [A comparative study of the faculties of memory of children from different ethnic groups aged 9 and 11 on the Qinghai Plateau]. Acta Psychologica Sinica, 17, *401-409. (In Chinese.)*

This article presents a comparative study of the memory development of children aged 9 and 11 years, of the Han, Sala, Hui, Mongolian, Tu, and Tibetan nationalities living in nine different regions of the Qinghai Plateau. The indicators included cognition speed, memory scope, recollection of pictures, and association memory. The study indicates that children's memory among the Han, Sala, and Hui nationalities show no distinctive differences, but marked dissimilarity to that among Mongolian, Tu, and Tibetan children. Also, the memory between Mongolian, Tu, and Tibetan children show marked distinctions, which stem from differences in culture, geographical and economic environments, language facility and, most importantly, educational backgrounds. Overall, the results show that there are certain common characteristics in children's memory between the nationalities studied.

1069

Wang, Y. M. (1986). [Children's comprehension of dative and instrumental sentences and their comprehension strategies]. Information on Psychological Sciences, *No. 2, 16-22. (In Chinese.)*

The author investigated children's comprehension strategies on dative and instrumental sentences. Sixty children aged 3 to 7.5 performed test sentences with toys. In interpreting the test sentences the younger children were found to employ more frequently the event probability strategy based on semantic relations while the older ones relied more on the word-order strategy of regarding the first noun as the actor. These results are similar to those obtained in other countries, suggesting that these strategies are of universal significance.

1070

Ward, B. (1980). The integration of children into a Chinese social world: A preliminary exploration of some non-literate village concepts. Hong Kong Psychological Society Bulletin, *No. 4, 7-17.*

Describes the socialization of children in a small village (population 500) in the New Territories of Hong Kong in the 1950's, by exploring the traditional usages and connotations of 3 Cantonese words. (1) "Kaau", meaning broadly "instruct", was important because instruction was the only recognized way of training children. Kaau also applied to instruction in social behavior, especially in the correct ritual forms of greeting. (2) "Yeung" expressed the concepts of nurturing--caring for plants, animals, and other people. Up to the age of 6 or 7 children were the recipients of "yeung"; thereafter, children bestowed it, the role change being sharper for boys than girls. (3) "Hok" also had a variety of connotations--to learn, copy, and imitate--in which the child is seen as the subject, rather than as the object of action as in "kaau" and "yeung". The author speculates on the effect of modern changes in nurturing practices on the development of young children in Hong Kong.

1071

Ward, B. E. (1970). Temper tantrums in Kau Sai: Some speculations upon their effects. In P. Mayer (Ed.), Socialization: The approach from social anthropology *(pp. 109-125). London: Tavistock.*

1072

Weeks, M. F., & Moore, R. P. (1981). Ethnicity-of-interviewer effects on ethnic respondents. Public Opinion Quarterly, 45, *245-249.*

Considerable research has been reported on race-of-interviewer effects in White/Black dichotomies. Little is known, however, about interviewer effects on respondents representing other ethnic groups. The present study reports on a 1975 study of ethnicity-of-interviewer effects among 4 ethnic minorities--Cubans, Chicanos, Native Americans, and Chinese. It is suggested that the findings for Blacks and Whites are generalizable to other ethnic groups.

1073

Wei, C., Hwang, H. Y., Sung, C. Y., & Wang, C. F. (1964). [The development of the ability to compare in primary school children]. Acta Psychologica Sinica, *No. 3, 274-280. (In Chinese.)*

The results of an experimental study indicated that the development of the ability to compare in primary school children was influenced by the nature of the objects compared and the methods of comparison. It was also found that the comparing ability of primary school children grew gradually in accordance with age and grade. Different stages of age had different rates of development.

1074

Wei, C., Xiong, Z. C., & Shi, W. L. (1983). [An experimental research on the conception of some common natural phenomena and objects by children]. Information on Psychological Sciences, *No. 5, 9-18. (In Chinese.)*

This is a study of children's the cognition concerning some common natural phenomena and objects. The subjects were of 6 to 10 year olds. The results indicated that: (1) Though their cognitive level increased with age, most of the children 6 to 8 years old remained at the level of describing objects from their external characteristics and apparent connections; most of 9 to 10 year olds could grasp some of the essential characteristics and intrinsic connections. (2) Children of the same age, or even the same child, could exhibit different cognitive levels due to differences in the complexity of natural objects and phenomena. (3) Cognitive level was influenced by the children's living environment and particularly school education.

1075

Weissbluth, M. (1982). Chinese-American infant temperament and sleep duration: An ethnic comparison. Journal of Developmental & Behavioral Pediatrics, 3, *99-102.*

Parents' responses to the Carey Infant Temperament Questionnaire and results of a standard interview regarding sleep duration were obtained for 23 Chinese-American and 60 non-Chinese infants. Chinese-American Ss were rated as significantly more withdrawing, less adaptable, and more negative in mood than the other Ss. Total sleep duration for the Chinese-American Ss was 13.2 hrs as compared to 14.2 hrs for the others. Night sleep duration had a significant negative correlation with mood ratings in the Chinese-American Ss. Findings suggest that there are ethnic differences in infant temperament and that the relationship between negative mood and brief sleep is present among different ethnic groups.

1076

Westbrook, C. H., & Yao, H. H. (1937). Emotional stability of Chinese adolescents as measured by the Woodworth-Cady-Mathews questionnaire. Journal of Social Psychology, 8, *401-410.*

The Chinese translation of the Woodworth-Cady-Mathews questionnaire was administered to over 1,000 students. When the results are compared with those secured by Brooks from American students, it is found that the most unfavorable age for responses is 18 with Chinese subjects, whereas it is 7 for Brooks' American subjects. At every age the unfavorable responses of Chinese adolescents exceed those of foreign children at the corresponding age. In Terman's study (with gifted children) no significant sex difference is noted, whereas the authors found that Chinese girls at all ages have higher scores than Chinese boys. Eight items elicited over 50% unfavorable responses from both sexes. Further experimentation with the translations of the questions is necessary to determine whether the results obtained show a real or approximate measure of emotional instability for these Chinese students.

1077

Wheelwright, J. B. (1959). Some comments on the aging process. Psychiatry, 22, *407-411.*

1078

Wilson, R. W. (1967). [Childhood political socialization on Taiwan]. *Unpublished doctoral dissertation, Princeton University, Princeton, NJ.*

1079

Wilson, R. W. (1970). Learning to be Chinese: The political socialization of children in Taiwan. *Cambridge, MA: MIT Press.*

Attempts to explain the often puzzling behavior of the Chinese in terms of the concept of "face" and how Chinese children acquire attitudes toward authority, group cohesiveness, acceptable targets for aggression, and other nonpolitical but relevant aspects of personality. Data from 3 large primary schools are presented, and the relationships of "face" to group loyalty, political hierarchies, and political stability and how this relationship affects the style of government in China are discussed.

1080

Winitz, H. (1981). Input considerations in the comprehension of first and second language. Annals of the New York Academy of Sciences, 379, *296-308.*

Investigated whether adults differ from children on phonetic distinctions with which they are unfamiliar. Phonetic elements from Mandarin Chinese were selected for analysis in a study with 48 monolingual English-speaking 3rd graders and 48 college students. Findings show that adults were significantly better than children in distinguishing among Mandarin tones and sounds. It is argued that nonlinear learning typifies the lst-language learner, in contrast to the quite different experiences of 2nd-language learners. Implications for the crossover effect (i.e., that adults show an initial superiority over children in the initial stages of language learning but a subsequent relinquishing of this dominance as the 2nd language is acquired) are considered.

1081

Wolf, A. P. (1966). Childhood association, sexual attraction, and the incest taboo: A Chinese case. American Anthropologist, 68, *883-898.*

Whereas most sociological and biological explanations of the incest taboo assume that intimate childhood association enhances sexual attraction, most psychological explanations assume that such association depresses it. In northern Taiwan one of several forms of marriage involves the introduction of the bride into her future husband's home as an infant; bride and groom are then raised as members of the same family, experiencing a prolonged period of intimate association. The responses of these couples to marriage and sexual relations support the psychological view of the effects of intimate association on sexual attraction and thereby challenge the basis of most sociological and biological explanations of the incest taboo.

1082

Wolf, M. (1964, January). Child training in a Hokkien village. *Paper presented at the seminar Personality and Motivation in Chinese Society, Bermuda.*

1083

Wolf, M. (1970). Child training and the Chinese family. In M. Freedman (Ed.), Family and kinship in Chinese society *(pp. 37-62). Stanford, CA: Stanford University Press. (Republished in A. P. Wolf, Ed.,* **Studies in Chinese society,** *pp. 221-246. Stanford, CA: Stanford University Press, 1978.)*

1084

Wolfenstein, M. (1955). Some variants in moral training of children. In M. Mead & M. Wolfenstein (Eds.), Childhood in contemporary cultures *(pp. 349-368). Chicago, IL: University of Chicago Press.*

1085

Wolff, P. H., Hurwitz, I., Imamura, S., & Lee, K. W. (1983). Sex differences and ethnic variations in speed of automatized namings. Neuropsychologia, 21, *283-288.*

130 American-Caucasian, 110 Japanese, 60 Korean, and 110 American-Chinese 6-12 yr olds were administered the Stroop Color-Word Test. Results show significant sex differences for Caucasians; in each case, girls outperformed boys. American-Chinese, Japanese, and Korean Ss did not differ from Caucasians in naming speed when scores for boys and girls were combined. It is suggested that biological as well as experiential factors contribute to behavioral sex differences and that biological (genetic) variables associated with mating-group membership modify the expression of cognitive sex differences.

1086

Wong, A. (1981). A study of the initial adjustment to the American society of six Chinese immigrant females in high school. Dissertation Abstracts International, 41, *B3204.*

1087

Wong, P. T., & Reker, G. T. (1985). Stress, coping, and well-being in Anglo and Chinese elderly. Canadian Journal on Aging, 4, *29-37.*

Ethnic differences related to the coping behaviors of 40 elderly Chinese living in Canada were compared with 40 Caucasian Canadians. Internal, external, and palliative coping strategies were examined with a perceived well-being scale and a coping inventory. Results indicated that while Chinese subjects employed more coping strategies, they found growing old a more stressful experience, reported lower psychological well-being, depended more heavily on external and palliative coping strategies, and felt less effective in coping as compared to Anglo counterparts. Findings support the double jeopardy hypothesis of ethnic minority aging, which postulates that normal biological constraints of aging are compounded by acculturational stress and disadvantages associated with being a minority.

1088

Wong, S. Y., & Lii, S. Y. (1982). [Hemispheric specialization and its relation to subjects' gender, creativity, and sex-role typing]. Acta Psychologica Taiwanica, 24, *85-100. (In Chinese.)*

The present study used 939 elementary and junior high school students as subjects to investigate hemispheric specialization as measured by Torrance' revised Your Styles of Learning and Thinking. In addition, the Torrance Test of Creative Thinking was administered to 384 subjects of the original sample. The main findings were: (1) The correlations between Right Hemisphere Specialization (RHS) and creativity were positive and significant. Those between Left Hemisphere Specialization (LHS) and creativity were negative and significant. There were no significant correlations between Integrative Style (IS) and creativity. (2) Male students scored significantly higher than female students on RHS and LHS; females scored significantly higher on IS than males. (3) Gifted students scored significantly higher than ordinary students on RHS and IS; however, ordinary students scored significantly higher on LHS than gifted students. (4) The male students' positive masculinity trait was highly and positively correlated with RHS. Their positive femininity trait was highly and negatively correlated with IS. (5) The female students' positive masculinity trait was highly and positively correlated with IS. The implications of these findings to the development of creativity were discussed.

1089

Workie, A. (1979). The effect of meaningfulness on short- and long-term recall among Ethiopians. Journal of Social Psychology, 108, *161-164.*

Sought to demonstrate, in a non-Western (Ethiopian) cultural setting, the hypothesis that greater meaningfulness of verbal material results in better recall under conditions of short- and long-term memory. Verbal material of 3 levels of meaningfulness was presented to 31 male Ethiopian 12th graders. The least meaningful material was made up of words taken from Zulu, Hausa, and Chinese languages, while the intermediate and high-meaningful material consisted of Geez and Amharic words, languages prevalent in Ethiopia. Ss performed significantly better in high than in intermediate or low, and in intermediate than in low, meaningfulness conditions. Results confirm the hypothesis and validate it cross-culturally.

1090

Wu, F. Y. (1975). Mandarin-speaking aged Chinese in the Los Angeles area. Gerontologist, 15, *271-275.*

Notes that for centuries care of the aged was not a major social problem in China because the Confucian teaching of the Hsiao Ching of responsibility was deeply ingrained in the Chinese culture. In this Los Angeles study, it was noted that Mandarin-speaking elderly are the victims of political, social, economic, and cultural changes, including the change in the concept of filial piety. Data were gathered from interviews with 50 6-85 yr olds, questionnaires from 50 middle-aged respondents, and interviews with 10 community leaders and 4 social agency personnel in Chinatown. Inability to speak or understand English was the most serious problem for the elderly, who immigrated at an old age. Language barriers and cultural shock alienated the Chinese elderly from the mainstream of American society and excluded them from receiving needed services.

1091

Wu, J. P., & Xue, H. F. (1985). [Divergent thinking ability in school children]. Information on Psychological Sciences, *No. 5, 25-30. (In Chinese.)*

1092

Wu, T. M. (1983). [Preliminary research on the enhancing of intelligence]. Acta Psychologica Sinica, 15, *250-255. (In Chinese.)*

1093

Wu, T. M., & Xu, Z. Y. (1979). [A preliminary analysis of language development in children during the first three years]. Acta Psychologica Sinica, 11, *153-165. (In Chinese.)*

Sound records of five children taken from birth through the first 3 years of age were analyzed. Three points concerning the development of language in children were made: (1) The development of language is a continuous, sequential, and regular process, with both quantitatively and qualitatively changes throughout. Development is also in 6 stages: simple vocalization from birth to 3 months, continued syllable repeating from 4 to 8 months, beginning of speech from 9 to 12 months, uttering one word sentences from 1 to 1 year and 6 months, uttering simple sentences from 1 to 2 years, and beginning to use compound sentences from 2 to 3 years. (2) The child's language development proceeds from the concrete to the abstract, as may be seen from grasping words and their parts of speech. (3) Individual differences are quite clear even among such a small group of infants.

1094

Wu, W. T. (1977). [Locus of control as related to achievement, self-concept, and social interaction in school children: A review]. Bulletin of Research Institute of Education *(Taiwan Normal University),* **19,** *163-178. (In Chinese.)*

1095

Wu, Y. F. (1978). [An investigation of university-student subculture in Taiwan, Republic of China]. Bulletin of Research Institute of Education *(Taiwan Normal University),* **20,** *613-622. (In Chinese.)*

1096

Wu, Y. H. (1966). [An anthropologist looks at Chinese child training method]. Thought and Word, 3, *3-7. (In Chinese.)*

This study is based on anthropological observations of the Paiwan tribe of aborigines in southern Taiwan, whose style of life, thinking, and social structure have remained basically unchanged in the last 200 years, despite obvious improvements in their material conditions of life. It is felt that the Paiwan patterns of child rearing share many features in common with those of the traditional Han Chinese: in the indulgence toward the infant and severe training of the older child, especially in the emphasis given to training for obedience and responsibility.

1097

Wu, Z. Y., Xu, S. L., & Sun, C. H. (1985). [Adult intelligence development through different age groups and its relationship with memory]. Acta Psychologica Sinica, 17, *243-249. (In Chinese.)*

The aging of adults' intelligence was tested with the Chinese version of the Wechsler Adult Intelligence Scale-Revised. There were 140 subjects, divided into 7 age groups from 20 to 90 years matched for sex and educational level. The results were essentially the same as those of the classical pattern of aging reported abroad, but with lower scores for the 20-year-old group. Intelligence significantly correlated with memory ($r = .55$). The aging tendency of memory was similar to that reflected in the intelligence test results.

1098

Xia, Z. Y., & Zhang, M. Y. (1981). [The development and present state of modern psychiatry in China]. Chinese Journal of Neurology & Psychiatry, 14, *170-173. (In Chinese.)*

1099

Xu, S. L., Sun, C. H., Wu, Z. Y., Wang, X. D., & Cai, X. J. (1985). [Changes in some memory activities of adults from 20 to 90 years of age]. Acta Psychologica Sinica, 17, *154-161. (In Chinese.)*

This is a follow-up of our earlier study of the effects of aging on memory. The subjects were 210 healthy adults 20-90 years of age, divided into 7 age groups, matched on sex and educational level. The Clinical Memory Test designed by the investigators and standardized by a nation-wide cooperative research group was used; 20 subjects in each group were also tested with the WAISRC. The results indicated: (1) Generally, memory decreased with age, beginning from 50 and becoming more marked after 70. (2) The same tendency of decrease was found in subjects of different age groups (20, 30, 50, 60, and 70) matched on intelligence. (3) Age differences were least apparent in the recognition of meaningless figures and in related-paired-association; they were most apparent in unrelated-paired-association and in the recall of surnames and hobby characteristics of individuals in pictures, indicating that the aged have great difficulty in establishing new associations. The authors suggest that memory difficulties of the aged result from interactions between encoding, storage, and retrieval.

1100

Xu, S. L., & Wu, Z. P. (1984). [A preliminary investigation of the psychosocial condition of the aged in Beijing Municipality]. Information on Psychological Sciences, *No. 6, 50-54. (In Chinese.)*

1101

Xu, Z. Q., & Song, B. L. (1981). [A study of the individual case of a child in mastering number concept: A follow-up study of a child at the age of 3-4 years]. Acta Psychologica Sinica, 13, *150-158. (In Chinese.)*

This report is based upon a follow-up study of the number-concept-mastering process of a child of 3-4 years old. The result of investigation shows that it is not only possible but also necessary for a 3-4 year-old child to master the concept of numerals. The development of numeral concept extension has a certain procedure. The level of number concept is raised through the practice of counting, taking things, comparing, calculating, reading and writing, with counting as the first step. The number concept cannot be mastered spontaneously, nor is it a result of training and learning. It plays an important part in overcoming difficulties in reading and memorizing the numeration table. To master number concept is to master numerical knowledge; it is a process of cognition, in which functions of actions and memory are the most prominent.

1102

Xu, Z. Q., & Song, B. L. (1982). [An individual case study of a child mastering number concepts: Vol. 2. A follow-up study of a child at the age of 4-5 years]. Acta Psychologica Sinica, 14, *56-69. (In Chinese.)*

This is a follow-up study on the development of the concept of number in a 4-5 year old child. The results showed that under conditions of effective training and adequate drilling, mastery of preliminary number concepts enters a critical year. Counting and writing numbers, and using numbers as signs to calculate are most prominent in this procedure. Trial and error, sudden realization, and counting fingers is transformed into the ability of oral counting. Counting according to different number order is the main content of oral counting. The the ability to count articles develops before the ability to count numbers. Reading and memorizing the different numeral tables will enable the child to understand the basic types of numbers, the combining of numbers and the relationship between them. Reading and writing numbers are the main methods that will enable the child to master and operate the "word-formation" of numbers, and promote the development of counting. It is also an essential method used by the child in developing number concepts. The pattern of development of calculating ability is: plus and minus one by one, plus and minus by groups, and plus and minus with dividing and grouping of numbers. Calculating numbers (plus, minus, multiplication and division) is the method used by the child in learning number formation, it is also an important method in raising his level of conception of numbers.

1103

Yan, Y. Y. (1983). [A preliminary study of the development of reasoning in children aged 3 to 7 years]. Information on Psychological Sciences, *No. 1, 28-36. (In Chinese.)*

The purpose of this study is to investigate, under play-like conditions, the development of children's reasoning process from age 3 to 7. Induction and deduction are considered as two unseparable aspects of the reasoning process. One hundred and seventy-five subjects were tested individually, and inquiries and suggestions were made when necessary. The results show that there are different forms and levels of children's reasoning process; that six types of reasoning reflect the gradual developmental process; and that the procedure of making inquiries and suggestions may facilitate the exploration of children's reasoning process.

1104

Yang, H., Gao, X., & Wang, W. (1980, October). [Let us all be concerned with only children]. Zhongguo Qingnian Bao [Chinese Youth News], *pp. 2. (In Chinese.)*

This is a study on the behavior of 1,743 children conducted by three students at Beijing Normal University. Only children were found to be better developed intellectually, academically, and physically, but were also more wilful, selfish, and lacking in a sense of responsibility and collective outlook.

1105

Yang, I. L. (1982). A longitudinal study of two Mandarin Chinese speaking children learning English as a second language. Dissertation Abstracts International, 42, *A3046-3047.*

1106

Yang, K. S. (1974). [The development and correlates of self-concept in Chinese children]. In K. S. Yang & C. H. Chang (Eds.), [Behavioral development of Chinese children*]. Taipei: Huan-yu Publishing Co. (In Chinese.)*

1107

Yang, K. S., & Chang, C. H. (Eds.). (1974). [Behavioral development of Chinese children*]. Taipei: Huan Yu. (In Chinese.)*

1108

Yang, K. S., & Yang, Y. W. (1974). [Language development in children during their preschool years]. In K. S. Yang & C. H. Chang (Eds.), [Behavioral development of Chinese children*]. Taipei: Huan-yu Pub. Co. (In Chinese.)*

1109

Yang, K. S., Yang, Y. W., & Hsiao, Y. F. (1974). [Language development and its correlates in Chinese children]. In K. S. Yang & C. H. Chang (Eds.), [Behavioral development Chinese children*]. Taipei: Huan-yu Publishing Co. (In Chinese.)*

1110

Yang, M. C. (1965). Child training and child behavior in varying family patterns in a changing Chinese society. *Paper presented at the 9th International Seminar on Family Research, Tokyo, Japan, Sept. 14-20.*

This is a study of the traditional ideals and practices of child training, and contemporary changes in these aspects during the process of modernization in China. An analysis of historical documents was made and interviews with experienced old people were conducted; survey methods were used to study changes in the last 30 years.

1111

Yang, M. M. C. (1967). [Child training and child behavior in varying family patterns in a changing Chinese society]. Journal of Sociology *(National Taiwan University),* **3,** *77-83. (In Chinese.)*

The data for this article was gathered by the author from over two hundred young male and female students in three universities in Taipei, Taiwan. An outline of information wanted was distributed to and discussed by the students and then written reports turned in to the author. These were analyzed and joined with materials from printed sources obtainable here in Taiwan. The traditional Chinese family has experienced many changes in the last sixty years and these changes were brought on by modern education, infiltration of Western culture, and development of occupations and industries different from the traditional farming and handicraft work. The changes produced new family patterns which may be classified as: (1) the fossilized extended family, (2) the three generation single trunk family, (3) the Western type nuclear family. By occupation, they may be classified as those of the intellectuals, those of government officials and business men, and those of farmers, workers and other low income groups. Child training differs somewhat in each of these categories.

1112

Yang, Q. Z., Wang, M. J., & Chen, S. (1981). [A preliminary study of the development of the size-discrimination ability of infants]. Information on Psychological Sciences, *No. 2, 14-20. (In Chinese.)*

1113

Yang, Z. L., Ye, Y. Q., Zhu, P. L., Gao, Y. M., & Li, M. (1981). [An approach to the optimal age of the recognitive ability: An evaluation with the signal detection theory]. Acta Psychologica Sinica, 13, *42-52. (In Chinese.)*

This study explored the relationship between age and recognition ability. Eight age groups were tested, each of which consisted of 24 subjects, with a total of 192 subjects in all. Three groups of test materials were used in the experiment; concrete pictures, abstract pictures, and words. The results showed that the best age for recognizing concrete pictures is eleven, and that middle school students aged 15 are the most able at recognizing abstract pictures and words. The advantages of signal detection theory as a research tool in the study of memory were also evaluated.

1114

Yang-Lee, P. H., & Yang, S. J. (1975). [The discrepancy between the university senior's perceptions of his major and his previous expectations]. Acta Psychologica Taiwanica, 17, *125-143. (In Chinese.)*

A survey of senior students' opinions about, and attitudes toward, their academic major was conducted at National Taiwan University. The total sample was comprised of 232 male and 404 female students, drawn from graduating classes of various departments. Only a moderate degree of congruence was found between students' perceptions of their present major and expectations they had before the College Joint Entrance Examination was taken. However, there was considerable variation along different dimensions of expectations.

1115

Ye, Y. D. (1985). [An analysis by signal detection theory of schoolchildren's ability to recognize Chinese idiomatic phrases in middle and higher grades]. Acta Psychologica Sinica, 17, *86-91. (In Chinese.)*

The is a study of the recognition of three different kinds of Chinese idiomatic phrases: homonyms, synonyms, and phrases similar in form. It was found that recognition of the last kind was the poorest; homonyms and synonyms were confused only when they appeared in the same sentence. Among four recognition methods, pictographic recognition was the best and general recognition was the poorest; semantic recognition and phonetic recognition varied between different grades. When the recognition method and materials were consistent, pupils in the third grade were the least capable. When pictographic recognition was employed, pupils in the fifth grade did well with any kind of material but were apparently better in semantic recognition.

1116

Yeh, H., & Fang, Y. C. (1958). [A preliminary experimental study in spatial orientation of preschool children]. Acta Psychologica Sinica, 2, *65-71. (In Chinese.)*

1117

Yeh, M. (1981). Canadian vs. Chinese cross-cultural developmental study of moral judgment. Dissertation Abstracts International, 42, *B360.*

1118

Ying, H. C. et al. (1983). [Characteristics of children's mastery of quantitative concepts]. Information on Psychological Sciences, *No. 6, 24-32. (In Chinese.)*

In the Chinese language, quantitatives are used not only for uncountable but also for countable objects, and there is no explicit rule about their collocation. Because of this, it is rather difficult for young children to master quantitatives. In this study, 179 children aged between 4 and 7 years were tested to investigate how they learned individual, collective, and temporary quantitatives. The results showed that there was a certain order in mastery. Children at 4 years of age could master only a few common individual quantitatives, and they tended to overuse them. There was a rapid increase in the rate of mastering individual quantitatives from 5 to 9 years; children in this age group began to master temporary and collective quantitatives. Children at 6 or 7 years had basically mastered common individual quantitatives, and rates of the correct use of temporary and collective quantitatives increased rapidly. This study shows that children's mastery of quantitatives is correlated with their levels of cognitive development and experiences.

1119

Young, N. F. (1972). Socialization patterns among the Chinese of Hawaii. Amerasia Journal, 1, *31-51.*

1120

Yuan, L. Z., & Li, R. W. (1966). [A preliminary study of stories about revolutionary heroes in forming the morale of students in primary school]. Acta Psychologica Sinica, *No. 2, 154-162. (In Chinese.)*

1121

Yuan, S. S. (1972). [Family authority patterns, rearing practices and children's sense of political efficacy]. Thought and Word, 10, *35-55. (In Chinese.)*

1122

Zeng, H. W. (1986). [Characteristics and development of color preference in Chinese schoolchildren]. Information on Psychological Sciences, *No. 1, 16-22. (In Chinese.)*

1123

Zha, Z. X. (1984). [A comparative study of the analogical reasoning of supernormal and normal children aged 3 to 6 years]. Acta Psychologica Sinica, 16, *373-382. (In Chinese.)*

This study compares superior children and normal children aged 3 to 6 years in analogical reasoning. Three experiments were conducted, using pictures of real objects and graphs as test materials. The subjects were 650 children, divided into four age groups. The results showed: (1) Analogical reasoning developed with age. (2) The scores of the overwhelming majority of the superior children differed from the scores of normal children of the same age group by at least two standard deviations; the superior children were even better than those two years their senior. (3) The developmental levels of their analogical reasoning were divided into 5 grades. The supernormal children surpassed normal children of the same age group by 1-2 grades, and were found to be quick in comprehension and alert and resourceful in grasping the interrelationships of bipartite situation.

1124

Zha, Z. X. (1985). [Comparative study of the analogical reasoning of only and non-only children aged 3 to 6 years]. Acta Psychologica Sinica, 17, *144-153. (In Chinese.)*

This paper compares the analogical thinking of only and the nononly children. The subjects were 400 children aged from 3 to 6 years, divided into four age groups. In each age group, the numbers of onlies and nononlies were either equal or proportional to the actual numbers of the two categories at that particular age. The results showed that there were no significant differences between only and nononly children in analogical reasoning test scores. However, there were obvious differences between children in the same category with different home backgrounds. Home factors such as family size, income, living standards, cultural life, educational level, and home education were important in affecting the children's intellectual development.

1125

Zha, Z. X. (1986). [A five-year study of the mental development of supernormal children]. Acta Psychologica Sinica, 18, *123-132. (In Chinese.)*

In step with China's four modernization programs, research on the development of supernormal children began in 1978 as a nationwide cooperative project. A dynamic longitudinal comparative study using multiple criteria and various methods was carried out, with emphasis on the child's thinking process and personality traits. The results of five years of study were: (1) The differences between supernormal and normal children were found not only in the pace and dimension of development, but also in the developmental process, mode, and characteristics. (2) There were many different types of supernormal children; they shared certain psychological characteristics and had the same need for support and assistance in connection to their development.

1126

Zhang, D. X. (1985). [An exploratory study of creative thinking in adolescents]. Information on Psychological Sciences, *No. 2, 20-25. (In Chinese.)*

The Test of Creative Thinking Potential was given to 874 adolescents. A high correlation was found between the standard scores and school achievements. Comparisons of thinking patterns showed less productivity associated with convergent thinking than with divergent thinking. In divergent thinking, the higher the grades, the better the answers to questions. Sex differences were less significant than individual differences. Moral judgment was related to creative thinking. Students who possessed higher creative abilities judged moral events more adequately.

1127

Zhang, H. C., Meng, Q. M., & Zheng, R. C. (1981). [Studies on cognitive styles: Role of the individual differences in field-dependence in learning and visual after-effect]. Acta Psychologica Sinica, 13, *299-304. (In Chinese.)*

Conducted 2 studies of individual differences in field dependence with 8-11 yrs old. In Study 1, 68 Ss' scores from the Group Embedded Figures Test were compared with their scores on the Test of Learning Ability for Children and their academic achievement. Results show that the degree of field independence was positively correlated with performance in mathematics, and there was no correlation between field independence and learning of Chinese. In Study 2, 24 Ss at both ends of the continuum for field dependence-independence participated in a tilted-line aftereffect study in a darkroom. Results show that the additional object for reference provided in the visual field produced an effect for the field dependents and no effect for the field independents. In both studies there was evidence of sex differences in cognitive style.

1128

Zhang, J. W. (1980). [A comparison of the characteristics of thinking development in reasoning between the Tibetan and Han primary school children]. Acta Psychologica Sinica, 12, *406-414. (In Chinese.)*

Studied similarities in analytical synthesis, comparison, and abstract reasoning abilities in Tibetan and Han children. Results indicate that although the general levels and characteristics of cognitive development are similar in the 2 groups, there are certain differences in reasoning by analogy and in generalization ability, most of which are related to environmental and cultural differences.

1129

Zhang, M. L. (1980). [An investigation in cognitive development of the relation between part and whole in children: Vol. 1. Experimental studies on the concept of class inclusion and number inclusion in children of 4-7 years]. Acta Psychologica Sinica, 12, *37-45. (In Chinese.)*

A study was made on kindergarten children 4-7 years of age in Beijing. Each child was asked to do some tasks on class inclusion and number inclusion. The results showed that: (1) In general, successful performance increased with age for. (2) Class inclusion could not be understood by children before 4 years and 6 months; understanding began by 5 years and was more obvious by 5-6 years. Understanding of number inclusion developed earlier, beginning from 4 years and basically mastered by 5 years and 6 months. (3) The children's responses could be classified into three different levels: inability to see the relation between parts and the whole, making increasing correct responses through representation, and showing understanding of the logical relationships involved and performing nearly without mistakes.

1130

Zhang, M. Y. et al. (1980). [A research into the developmental potentials of children in thinking]. Acta Psychologica Sinica, 12, *397-405. (In Chinese.)*

1131

Zhang, S. F. (1984). [A research on the development of adolescent morality among Lahu and Hani nationalities in Xishuangbanna in Yunnan province]. Acta Psychologica Sinica, 16, *447-454. (In Chinese.)*

The moral education for adolescents of the Lahu and Hani nationalities in Xishuangbanna was studied. In the process of social integration and transition from adolescence to adulthood, the adolescents' sense of independence and maturity enjoy the recognition from and respect of their own people. They are trusted in productive work and more generally in social life. Their small peer group activities not only enhance their sense of belonging, but also help them to conform to the moral and behavioral norms of their own nationalities. These two nationalities use every opportunity and means to help adolescents to develop their morality. Learning from models and from their own direct experiences has been found to be most rewarding.

1132

Zhang, Z. H., & Lin, Z. X. (1982). [Studies of preschool children's naming and recognition of colors]. Information on Psychological Sciences, *No. 2, 17-22. (In Chinese.)*

One hundred and twenty preschool children aged 3-6 years were investigated as to their ability to name and recognize colors. Eight different colored chips were used to test color naming, and twelve colors were used to study the recognition of colors. It was found that the ability of naming and recognizing of colors increased with age. A critical period in the development of this ability was about 5 years of age.

1133

Zhang, Z. H., & Lin, Z. X. (1983). [Experimental research on color and figure discrimination of 3-6 years old children]. Acta Psychologica Sinica, 15, *461-468. (In Chinese.)*

Perceptual discriminations of 12 colors and 12 figures by children 3-6 years old were studied. Three exposure times (0.01 sec, 0.05 sec, and 0.1 sec) for each color and each figure were presented in random order. The results showed that exposure time had significant effects on color and figure discrimination. The effect of exposure time on figure discrimination was more pronounced for younger children. Discrimination ability increased with age step by step. The percentage of correct discrimination was the highest for yellow, red, and green.

1134

Zhang, Z. H., Lin, Z. X., & Mao, Y. Y. (1984). [Color matching, color preference and color naming in young children aged 1.5 - 3 years]. Information on Psychological Sciences, *No. 1, 7-13. (In Chinese.)*

This is a preliminary study on color matching, color preference, and color naming in young children. The subjects were 120 children selected from a nursery. They were divided into four age groups (1.5, 2, 2.5, and 3 years), with 30 in each group. The results were: (1) A "leap" in the ability of color matching ability seemed to occur at 2.5 years of age. The children at 1.5 years could not express their color preferences by overt behavioral indications, and none could name any of eight colors correctly. (2) The children from 2 to 3 years old were able to express their color preferences; some were able to name a few colors correctly. The order of their color preference was: red, yellow, green, orange, blue, white, black, and purple.

1135

Zhang, Z. J. (1985). [Experiments on children aged 5 - 15 in grasping the concept of probability]. Information on Psychological Sciences, *No. 6, 1-6. (In Chinese.)*

The development of 5 to 15-year-old children's concept of probabilities of 1/2, 1/3, 1/6 and 2/3 was experimentally tested. The results showed: (1) The development of the concept of probability depended on the degree of complexity of the task. Children's concept of simple probability developed more rapidly from about the tenth year on. (2) Generally speaking, children acquired the knowledge of probability through three successive steps: knowing the possibility of the occurrence of events and the random distribution of objects, the relative magnitude of possibilities, and finally the concept of probability itself. (3) Suggestions with speech, relevant drawings or physical objects promoted children's knowledge of probability to a certain degree. (4) The cognitive behavior of children's solving probability problems could be divided into five levels.

1136

Zhao, S. W., & Liu, F. (1982). [An experimental study of children's cognition of some common natural phenomena]. Acta Psychologica Sinica, 14, *397-406. (In Chinese.)*

The development of children's cognition of natural phenomena was explored. The subjects were 100 children aged 6-10 years. They answered three kinds of questions concerning 19 natural phenomena (e.g., the sun, the moon, air, clouds and rain): (a) "What is it?", (b) "Do they share some common characteristics?", and (c) "Why does it comes about?" The results were: (1) Cognition of natural phenomena may be divided into two stages: lack of clear understanding, and a stage of transition. Most of the children tested were at the latter stage. The period from 8 to 10 years showed much development in this area. (2) Children tended to rely on personal experiences to explain natural phenomena. Their cognition of these phenomena developed according to a sequence: formation of concepts, generalization from similarities, and understanding of causal relations.

1137

Zhao, S. W., & Liu, F. (1983). [Development of the concept of volume in children and adolescents -- A study on the development of children's cognitive structure Vol. 2]. Information on Psychological Sciences, *No. 4, 21-27. (In Chinese.)*

This is an investigation of the development of the concept of volume in children and adolescents. In order to control for the influence of the shape, size, area, and quantity of the container, a fixed container was used. The results indicated that: (1) the period between 12-15 years of age was one of speedy development of the concept of volume; (2) there were four levels of cognition of volume changes: arbitrary, sensorimotor dominance, mental-image dominance; and conceptual dominance; and (3) errors concerning volume changes were principally due to the confusion of area with volume, failure to differentiate between volume and height, and inability to identify the correspondence between space and quantity.

1138

Zheng, D. C. (1982). [An experimental study of children's conceptions of left and right]. Information on Psychological Sciences, *No. 6, 29-33. (In Chinese.)*

In this experiment the development of children's conceptions of left and right was explored. The results showed that children from 8 to 9 years old could master the conception of left and right exactly and flexibly. The leap in the development could be found between the age of 6-7. These results are different from the conclusions reached in previous experiments conducted in China.

1139

Zheng, X., & Wen, Y. (1984). [The development of visual-motor coordination and cognition in Li-Han children on Hainan Island]. Information on Psychological Sciences, *No. 1, 23-30. (In Chinese.)*

This is a study of the development of visual-motor coordination in two groups of minority children in the Lishui and Baoting counties on Hainan island. Two tests were used: the visual-motor test by Berry and Buktenica and the classic cognitive test of the Geneva School. The subjects were 180 children from 7 to 10 years of age. The results were: (1) No difference in the development of visual-motor coordination was found between the two minority groups. (2) The rate of development was uneven--rapid development between 7 and 9 years of age, and stagnation around 9 to 10 years. (3) Girls surpassed boys at around 7 to 8 years, but the boys caught up at around 9 to 10 years. (4) A correlation coefficient of .39 was obtained between scores of the two tests.

1140

Zhu, M. S. et al. (1985). [Spatial concepts in Chinese and Canadian children]. Information on Psychological Sciences, *No. 3, 14-18. (In Chinese.)*

Chinese and Canadian children (4 to 6 years old) were presented with a series of 11 graphic models, and asked to draw them. The data indicated that drawing performance increased over the age span surveyed, that performance on the topological dimension was better than that on the Euclidean dimension, and that there were neither sex nor cultural differences in performance. The research offers strong support for a main effect of biological or maturational factors as the foundation for the developmental influences in the acquisition of spatial conceptions.

1141

Zhu, M. S. et al. (1986). [Young children's interpretation of demonstrative pronouns]. Information on Psychological Sciences, *No. 3, 1-6. (In Chinese.)*

Children aged 3 to 7 years were requested to choose proper toys and place them at proper places in the model of a zoo in accordance with instructions using demonstrative pronouns including "this", "that". Three conditions were mainpulated: (1) As the receiver of instructions the subject sat close by the experimenter (speaker) with the "zoo" in their front. (2) The subject sat on the other side of the zoo and acted as the listener of the conversation between two experimenters sitting face to face with the "zoo" in the middle. (3) As the receiver of instructions given through the conversation between two experimenters, the subject sat face to face with one of the experimenters. The "zoo" was sandwiched in between the subject and the experimenter. The results were: (1) Children's scores for the interpretation of demonstrative pronouns were highest in the first condition followed respectively by the second and third conditions. (2) Although the scores in each age group were in direct proportion with age, the oldest age group failed to fulfill the task satisfactorily in the third condition.

1142

Zhu, M. S., & Wu, J. Z. (1982). [A comparative study of normal, deaf-mute and blind children -- on the relationship between language and thought]. Information on Psychological Sciences, *No. 1, 15-21. (In Chinese.)*

1143

Zhu, M. S., & Wu, J. Z. (1984). Chinese children's comprehension and production of passive voice and double negative sentences. International Journal of Behavioral Development, *7, 67-76.*

Two experiments examined the abilities of 36 normal 5-7 yr olds and 13 deaf-mute 11-18 yr olds in tasks demanding comprehension, production, and imitation of passive voice and double negative sentences. Results show that comprehension preceded production and, while imitation can improve production, it only did so for Ss showing some initial levels of comprehension. It is suggested that in productive learning, imitation has little effect on the performances of Ss who display no ability for comprehension of the syntactic structures employed. On the basis of these data, it is argued that the acquisition of syntactic structures is determined by levels of cognitive ability. A comparison of deaf and hearing Ss revealed that while the former were delayed in the acquisition of these syntactic structures, some did eventually succeed in mastering them. Implications for the role of language in the development of cognitive abilities are explored.

1144

Zhu, M. S., Wu, J. Z., & Miao, X. C. (1979). [An investigation of the development of oral speech in preschool children: Vol. 1. Analysis of the structure of simple declarative sentences in preschool children]. Acta Psychologica Sinica, 11, *281-286. (In Chinese.)*

This paper is one of a series on the speech development of preschool children. It analyses the structure types of the most fundamental sentences: simple, affirmative, active, and declarative. The subjects were 70 preschool children (33 males and 37 females) randomly drawn from two kindergartens and two nurseries. They were divided into seven age groups (2, 2-1/2, 3, 3-1/2, 4, 5, and 6 years), with 10 subjects in each. The spontaneous speech of each subject was recorded with a tape recorder twice within a period of 2 weeks, each time for half an hour. A total of 3,459 simple declarative sentences were recorded and 9 structure types ranging from simple to complex were found. The distribution of these types at different age groups showed that the structure of the children's fundamental sentences developed with increasing differentiation, organization, and flexibility.

1145

Zhu, M. S., Wu, J. Z., Zhuang, X. J. et al. (1982). [Children's comprehension of several kinds of temporal words in sentences]. Acta Psychologica Sinica, 14, *294-301. (In Chinese.)*

This study showed: (1) Children's comprehension of temporal words in sentences developed rather slowly. (2) Children's comprehension of temporal words developed in a steady sequence; this has been shown by both longitudinal and cross-sectional studies. However, there were obvious individual differences in the speed of development. Both the levels and stages of comprehending temporal words expressing the order of activities varied with the nature of the temporal words presented, word order, sentence structure, and the number of the objects to be acted upon. In comprehending words about temporal units (or periods), children first understood "today," "yesterday," and "tomorrow"; they then gradually learned smaller units such as "morning," "afternoon," "evening," "at x in the morning," "at x in the afternoon," and "at x in the evening," or bigger units such as "this year," "last year," and "next year." In comprehending tenses, children learned the progressive tense first, the perfect tense next, and the future tense last.

1146

Zhu, W. B., & Tan, M. Z. (1979). [A psychological analysis of the formation of moral character among pupils under the influence of the class collective]. Acta Psychologica Sinica, 11, *175-183. (In Chinese.)*

This study follows the work experience of Mr. Liu Chun-pu, a national outstanding teacher, and gives a tentative analysis on the psychological processes of the formation of moral character among primary middle school pupils under the influences of class collective. The findings showed that the formation of pupils' moral character is a process of struggle and resolution of the contradiction between new moral demands and old behavioral habits. In this process, the pupil's attitudes have to be modified so that they can receive instructions conscientiously. A class collective should be established as the central orientation; rich and varied educational activities should be launched, and special attention paid to the transformation of those who lagged behind. Teachers must take educational measures effectively in accordance with the peculiarities of their pupils at different developmental stages in order to solve different problems characteristic of a given stage. In doing so, the teachers may be able to guide the formation and development of the pupils' communist morality.

1147

Zhu, Y. Y., & Yuan, W. C. (1985). [Primary schoolchildren's difficulties in grasping the concept of direct and inverse proportions and their psychological analysis]. Information on Psychological Sciences, *No. 5, 18-24. (In Chinese.)*

1148

Zhu, Z. X. (1979). Child psychology instruction and research in the People's Republic of China. School Psychology International, 1, *3-5.*

Discusses the introduction of child psychology to China, emphasizing the following areas: role of heredity, environment, and education in child development; interplay between internal and external factors; effects of education on child development; and age and individual differences among children. Areas of current research are briefly reviewed.

1149

Zhu, Z. X., Qian, M. J., Wu, F. G., & Clin, H. D. (1982). [An experimental study of the synthetical classification of word concepts in schoolchildren]. Acta Psychologica Sinica, 14, *302-310. (In Chinese.)*

This study investigated schoolchildren's ability in the synthetical classification of word concepts. It was shown that classification ability was better than the ability to explain the grounds for classification. Differences in classification material, cultural background, individual experiences, and the quality of instruction affected the level of classification ability.

1150

Zhu, Z. X., Qian, M. J., Wu, F. G., & Lin, C. D. (1982). [A study of the development of word concepts in elementary school children]. Information on Psychological Sciences, *No. 3, 23-29. (In Chinese.)*

1151

Zon, M. L. (1983). [A cross-cultural study of children's cognitive development]. Information on Psychological Sciences, *No. 3, 14-20. (In Chinese.)*

The purpose of this experiment is to study the influence of culture, nationality and language on children's cognitive development. The subjects included 540 children (5 to 11 years old) from five different nationalities, residing in various parts of Yunnan province. Seven items of "Piagetian" concepts including conservation, class inclusion, and seriation were studied. The results show that children with different cultural backgrounds acquire the conservation concepts at different ages due to the differences in their education and culture. With children who come from different nationalities but have a similar cultural background, there is no significant difference in acquiring the conservation concept. Difference in speech proficiency of children among the different nationalities has no marked influence on their acquiring the conservation concept.

1152

Zuo, M. L., Liu, J. X. et al. (1984). [A study of the development of the concept of number series in children 5-11 years old in five districts in China]. Acta Psychologica Sinica, 16, *174-181. (In Chinese.)*

1153

Zuo, M. L., Wei, C., & Fu, J. Z. (1986). [Comparison of cognitive development between Han and Dai children aged 10-15]. Information on Psychological Sciences, *No. 2, 1-8. (In Chinese.)*

Based on a study of the cognitive development of Han and Dai children aged 10 to 15 years, it was found that: (1) The age of 13 years was critical for cognitive development to change from concrete to formal operations. (2) No obvious difference was found between Han and Dai children.

1154

Zuo, Q. P. (1985). [Analysis of the developmental stages of self-consciousness and the characteristics in the juvenile period]. Acta Psychologica Sinica, *17, 257-263. (In Chinese.)*

The author holds that self-consciousness includes two dimensions in dialectical unity--self-intention and self-cognition. It proposes three bases for identifying developmental stages according to the characteristics of contradictory movements dictated by the two aspects of self-consciousness: (a) interchange in the degree of dependency and independency; (b) depth of the development of self-cognition from the perceptual to the rational, and from the concrete to the abstract; and (c) the imbalance in the development of self-intention and self-cognition. On this basis, the development of self-consciousness is divided into four stages with particular emphasis on the analysis of the characteristics of the juvenile period. Understanding these characteristics will help further investigation of the developmental laws of self-consciousness and improve the education of juveniles.

The following references are also relevant to this chapter:

206, 213, 237, 244, 254, 305, 384, 597, 640, 643, 648, 649, 650, 669, 1157, 1164, 1196, 1333, 1375, 1401, 1512, 1666, 1775, 1844, 1965, 2008, 2153, 2209, 2213, 2240, 2343, 2349, 2350, 2358, 2374, 2414, 2491, 2564, 2715, 2837, 2878.

PERSONALITY 8

Citations in personality (in the present chapter) constitute 6.5% of the total in the present volume, ranking 6th out of 13 content classification categories (see Table 1). (To some extent, the relatively low percentage is due to the fact that most personality studies involving children have been classified as belonging to developmental psychology.) However, in actuality personality is pertinent to a larger number of studies. This is indicated by the fact that the subject term *personality* is used for indexing as many as 9.1% or 322 of the total of 3,548 citations (see data presented in the Introduction).

Subject terms used for indexing citations related to personality are grouped according to geographical area, subject population, and topic. These are presented below, in a descending order of frequency. (The frequency of single-word subject terms includes those of compound terms in which the single word appears. Subjects terms used for indexing citations from other chapters may have been included. Terms with a frequency of less than 10 are not shown.)

Geographical area

128 Taiwan
82 Asia
30 Peoples Republic of China
18 Hong Kong
10 United States

Subject population

86 students
50 adults
45 college students
36 children
34 adolescents
19 Asians
13 high school students
11 Asian Americans
10 junior high school studentsl

Topic

150	personality
52	personality traits
44	cross cultural differences
40	sex
39	intelligence
24	personality measures
19	adulthood
18	Rorschach test
17	self concept
16	attitudes
16	internal external locus of control
16	test validity
15	achievement
15	sociocultural factors
14	human sex differences
13	ethnic groups
13	health
13	intelligence measures
13	projective techniques
11	mental health
10	development
10	test construction

It may be observed that studies relevant to personality conducted in Taiwan are the most numerous, exceeding those in the PRC and Hong Kong by far. There is clearly a lack of research attention paid to personality in the PRC.

Researchers seem to be preoccupied with personality traits, intelligence in particular; personality processes are neglected. One may question the wisdom of this overreliance on the dispositional strategy in research. Again, as discussed in the Introduction, this strategy appears to be based more on the mere availability of measuring instruments than on theoretical considerations.

Book-length contributions devoted to Chinese character (Li and Yang 1988) and to personality change in the face of modernization (Yang 1988) have appeared. Literature reviews may be found in Hwang (1982) and Yang (1986).

REFERENCES

Hwang, C. H. (1982). Studies in Chinese personality: A critical review. *Bulletin of Educational Psychology, 15*, 227-241.

Li, Y. Y., & Yang, K. S. (Eds.) (1988). [*The character of Chinese people*]. Taipei: Kuei Kuan. (Originally published under the title: [Symposium on the character of the Chinese: An interdisciplinary approach]. Taipei: Institute of Ethnology, Academia Sinica, 1972.) (In Chinese.)

Yang, K. S. (1986). Chinese personality and its change. In M. H. Bond (Ed.), *The psychology of the Chinese people* (pp. 106- 170). Hong Kong: Oxford University Press.

Yang, K. S. (1988). [*The changing Chinese personality*]. Taipei: Kuei Kuan. (In Chinese.)

1155

Abel, T. M. (1950). *Columbia University Research in Contemporary Cultures* **(CH-610). Unpublished document, American Museum of Natural History, New York.**

1156

Abel, T. M., & Hsu, F. L. K. (1949). Some aspects of personality of Chinese as revealed by the Rorschach Test. *Rorschach Research Exchange and Journal of Projective Techniques, 13,* **285-301. (Reprinted in M. Mead & R. Metraux (Eds.),** *The study of culture at a distance.* **Chicago, IL: University of Chicago Press, 1953.)**

1157

Bierbryer, B. (1973). Conceptual tempo, sex, and creative thinking. *Dissertation Abstracts International, 33,* **A6168.**

1158

Boey, K. W. (1976). *Rigidity and cognitive complexity: An empirical investigation in the interpersonal, physical, and numerical domains under task-oriented and ego-involved conditions.* **Unpublished doctoral dissertation, University of Hong Kong, Hong Kong.**

1159

Boey, K. W. (1985). [The MMPI response pattern of Singapore Chinese]. *Acta Psychologica Sinica, 17,* **377-383.** (In Chinese.)

This study showed that the Chinese and the English Minnesota Multiphasic Personality Inventory (MMPI) were highly equivalent. Their average scale reliabilities were satisfactory, reaching .85 and .78 respectively. When scales scores were ranked, Singapore Chinese ranked appreciably higher on Scale Ma and lower on Scale Pa when compared with Mainland Chinese. Their ranking on Scale Si was slightly higher when compared with Hong Kong Chinese. Significant rank order correlations were found between Chinese-educated Chinese in Singapore and the Chinese in Mainland China and Hong Kong. For the English-educated Chinese in Singapore, only the profiles of males were similar to their counterparts in Hong Kong. In terms of endorsement pattern, correlations of the English educated were higher with six American samples than with Chinese in Hong Kong; whereas for the Chinese educated, the reverse was found. These findings showed that the English educated and the Chinese educated could not be considered as homogeneous. The research meets the need for a local norm and makes cross-cultural comparisons possible.

1160

Bond, M. H., & Cheung, T. S. (1983). College students' spontaneous self-concept: The effect of culture among respondents in Hong Kong, Japan, and the United States. *Journal of Cross-Cultural Psychology, 14,* **153-171.**

Cross-cultural comparisons of self-concept have typically used structured inventories created in the US, although importing and using such methodology may prevent culturally unique dimensions and contents from appearing. To overcome this problem, the Twenty Statements Test was administered to 633 university students in Japan, the US, and Hong Kong to assess cultural influences on the self-concept assessed from this open-ended inventory. Numerous cultural differences were found in the frequency of categories and subcategories used for self-statements (such as social identity and personal attributes, including aspirations and psychological characteristics) and in the level of self-esteem. These differences are related to previous research on self-concept, socialization practices, and central concerns in these cultural groups.

1161

Chai, C. (1959). Chinese humanism: A study of Chinese mentality and temperament. *Social Research, 26,* **31-46.**

1162

Chan, Y. K., & Lee, R. P. L. (1978). Personal happiness in Hong Kong. *The Bulletin of the Society of Community Medicine* **(Hong Kong),** *9.*

1163

Chang, C. J., & Lee, S. C. (1974). [A study of musical ability in Chinese students]. *Acta Psychologica Taiwanica, 16,* **155-161.** (In Chinese.)

Four musical ability tests--Tonal Discrimination Test, Tonal Memory Test, Consonance Analysis Test, and Rhythm Memory Test--were administered to 117 undergraduate students, who were divided into music-major and general groups, and 223 junior high school students, who were divided into chorus and general groups. The musical ability of junior high school students was found to be inferior to that of undergraduate students. Among undergraduate students the music-major group showed better musical ability than the general group. Among junior high school students, the musical ability of the chorus group was superior to that of the general group.

1164

Chang, R. H., & Dodder, R. A. (1985). Activity and affect among the aged. *Journal of Social Psychology, 125,* **127-128.**

The authors investigated the scores of 177 retired teachers from Oklahoma and 202 retired teachers in

Taipei, Taiwan on the Affect Balance Scale developed by N. M. Bradburn (1969) and measured the subjects' activity levels. Findings showed that contrary to disengagement theory, activity was not highly related to psychological well-being, although higher levels of activity were somewhat more related to successful aging in terms of psychological well-being among the Taiwan subjects.

1165

Chang, S. S., Hsiao, S. L., & Huang, P. Y. (1960). [The interest patterns of students in departments in the colleges of science and agriculture]. *Acta Psychologica Taiwanica,* **No. 2, 43-49.** (In Chinese.)

1166

Chang, S. S., Hsiao, S. L., Wu, C. H., & Chang, S. (1958). [A study of the interests of the 1957 Freshmen Class of National Taiwan University]. *Acta Psychologica Taiwanica,* **No. 1, 85-98.** (In Chinese.)

In this tentative study, the Specific Interest Inventory was translated into Chinese and revised to adapt to Chinese cultural conditions. The aim was to survey the interests of freshmen students and to study the applicability of the Inventory in Chinese culture. Attention was especially centered on the interest differences among the students of the six colleges of National Taiwan University, and how particular interest patterns guide one's choice of college. The following results were obtained: (1) For the different colleges studied, there were specific interest patterns which could be used as a guide for choice of college. (2) For some of the colleges, low consistency was found between actual choice of college and suggested college on the basis of professed interests. (3) Male students were more interested in objective matters whereas females were more interested in matters of a subjective and personal nature. The number of common interests among female students was greater than that among male students.

1167

Chang, S. S., & Lu, C. Y. (1969). [A report on the Guilford-Zimmermann Temperament Survey]. *Acta Psychologica Taiwanica, 11,* **13-23.** (In Chinese.)

1168

Chang, S. T., & Shen, D. L. (1964). [An experimental study on some personality characteristics of children's intellectual activities]. *Acta Psychologica Sinica,* **No. 1, 49-56.** (In Chinese.)

The stability and flexibility of "task consciousness" of 10 second grade children (five more intelligent and five less intelligent) were investigated using experiment, group test and interview. The results showed: (1) In more intelligent children, the stability and flexibility of "task consciousness" were mostly of a higher degree, compared with children of lower intellectual level. (2) Comparing individual subjects revealed that, in some cases, the level of intellectual activities and the degree of stability and flexibility of "task consciousness" were not always in accordance. (3) The traits, stability and flexibility, were neither exclusive of one another nor perfectly related to each other.

1169

Chang, W. H. (1975). [A study of the personal preferences of Tunghai University students]. *Psychological Testing, 22,* **59-63.** (In Chinese.)

1170

Chao, H. L. (1978). [Self-concept and anxiety in gifted children]. *Research in Education & Psychology, 2,* **234-235.** (In Chinese.)

1171

Chen, C. N. (1982). The gradual metamorphosis of psychiatry. *Chinese University Bulletin,* **Supplement No. 10.**

1172

Chen, Z. G., Wu, G. C., & Peng, K. P. (1985). [Extraversion, neuroticism and psychoticism of some school-age children in Beijing]. *Acta Psychologica Sinica, 17,* **250-256.** (In Chinese.)

Items of the Eysenck Personality Questionnaire (EPQ) were translated into Chinese and analyzed. A slightly modified EPQ (junior) in Chinese was given to 370 school children aged 7-15 years. The data showed that: (1) Boys scored higher on extraversion and psychoticism than girls; girls had higher neuroticism and lie scores than boys. (2) The intercorrelation of PL was negative and very high, and those of PE, PN, and EN were all below .30. (3) Age trends were inverse to those observed in adults, and the ENL trends were to some extent in accord with Eysenck's. (4) The results of three scales combined suggested high percentages of low psychoticism, of low psychoticism and neuroticism, and of introversion, especially in girls. (5) Most children showed a tendency of having wide interests; boys appeared more venturesome and girls appeared more active than before.

1173

Chen, Z. Y. (1986). [A factor analytic study of three children's intelligence scales]. *Information on Psychological Sciences,* **No. 4, 17-23.** (In Chinese.)

In this synthetic factor analytic study of the Chinese Binet Scale (3rd revision), Wechsler Intelligence Scale for Children (WISC, first revision), and Raven's Progressive Matrices, six common factors were found and were respectively named Verbal Understanding and Reasoning, Figural Relation Reasoning, Perceptual Organization, Numerical Reasoning, Memory, and Hand Operation. The results showed that abilities measured by these scales were not identical; children having the same full scale scores or IQs were considerably different from each other when various factors were compared. There existed one main factor indicating handicap among children with low IQs, and not all the factors were low.

1174

Cheng, C. K. (1946). Characteristic traits of the Chinese people. *Social Forces, 25,* **146-155.**

1175

Cheng, F. M. (1956). [An appraisal of the psychology of Chinese youth]. *Psychological Testing, 4,* **253-263.** (In Chinese.)

1176

Cheng, F. M. (1975). [A study of interest patterns of senior high school students in China]. *Psychological Testing, 22,* **20-29.** (In Chinese.)

1177

Cheng, F. M., & Fong, Y. J. (1973). [A study of the Meier Art Judgment Test]. *Psychological Testing, 20,* **1073-1114.** (In Chinese.)

1178

Cheng, F. M., Kao, L. Y., & Chen, Y. H. (1965). [A report on personality test results of the overseas Chinese students]. *Psychological Testing, 12,* **144-157.** (In Chinese.)

1179

Cheng, F. Y. (1974). Confucian concept of human nature. In Science Council of Japan, *Proceedings of the Twentieth International Congress of Psychology* **(pp. 86-90), Tokyo, August 1972. Tokyo: University of Tokyo Press.**

1180

Cheng, F. Y., Chen, C. C., & Rin, H. (1958). A personality analysis of the Ami and its three subgroups by Rorschach Test. *Acta Psychologica Taiwanica,* **No. 1, 131-143.**

1181

Cherng, L. L. (1986). The Chinese college students' help-seeking and receiving processes. *Dissertation Abstracts International, 46,* **A2967.**

1182

Chiu, W. C. (1963). [Sex differences in level of aspiration on the Ring Throwing Test]. *Psychological Testing, 10,* **763-768.** (In Chinese.)

1183

Chiu, W. C. (1965). [Sex differences in the level of aspiration]. *Psychological Testing, 12,* **183-188.** (In Chinese.)

1184

Chiu, W. C. (1967). [Survey of social interests: A preliminary report]. *Psychological Testing, 14,* **45-50.** (In Chinese.)

1185

Chu, C. L. (1973). [On the shame orientation of the Chinese]. In Y. Y. Li & K. S. Yang (Eds.), [*Symposium on the Character of the Chinese: An Interdisciplinary Approach*] **(pp. 85-117). Taipei: Academic Sinica, Institute of Ethnology.** (In Chinese.)

1186

Chu, C. P. (1968). The remodification of TAT adapted to Chinese primary school children: II. The application and evaluation of pictures. *Acta Psychologica Taiwanica, 10,* **74-89.**

Presents a 4-part study of the remodification of TAT adapted for Chinese primary school children: (a) the remodification of a new set of pictures, (b) the setting up the objective scoring methods, (c) the application of a new set of pictures in the developmental and comparative studies of children's TAT responses, and (d) the evaluations of each picture. These newly developed pictures and scoring methods will be useful for personality studies of children.

1187

Chu, C. P. (1968). The remodification of TAT adapted to Chinese primary school children: I. Remodification of the pictures and setting up the objective scoring methods. *Acta Psychologica Taiwanica, 10,* **59-73.**

Discusses the 1st part of a study on remodification of TAT for Chinese primary school children. This involved preparing a set of applicable TAT pictures, and setting up objective administering and scoring methods in order to have a standardized test. The developing of TAT pictures is based on rationales which may provide a broader meaning in understanding personalities. The setting up of objective scoring methods has benefits in studies of larger samples or group comparisons. Most of the contents of scoring methods are developed from other studies and are checked by 12 representative Chinese primary school children's responses. The final scoring sheets are included.

1188

Chu, G. C. (1966). Culture, personality, and persuasibility: A comparison of Chinese and Americans. *Sociometry, 29,* **169-174.**

Studies of general persuasibility and personality by Janis and Field were replicated in a Chinese culture, and differences in persuasibility between Americans and Chinese investigated. The persuasibility test and personality inventory used by Janis and Field were adapted. Intercorrelations among opinion changes on different topics showed some individual consistency in persuasibility, but factor analysis indicated that a general persuasibility factor, as such, was not prominent in inducing responses to persuasive communications. From correlational analysis, low persuasibility appeared indicative of a neurotic personality. The Chinese subjects were significantly more persuasible than the American subjects.

1189

Chu, G. C. (1967). Sex differences in persuasibility factors among Chinese. *International Journal of Psychology, 2,* **283-288.**

1190

Chyau, H. S. (1957). [Distribution curves of pure color reactions on the Rorschach]. *Psychological Testing, 5,* **367-369.** (In Chinese.)

1191

Colodzin, B. M. (1984). Self-identity and the open-system self: A Taoist/systems paradigm. *Dissertation Abstracts International, 45,* **A1072.**

1192

Committee for Education, Ministry of Education, Republic of China. (1983). [*Values and their correlates among Chinese adolescents*]. **Taipei: Ministry of Education.** (In Chinese.)

1193

Courtney, A. J. (1986). Chinese population stereotypes: Color associations. *Human Factors, 28,* **97-99.**

The author investigated population stereotypes for color using a paper-and-pencil test. Seven hundred and eighty-four 20-60 yr old Yunnan Province Chinese subjects of both sexes from a wide range of backgrounds were asked to indicate color associations for nine concepts, such as go, off, and stop, using eight colors. The results indicated that the subects did not yield such clear-cut associations as those found with U.S. subjects. Red for stop and green for go, which have virtually perfect association for U.S. subjects, were not particularly strong associations for the Chinese subjects. Also, the Chinese chose green for on, whereas U.S. subjects were more likely to choose red.

1194

Creighton, J. W. (1917). The Chinese mind: A study in race psychology. Doctoral dissertation, University of Missouri.

1195

Derogatis, L. R., Gorham, D. R., & Moseley, E. C. (1968). Structural vs. interpretive ambiguity: A cross-cultural study with the Holtzman Inkblots. *Journal of Projective Techniques & Personality Assessment, 32,* **66-73.**

Examined the concepts of structural vs. Interpretive ambiguity and defines the measures of each using the 45 blots of the Holtzman Inkblot Test. the ambiguity measures were taken from 2 distinct sets of 4 student samples with diverse cultural backgrounds. Structural ambiguity ratings were also made by a sample of 20 professional psychologists. The nature and degree of relationship between the structural and interpretive ambiguity measures was determined for each of the 4 cultural groups, and the extent of agreement among the groups was obtained for both measures. Findings indicated that the nature of the relationship between the 2 measures is an inverse one, with blots rated low in structural ambiguity receiving high interpretive scores and vice versa. Results showed high agreement among the student samples, and among the sample of psychologists, regarding the structural measure. Substantial agreement was also found among the student samples on the interpretive measure of ambiguity.

1196

Dien, D. S. (1983). Big me and little me: A Chinese perspective on self. *Psychiatry, 46,* **281-286.**

A child in China is born into a family and placed in a network of interrelated persons. The self does not develop in a process of gradual separation and individuation, as is often conceptualized in Western psychological theories. Instead, a "little me" maintains its interdependency within the context of the "big me" (i.e., the family, the state, the world) throughout the life span. This view of self-hood is found in the dominant philosophical traditions of Taoism and Confucianism as well as in the present-day socialist ideology. In light of the health notion of psychological balance and emotional tranquility, combined with the conception of big me and little me, when a person is troubled or emotionally distraught in China, he/she is usually advised to "think it through" or to "view things clearly." This means that the individual should put things in a wider and broader context, view oneself in relation to the total scheme of things, and exert more self-control. This is different from the concept of catharsis, widely practiced in the West. The troubled individual in China is generally advised to think about the present and the future rather than dwell on the past.

1197

Dubbin, S. M. (1978). Ego and self in consciousness: A study in East-West perspectives. *Dissertation Abstracts International, 39,* **B2979.**

1198

Dugdale, A. E., & Chen, S. T. (1979). Ethnic differences in the Goodenough-Harris draw-a-man and draw-a-woman tests. *Archives Dis. Children, 54,* **880-885.**

The draw-a-man (DAM) and draw-a-woman (DAW) tests were given to 307 school-children in Petaling Jaya, Malaysia. The children were ethnically Malay, Chinese, or Indian (Tamil), and all came from lower socioeconomic groups. The standard scores of the Chinese children averaged 118 in the DAM and 112 in the DAW tests. These scores were significantly better than the American standards. Malay children scored significantly lower than Chinese, and Tamil children scored lower again. The nutritional status of the children had no influence on the scores. Chinese and Tamil children scored better in the DAM than the DAW, while in Malay boys the reverse was true. Malay children tended to emphasize clothing in the DAM, but Chinese and Tamil children scored better on items relating to facial features and body proportions. The Goodenough-Harris draw-a-person tests are obviously not culture-free, but the causes of ethnic differences have not been elucidated.

1199

Fan, D. H. (1978). [Relationship between personality traits and nominated leadership position of middle school students]. *Bulletin of Educational Psychology, 11,* **123-130.** (In Chinese.)

The purpose of this study is to investigate the relationship between personality traits and nominated leadership position among middle school students. The Revised Gorden Personal Profile, Gorden Personal Inventory, Survey Interpersonal Value, and a sociometric measure of leadership were administered to 349 ninth graders from six middle schools. Both boys and girls were classified into three groups, according to their sociometric scores: the top 27% as the high leadership group (H-L), the middle 46% as the middle leadership group, and the lower 27% as the low leadership group (L-L). It was found that: (1) Among boys, the H-L group had significantly higher scores in ascendency and cautiousness than the L-L group. (2) Among girls, the H-L group had significantly higher scores in responsibility, emotional stability, and benevolence, but lower scores in expressed leadership and recognition, than the L-L group. (3) H-L boys showed a stronger tendency in ascendency, recognition, and leadership than H-L girls. However, among the entire group of subjects, boys obtained higher scores in original thinking and expressed leadership than girls, but lower scores in personal relations and benevolence. (4) Sociometric leadership scores were significantly correlated with scores in ascendency, support, cautiousness, recognition, and benevolence.

1200

Fan, D. S. (1977). [Personality traits of primary-school pupils in urban and rural Taiwan]. *Testing and Guidance* **(Taipei),** *23,* **366-367.** (In Chinese.)

1201

Fan, D. S. (1978). [Ordinal position and personality traits among Chinese secondary school students in Taiwan]. *Testing and Guidance^ (Taipei),* **30,** *474-477. (In Chinese.)*

1202

Feng, T. Y. (Ed.) (1983). [Chinese thinkers on intelligence*]. Wuhan: Hubei People's Press. (In Chinese.)*

1203

Fenz, W. D., & Arkoff, A. (1962). Comparative need patterns of five ancestry groups in Hawaii. Journal of Social Psychology, 58, *67-89.*

The purpose of the present study was to evaluate current personality patterns of five major ethnic groups in Hawaii. The 1,015 subjects were drawn by means of ethnic questionnaires from the senior bodies of the five largest high schools on the island of Oahu. The sample included: 146 Caucasians, 155 Chinese, 67 Filipinos, 87 Hawaiians and Part-Hawaiians and 560 Japanese; the Japanese were further classified as second generation (84) and third generation (476) Americans. The research instrument was the Edwards Personal Preference Schedule. The results indicated that the Caucasian profile was singular. Differences appeared among the other groups but, in general, they resembled each other more than they did the Caucasians. For many of the needs there seemed to be a Caucasian and a non-Caucasian level of expression. The results also indicated that the female groups were more similar to each other than were the male groups. There was some suggestion of an acculturational process among the Japanese-Americans.

1204

Fisher, D. E. (1981). Chou En-lai, a life style analysis based on Adlerian psychological theory. Dissertation Abstracts International, 42, *B765-766.*

1205

Foley, P. (1976). Programming people for what? Mental Health in Australia, 1, *156-161.*

Discusses the personal characteristics consistent with mental health and the ways in which cultural and family structures affect the development of these characteristics and determine what is and is not acceptable behavior. Personal characteristics and associated child-rearing practices in Israel, Western cultures, Japan, India, Russia, and China are surveyed. It is difficult to determine whether or not these systems suggest that there are overriding, general components of mental health. Consideration of characteristics likely to have survival value are recommended. Mechanisms for meeting security needs vary considerably, and the development of survival capabilities is an area in which there is room for personal growth across cultures.

1206

Gong, Y. X. (1984). Use of the Eysenck Personality Questionnaire in China. Personality and Individual Differences, 5, *431-438.*

The Eysenck Personality Questionnaire (EPQ) was administered to 6,418 subjects (2,517 adults and 3,901 school children) in 13 of China's provinces. Results were compared to those from English and Greek samples, using the British scoring key. Personality traits measured by the EPQ showed significant variation cross-culturally. Items suggestive of prepsychotic traits were more commonly affirmed by Chinese and Greek subjects than by English subjects; the English and Greeks were more extroverted than the Chinese; the Greeks were more neurotic and emotionally labile than the English and the Chinese; and the Chinese and Greeks had higher Lie scale scores than the English. In order to develop a culturally appropriate version of the EPQ, 1,000 adults and 1,000 students were chosen from the original 6,418 subjects for a standardization sample. The resultant Chinese scoring key included most of the items used in the British version, with some items dropped and others added. Test-retest reliability coefficients of the junior EPQ based on 87 primary school and 49 middle school students were high. It is concluded that the EPQ measures three dimensions of personality, the majority of its items are suitable cross-culturally, and it has value in clinical applications, in addition to research.

1207

Goodnow, R. E. (1961). Study of Chinese personality *(July Report, pp. 33-35). Washington, DC: Human Ecology Fund.*

1208

Gorham, D. R., Moseley, E. C., & Holtzman, W. H. (1968). Norms for the computer-scored Holtzman inkblot technique. Perceptual & Motor Skills, 26, *1279-1305.*

Validated a computer scoring system for scoring 17 Holtzman inkblot technique (hit) variables: location, rejection, form definiteness, color, shading, movement, integration, human, animal, anatomy, sex, abstract, anxiety, hostility, barrier, penetration, and popular. The HIT was group administered to a basic sample of 145 college students. An expert scorer's values were the criteria for validating computer scores. Validity of computer scoring was attested by comparability of means and standard deviations, by acceptable correlations between the 2 methods, and by identical factor structure among 8 rotated factors. The correlation of the computer with the mean of 3 hand scorers equaled or approached the interscorer reliability of the scorers. This report presents norms for over 5000 ss. Normal ss include high school and college students and navy enlistees. Clinical ss include veterans administration and state hospital schizophrenics, depressives, psychoneurotics, alcoholics, and chronic brain syndrome patients. Cultural samples include university students from Argentina, Australia, Columbia, Denmark, Germany, Hong Kong, Hungary, India, Japan, Lebanon, Mexico, Nigeria, Panama, Turkey, Venezuela, and Yugoslavia.

1209

Graham, V. T. (1926). The intelligence of Chinese children in San Francisco. Journal of Comparative Psychology, 6, *43-72.*

1210

Granberg, D. (1972). Authoritarianism and the assumption of similarity to self. Journal of Experimental Research in Personality, 6, *1-4.*

Conducted a 2 * 2 design study in which 236 undergraduates high or low in authoritarianism (A) responded to 20 opinion items themselves and then again as they thought the average college student in either the U.S. or Communist China would. For both referents, high As assumed greater similarity to self than did low As, and the U.S. referent was judged more similar than the Communist Chinese referent. The predicted interaction effect did not occur. Results support a pervasive assimilation effect on the part of high As.

1211

Han, E. Y. H. (1974). Responses of Chinese university students to the Thematic Apperception Test. Journal of Social Psychology, 92, *315-316. (Original work published* **Psychological Testing^ (Taiwan), 1965,** *12,* **52-70, in Chinese.)**

1212

Han, Y. H. (1956). [A study of the intelligence of schoolchildren in Pintung Aboriginal Districts]. *Psychological Testing, 4,* **272-275.** (In Chinese.)

1213

Han, Y. H. (1959). [A study of problem solving rigidity]. *Psychological Testing,* 7, **512-525.** (In Chinese.)

1214

Han, Y. H. (1967). [A comparison of the responses of the university students, criminals, and psychiatric patients to the Thematic Apperception Test]. *Psychological Testing, 14,* **346-359.** (In Chinese.)

1215

Han, Y. H. (1968). [A study of personality characteristics and parental image in institutionalized children]. *Psychological Testing, 15,* **502-520.** (In Chinese.)

1216

Han, Y. H. (1969). [The draw a person test and personality]. *Psychology and Education, 3,* **69-88.** (In Chinese.)

The purpose of this study was to investigate the use of the human figure drawing test (same sex) and the Eysenck's Maudsley Personality Inventory. The subjects were 1,227 male and female students from seven universities in Taipei. The major results were: (1) In their drawings, extreme introverts showed more frequently than extreme extraverts: profile and midline emphasis (by both male and female students), and anxiety indicators (shading and special line forms; by male students); extreme extraverts drew more frequently than extreme introverts: only the head or upper torso (by male students) and large-size figures (by female students). (2) Low-neurotic male and female students drew more frequently than high-neurotic students small-size figures and on the left side of the page; more frequently than low-neurotic females, high-neurotic female students drew legs and feet which were small, cut off by the edge of the page, or omitted altogether. (3) No significant differences in extraversion-introversion or neuroticism were found between those who exhibited a particular drawing characteristic and those who did not. (4) About half of the subjects identified the figures drawn as either themselves or someone similar to their age, sex, or social status. The figure identities mentioned by males were much more varied than those by females.

1217

Hang, T. C. (1966). *[Chinese national character].* **Taipei: Shang Wu.** (In Chinese.)

1218

Hchu, H. Y., & Yang, K. S. (1972). [Individual modernity and psychogenic needs]. In Y. Y. Li & K. S. Yang (Eds.), *Symposium on the character of the Chinese: An interdisciplinary approach* **(pp. 381-410). Taipei: Academia Sinica, Institute of Ethnology.** (In Chinese.)

1219

Hellersberg, E. F. (1953). Visual perception and spatial organization: A study of performance on the Horn-Hellersberg Test by Chinese subjects. In M. Mead & R. Metraux (Eds.), *The study of culture at a distance* **(pp. 320-328). Chicago: University of Chicago Press.**

1220

Heyer, V., & Muensterberger, W. (1948). *A character analysis of Chinese men from a thematic study of folk and literacy tales.* **Unpublished manuscript, Columbia University Research in Contemporary Cultures.**

1221

Ho, D. Y. F. (1969). [Authority and personality in Chinese society]. *Characters and Ideas, 30,* **4-6.** (In Chinese.)

1222

Ho, D. Y. F. (1977). Culture-specific belief stereotypy and some of its personality, attitudinal, and intellective correlates. In Y. H. Poortinga (Ed.), *Basic problems in cross-cultural psychology* **(pp. 289-298). Amsterdam: Swets & Zeitlinger.**

A scale for measuring belief stereotypy was developed, using popular Chinese sayings expressing descriptive or existential beliefs. This scale was administered to 230 university students in Hong Kong. It was found that belief stereotypy correlated positively with authoritarianism, rigidity, dogmatism, conformity, culturocentrism, traditionalism, prejudice against women, and compulsive study orientation, but negatively with English language skills and academic performance. The research has demonstrated the methodological efficacy of using materials that are already available in the culture, rather than imported or "invented" materials, for constructing measuring tools.

1223

Ho, D. Y. F. (1986). Review of *Culture and self: Asian and Western perspectives. International Psychologist, 27,* **20-22. (Republished in** *Bulletin of the Hong Kong Psychological Society,* **No. 18, 70-75.)**

1224

Ho, Y. C. (1982). [The factor structure of values among college students]. *Bulletin of Educational Psychology, 15,* **205-213.** (In Chinese.)

419 college students stated how proud or ashamed they would be of 96 behaviors. The ratings by each sex were then factor analyzed. Results suggest an organization of values that distinguished between competence and moral values. Personal accomplishment was the primary factor and Academic Failure the 2nd factor for males and females. There were more morality-related factors for females than for males,

suggesting that morality is more differentiated for females. In addition, females rated "ashamed" behaviors more severely than did males. The cross-cultural comparison of the factor structure for American and Chinese college students is discussed.

1225

Ho, Y. F., & Lee, L. Y. (1974). Authoritarianism and attitude toward filial piety in Chinese teachers. *Journal of Social Psychology, 92,* **305-306.**

A moderate correlation (.50) was obtained between authoritarianism and attitude toward filial piety among teachers in Taiwan. This finding lends support to the contention that, as the precepts of filial piety are internalized, they will result in a greater tendency toward authoritarianism.

1226

Hsiao, H. H. (1929). The mentality of the Chinese and Japanese. *Journal of Applied Psychology, 13,* **9-31.**

1227

Hsu, C. Y. (1965). [Chinese traditional personality stereotype and moral norms]. *Thought and Word, 2,* **407-408.** (In Chinese.)

1228

Hsueh, C. C. (1956). [A comparison of theories on temperament in Chinese medicine, nervous system typologies in dialectical materialism, personality typologies in mentalism and mechanistic materialism]. *Chinese Journal of Neurology and Psychiatry, 2,* **313-321.** (In Chinese.)

1229

Hsueh, S. W. C. (1978). Adolescent perceptions of television heroes: A cross-cultural study. *Dissertation Abstracts International, 38,* **A4428.**

1230

Huang, K. L. (1983). [The relationships of stereotype to attribution, dogmatism and demographic variables]. *Journal of Education & Psychology, 6,* **75-98.** (In Chinese.)

This study investigated students' stereotypes of ordinary Americans, white Americans, black Americans, and President Reagan and his administrative officials. The relationships of stereotype to attribution, dogmatism and demographic variables were also explored. Subjects were 610 students. The results showed that: (1) Stereotypes of ordinary Americans and white Americans were quite favorable; those of black Americans were neither favorable nor unfavorable. (2) Stereotypes of President Reagan and his administrative officials were more favorable than those of Carter and his administrative officials. (3) Age and education were related to impressions of white Americans, black Americans and President Reagan. (4) The higher the students' disposition to attribute their failure to fate, the more favorable were their impressions of white Americans and President Reagan, and the less favorable were their impressions of black Americans. (5) Females had more favorable impressions of Reagan's administrative officials, ordinary Americans and white Americans than male subjects did. The significance and the implications of these findings were discussed.

1231

Huang, L. J. (1971). Sex role stereotypes and self-concepts among American and Chinese students. *Journal of Comparative Family Studies, 2,* **215-234.**

Administered to male and female American and Chinese college students a 122-item questionnaire developed by P. Rosenkrantz et al. to measure sex-role stereotypes and self-concepts. 58 American and 43 Chinese male Ss rated American and Chinese male characteristics, respectively, while 54 American and 78 Chinese males rated American and Chinese female characteristics. 79 American and 62 Chinese females rated American and Chinese male characteristics, while 92 American and 50 Chinese females rated American and Chinese female characteristics. Results show that a pervasive double standard exists in both Chinese and American males' perception of females. Significant differences were also found in self-concepts of American and Chinese Ss. Females had significantly different concepts of males than males had of themselves. Specific differences between groups are analyzed. The role of the Chinese student on an American campus is discussed.

1232

Huang, Y. H. (1973). [Resistance to temptation as related to the level of anxiety]. *Bulletin of Educational Psychology, 6,* **45-56.** (In Chinese.)

The purpose of this experiment was to examine the relationship between anxiety level (AL) and resistance to temptation (RT). According to escape training and avoidance conditioning, escape or avoidance behavior is aroused by the fear of an organism for that event, either signaled or not; the distance of the organism to that event is related to the strength of the fear. Therefore, it was hypothesized that: (a) A negative correlation exists between AL and RT, and (b) a significant difference exists between AL and RT. The two hypotheses were confirmed in the test self-rating situation. In order to eliminate effects other than AL, the Teacher's Rating Score (TRS) was kept constant, and tested, and the combination effect of variance of AL and TRS on RT was also tested. Both were found to be significant. It was assumed that an interaction might exist between AL and TRS on RT.

1233

Hung, K. Y., & Yang, K. S. (1979). [Attributional variables as cognitive traits: Measurement and validation]. *Bulletin of The Institute of Ethnology* **(Academia Sinica), No. 48, 89-154.** (In Chinese.)

In the present study, a serious attempt was made to measure some major causal attributional variables (i.e., ability, effort, fate, and luck) as separate cognitive traits, using junior high school students as subjects. A 30-item attribution scale was constructed and evaluated against some common psychometric requirements. The scale was so designed that it was able to provide scores on 18 basic and composite attributional variables. Based upon the basic variables, 16 attributional patterns were defined and identified. In order to demonstrate the construct validity of the scale, the relationships of these attributional variables and patterns to 12 child-parent-relations variables (as antecedent variables) and 8 scholastic-achievement variables (as consequent variables) were empirically explored. In general, the results indicated that the major attributional variables derived from the scale responses had a satisfactory internal-consistency reliability and a promising construct validity.

1234

Hung, Y. Y. (1974). [Socio-cultural environment and locus of control]. *Acta Psychologica Taiwanica, 16,* **187-198.** (In Chinese.)

The present study investigated internal versus external control as related to social environment and cultural factors. Four groups of students were used as subjects: (1) 57 Chinese graduate students in Taiwan; (2) 57 Chinese graduate students studying in the United States; (3) 481 Chinese undergraduate students in Taiwan; and (4) 159 American undergraduate students. Rotter's Internal-External (I-E) Scale was used as the main measuring instrument. The results indicated that the Chinese graduate students studying in the United States had significantly higher external scores than those in their home land. However, there were no significant differences between Chinese and American undergraduate students. In addition, analysis of the content subscales of I-E Scale revealed: (a) the Chinese overseas graduate students were more external than their home counterparts on the Luck-Fate subscale; (b) on the Academic subscale, female Chinese overseas graduate students were more external than males in the same group and female graduate students in the home group; and (c) on the Respect subscale, Chinese undergraduate students were more internal than American undergraduate students.

1235

Hung, Y. Y. (1975). [Internal-external control and adjustment problems among college students]. *Bulletin of Educational Psychology, 8,* **81-94.** (In Chinese.)

To investigate the relationship between locus of control and adjustment problems, 275 college students were given the Rotter's Internal-External (I-E) Scale and the Mooney Problem Check List (College Form). Subjects scoring higher than one standard deviation above the mean on I-E Scale were assigned to the external control group (ECG), those scoring lower than one standard deviation below the mean were the internal control group (ICG), and those whose scores were between +/-.30 standard deviations from the mean were the moderate control group (MCG). There were 40 students (20 males and 20 females) in each group. The results indicated: (1) ECG reported more total problems of concern than ICG and MCG, but no significant differences between ICG and MCG and no significant sex differences were found. (2) The finding of this study, which indicates that the higher the scores of externality are, the higher the number of problems, is suggestive of a linear rather than U-shaped curvilinear relationship between locus of control and adjustment. (3) The major problem areas were similar for the three groups.

1236

Hung, Y. Y. (1977). Internal-external locus of control and adjustment problems among junior high school students. *Bulletin of Educational Psychology,* *10,* **107-122.**

To investigate the relationship between locus of control and adjustment problems, 180 junior high school students were given the Nowicki-Strickland's Locus of Control Scale and the Mooney Problem Check List (Junior High School Form). Subjects scoring one standard deviation above the mean were considered as belonging to the external control group (ECG), those scoring one standard deviation below the mean the internal control group (ICG), and those scoring half a standard deviation above or below the mean the moderate control group (MCG). Each group consisted of 60 students (30 boys and 30 girls). The results indicated: (1) The ECG group reported more problems than the ICG and MCG groups, but no significant sex differences were found. (2) The result is suggestive of a linear rather than a U-shaped curvilinear relationship between locus of control and adjustment. (3) There is agreement among the three groups in the ranking of problem areas. (4) The major problem areas reported were "Self-Centered Concerns," "School," and "Money-Work-the Future."

1237

Hwang, C. H. (1955). [Rorschach "popular" responses in Chinese subjects]. *Psychological Testing, 3,* **63-70.** (In Chinese.)

1238

Hwang, C. H. (1964). [The application of Raven's Progressive Matrices in Taiwan]. *Psychological Testing, 11,* **20-23.** (In Chinese.)

1239

Hwang, C. H. (1967). A study of the personal preferences of Chinese university students by the Edwards Personal Preference Schedule. *Psychology and Education, 1,* **52-68.**

1240

Hwang, C. H. (1967). The Rorschach as a test of creativity. *Psychological Testing, 14,* **360-370.**

1241

Hwang, C. H. (1968). Reactions of Chinese university students to Rosenzweig's picture-frustration test. *Psychology and Education, 2,* **37-48.**

1242

Hwang, C. H. (1969). Parent-child resemblance in psychological characteristics. *Psychology and Education, 3,* **29-37.**

1243

Hwang, C. H. (1976). Change of psychological needs over thirteen years. *Bulletin of Educational Psychology, 9,* **85-94.**

Studied changes in scores on the EPPS of 160 male and female Ss who were surveyed in 1963 and in 1976. Results indicate significant increases in the 1976 measures of Achievement, Order, Autonomy, Dominance, Heterosexuality, and Aggression and significant decreases in Affiliation, Introception, Succorance, and Abasement. Men and women showed similar trends in need changes but differed in the magnitude of the changes. These changes appeared to be a result of personal development rather than of social changes.

1244

Hwang, C. H. (1976). [Changes of psychological needs of Chinese university students from 1963-1975]. *Psychological Testing, 23,* **46-52.** (In Chinese.)

The Chinese revision of Edwards Personal Preference Scale (EPPS) was administered to 269 Chinese university students (128 males and 141 females) and the results were compared with those obtained from students of the same institution who took the test twelve years ago. Significant differences were found on nine of the fifteen EPPS scales. Subjects in the present study got significantly higher scores than the 1963 sample on Exhibition, Autonomy, Introspection, Change, and Heterosexuality; and lower scores on Deference, Order, Nurturance, and Endurance. The differences were attributed to the general cultural changes over these years. Based on these findings, it was suggested that: (a) the social desirability (SD) value of the EPPS items be rechecked to determine if items in each pair are still matched in SD value; and (b) norms of personality tests be restandardized from time to time. The crucial question of how changes of psychological needs should be dealt with was also brought up.

1245

Hwang, C. H. (1982). Studies in Chinese personality: A critical review. *Bulletin of Educational Psychology, 15,* **227-241.**

In this speech presented at the International Association of Cross Cultural Psychology and the International Council of Psychologists Joint Asian Regional Conference in Taipei in 1981, the author demonstrates that recent Taiwanese personality studies have emphasized 3 stereotypically Chinese traits: conformity and self-restraint, humility, and holism. Studies have found a far greater tendency in Chinese Ss than in American Ss toward conformity. Studies have also found support for the time-honored virtue of humility as it is taught in Taiwanese culture. Holism refers to the global perspective taught in this culture. Holism is manifested and reinforced in the ethic of togetherness and the emphasis of one's membership in a larger unit. However, longitudinal studies have found that the people of Taiwan are responding to their country's industrialization by moving away from their social orientation toward a more Western self-orientation. Signs of this change are found in the greater equality in sex roles, increased internal control, an orientation to the future rather than to the past, an increased tolerance of difference rather than conformity, and an emphasis on action and achievement rather than meditation.

1246

Hwang, C. H. (1985). [Social interest: Its measurement and its correlations with other personality attributes]. *Bulletin of Educational Psychology, 18,* **1-16.** (In Chinese.)

The author developed a scale (Crandall Social Interest Scale, CSIS) to measure the social interest of Chinese university and college students. The scale was found to have adequate reliability and validity. The mean score of 529 university subjects was 8.43, with neither sex difference nor age difference. However, students in the College of Education had a mean CSIS score higher than that of their counterparts in the College of Science. The CSIS score of subjects with adjustment difficulties at a junior college was significantly lower than that of the well adjusted students in the same institution. Among the university subjects, no correlation was found between CSIS scores and those of Internal-External (I-E) control, self-concept, extraversion and neuroticism.

1247

Hwang, C. H., & Chang, C. W. (1965). [Revision of the GATB paper-pencil tests]. *Psychological Testing, 12,* **235-238.** (In Chinese.)

1248

Hwang, C. H., & Lu, C. M. (1965). [Attitudes of high school boy's toward thirteen behavioral traits]. *Psychological Testing, 12,* **158-163.** (In Chinese.)

1249

Hwang, K. K. (1980). [Perception of life events: The application of non-metric multi-dimensional scaling]. *Acta Psychologica Taiwanica, 22,* **25-32.** (In Chinese.)

The purpose of this study was to investigate the dimensions along which subjects perceive life events and the scatter configuration of life events in the subjects' perceptual space. Twenty male college students were asked to fill out the Social Readjustment Rating Scale; their responses were arranged according to the rank orders of the magnitudes of stresses resulting from life events. The data were analyzed by the method of multi-dimensional scaling; three dimensions which constitute the perceptual space for perceiving the life events were obtained. They were labelled as magnitude, uncontrollability and stability. On both the plane formed by the axes of magnitude and stability, and that formed by the axes of uncontrollability and stability, the scatter configuration of the life events comprised three clusters: those related to one's family, those related to one's career, and those related to changes of one's life habits.

1250

Hwang, K. K., & Marsella, A. J. (1977). The meaning and measurement of Machiavellianism in Chinese and American college students. *Journal of Social Psychology, 101,* **165-173.**

Although there has been considerable cross-cultural research on Machiavellianism in recent years, researchers have failed to examine the conceptual equivalence of the concept across cultural boundaries. Researchers have used measures of Machiavellianism (Mach IV) which were derived from Western concepts and which may not have similar meanings when applied to non-Western groups. The purpose of the present study was to examine the factorial structure of the Mach IV scale in matched samples (age, sex, education, social desirability) of 128 male and female Chinese and American college students. It was hypothesized that the groups would differ with respect to the factorial structure of the Mach IV because of ethnocultural differences in meaning of the factorial terms and in their behavioral referents, correlates, and functional implications. The results supported the hypothesis. It was concluded that researchers must exercise considerable care in cross-cultural personality research, since constructs may lack conceptual and behavioral equivalency.

1251

Kao, D. F., Su, T. T., & Chen, C. I. (1975). [The relationships of field independence to sex, general intelligence, and self acceptance]. *Acta Psychologica Taiwanica, 17,* **105-108.** (In Chinese.)

Investigated the relationships of field-independence to sex, general intelligence, and self-acceptance among 155 Chinese junior high school students. Field-independence was found to be significantly higher in male than in females. It was also found that field-independence positively correlated with intelligence and had no significant correlation with self-acceptance. Furthermore, the partial correlation between field-independence and intelligence remained unchanged with self-acceptance statistically controlled.

1252

King, L. M. (1927). *China in turmoil: Studies in personality.* **London: Heath Cranton.**

1253

Klopf, D., & Cambra, R. (1980). Apprehension about speaking among college students in the People's Republic of China. *Psychological Reports, 46,* **1194.**

Administered the Personal Report of Communication Apprehension for College Students to 275 Chinese students. Although 20.2% of the Ss were apprehensive, data support the hypothesis that there would be no significant difference in the incidence of apprehension about speaking between the Chinese and the 2,479 American university students who were used to generate the inventory.

1254

Ko, Y. H. (1962). [A scoring system for the Bender-Gestalt Test and its relation to intelligence]. *Psychological Testing, 9,* **652.** (In Chinese.)

1255

Ko, Y. H. (1963). [A study of intelligence and personality with the Bender-Gestalt Test]. *Psychological Testing, 10,* **829-833.** (In Chinese.)

1256

Ko, Y. H. (1973). Birth order and psychological needs. *Acta Psychologica Taiwanica, 15,* **68-80.**

Compared the Edwards Personal Preference Schedule scores of 4 groups of 32 university students who were only sons, eldest sons, 2nd-born sons, and youngest sons. Each group was similar on age, family socioeconomic status, father's education, and the degree of urbanization. Results provide partial support for the findings of a previous study by Y. H. Ko and L. H. Lin. Findings concerning the need for achievement and dominance contradict US findings about the eldest son and support US findings about the only son.

1257

Ko, Y. H. (1976). The mental health of junior and senior high school boys. *Acta Psychologica Taiwanica, 18,* **37-52.**

Compared the scores of 313 junior high school, 741 senior high school, and 1,291 university male students on Ko's Mental Health Questionnaire. Results indicate that the mental health of the senior high school group was the worst and that of the junior high school group was not significantly different from that of the university group. Although the mental health of the 3rd-yr senior high school students was significantly poorer than that of the 1st- and 2nd-yr senior high school students, and that of the 3rd-yr junior high school students poorer than that of the 2nd-yr junior high school students, the mental health and personality of the 3rd-yr teachers' college students were slightly better and more mature than those of the 1st- and 2nd-yr teachers' college students. This finding suggests the noxious influence of the joint entrance examination to universities on the mental health of the adolescents.

1258

Ko, Y. H. (1976). [The influence of purpose of testing on EPPS and KMHQ responses]. *Psychological Testing, 23,* **53-56.** (In Chinese.)

1259

Ko, Y. H. (1979). [A psychological study on the delinquent behavior of adolescence]. *Acta Psychologica Taiwanica, 21,* **75-83.** (In Chinese.)

A delinquent group was compared with a normal group on five test scores. The former group consisted of ninety delinquent boys of a Taipei reformatory school and the latter of ninety male students of several junior or senior high schools in Taipei city. The following results were obtained: (1) The results of the Wechsler Adult Intelligence Scale (WAIS), Bender-Gestalt, and the Rorschach tests showed that although the verbal abilities of the delinquent group were lower than that of the normal group, the non-verbal abilities of the former were higher than those of the latter. (2) The results of attention test showed that the delinquent group had a significantly higher attention speed and a better concentration than the normal group. (3) The Ko Mental Health Questionnaire results showed that the delinquent group was psychologically less healthy than the normal group, the former being significantly more hypochondriac, depressive, hostile and dissatisfied with life. It was pointed out that the above mentioned significant differences might be partially attributed to the significant age and education differences.

1260

Ko, Y. H., & Lin, L. H. (1966). The relationships between personality and ordinal positions among university students. *Acta Psychologica Taiwanica, 8,* **29-37.**

To study the relationship between birth order and personality, the Edwards Personal Preference Schedule (EPPS) was administered by the group method to 337 male university students. Out of 15 EPPS needs, 6 were found to be significantly related to birth order. Necessities of a cross-validational study and a more detailed scheme for classification of birth order were emphasized.

1261

Koh, T. H., & Liang, H. H. (1965). [A scoring system of Rorschach responses for quantitative evaluation of intelligence]. *Psychological Testing, 12,* **127-131.** (In Chinese.)

1262

Koh, Y. H. (1960). [Size of Bender-Gestalt Test figures and the personality of subjects]. *Psychological Testing, 8,* **574-578.** (In Chinese.)

1263

Kuo, Z. Y. (1961). *Behavioral characteristics of the Chinese^ (July Report). Hong Kong: Human Ecology Fund. (Reviewed Newsletter, Hong Kong Mental Health Association, 1962).*

1264

La Barre, W. (1946). Some observations on character structure in the Orient: II. The Chinese, Pt. 1 and 2. Psychiatry, 9, *215-237 & 375-395.*

1265

LaBarre, W. (1945). Some observations on character structure in the Orient. Psychiatry, 8, *319-342.*

1266

Lai, C. C. (1978). Culture and control orientation: A study of internal-external locus of control in Chinese and American-Chinese women. Dissertation Abstracts International, 39, *A770.*

1267

Lao, R. C., Chuang, C. J., & Yang, K. S. (1977). Locus of control and Chinese college students. Journal of Cross-Cultural Psychology, 8, *299-313.*

Examined the cross-cultural feasibility of the internality-externality (I-E) construct by administering a Chinese translation of the Internality, Powerful Others, and Chance Scales (IPC; H. Levenson, 1972) to 243 male and 274 female Chinese undergraduates in Taiwan. Ss were also administered a questionnaire assessing background, socioeconomic status, academic performance, and educational and occupational expectancies. Results indicate that (a) compared to females, males felt they had more control over their lives on the general internality factor; (b) the relationships among the various components of the I-E presented the same pattern for the Chinese as they did for Americans; and (c) I-E related to other important variables for the Chinese. These findings are similar to previous findings in the US and some other countries, indicating that I-E seems to be a potentially meaningful variable across cultures. Some cultural specific characteristics were also unveiled. It is concluded that future research should be directed at testing I-E in other cultures and looking further into the dynamics, uses, and limitations of the I-E construct for the Chinese.

1268

Lee, H. (1954). [An analysis of the personality traits of police]. Psychological Testing, 2, *112-115. (In Chinese.)*

1269

Lee, P. L. M., Priester, H. J., & Yung, G. Y. M. (1983). Factor analysis and construct validity of the Hong Kong-Wechsler Intelligence Scale for children (HK-WISC). *Unpublished manuscript, Education Department, Committee on Research of HK-WISC, Hong Kong.*

1270

Lesser, G. S., Fifer, G., & Clark, D. H. (1965). Mental abilities of children from different social class and cultural groups. Monographs of the Society for Social Research in Child Development, 30, *(Serial No 102).*

1271

Li, C. K. (1979). Conflict -- a Personal Construct Theory exploration of Chinese parent-youth relationships. *Unpublished master's thesis, University of Hong Kong.*

In a Repertory Grid exploration, the significance of core role structure (the self) and the experience of threat as a conflict correlate have been demonstrated. However, no correlations between pre-emptive construing (operationalized as extreme response style) and conflict or between constellatory construing (operationalized as the explanatory power of the first component) and conflict have been obtained. The problem may lie in the operationalization of these variables. Structural measures of the Repertory Grid may not be good indicators of the dynamic process of construing. Nevertheless, qualitative analysis of the Repertory Grid, with the help of graphic methods, has proved to be useful in understanding parent-youth conflict idiographically. The Chinese emphasis on interpersonal harmony and filial piety may lead to the avoidance of open confrontation with parents. Thus conflict may exist as a tension in the parent-youth relationship.

1272

Li, D. M. (1985). [A study on the relationship between sleep quality and some psychological functions of college students]. Acta Psychologica Sinica, 17, *418-422. (In Chinese.)*

The sleep patterns of 268 college students were investigated, using a questionnaire. Then, 20 good sleepers and 20 poor sleepers were given four tests of psychological functions: digit span, digit symbol, cube figure, and digit cancellation. The results showed that the short-term memory of digit span of the good sleepers was markedly better than that of the poor sleepers. This indicates that sleep quality may be closely related to short-term memory.

1273

Li, I. Y. (1965). [Social structure, value system and the formation of character]. Thought and Word, 2, *409-414. (In Chinese.)*

This paper presents a social-anthropological analysis of relations among social structure, value system, and personality formation in traditional China. This analysis was based partly on previous research findings on Chinese personality.

1274

Li, M. C., & Yang, K. S. (1972). [A study of values among Chinese college students]. In Y. Y. Li & K. S. Yang (Eds.), Symposium on the character of the Chinese: An interdisciplinary approach *(pp. 313-332). Taipei: Academia Sinica, Institute of Ethnology. (In Chinese.)*

1275

Li, Y. Y., & Yang, K. S. (Eds.). (1972). [Symposium on the character of the Chinese: An interdisciplinary approach] *(Monograph Series B, No. 4). Taipei: Academia Sinica, Institute of Ethnology. (In Chinese.)*

1276

Li, Z. (1982). [Survey and analysis on temperament and character of 306 university students]. Acta Psychologica Sinica, 14, *120-125. (In Chinese.)*

1277

Lii, S. Y. (1982). [The psychological characteristics of gifted children]. Journal of Education and Psychology, 5, *225-250. (In Chinese.)*

Data were obtained from 491 gifted and ordinary students of elementary school on the following variables: parental educational and occupational level; general anxiety scale for Chinese children; attributes of positive masculinity, negative masculinity, positive femininity, and negative femininity; and eight measures of self-concept. The main findings were: (1) The gifted students' family background was better than that of ordinary students. (2) The gifted female students had lower anxiety and higher self concept scores than the ordinary female students. (3) The gifted female students had higher self-concept scores than the gifted male students. (4) The gifted male students had higher masculine attributes than the ordinary male students. The gifted female students had higher positive masculine attributes than the ordinary female students. (5) The gifted male students with positive androgynous or negative undifferentiated attributes and the gifted female students with higher positive feminine attributes had higher self-concept and self defensiveness scores.

1278

Lin, C. S. (1976). [Locus of control and control of emotion: An interaction study on the differences of emotional changes between internals and externals]. Bulletin of Educational Psychology, 9, *43-56. (In Chinese.)*

An experiment was designed to investigate the relation between locus of control and the trend of emotional changes. Based on Rotter's theory, it was hypothesized that internals would achieve a better control of emotions than externals when instructed to be calm and relaxed as soon as possible, and that consequently there would be an Internal-External times Time-Block interaction effect as the experiment continued. Heart rate and skin resistance were simultaneously recorded during four time blocks. The subjects were 20 internals and 20 externals, counterbalanced for sex. The data were analyzed by multivariate techniques and showed that there was no significant interaction effect as predicted. Both internals and externals showed the same trend in lowering their heart rate and skin conductance. The results did not seem to support the notion that heart rate and skin resistance could be intentionally controlled.

1279

Lin, P. C. (1978). [Reflection-impulsivity, personality traits, and learning attitude in junior high school children]. Psychological Testing, 25, *38-53. (In Chinese.)*

1280

Lin, P. C. (1982). [The relationship of field independence to concrete operations and formal operations]. Acta Psychologica Taiwanica, 24, *101-110. (In Chinese.)*

In the present study 464 junior high school students in Taipei county were used as subjects. Data were obtained on six variables: Piagetian formal operational thought and concrete operational thought, field independence, locus of control, interpersonal relations, parents' education and occupational prestige, and academic achievement. Multivariate analysis of variance and canonical correlation analysis were used to analyze relations among field independence, concrete operations and formal operations, and other variables. The main findings were: (1) The field independent individual had better formal operations than the field dependent. (2) Boys had better performance on tests of field independence, propositional logic and combinatorial reasoning than girls. (3) Parents' education was positively correlated with field independence, propositional logic and combinatorial reasoning. (4) Formal operations and field independence overlapped with academic achievement but not with interpersonal relation. (5) Concrete operations of junior high school students were not correlated with sex, field independence, interpersonal relations, or parents' education and occupation prestige.

1281

Lin, Y. N. (1978). [A study of the value orientations of junior high school students in the Republic of China]. Guidance Journal ^ (Changhua, Taiwan), *1,* **291-244.** (In Chinese.)

1282

Liu, C. Y., & Shiao, W. S. (1985). [Characteristics of modern rural youth]. *Chinese Journal of Mental Health, 2,* **33-40.** (In Chinese.)

This study investigates the modern characteristics of young people from farms and fisheries and the relationship between these characteristics and other individual variables and social behavior. The data were collected from a sample of 655 young people, using questionnaires. Analysis showed that most of the rural youth have changed their psychological characteristics from traditional states to modernity. Young adults from farms seemed to show higher modernity than those from fisheries.

1283

Liu, P. Y., & Meredith, G. M. (1966). Personality structure of Chinese college students in Taiwan and Hong Kong. *Journal of Social Psychology, 70,* **165-166.**

A study to investigate personality differences between Taiwan and Hong Kong college students. A newly translated Chinese version of the 16 PF Questionnaire was administered to 556 subjects and significant location differences were observed.

1284

Lo, M. Y. (1965). [An application of the Multiple Choice Rorschach Test to college students]. *Psychological Testing, 12,* **203-220.** (In Chinese.)

1285

Low, D. N. L. (1974). Dimensions in the identity profile of the American educated Hong Kong Chinese. *Dissertation Abstracts International, 35,* **B2408-2409.**

1286

Lu, C. M. (1969). [A study of adult intelligence and age by the Revised WAIS]. *Psychological Testing, 16,* **617-679.** (In Chinese.)

1287

Lu, C. M. (1975). [Academic performance and personality characteristics of bright high school students]. *Psychological Testing, 22,* **46-51.** (In Chinese.)

1288

Lu, C. Y. (1968). [The preparation of the Chinese juvenile personality inventory]. *Psychology and Education, 2,* **23-36.** (In Chinese.)

The Juvenile Personality Inventory which mainly follows the pattern of the California Test of Personality has been developed as an instrument for personality studies in Chinese junior middle schools. 662 junior middle school students in Taiwan, equally divided by sex, were given this test. It was found that these students, like their American counterparts, obtained the highest score on the Social Standard scale; however, they obtained very low scores on all other scales, due probably to cultural and social factors. The results suggested that the Juvenile Personality Inventory was useful for detecting and identifying personality adjustment problems among junior middle school students in Taiwan.

1289

Luh, C. W., & Sailer, R. C. (1933). The self-estimation of Chinese students. *Journal of Social Psychology, 4,* **245-249.**

1290

Luh, C. W., & Wu, T. M. (1931). A comparative study of the intelligence of Chinese children on the pinter performance and the Binet Tests. *Journal of Social Psychology, 2,* **402-408.**

1291

Ma, L. C., & Smith, K. B. (1985). Individual and social correlates of the Just World Belief: A study of Taiwanese college students. *Psychological Reports, 57,* **35-38.**

One thousand and ninety-one Taiwanese undergraduates indicated that the average Just World Scale score fell almost at the midpoint of the acceptance-rejection attitudinal continuum; there were strong correlations between belief scores and scores on work ethic and alienation scales; weak correlations were found for belief scores with authoritarianism, sex, religiosity, subjective social class location, and parents' education.

1292

Marsella, A. J., Shizuru, L., Brennan, J., & Kameoka, V. (1981). Depression and body image satisfaction. *Journal of Cross-Cultural Psychology, 12,* **360-371.**

Investigated the relationship between depression and body-image satisfaction in different ethnic groups by comparing 256 depressed and nondepressed (as measured by the Zung Self-Rating Depression Scale) Caucasian-American, Chinese-American, and Japanese-American undergraduates. It was hypothesized that depressed Ss would manifest significantly higher levels of body-image dissatisfaction than nondepressed respondents, regardless of ethnicity and gender. Results support the hypothesis. As a function of the depression condition, however, there were numerous ethnic and gender differences with regard to dissatisfaction with specific body parts. It is concluded that depression exacerbates levels of existing body-image dissatisfaction for some groups, introduces new areas of body-image dissatisfaction for others, and does not alter the image for yet others. It is further noted that research in this area could help improve understanding about the etiology and expression of depression.

1293

McCartney, J. L. (1927). Psycho-analysis and Chinese characters. *China Journal* **(Shanghai),** *6,* **145-150.**

1294

Miao, E. S. C. (1983). Concept of a mentally healthy person: A comparison of Confucius, Maslow, and Selye's theories. *Acta Psychologica Taiwanica, 25,* **75-84.**

The present study investigated aspects of Confucius', Maslow's, and Selye's Theories which have relevance for the concept of a mentally healthy person. Four questions were formulated: (1) What is the essence of Confucius', Maslow's and Selye's theories? (2) How should psychologists and educators look at the solid values that great civilizations espoused? (3) How to prevent the degeneration of modern society amidst materialistic and technological advances? (4) What kind of people could enhance the quality of life? Though Maslow and Selye lived 2,500 years after Confucius' time, the positive intrinsic values they all espouse are similar and deeply embedded in human nature.

1295

Miao, E. S. C. (1985). The Luscher Short Test: Color preference and rejection of some outstanding woman in Taiwan. *Chinese Journal of Psychology, 27,* **13-25.**

1296

Muensterberger, W. (1951). Orality and dependence: Characteristics of southern Chinese. In G. Roheim et al. (Eds.), *Psychoanalysis and the social sciences* **(Vol. 3, pp. 37-69). New York: International Universities Press.**

1297

Munro, D. J. (1969). *The concept of man in early China.* **Stanford, CA: Stanford University Press.**

1298

Nagoshi, C. T. et al. (1984). Group differences and first principal-component loadings in the Hawaii Family Study of Cognition: A test of the generality of "Spearman's hypothesis". *Personality & Individual Differences, 5,* **751-753.**

Tested the generality of C. Spearman's hypothesis that varying differences between Whites and Blacks on various tests of mental ability are correlated with their general factor loadings (g-loadings) by analyzing group data from the Hawaii Family Study of Cognition. Data from 5,333 Americans of Japanese, Chinese, or European ancestry tested in the Hawaii study were subjected to a principal-component (PC) analysis and the 1st PC was used as a measure of g. Ethnic group and generation (parent-offspring) differences on 15 tests of specific cognitive abilities were then correlated with their 1st PC loadings. Findings suggested that Spearman's hypothesis does not generalize to other racial/ethnic groups.

1299

Ng, W. W. C (1979). *An examination of the relationships between field dependence reasoning abilities and the independent personality.* **Unpublished master's thesis, University of Hong Kong.**

This study found that the correlation between field-dependence-independence and personality was not significantly different from that between reasoning ability and personality. Considered together with the inadequacy of the concept of field-dependence-independence discussed, this finding suggested that the theoretical significance attached to it is unwarranted.

1300

Nie, S. M. (1966). [The function of emulation in young people's self-criticism]. *Acta Psychologica Sinica,* **No. 2, 146-153.** (In Chinese.)

1301

Nih, L., Chen, F. Y., & Chang, H. H. (1954). [Application of the Rorschach Test in China's high schools]. *Psychological Testing, 2,* **33-39.** (In Chinese.)

1302

Oksenberg, L. (1970). Machiavellianism in traditional and westernized Chinese students. In W. Lambert & R. Weisbrod (Eds.), *Comparative perspectives in social psychology* **(pp. 92-99). Boston: Little, Brown.**

1303

Pai, T., Sung, S. M., & Hsu, E. H. (1937). The application of Thurstone's personality schedule to Chinese subjects. *Journal of Social Psychology, 8,* **47-72.**

The Thurstone personality schedule in Chinese translation was given orally and individually to 617 Chinese male subjects, including 127 medical patients, 224 neurological patients, 62 applicants for nonprofessional work, 101 mental patients, and 103 drug addicts. The mean score for all cases was 51.82. The score of the neurological patients was significantly higher than that of the medical patients, applicants, and addicts; the scores of the mental patients and those of the addicts and medical patients were higher than those of the applicants. When the subjects were regrouped according to their occupations, the scores of the student, teacher, and clerk groups were significantly higher than those of the coolie group. The schizophrenic group and psychopathic patients without demonstrable organic basis showed a higher score than that of the addicts and manic patients. The coefficient of contingency between clinical diagnosis and neurotic score was .47. A high proportion of similarity between the American and Chinese was found in the most diagnostic items.

1304

Pan, J. et al. (1983). [A research on divergent thinking in university students in Shanghai]. *Information on Psychological Sciences,* **No. 4, 28-36.** (In Chinese.)

This is a report on a study of the divergent thinking of university students in Shanghai. Their responses to 18 figural, symbolic, and semantic test problems were analysed. The results showed obvious individual differences in fluency, flexibility, and originality. Obtained fluency scores were the highest, followed by flexibility scores; originality scores were the lowest, reflecting that only a few subjects did well on tests of originality.

1305

Paschal, B. J., & Kuo, Y. Y. (1973). Anxiety and self-concept among American and Chinese college students. *College Student Journal, 7,* **7-13.**

Conducted a cross-cultural study of test anxiety, manifest anxiety, and self-esteem factors in the self-concept among American and Chinese college students. 60 Ss were selected from students at Ball State University and 60 Ss from the National Chengshi University in Taiwan. 23 males and 37 females constituted each group. Ss were matched with respect to age, sex, grade equivalents, and birth order. They responded to the Tennessee Self Concept Scale and its translation. A 2 * 2 * 3 factorial multivariate analysis of variance tested the mean differences of 7 null hypotheses. The 7 dependent variables were number of deviant signs, manifest anxiety, self-esteem, net conflict, total conflict, variability, and test anxiety. The hypotheses that indicated significant differences were rejected. The differences in the variables self-esteem and test anxiety were not rejected. Results indicate that Chinese Ss were considerably more anxious, more variable, more compartmentalized, and had more conflicts than American Ss. The variability in self-esteem seemed to cancel out the gross differences between S groups.

1306

Pedersen, P. B. (1983). Asian theories of personality. In R. J. Corsini & A. J. Marsella (Eds.), *Contemporary theories of personality* **(rev. ed.) (pp. 537-582). Itasca, IL: Peacock.**

1307

Porteus, S. D. (1939). Racial group differences in mentality. *Tabulac Biologicae, 18,* **66-75.**

1308

Pyle, W. H. (1918). A study of the mental and physical characteristics of the Chinese. *School and Society, 8,* **264-269.**

1309

Qiu, Y. J., & Bei, E. B. (1986). [A preliminary study of the personality characteristics of excellent Chinese sprinters]. *Information on Psychological Sciences,* **No. 3, 20-26.** (In Chinese.)

This paper is a comparative study of the indexes concerning mental movement characteristics, field-dependence/field-independence, Eysenck Personality Questionnaire (EPQ) and Sixteen Personality Factor Questionnaire (16 PF) which were obtained from 129 subjects (64 excellent male and female sprinters and 65 ordinary students who formed a control group). The results indicated the distribution of the characteristics of the types of mental movement of the excellent Chinese sprinters was related to their performances and the problems as found in their current training. The characteristics of field-dependence, field-independence, emotional stability and tendency of the sprinters bore similarities and dissimilarities to those of the control group. These findings can be used as testing tools and parameters for the psychological diagnosis and selection of elite sportsmen and their mental training.

1310

Razavi, M. Z. (1975). Personality correlates relating to the brain drain among foreign students from Far Eastern and South American countries. *Dissertation Abstracts International, 36,* **A136-137.**

1311

Richard, T. W. (1954). The Chinese in Hawaii: A Rorschach report. In F. L. K. Hsu (Ed.), *Aspects of culture and personality.* **New York: Abelard-Schuman.**

1312

Richards, T. W. (1954). The Chinese in Hawaii: A Rorschach report. In F. L. K. Hsu (Ed.), *Aspects of culture and personality* **(pp. 67-89). New York: Abelard-Schuman.**

1313

Ruch, L. O. (1984). Dimensionality of the Bem Sex Role Inventory: A multidimensional analysis. *Sex Roles, 10,* **99-117.**

Administered the Bem Sex-Role Inventory to 270 ethnically diverse undergraduates (Japanese, White, Hawaiian, and Chinese) to partially replicate findings by E. J. Pedhazur and T. J. Tetenbaum, who raised questions about the unidimensionality of the Feminine and Masculine subscales in the inventory. Factor and smallest-space analyses were applied to the data. Results of both techniques show that the feminine and masculine subsets on the inventory were not unidimensional and yielded different results concerning the nature of the dimensions. Factor analysis showed that feminine and masculine items were dispersed over 4 factors; the 2 items feminine and masculine loaded on their own bipolar factor; other traits failed to load at all. Smallest-space analysis located the primary dimension in the data on the horizontal axis and suggested that Feminine-Masculine is the most important dimension in the inventory. Factor-analysis results are consistent with Pedhazur and Tetenbaum's findings, thus yielding mixed evidence about the validity of their conclusions based solely on factor-analyzed data.

1314

Sanders, B., Wilson, J. R., & Vandenberg, S. G. (1982). Handedness and spatial ability. *Cortex, 18,* **79-89.**

Administered 15 cognitive tests, including 2 that contributed strongly to the spatial factor (the Shepard-Metzler Mental Rotations Test and the ETS Card Rotations Test), to 879 adults and their adolescent offspring in the Hawaii Family Study of Cognition. Analyses revealed a Sex * Handedness * Ethnicity interaction on the Spatial factor and no significant handedness-related differences on the Verbal factor. In all ethnic groups (European, Japanese, and Chinese), strongly left-handed males had higher Spatial scores than strongly right-handed males, whereas strongly left-handed females had lower Spatial scores than strongly right-handed females. Among Ss of Japanese or Chinese ancestry, strongly left-handed Ss differed from ambidextrous Ss as well as from right-handed Ss, and these differences were also of opposite sign for males and females. It is suggested that the use of spatial abilities measures that are relatively insensitive to differences in right hemisphere ability, as well as failure to attend to degree of handedness, ethnicity, and particularly gender, may be responsible for the negative findings in this area of research.

1315

Sandiford, P., & Kerr, R. (1926). Intelligence of Chinese and Japanese children. *Journal of Educational Psychology, 17,* **361-367.**

1316

Shen, E. (1936). Differences between Chinese and American reactions to the Bernreuter Personality Inventory. *Journal of Social Psychology, 7,* **471-474.**

The author found that the Chinese boys and girls had higher B1-N and B3-I, and lower B2-S and B4-D scores, in comparison with American boys and girls. This was so even when Chinese boys were compared with American girls. A discussion of these differences was given.

1317

Shen, E. C., & Liu, C. C. (1935). [The norms for Bernreuter's Personality Inventory in China]. *Education and Vocation,* **No. 161, 11-13.** (In Chinese.)

1318

Shi, R. H., & Wang, W. (1985). [A study of students' self -evaluation of their moral character]. *Acta Psychologica Sinica, 17,* **129-136.** (In Chinese.)

This is a study of students' self-evaluation of their moral character. The subjects were 320 students of different ages (8, 11, 14, 17, 20). They made self-evaluations as well as criticisms of others relating to eight aspects of moral character. The result shows that self-evaluations generally tended to overestimate one's strong points when compared with evaluations made by others. However, self-criticisms of weak points were generally stronger than self-evaluations of strong points. Self-evaluations varied with age and sex. The fifth grade in primary school appeared to be a turning point, beginning from which the pattern of self-evaluation tended to depart from that of children in the lower grades and to follow that of children in the higher grades.

1319

Shryock, J. (1937). *The study of human abilities: The Jen Wu Chih by Liu Shao (3rd Century, A.D.).* **(American Oriental Series No. 11). New Haven: American Oriental Society.**

1320

Singh, P. N., Huang, S. G., & Thompson, G. G. (1962). A comparative study of selected attitudes, values, and personality characteristics of American, Chinese, and Indian students. *Journal of Social Psychology, 57,* **123-132.**

1321

Smith, W. C. (1928). Changing personality traits of second generation Orientals of America. *American Journal of Sociology, 33,* **922-929.**

1322

Song, W. Z. et al. (1980). [Report of a trial of Minnesota Multiphasic Personality Inventory (MMPI) in some districts of our country]. *Chinese Journal of Neurology & Psychiatry, 13,* **157-160.** (In Chinese.)

1323

Song, W. Z. (1985). [An analysis of MMPI results of normal Chinese subjects]. *Acta Psychologica Sinica, 17,* **346-355.** (In Chinese.)

The Minnesota Multiphasic Personality Inventory (MMPI) has now been in use in China for 3 years. Previous research indicates its use in China has a certain reliability and validity, especially for psychiatric clinical use. However, there are many deficiencies in the results of this research. The main problem is that the MMPI was produced by foreign psychologists, so that many items and standards are not suitable for the Chinese. This paper introduces our studies in analyzing the items of the MMPI and provides our formulations for our own standards according to the condition of our country. The results showed: (1) Chinese subjects scores were higher than the original MMPI scores in all the clinical scales. (2) The test results on the clinical scales changed with the advancement of age. (3) 76% of males and 71% females have the same scores in 399 items of the MMPI as the American standards. Other items have greater differences. (4) In-depth analysis of the clinical data needs to be made for the determination of a standard for normal subjects.

1324

Sue, D. W., & Kirk, B. A. (1972). Psychological characteristics of Chinese-American students. *Journal of Counseling Psychology, 19,* **471-478.**

Administered the School and College Ability Test, the Omnibus Personality Inventory, and SVIB to 3,053 University of California entering freshmen. 236 Chinese-American Ss were identified and compared to all other Ss. Results indicate that Chinese-American students (a) scored higher on quantitative and lower on verbal and combined sections of the ability test; (b) tended to be more interested in physical sciences, applied technical fields, and business occupations, and less interested in social sciences, aesthetic-cultural fields, and verbal-linguistic vocations; and (c) were more conforming, less socially extroverted, preferred concrete-tangible approaches to life, and experienced greater emotional distress than other students. These differences are discussed in relationship to the subcultural values of the Chinese-American.

1325

Sue, S., & Sue, D. W. (1971). Chinese-American personality and mental health. *Amerasia Journal, 1,* **36-49.**

1326

Sun, C. W. (1960). [A comparative study of Chinese and American college students on the Cattell Sixteen Personality Factor Questionnaire]. *Psychological Testing, 8,* **33-37.** (In Chinese.)

1327

Symonds, P. M. (1924). The intelligence of the Chinese in Hawaii. *School and Society, 19,* **442.**

1328

Takigami, Y. (1975). [Sex differences in field dependence]. *Japanese Psychological Review, 18,* **14-24.** (In other language.)

A review of the literature on sex differences in field dependence indicates that among children and adults, males are more field dependent. This consistent and pervasive finding was observed in most populations from the US, France, Holland, Italy, Israel, Hong Kong, and Japan. Only in Canadian Eskimos did these sex differences not appear. In preschool children, females tended to be more field independent than males. No sex differences were found in geriatric populations.

1329

Tang, S. C., & Cheng, F. Y. (1959). [A comparative study of personality traits of three groups of students in Taiwan]. *Psychological Testing* **(Taipei),** *7,* **38-42.** (In Chinese.)

1330

Ting, H. L. (1971). [A critique of Liu Shao-chi's reactionary theory of human nature]. *Red Flag, 11,* **33-42.** (In Chinese.)

1331

Traver, H. (1984). Orientations toward privacy in Hong Kong. *Perceptual & Motor Skills, 59,* **635-644.**

Factor analysis was used to determine orientations toward privacy among the urban adult Chinese population of Hong Kong. A 60-item questionnaire dealing with different possible types of privacy was administered to a random sample of 355 adult subjects. Five major factors based on 21 of these 60 items emerged from the factor analysis. The context of these factors centered on a desire for solitude, a concern for information collecting by the government, a need to escape the presence of friends and relatives, the control of domestic living space, and regulation of the flow of personal information to outsiders. The nature of the relationship between preferences for these types of privacy and indicators of density, age of respondents, length of residence in Hong Kong, and experience of living in a rural environment was examined by multiple regression analysis. Results supported the notion that high density acts to reduce the preference for privacy. Other socioenvironmental factors, including Chinese cultural emphases, were examined.

1332

Trow, W. C., & Pu, A. S. T. (1927). Self-ratings of the Chinese. *School and Society, 26,* **213-216.**

1333

Tsai, S. L. (1984). [The relationships among family factors, educational backgrounds, and assertiveness of college students, and the effects of assertion training]. *Bulletin of Educational Psychology, 17,* **197-230.** (In Chinese.)

This is a report on two studies. The first study investigated relations among family factors, educational backgrounds, and assertiveness of college students. The second study examined the effects of assertiveness training. In the first study, the subjects were 661 students from National Taiwan Normal University, varying in sex, educational backgrounds, and family factors. Measures of assertiveness, irrational beliefs, social anxiety, and self-esteem scales were obtained. The results indicated that educational backgrounds, sex, and two family factors were significantly correlated with assertiveness, but their predictive power was low. Social anxiety, three irrational beliefs, social avoidance and distress together effectively predicted assertiveness. In the second study, the pretest-midtest-posttest control group design was adopted. The subjects were 24 volunteer undergraduates who had low levels of assertiveness. The treatment group received weekly cognitive-behavioral group assertiveness training for 10 weeks, and the control group received no treatment. A final follow-up meeting was held 2 months after the last treatment session. Scores on assertiveness, irrational beliefs, social anxiety, self-esteem, and self-efficacy scales were obtained. The results indicated that there were significant differences between the treatment group and the control group, excepting the pretest. It was, therefore, concluded that the treatment used was effective in increasing assertive behavior and self-esteem and in reducing irrational beliefs and social anxiety.

1334

Tsai, S. L. (1986). [Relationship between assertiveness and social interest, and differential reactions to males' versus females' assertiveness and nonassertiveness]. *Bulletin of Educational Psychology, 19,* **149-176.** (In Chinese.)

The relationship between assertiveness and social interest was examined and differences in assertiveness and reactions to assertiveness were investigated. The subjects were 663 subjects junior high school students. The dependent variables were scores on assertiveness, social interest and interpersonal attraction scales. The independent variables were sex, levels of social interest, types of situation (refusal and commendatory), and model's behavior (assertive and nonassertive). The results indicated a difference between males and females in different situational assertions. There was an interaction between sex and levels of social interest on interpersonal conflict resolution/negative expression. Assertiveness was significantly negatively correlated with social interest.

1335

Tseng, I. H. (1977). [Some correlating factors concerning the formation of Taiwan's national middle school students' belief in internal-external controls]. *Bulletin of Research Institute of Education* **(Taiwan Normal University),** *19,* **495-506.** (In Chinese.)

1336

Tseng, W. S. (1972). [On Chinese national character from the viewpoint of personality development]. In Y. Y. Li & K. S. Yang (Eds.), *[Symposium on the character of the Chinese: An interdisciplinary approach]* **(Monograph Series B, No. 4, pp. 227-250). Taipei: Academia Sinica, Institute of Ethnology.** (In Chinese.)

1337

Tseng, W. S. (1973). The concept of personality in Confucian thought. *Psychiatry, 36,* **191-202.**

1338

Tseng, W. S., & Wu, D. Y. H. (Eds.). (1985). *Chinese culture and mental health.* **Orlando, FL: Academic Press.**

1339

Tsui, C. L. C. (1978). Culture and control orientation: A study of internal-external locus of control in Chinese and American-Chinese women. (Doctoral dissertation, University of California, Berkeley, 1977). *Dissertation Abstracts International, 39,* **A770.**

1340

Tsung, L. T., & Han, Y. H. (1953). [A study of the intelligence of school children in aboriginal districts in Taiwan]. *Psychological Testing, 1,* **26-32.** (In Chinese.)

1341

Upmanyu, V. V., & Vasudeva, P. N. (1982). National stereotypes of university students in Northern India. *Asian Journal of Psychology & Education, 9,* **1-2.**

100 male and 100 female university students chose from a list of 48 adjectives those most characteristic of 8 nationalities. The English, Russians, Japanese, and Americans were rated most favorably; all were characterized as intelligent, industrious, progressive, efficient, and practical--although the English and Americans were also characterized as materialistic. The Chinese and Pakistanis were rated extremely unfavorably, probably due to previous military conflict with India, suggesting a basis of national stereotypes in socio-political factors. No sex differences were found.

1342

Vandenberg, S. G. (1959). The primary mental abilities of Chinese students: A comparative study of the stability of a factor structure. *Annals of the New York Academy of Sciences, 79,* **257-304.**

Scores on 35 tests, including 20 identical to those in Thurstone's Primary Mental Ability study of United States college students, administered to 92 Chinese students studying at United States universities were factor analyzed and yielded 13 factors. Analysis of the 20 identical tests yielded congruent factors of spatial, verbal, numerical, memory, and perceptual speed. Only the verbal factor correlated significantly with acculturation measures. Cultural influences help shape some of the underlying abilities, but other potentialities exist independent of one another and cultural milieu.

1343

Walcott, G. D. (1920). The intelligence of Chinese students. *School and Society, 11,* **474-480.**

1344

Wang, D., Qi, S. P., & Chen, Z. P. (1986). [A preliminary report on the clinical use of the "Chinese-Binet Scale"]. *Information on Psychological Sciences,* **No. 3, 39-43.** (In Chinese.)

The Chinese Binet Scale was used to test children in the iodine-deficient regions of Shanxi and Hebei Provinces, where endemic goiter and endemic cretinism are prevalent. The average IQ of these children was found to be distinctly lower than that in non-iodine-deficient regions; 15.4-16.7% had slight feeble mindedness which was apparently associated with iodine deficiency. It is maintained that there are a considerable number of subclinical cretins among so-called normal children. The validity and reliability of the Chinese Binet Scale appear satisfactory enough to meet the needs for clinical assessment.

1345

Wang, M. J. (1969). Report on the revision of the Thematic Apperception Test. *Acta Psychologica Taiwanica, 11,* **24-41.**

Revised the TAT for the Chinese culture by developing an alternate set of cards designed by a Chinese artist. Preliminary tests were made involving university students, and the pictures were analyzed and modified until a satisfactory series evolved. The new cards were administered to 100 student Ss and 20 schizophrenic patients equally divided in terms of sex and educational level. Their protocols were analyzed in terms of needs for achievement, affiliation, power, and aggression. The intrascore reliabilities for 20 Ss were .93, .82, .86, and .95, respectively.

1346

Wang, S. L. (1926). A demonstration of the language difficulty involved in comparing racial groups by means of verbal intelligence tests. *Journal of Applied Psychology, 10,* **102-106.**

1347

Watrous, B. G., & Hsu, F. L. K. (1963). A thematic apperception test study of Chinese, Hindu, and American college students. In F. L. K. Hsu (Ed.), *Clan, caste and club* **(pp. 263-311). New York: van Nostrand.**

1348

Wei, C. T. (1972). [The ideal character of the traditional Chinese]. In Y. Y. Li & K. S. Yang (Eds.), *[Symposium on the character of the Chinese: An interdisciplinary approach]* **(pp. 1-45). Taipei: Academia Sinica, Institute of Ethnology.** (In Chinese.)

1349

Wen, C. I. (1972). [Chinese national character as revealed in value orientations]. In Y. Y. Li & K. S. Yang (Eds.), *[Symposium on the character of the Chinese: An interdisciplinary approach]* **(pp. 47-84). Taipei: Academia Sinica, Institute of Ethnology.** (In Chinese.)

1350

White, W. G., & Chan, E. (1983). A comparison of self-concept scores of Chinese and White graduate students and professionals. *Journal of Non-White Concerns in Personnel & Guidance, 11,* **138-141.**

50 Chinese-American graduate students and professionals (34 males, 16 females) and 50 White graduate students and professionals (8 males, 42 females) were administered the Wallace Self-Concept Scale (WSCS). MANOVA produced a significant overall race effect, a nonsignificant overall sex effect, and a significant overall sex-by-race effect. Chinese-Americans reported themselves as less active, flexible, attractive, sharp, and beautiful than did Whites. They also scored lower than Whites on the total score. Significant sex-by-race interactions were the result of Chinese-American males reporting themselves less flexible, attractive, and beautiful than Whites. A traditional interpretation of results (i.e., Chinese-Americans are less well-adjusted than their White counterparts) is rejected in favor of one that regards the Chinese culture as a factor. Considered within the context of Chinese culture, results reflect the same behavioral correlates but lose the negative connotations. The Chinese culture emphasizes humility; modesty; treating oneself strictly while treating others more leniently; obligation to family; conformity, obedience, and subordination to authority. These characteristics make one less independent and autonomous. Emphasis on reserve and formality in interpersonal relationships, restraint, inhibition of strong feelings, and the use of shame and guilt to control behavior further influence the way a Chinese person would respond to WSCS items.

1351

Wilson, V. W. (1960). The use of the Rorschach with Asian people. *Australian Journal of Psychology, 12,* **199-202.**

1352

Wright, G. N., & Phillips, L. D. (1980). Cultural variation in probabilistic thinking: Alternative ways of dealing with uncertainty. *International Journal of Psychology, 15,* **239-257.**

Presents cross-cultural data from Malay, Indian, Chinese Malaysian, and Moslem and Christian Indonesian college students and British, Hong Kong, and Indonesian managers. Differences were found between Ss raised under Asian and British cultures on measures of this ability (a probability assessment questionnaire and a view-of-uncertainty questionnaire). These differences were found to outweigh any influence of subculture, religion, occupation, arts/science orientation, and sex. Generally, Asians adopted a less finely differentiated view of uncertainty both numerically and verbally than the British. Numerical probabilities assessed by the Asians were more extreme and less realistic than those of the

British sample. Possible antecedents of these differences are outlined, and cultural differences in probabilistic thinking are shown to be compatible with descriptions of cultural differences in business decision making.

1353

Wu, H. Y. (1984). [*A comparative study of value patterns of medical and non-medical students in Taiwan*]. Taipei: Chung-Shung. (In Chinese.)

1354

Wu, J. J., Ting, S. S., Wang, J. J., Su, H. L., & Dai, L. M. (1979). [Development of field-independence and its correlates among Chinese students]. *Journal of Education & Psychology*, *3*, **118-140.** (In Chinese.)

This is a longitudinal study of the development and correlates of field-independence among school children in Taiwan. The subjects were 198 elementary, junior and senior high school boys and girls. The Hidden Figures Test was administered to these subjects in Grades 4, 7, and 10 successively and again 2 years later. The results were: (1) Posttest scores were significantly higher than pretest scores. (2) High school students scored significantly higher than junior high school students, who in turn scored significantly higher than elementary school children. (3) There was no significant sex difference in field-independence. (4) In general, field-independence was significantly related to academic achievement at elementary and junior high school levels but not at the senior high school level. (5) For high school subjects, field-independence was significantly related to nonverbal IQs for girls, and to occupational preference for both boys and girls.

1355

Yang, H. L. (1978). [The mental health of junior high school students in the urban, county, and city areas]. *Acta Psychologica Taiwanica*, *20*, **35-39.** (In Chinese.)

The Ko Mental Health Questionnaire was administered to several groups of junior high school students to investigate their mental health. The subjects were divided into an urban group, a town group and a county group. The result showed that mental health is related to environment. The mental health of junior high school male students in the urban area was found to be poorer than that of the junior high school male students in the county area, but the maturity of personality of the former was found to be better than that of the latter. The junior high school male students in the town area had better mental health than the students in the county or the urban areas. The mental health of junior high school female students in the urban area was superior to that of the female students in the county area, and the town female students had better mental health than the county and urban female students. Compared with the urban female students, the county female students were more independent and elated emotionally.

1356

Yang, K. S. (1965). [Psychological studies on Chinese national character: A literature review]. *Thought and Word*, *2*, **3-19.** (In Chinese.)

1357

Yang, K. S. (1966). A comparative study on motivational and temperamental characteristics of Malaya and Singapore overseas Chinese students. *Bulletin of the Institute of Ethnology* **(Academia Sinica), No. 22, 139-168.**

1358

Yang, K. S. (1967). Need patterns of overseas Chinese students in Taiwan from different Southeast Asian countries. *Acta Psychologica Taiwanica*, *9*, **1-23.**

The purpose of the present study was to appraise current need patterns of the overseas Chinese students in Taiwan. About 2,000 overseas and nonoverseas students were drawn from three universities and two high schools. The subjects retained for the final comparisons were divided into six groups--five overseas and one nonoverseas. The five overseas groups were from Indonesia, Malaya-Singapore, Vietnam, Burma, and Hong Kong. The research instrument used was the Edwards Personal Preference Schedule. The results revealed that the Hong Kong group was most singular in its need profile. Differences appeared among the other groups but, in general, subjects in these other groups resembled each other more than they did the Hong Kong subjects. It was also found that the need patterns of subjects in the Indonesia, Malaya-Singapore, and Burma groups were most, and those in the Hong Kong and Vietnam groups least, similar to those of the traditional Chinese. The need patterns of subjects in the nonoverseas group were between these two extremes. In addition, the results indicated that female subjects were more similar to each other than were male subjects.

1359

Yang, K. S. (1970). Authoritarianism and evaluation of appropriateness of role behavior. *Journal of Social Psychology*, *80*, **171-181.**

A revised California F Scale was used to measure the personality variable, and an adaptation of the Triandis Role Differential was employed to assess the role perceptions of 227 Chinese university students. The main findings are: (a) The high- and low-authoritarian Ss did not differ from each other in the number, nature, and relative weights of the meaningful role-behavior factors extracted, of which the largest were Nurturance, Hostility, Superordination, Acquiescence, Subordination, and Dependency. (b) For the low-high and equal role pairs, authoritarianism correlated positively with the appropriateness of the Nurturance, Acquiescence, Subordination, and Dependency factors; for the high-low role pairs it correlated positively with the appropriateness of Superordination only.

1360

Yang, K. S. (1972). [Expressed values of Chinese college students]. In Y. Y. Li & K. S. Yang (Eds.), *[Symposium on the character of the Chinese: An interdisciplinary approach]* **(pp. 257-312). Taipei: Academia Sinica, Institute of Ethnology.** (In Chinese.)

1361

Yang, K. S. (1979). [Inconsistencies in personality and behavior of Chinese people in an industrializing society]. In K. S. Yang & C. C. Yeh (Eds.), *[Contemporary social problems in Taiwan]*. **Taipei: Great Stream Publishing.** (In Chinese.)

1362

Yang, K. S. (1981). Social orientation and individual modernity among Chinese students in Taiwan: Further empirical evidence. *Journal of Social Psychology, 113,* **159-170.**

Reviews a series of studies that has already been published in Chinese on the relationship between social orientation and individual modernity among Chinese students in Taiwan. The present paper also reports results from another study in the series. 92 Taiwanese undergraduates served as Ss. 46 high and 46 low scorers on an individual modernity scale were administered the Rorschach. More modernized Ss had a larger total number of responses and a smaller number of popular responses. They also used a shorter amount of time to produce the 1st and subsequent responses. Findings support a negative covariation between social orientation and individual modernity.

1363

Yang, K. S. (1981). [The formation and change of Chinese personality: A cultural-ecological perspective]. *Acta Psychologica Taiwanica, 23,* **39-55.** (In Chinese.)

This paper aimed to understand the formation and change of Chinese personality from a cultural-ecological perspective. In the last 30 years, Taiwan has undergone a rapid change from an agricultural society to an industrial society. The resulting transformation of social structure has considerably modified socialization practices as well as people's attitudes, thoughts, and behaviors. Due to modernization, changes in Chinese personality are directed from: (1) group-other orientation to individual-self orientation; (2) authoritarian character to equalitarian character; (3) external control to internal control; (4) autoplastic adaptation to alloplastic adaptation; (5) past perspective to present and future perspectives; (6) mediation and inner development to action and achievement; (7) dependence to independence; (8) preference for conformity to tolerance of differences; (9) particularism to universalism; and (10) suspecting others to trusting others. A conceptual scheme is proposed to describe and explain the determinants and characteristics of these changes.

1364

Yang, K. S. (1985). [Changes in personality and behavior among the people in Taiwan]. In *Collected Papers of the Fourth Social Science Conference.* **Nankang, Taiwan: Academia Sinica, The Institute for the Study of the Three Principles.** (In Chinese.)

1365

Yang, K. S., Chen, W. Y., & Hsu, C. Y. (1965). Rorschach responses of normal Chinese adults: Vol. 4. The speed of production. *Acta Psychologica Taiwanica, 7,* **34-51.**

1366

Yang, K. S., & Chiu, H. Y. (1974). [Determinants, correlates, and consequences of Chinese individual modernity]. *Bulletin of the Institute of Ethnology* **(Academia Sinica),** *37,* **1-38.** (In Chinese.)

1367

Yang, K. S., Ko, Y. H., & Yang-Lee, P. H. (1973). [Personality correlates of scholastic achievement among Chinese junior high-school students]. *Bulletin of the Institute of Ethnology* **(Academia Sinica), No. 35, 41-86.** (In Chinese.)

This investigation was concerned with the relationships of scholastic achievement to such personality variables as general intelligence, need for achievement, test anxiety, study attitudes, and self-concept as measured by the California Psychological Inventory. The subjects were 608 Chinese students from two junior high schools in Taipei. The major findings were: (1) Scholastic achievement was negatively correlated with test anxiety, and positively correlated with intelligence, achievement motivation, study attitudes, and ideal self-concept. These correlations tended to decrease in absolute size when intelligence was statistically partialled out. (2) Scholastic achievement was positively correlated with communality, responsibility, capacity for status, intellectual efficiency, socialization, and sense of well-being. However, when intelligence was controlled, only the partial correlations with the first four variables were statistically significant. (3) Intelligence functioned as a moderator variable in the relationships between scholastic achievement and need for achievement, test anxiety, and ideal self-concept. (4) Separate regression equations for males and females with five to seven personality variables selected as predictors accounted for an average of 54% of the total variance of the dependent variable.

1368

Yang, K. S., & Lee, B. H. (1962). [Preference order of the ten Rorschach Cards: An experimental identification]. *Psychological Testing, 9,* **695-699.** (In Chinese.)

1369

Yang, K. S., & Liang, W. H. (1973). Some correlates of achievement motivation among Chinese high-school boys. *Acta Psychologica Taiwanica, 15,* **59-67.**

Studied the relationship of several psychological and sociological variables' to achievement motivation, as measured by the Thematic Apperception Test, among 96 Chinese high school boys. The need for achievement was found to be positively correlated with individual modernity and was an inverted-U function of father's socioeconomic status. Firstborns scored significantly higher in need achievement than the youngest, with the mean scores of middle children in between.

1370

Yang, K. S., & Lin, N. P. F. (1964). [Chinese handwriting and personality: An exploratory investigation]. *Acta Psychologica Taiwanica, 6,* **39-62.** (In Chinese.)

1371

Yang, K. S., Tsui, S. G., & Hwang, M. L. (1963). [Rorschach responses of normal Chinese adults: Vol. 3. Number of responses and number of refusals]. *Psychological Testing, 10,* **127-136.** (In Chinese.)

1372

Yang, K. S., & Yang, P. H. L. (1974). Relationship of repression-sensitization to self-evaluation, neuroticism, and extraversion among Chinese senior high-school boys. *Acta Psychologica Taiwanica, 16,* **111-118.**

This study investigates correlates of repression sensitization in Chinese culture. The subjects were 146 senior high school boys in Taiwan. Repression sensitization, as measured by the Bryne Scale, was positively correlated with self-ideal discrepancy, value-feeling incongruence, and neuroticism, and negatively correlated with actual self-concept and extraversion; it had no linear relation with ideal self-concept. This pattern of correlations is similar to that found for American subjects, and is interpreted as evidence for the construct validity of the Byrne Scale as a measure of repression sensitization cross-culturally.

1373

Yang, L. N., & Sun, Z. X. (1986). [The evaluation and preliminary analysis of test anxiety victims among middle school students on MMPI]. *Information on Psychological Sciences,* **No. 3, 36-38.** (In Chinese.)

1374

Yang-Lee, P. H. (1973). [Some personality correlates of individual modernity in Chinese college students]. *Acta Psychologica Taiwanica, 15,* **46-53.** (In Chinese.)

Studied the relationship between 45 personality variables and individual modernity in 374 male and 673 female Chinese college students. Personality variables were assessed by the Chinese versions of the 16 Personality Factor Questionnaire (16 PF), Guilford-Zimmerman Temperament Survey (GZTS), California Personaity Inventory (CPI), and Taylor's Manifest Anxiety scale. Modernity was measured by the Individual Traditionality-Modernity Scale, a test specifically constructed for use with Chinese Ss. It was found that individual modernity was positively correlated with CPI scales measuring spontaneity and flexibility and, for females only, with CPI scales reflecting well-being, tolerance, and achievement via conformance. Modernity was negatively correlated with the GZTS scale assessing personal relations for both sexes, and with constraint and friendliness for females. Modernity was positively correlated for females with GZTS ascendance and masculinity scales. Positive correlations were obtained with 5 factors of the 16 PF and modernity was negatively correlated with 2 16 PF scales.

1375

Yang, S. J., & Yang, K. S. (1976). [Antecedents, and consequents, and correlates of children's beliefs in internal-external control]. *Acta Psychologica Taiwanica, 18,* **105-119.** (In Chinese.)

The purpose of the present study was to explore the role of childrearing practices as perceived by children in the development of their beliefs in locus of control, and to study the relationship of these beliefs to scholastic performance, level of aspiration, and popularity. Fourth-grade pupils were administered a scale of internal-external control for children and extreme groups were formed on the basis of their scores, each consisting of 40 boys and girls. The groups were compared in terms of variables of perceived childrearing practices, as measured by a parent-child relations questionnaire, and variables of performance, aspiration, and popularity. The major findings were: (1) Externals, as compared with internals, perceived their parents as more rejecting, neglecting, casual, and demanding and as using more symbolic-love and direct-object reward, but lacking principles in rewarding and punishing children. (2) Externals tended to have lower scholastic aspirations than internals and there were no significant differences in performance and popularity between the two groups.

1376

Yang, S. T. (1977). A study of the personal psychological needs of the freshmen students at the Taiwan Provincial College of Education. *Journal of the Taiwan Provincial College of Education*, *2*, **493-499.**

1377

Yee, D. H. (1984). [Relationship between coping cognition and test emotionality along a temporal variable]. *Chinese Journal of Mental Health*, *1*, **57-65.** (In Chinese.)

Coping process under test stress was assumed to contain two components: (a) the tendency toward information processing; attending to test information, and handling difficult information needed for processing; and (b) the tendency toward self-evaluation; appraising the threatening information about self while processing. These two components were measured in 124 college students, 5 days and 1 day before an exam, and the day before the next exam. Subjects' somatic anxiety, depressive mood and coping cognition were measured on each occasion. The results showed that negative appraisal about self was the most important variable covariated with test emotionality. The information processing factor was not related to test emotionality along a temporal variable. It was suggested that during test stress, information processing and self-appraisal were two relatively independent processes; the former was related to situational demands, and the latter to an internal stable factor.

1378

Yeh, E. K. (1976). Cross-cultural adaptation and personal growth: The case of Chinese students. *Acta Psychologica Taiwanica*, *18*, **95-104.**

Cross-cultural contact has become one of the increasingly popular experiences for the modern individual. Adaptation in the new cultural environment provides opportunities for self-realization and reevaluation of ego identity but often provokes "identity-crisis". Though psychological turmoil in identity-crisis may become a threat to the integration of ego for those who are vulnerable to this kind of stress, for the average young person to undergo and to work out these crises are worthwhile experiences in strengthening ego identity and psychosocial maturity. Some findings of the author's study on Chinese students in the US and American students in Taiwan are presented for discussion.

1379

Yeung, K. T. (1921). Intelligence of Chinese children in San Francisco and vicinity. *Journal of Applied Psychology*, *5*, **267-274.**

1380

Yu, E. S. H. (1980). Chinese collective orientation and need for achievement. *International Journal of Social Psychiatry*, *26*, **184-189.**

This is an attempt to replicate the findings of McClelland et al. on the arousal of need for achievement (nAch) motive by means of the TAT, and contrasted the effectiveness of individual versus collective orientation in eliciting the nAch of 401 Chinese 14-16 year olds. The subjects were given a poem transposition task and the TAT, and four types of experimental conditions were induced among the subjects: relaxed, neutral, individual failure, and collective failure. The results indicated that the individual failure condition, as employed by McClelland et al., was not particularly salient in arousing nAch in the present subjects. Instead, they responded most favorably when the achievement demands were least overt, and when they were impressed with the significance of their performance on a larger collectivity than oneself. It is concluded that the concepts of independence and individualism, so strongly emphasized and highly valued in the American culture, are alien to Chinese students socialized in the traditional manner to stress interdependence and affiliation.

1381

Yuen, R. K. (1985). A cross-cultural study of Chinese core personality characteristics. *Dissertation Abstracts International*, *46*, **B974-975.**

1382

Zhang, H. C., & Zheng, R. C. et al. (1982). [A research study of cognitive style]. *Information on Psychological Sciences*, **No. 2, 12-16.** (In Chinese.)

1383

Zhang, S. F. (1982). [Formation of character in Kemu and Ji-no youth in Xishuang-ban-na of Yunnan province]. *Acta Psychologica Sinica*, *14*, **459-465.** (In Chinese.)

1384

Zhang, Z. G., Wang, G. C. et al. (1982). [Psychological analysis of the position of the individual in the class group and its influence on moral character]. *Acta Psychologica Sinica*, *14*, **190-198.** (In Chinese.)

The following references are also relevant to this chapter:

74, 156, 205, 211, 214, 216, 226, 234, 239, 242, 243, 251, 252, 259, 262, 267, 271, 275, 277, 278, 283, 285, 291, 295, 296, 298, 314, 317, 478, 694, 751, 846, 854, 951, 995, 1024, 1053, 1061, 1094, 1097, 1469, 1494, 1626, 1688, 1692, 1795, 1989, 2093, 2116, 2164, 2299, 2464, 2584, 2745, 3157.

SOCIAL PSYCHOLOGY 9

The number of citations in social psychology ranks first among the 13 major content classification categories. Frequency data on citations in this chapter, in terms of two main categories and subcategories, are presented in Table 8. (According to PsycINFO, the category social processes and social issues includes studies which examine social phenomena in a natural setting from a psychological perspective. The category experimental social psychology involves the study of social behavior in an experimental setting; it focuses on the dynamics and processes involved in interpersonal relations, but does not include relations between societies or countries.)

Table 8: *Number of Citations by Content Classification, Language, and Geographical Area*

Content classification	Total	CL	EL	OL	PRC	T	HK	US
Social processes and social issues	214	19	193	2	29	31	19	13
Social structure and social roles	16	1	15	0	2	3	0	2
Culture, ethnology, and religion	150	8	141	1	14	19	22	18
Political and legal processes	43	6	37	0	17	9	5	1
Marriage and family	104	17	87	0	15	21	24	2
Psychosexual behavior and sex roles	53	9	43	1	6	16	9	3
Drug and alcohol usage	30	0	30	0	3	2	4	1
Experimental social psychology	20	1	18	1	0	2	3	1
Group and interpersonal processes	47	22	25	0	1	20	4	2
Social perception and motivation	69	24	45	0	3	20	14	2
Total	746	107	634	5	90	143	104	45

Note: CL = Chinese language; EL = English language; OL = other languages. PRC = People's Republic of China; T = Taiwan; HK = Hong Kong; US = United States (Chinese Americans--according to the frequency of the subject term Asian Americans).

Subject terms used for indexing citations related to social psychology are grouped according to geographical area, subject population, and topic. These are presented below, in a descending order of frequency. (The frequency of single-word subject terms includes those of compound terms in which the single word appears. Subjects terms used for indexing citations from other chapters may have been included. Terms with a frequency of less than 20 are not shown.)

Geographical area

171	Taiwan
121	Peoples Republic of China
120	Hong Kong
81	United States

Subject population

117	students
83	Asians
83	college students
68	adults
58	children
57	Asian Americans
43	adolescents
37	human females
23	school age children

Topic

191	cross cultural differences
177	attitudes
101	family
87	ethnic groups
81	sex
79	personality
73	sociocultural factors
65	adulthood
61	values
58	perception
43	stereotyped attitudes
40	social perception
37	countries
36	social change
34	social behavior
33	cultural assimilation
33	health
33	human sex differences
30	family relations
29	sex roles
28	adjustment
26	personality traits
25	culture (anthropological)
25	history
23	attribution
23	education
23	ethnic identity
23	parent child relations
23	socialization
22	development
22	political attitudes
22	social values
21	acculturation
21	childrearing practices
20	politics
20	racial and ethnic attitudes
20	stress

Table 8 shows that citations in social processes and social issues (inclusive subcategories) constitute the majority, amounting to 81.8% of the total; the most numerous are in the subcategories: culture, ethnology, and religion; and marriage and family. Concerning experimental social psychology, citations in the subcategory social perception and motivation exceed those in group and interpersonal processes.

It is most revealing to note that citations pertaining to Hong Kong outnumber those pertaining to the PRC. Moreover, there are only four experimental studies pertaining to the PRC--substantiating the verdict that at present experimental social psychology in the PRC is embryonic at most.

Frequencies of subject terms indicate that attitudes and values occupy leading positions in terms of the attention they receive in social psychological research.

1385

Abbott, K. (1974). Psychosocial functioning, delinquency, and family in San Francisco and Taipei. In W. P. Lebra (Ed.), *Mental health research in Asia and the Pacific: Vol. 3. Youth, socialization, and mental health* **(pp. 121-152). Honolulu, HI: University Press of Hawaii.**

1386

Abbott, K. A. (1970). Harmony and individualism: Changing Chinese psycho-social functioning in Taipei and San Francisco. In T. K. Lou (Ed.), *Asian Folklore and social life monographs* **(Vol. 12). Taipei: Oriental Cultural Service.**

1387

Abbott, K. A. (1976). Culture change and the persistence of the Chinese. In G. A. De Vos (Ed.), *Response to change: Society, culture, and personality* **(pp. 74-103). New York: van Nostrand.**

1388

Ahern, F. M., Johnson, R. C., & Cole, R. E. (1983). Generational differences in spouse similarity in educational attainment. *Behavior Genetics, 13,* **95-98.**

Reports a lesser degree of assortative mating for educational attainment for parents than for maternal and paternal grandparents of the 3 major racial/ethnic groups (persons of Chinese, European, and Japanese ancestries) who took part in the Hawaii Family Study of Cognition (J. C. DeFries et al, also J. R. Wilson et al, 1975). Differences across generations were significant for persons of European and of Japanese ancestries but not for persons of Chinese ancestry. Data support the belief that there has been a secular change toward decreased homogamy.

1389

Anant, S. S. (1971). Stereotypes of educated North Indians about different ethnic groups. *International Journal of Psychology, 6,* **313-321.**

Asked 137 college educated males, drawn by stratified quota sampling from 3 urban centers in North India, to choose 5 traits that they considered to be most characteristic of 15 foreign nationalities from a list of 88 favorable, unfavorable, and neutral traits. The top 10 traits checked for each nationality were rank ordered. Germans, Canadians, and Russians were most favorably rated, while Chinese and Pakistanis received the least favorable ratings. An earlier conclusion, that frequency of contact is related to direction of stereotype, was not confirmed. Results do confirm, however, the contention that attributes associated with groups placed in acceptable categories are predominantly favorable, while those associated with rejected groups are largely unfavorable.

1390

Anant, S. S. (1971). Ethnic stereotypes of educated North Indians. *Journal of Social Psychology, 85,* **137-138.**

Results of a study of ethnic stereotypes of 137 educated Indians indicate that Germans, Russians, and Canadians were most favored and Chinese and Pakistanis the most rejected groups. The results tend to put the hypotheses and findings of H. C. Triandis and V. Vassiliou about the relationship between frequency of contact and favorability-unfavorability of stereotypes in doubt. They rather confirm M. Sherif and C. I. Hovland's theory that the favorability of stereotypes may be a function of the degree of acceptability of the group. Sociopolitical factors are seen as determinants of acceptability or nonacceptability.

1391

Ando, N. (1965). A cross-cultural study on value pattern of seven cultural samples. *Psychologia: An International Journal of Psychology in the Orient, 8,* **177-186.**

"a cross-cultural study was made concerning 7 cultural samples' value patterns on the basis of the data from 4 studies by means of Morris' value scale . . . . 2 Kinds of pattern similarity indexes, Cattell's r and Morris' d', were used to categorize 7 value patterns into fewer clusters . . . . As a result of analysis concerning pattern similarity of value factor profile mainly on the basis of r |, 4 clusters . . . ." Appeared: (1) patterns shown by the respondents in india and the Philippines, (2) those in Japan and Norway, (3) China, and (4) in the United States.

1392

Appleton, S. (1970, Oct.-Dec.). Taiwanese and Mainlanders on Taiwan: A survey of student attitudes. *China Quarterly.*

1393

Appleton, S. (1970, April-June). Surveying the values of Chinese college students. *Asian Forum,* **75-88.**

1394

Appleton, S. (1979). Sex, values, and change in Taiwan. In R. W. Wilson, A. A. Wilson & S. L. Greenblatt (Eds.), *Value change in Chinese society* **(pp. 185-202). New York: Praeger.**

1395

Arnold, F., & Kuo, E. C. (1984). The value of daughters and sons: A comparative study of the gender preferences of parents. *Journal of Comparative Family Studies, 15,* **299-318.**

The authors surveyed 1,000 to 3,000 wives and 25% to 50% of their husbands in each country (Turkey, Indonesia, the Philippines, Thailand, Korea, Taiwan,

Singapore, and the U.S.) about the preference for sons and daughters and their distribution if they were to have three children. Gender preference was operationalized using a scale measure and the percentage of males out of the total number of children in the ideal family. Resultsed show a male preference in a wide variety of countries. Sons were wanted to continue the family name, for a variety of economic reasons, and for companionship for fathers. Daughters were wanted to help in household chores and for a variety of desirable personality characteristics. The variable most strongly related to son preference was the sex composition of the children a couple already had.

1396

Ball, J. C., & Lau, M. P. (1966). The Chinese narcotic addict in the United States. *Social Forces, 45,* **68-72.**

1397

Barlow, J. A. (1981). Mass line leadership and thought reform in China. *American Psychologist, 36,* **300-309.**

Mass line leadership (similar to Lewinian (K. Lewin et al, 1939) "democratic" leadership and involving operant conditioning) played a critical part in Chinese Communist practice and its success in changing China. Mass line leadership, which may lead to thought reform, was implemented in small study groups by consciousness raising, study/thought revealing, and self-criticism/criticism. Mass line leadership and thought reform have significant new and unprecedented aspects.

1398

Barlow, J. A. (1982). Attitudes and purposes: A reply to the Freedmans. *American Psychologist, 37,* **105-106.**

Replies to A. Freedman and P. E. Freedman's charge that an earlier article by the present author is a "one-sided and highly misleading portrait of Mao's China". Barlow contends that it was not intended to be a portrait of China but a presentation of some of the writing concerning leadership by Mao, K. Lewin, and B. F. Skinner and a description of some examples of mass-line leadership in China. It is argued that physical punishment and outright terror are neither mass-line leadership nor overlooked in the article and that the confusion results from discrepancies between the attitudes and purposes of Freedman and Freedman and those of the author.

1399

Barnett, M. L. (1958). Some Cantonese-American problems of status adjustment. *Phylon, 18,* **420-427.**

1400

Barney, R. D., & Chu, G. G. (1976). Differences between Mormon missionaries' perceptions and Chinese natives' expectations in intercultural transactions. *Journal of Social Psychology, 98,* **135-136.**

30 former Mormon missionaries who served 2 yrs in Taiwan and Hong Kong and 30 native Chinese sorted 70 cultural statements involving 6 interaction concept areas (personal appearance, tradition, language, personal manners, church behavior, and personal space) into a rank-ordered scale ranging from strongly agree to strongly disagree. Significant differences in views between the 2 groups were found on 29 of the 70 statements and in 4 of the 6 interaction concept areas.

1401

Basow, S. A. (1984). Cultural variations in sex-typing. *Sex Roles, 10,* **577-585.**

Measured sex-typing of 581 Fiji secondary school and 240 university students using the Personal Attributes Questionnaire (PAQ). The Fiji sample (mean age 15.2 yrs) consisted of 87 male and 108 female Fijians, 118 male and 80 female Indo-Fijians, 34 male and 39 female part-Europeans, 19 male and 19 female Chinese, and 40 male and 37 female others. The university sample consisted of 23 male and 26 female Fijians, 80 male and 61 female Indo-Fijians, and 31 male and 19 female others. These samples were compared with US samples tested by J. T. Spence and R. L. Helmreich (1978). Results show that same-sex-typing was less marked in Fiji than in the US, and there were no differences between the sexes in sex-typing patterns. Minor ethnic group variations among Fiji students occurred. University students, especially females, were more similar to their US counterparts than were secondary school students. The pattern of intercorrelations of PAQ scales suggested a different definition of sex roles in the 2 countries. The use of the PAQ to tap meaningful cultural differences is discussed.

1402

Baum, C. L., & Baum, R. (1979). Creating the new communist child: Continuity and change in Chinese styles of early childhood socialization. In R. W. Wilson, A. A. Wilson, & S. L. Greenblatt (Eds.), *Value change in Chinese society* **(pp. 98-121). New York: Praeger.**

1403

Bayer, I. (1973). The world drug situation. *Unesco Courier, 26,* **16-22.**

1404

Beaudry, J. A. (1967). Acculturation and assimilation: Chinese professionals in upstate New York. *Dissertation Abstracts International, 27,* **A4366.**

1405

Bellah, R. N. (1948). Father and son in Christianity and Confucianism. *Psychoanalytic Review, 68,* **124-126.**

1406

Bergesen, A. J. (1978). A Durkheimian theory of "witch-hunts" with the Chinese Cultural Revolution of 1966-1969 as an example. *Journal for the Scientific Study of Religion, 17,* **19-29.**

Combines ideas from K. T. Erikson (1966) and G. E. Swanson (1964, 1967) to account for the appearance of political witch-hunts like the Chinese Cultural revolution. Erikson's idea of a boundary crisis and Swanson's notion of immanence are used to account for the highly religious overtones to these events. The American threat in Vietnam is identified as a threat to the Chinese and the purges and rectification campaigns of the Cultural Revolution are seen as Durkheimian efforts at reaffirming the collective identity of the Chinese nation. The idea of the sacred and the profane is shown to be similar to the notion of deviant and normal.

1407

Bernstein, I. H., Lin, T. D., & McClellan, P. (1982). Cross- vs. within-racial judgments of attractiveness. *Perception & Psychophysics, 32,* **495-503.**

Ss from 2 pairs of ethnic groups (30 Chinese and 30 White in Exp I, 30 Black and 30 White in Exp II) judged the attractiveness of faces in yearbook pictures of persons that belonged to their own or to the other ethnic group. This was to see whether (1) a given group would perceive more variation in the attractiveness of faces belonging to its own vs the other ethnic group, as suggested by the cross-racial literature, and (2) the 2 groups would use the same or different rules to define attractiveness. There were essentially no differences in perceived variation for cross- vs within-racial judgments, but there were differences in the criteria used to define attractiveness. As expected, Black and White aesthetic criteria were more like one another than were Chinese and White criteria. Discussion centered around reconciling these findings with the recognition literature.

1408

Berrien, F. K. (1969). Stereotype similarities and contrasts. *Journal of Social Psychology, 78,* **173-183.**

A cross-cultural test of mirror imaging employed Japanese and American students who stereotyped Russian, Chinese, and each other using an identical list of characteristics. Measures of friendliness toward and knowledge about target nationalities were analyzed along with the social desirability of the descriptive characteristics. Results show that the Japanese do not conform to mirror-image hypothesis. Cognitive balance cannot account for the data in this and related studies of foreign respondents. Cultural distance, a new hypothesized dimension, may account for the findings.

1409

Binnie-Dawson, J. L. M. (1980). The effects of economic development and modernization in resolving traditional modern attitudinal conflict. *International Journal of Inter-cultural Relations, 4,* **1-32.**

1410

Binnie-Dawson, J. L. M., Blowers, G. H., & Hoosain, R. (Eds.). (1981). *Perspectives in Asian cross-cultural psychology.* **Lisse, Netherlands: Swets & Zeitlinger.**

1411

Birch, C. (1961). *Chinese myths and fantasies.* **New York: H. Z. Walck.**

1412

Bloom, A. H. (1977). Two dimensions of moral reasoning: Social principledness and social humanism in cross-cultural perspective. *Journal of Social Psychology, 101,* **29-44.**

Attempted (a) to provide evidence from 3 contrasting cultural contexts for the cross-cultural operativity of 2 proposed underlying dimensions of moral reasoning, and (b) to examine the relationship between the 2 dimensions. The 1st dimension, social principledness, relates to a readiness to make sociopolitical decisions to differentiate between a conventional and a personal standard of morality; while the 2nd, social humanism, relates to a readiness to grant priority to the human implications of such decisions. Questionnaires distributed to 336 Hong Kong residents and 76 French and 52 American university students provide strong evidence of internal consistency in each dimension in each culture, or uniformity in the operation of each dimension cross-culturally, and of validity for each dimension as defined. Correlational analysis indicated the lack of any necessary interdependence between the dimensions. Results challenge L. Kohlberg's (1971) assumption of a necessary link between moral autonomy and humanistic values. They suggest a resolution of the problem of retrogression in the stage-sequence, and they point more generally to the role of underlying cognitive dimensions in influencing sociopolitical reasoning and behavior.

1413

Bloom, A. H. (1977). A cognitive dimension of social control: The Hong Kong Chinese in cross-cultural perspective. In A. A. Wilson, S. L. Greenblatt, & R. W. Wilson (Eds.), *Deviance and social control in Chinese society* **(pp. 67-81). New York: Praeger.**

1414

Blowers, G. H., & McCoy, M. M. (1986). Perceiving cinematic episodes: A cross-cultural repertory grid study of a narrative film segment. *International Journal of Psychology, 21,* **317-332.**

Film theory has advanced concepts for explaining how it is possible for film viewers to understand what they are seeing. Many of these concepts strongly imply that the production of meaning of a film lies within the film itself - the viewer's role being reduced to that of passive spectator. This study tested that assumption using a repertory grid analysis of constructs elicited from Australian and Hong Kong Chinese subjects as they interpreted a segment of a commercial film. The results showed that the Australian sample construed more emotionally than did the Hong Kong Chinese, who responded more at the level of the film's characterization. They were also more specific in their construals while the Australians were more diffuse. Further analysis suggested that differences between the two groups were the result of judgments about different attributes of the film, rather than because of different patterns of construing. It was concluded that since there are major differences in the two groups' interpretations of the same film, in the field of film/spectator studies where semiotics and psychology come together, the repertory grid analysis is a useful research tool.

1415

Bogardus, E. S. (1933). Racial stereotypes of 100 college students. *Journal of Abnormal and Social Psychology, 28,* **280-290.**

1416

Bogardus, E. S. (1935). Racial prejudice and racial stereotypes. *Journal of Abnormal and Social Psychology, 33,* **175-193.**

1417

Bohmer, C., & Lebow, R. N. (1978). Divorce comparative style: A paradigm of divorce patterns. *Journal of Divorce, 2,* **157-173.**

Examines the social conditions that bring about changes in divorce law and behavior. Modernization has had an important effect on divorce patterns, but depending on other social variables, it may make divorce easier or more difficult. The other variables that appear to influence patterns of divorce are the kinship system (e.g., in Arab countries), attitudes toward property (e.g., among the Zuni), the status of women (certain Muslim countries), religion and its political influence (the Soviet Union and certain Catholic countries), social class (Mexico and the Carribean), the social meaning of marriage (Japan), and the role of the state (People's Republic of China).

1418

Bond, M. H. (1979). Dimensions of personality used in perceiving peers: Cross-cultural comparisons of Hong Kong, Japanese, American and Filipino university students. *International Journal of Psychology, 14,* **47-56. (Also The Chinese University of Hong Kong, Social Research Centre, 1978.)**

20 bipolar descriptions from R. B. Cattell's (1957) reduced personality sphere were presented to 192 university students in Hong Kong. Each S used the scales to assess other students who were convened in same-sex groups of 6-10 members. Responses were then scored and factor analyzed. The resulting factor analysis was compared with that derived from American, Filipino, and Japanese university students using the same materials and procedures. The composition of the 1st 4 factors of person perception was highly similar across the 4 cultures. Results suggest the importance of perception in guiding fundamental interpersonal behavior in all cultures.

1419

Bond, M. H. (1983). How language variation affects inter-cultural differentiation of values by Hong Kong bilinguals. *Journal of Language & Social Psychology, 2,* **57-66.**

60 male Chinese bilingual undergraduates from Hong Kong responded to an expanded version of the Rokeach Value Survey written in either Chinese or English. Their task was to rate the perceived positions of a typical Hong Kong Chinese (autostereotype) and a typical English-speaking Westerner (heterostereotype). There was considerable differentiation between the 2 groups, with 18 values showing differences at the 0.01 confidence level. The size of this difference interacted with questionnaire language or task order for 6 of the discriminating values. A composite of the 17 Western "favoring" values was then analyzed. Results yielded interactions between the size of stereotype difference and both language and task order, with the difference smaller in English and when the outgroup was rated first. Correlational evidence about the size of the language effect supports derivations from social identity theory.

1420

Bond, M. H. (1983). Linking person perception dimensions to behavioral intention dimensions: The Chinese connection. *Journal of Cross-Cultural Psychology, 14,* **41-63.**

Using W. T. Norman's procedures and materials, 4 independent dimensions of person perception (extroversion, good-naturedness, conscientiousness, and emotional stability) have been isolated in a number of different cultures. In addition, H. C. Triandis (1977) had identified 4 universal dimensions of interpersonal behavior: overtness, association, subordination, and formality. In the present study, to explore the connection between these domains, 256 male Hong Kong undergraduates read about a same-sex peer whose description varied across the 4 dimensions of person perception. Half of the Ss anticipated the possibility of meeting this target person. Ss then indicated their behavior intentions toward the target person. As predicted, the behavioral factors of association, subordination, and formality were most highly influenced by variations across the perceptual dimensions of good-naturedness, conscientiousness, and emotional stability, respectively. Results also indicate the extensive influence of the good-naturedness variable and the unimportance of possible future interaction in this judgment task. The universality and cultural specificity of these results are discussed.

1421

Bond, M. H. (1985). *Inter-group relations in Hong Kong.* **Paper presented at the Conference on Inter-ethnic Conflict and Aggression, East-West Centre, Honolulu.**

1422

Bond, M. H. (1985). Language as a carrier of ethnic stereotypes in Hong Kong. *Journal of Social Psychology, 125,* **53-62.**

The author investigated whether language use contributes to group stereotypes independent of the target's ethnic-group identity. Seventy-one Chinese bilinguals from a Hong Kong high school were randomly assigned to 1 of 12 experimental conditions and examined by a different Chinese experimenter. All experimenters used Cantonese when addressing the subjects. Three Hong Kong Chinese and three Westerners (one American, one Irish, and one French) recorded both Cantonese and English presentations. Subjects were asked to listen to one presentation (a person described as either Chinese or British) and to make comments in either Cantonese or English. Rating scales were given to each subject after the tapes were presented. Results indicated that language carried the burden of the benevolence stereotype normally associated with the ethnic groups by Chinese bilinguals in Hong Kong. A Cantonese speaker was specifically rated as more humble, honest, and friendly than an English speaker, regardless of the speaker's ethnicity.

1423

Bond, M. H., & Cheung, M. K. (1984). Experimenter language choice and ethnic affirmation by Chinese trilinguals in Hong Kong. *International Journal of Intercultural Relations, 8,* **347-356.**

When communicating with a member of his or her ethnic in-group, a multilingual typically uses his common first language. If, however, the multilingual uses a common second or third language, we believe this choice will indicate his or her endorsement of attitudes believed to be held by that language out-group. An audience will respond to this implicit statement by a shift in its ethnically relevant attitudes either towards or away from the position of the speaker. Convergence is assumed to occur if relations between the language communities are harmonious, ethnic affirmation if relations are hostile. To explore this reasoning, experimenters addressed Chinese trilinguals in their first language of Cantonese, their second language of English, or their third language of Mandarin. When instructed in Mandarin, subjects assumed their experimenter held more traditional Chinese beliefs and they themselves completed a measure of traditional Chinese beliefs in a more Western direction. Although most Hong Kong students at university are ambivalent about their colonial status under Great Britain, they oppose Hong Kong's reversion to China in 1997 and are threatened by this prospect. Consequently, we believe that they responded to an experimenter speaking the Mandarin language of China by affirming a more Western identity.

1424

Bond, M. H., & Forgas, J. P. (1984). Linking person perception to behavior intention across cultures: The role of cultural collectivism. *Journal of Cross-Cultural Psychology, 15,* **337-352.**

The present study was an investigation of the potentially universal links between the dimensions of person perception and those of behavior intention, and dimensions of person perception that are most salient in collectivist as opposed to individualistic cultures. One hundred and twenty-eight male undergraduates from Hong Kong and 128 male undergraduates from Australia read a description of a target person (TP) varying across the universal dimensions of extraversion, agreeableness, conscientiousness, and emotional stability. They then indicated their behavior intentions toward that TP. Findings indicated that, across both cultures, TP conscientiousness was linked to intentions of trust, and TP extraversion and agreeableness to intentions of association. As predicted from the dynamics of cultural collectivism, the Chinese subjects were more responsive than the Australian subjects to TP conscientiousness in forming trust intentions and to TP agreeableness in forming associative intentions.

1425

Bond, M. H., Hewstone, M., Wan, K. C., & Chiu, C. K. (1985). Group-serving attributions across intergroup contexts: Cultural differences in the explanation of sex-typed behaviours. *European Journal of Social Psychology, 15,* **435-451.**

The authors attempted to integrate H. Tajfel's social identity theory with self-presentational concerns by exploring group-level attributions about perceived group differences in behavior (i.e., whether bias in making such verbal attributions varied as a function of the interviewer's group identity and the presence of an in-group audience). Sixty-eight undergraduates at a university in Hong Kong rated the appropriateness of in- and out-group-favoring explanations for male- and female-typed behaviors in a face-to-face interview. A group-serving bias was found for female-typed behaviors, but only when the same-sex audience was absent. A conceptual replication of the experiment was run in the U.S. with 98 undergraduates to examine the possible cultural basis for the Chinese moderation of favoritism in the audience condition. The group-serving bias was more robust for the American undergraduates, extending across male- and female-typed behaviors and also across audience conditions. These cultural differences in attributional bias appeared to reflect the strength of the movement for women's liberation and norms surrounding the avoidance of conflict in the U.S. and Hong Kong.

1426

Bond, M. H., & Lee, P. W. H. (1981). Face saving in Chinese culture: A discussion and experimental study of Hong Kong students. In R. P. L. Lee, & A. Y. C. King (Eds.), *Social life and development in Hong Kong* **(pp. 289-384). Hong Kong: Chinese University Press.**

1427

Bond, M. H., Leung, K., & Wan, K. C. (1982). The social impact of self-effacing attributions: The Chinese case. *Journal of Social Psychology, 118,* **157-166.**

Argued that a person in Chinese societies who makes self-effacing attributions for his performance should be better liked because his self-effacing attributions support norms whose function is to maintain harmonious interpersonal relationships. To test this hypothesis, 56 Chinese undergraduates watched 2 confederates (Cs) working on an intellectual task. These Cs were either competent or incompetent and subsequently made either self-effacing or self-enhancing attributions for their performance. Ss then rated them on 12 7-point bipolar scales tapping likability, competence, and anxiety. Results indicate that a self-effacing C was better liked but rated as less competent than a self-enhancing C. Although in the US competent persons are better liked, such a finding was not replicated in the present study. Consistent with a self-presentational analysis, incompetent performers who made self-enhancing attributions were perceived as more anxious than performers in the other conditions. The role of culture in producing the attribution results for likability and competence was analyzed.

1428

Bond, M. H., Leung, K., & Wan, K. C. (1982). How does cultural collectivism operate? The impact of task and maintenance contributions on reward distribution. *Journal of Cross-Cultural Psychology, 13,* **186-200.**

207 Chinese and American male undergraduates were asked to read a scenario describing a group member who made high, medium, or low task and maintenance contributions toward a group project for a university course. Ss then rated their perceptions of, and behavioral intentions toward, this target person. Task and maintenance contributions were linearly related to both types of dependent variable in each cultural group. However, the slope of this regression was more moderate for the Chinese than for the Americans where intentions to reward were concerned. This more egalitarian distribution of resources probably functions to promote the group cohesiveness valued by more collective cultures.

1429

Bond, M. H., Wan, K. C., Leung, K., & Giacalone, R. A. (1985). How are responses to verbal insult related to cultural collectivism and power distance? *Journal of Cross-Cultural Psychology, 16,* **111-127.**

It is assumed that an act is construed as aggressive and the actor thus negatively evaluated when that act falls outside legitimate modes of social control. If true, then cultural variations in the use of social control should be related to perceptions of an insult and of the insulter. In a scenario study, responses of Hong Kong Chinese, who are high in collectivism and power distance, were compared with those of Americans, who are low in collectivism and moderately low in power distance. In confirmation of this reasoning, the Chinese were found to be less critical of an insulter and of his or her action as long as he or she had higher status than the in-group target. Americans made no consistent distinctions as a function of the insulter's status or group membership.

1430

Bond, M. H., & Wang, S. H. (1982). Aggressive behavior in Chinese society: The problem of maintaining order and harmony. In R. P. Goldstein & M. Segall (Eds.), *Global perspectives on aggression^ (pp. 58-74). New York: Plenum. (Also in* **Hong Kong Psychological Society Bulletin,** *1982, No. 8, 5-25; and in* **Acta Psychologica Taiwanica,** *1981,* **23,** *57-73.)*

Confucian social philosophy was outlined and genetic and Chinese socialization influences on aggressive behavior were explored. It was contended that the Confucian construction discourages aggressive behavior because aggression often functions to challenge existing hierarchical arrangements and disrupts group harmony. If violence is suppressed, families remain intact, neighborhood relations are peaceful, and the wider social order will be protected. When directed toward a stigmatized out-group, however, collective acts of aggression are enhanced since they are group-serving. Evidence from folk wisdom; anthropological observations; sociological surveys; and psychological experiments investigating competition, conformity, and distribution of resources supported this hypothesis.

1431

Bond, M. H., & Yang, K. S. (1982). Ethnic affirmation versus cross-cultural accommodation: The variable impact of questionnaire language on Chinese bilinguals from Hong Kong. Journal of Cross-Cultural Psychology, 13, *169-185.*

184 Chinese bilingual undergraduates responded to 3 questionnaires in their 1st or 2nd language (Chinese or English, respectively). On some questionnaire items their answers to the English version differed from those to the Chinese version in a more "Western" direction (cross-cultural accommodation); for others, in a more Chinese direction (ethnic affirmation). These outcomes were unaffected by Ss' level of identification with traditional Chinese culture or by their degree of anonymity vis-a-vis the experimenter conducting the research. An internal analysis of responses to the Rokeach Value Survey revealed that the more important the value to Ss, the less likely they were to show cross-cultural accommodation. It appears that affirmation occurs on important issues to buttress the individual's feelings of psychological distinctiveness from other groups; compromise is possible on less important matters, presumably more peripheral to the individual's cultural self-concept.

1432

Borke, H., & Su, S. (1972). Perception of emotional responses to social interactions by Chinese and American children. Journal of Cross-Cultural Psychology, 3, *309-314.*

Asked 70 American and 80 Taiwan middle-class kindergarteners to describe situations which made them feel happy, sad, afraid, or angry. These situations were then written up as short stories for 2nd graders of each country who saw the situations identical to the younger Ss. It was found that older Chinese Ss saw more anger and American Ss more sadness. This finding is related to comparative childrearing practices.

1433

Borresen, C. R. (1982). An exploratory survey of the development of a Vietnamese stereotype. Psychological Reports, 50, *159-166.*

Surveyed 1,400 undergraduates and 180 factory and construction workers as to their knowledge about, responsibility toward, and attitudes toward the Vietnamese. With regard to knowledge about the Vietnamese, none of the items predicted attitudes. However, concerning responsibility toward the Vietnamese, 3 items significantly predicted attitudes. These items related to a general factor of social concern rather than a sense of responsibility toward the Vietnamese. The attitudinal data indicated a relatively positive attitude toward the Vietnamese, much like attitudes toward Chinese and Japanese individuals.

1434

Bourgeois, M. (1979). [The shunning of incest in human and non-human primates: A preliminary remark]. Annales Medico-Psychologiques, 137, *612-620. (In other language.)*

Although the incest taboo is still considered a strictly human phenomenon that accompanies the evolution of civilization, studies of macaques, baboons, and other monkeys indicate that nonhuman primates also observe the incest taboo. Furthermore, children who have grown up together frequently experience no sexual attraction toward each other even if they have no blood ties. If marriage is forced on them (as in traditional Chinese marriages), the union tends to result in sexual failure. It is argued that traditional interpretations of the incest taboo and psychiatric treatment of incest patients--both of which frequently consider incest as a regression to a "natural", "primitive" stage of existence--must be modified in the light of these findings.

1435

Braun, J. S., & Chao, H. M. (1978). Attitudes toward women: A comparison of Asian-born Chinese and American Caucasians. Psychology of Women Quarterly, 2, *195-201.*

Asian-born Chinese and Caucasian American men and women were compared on the Attitude Toward Women Scale. All Ss--74 Americans, 85 Chinese--were between 30 and 55 yrs of age and had at least a bachelor's degree. Chinese Ss were Mandarin in origin. The prediction that Chinese Ss would be more liberal was not confirmed. Women were more liberal than men on 2 factors: vocational, educational, and intellectual roles, and marital relations and obligations. Ethnic differences were not a main effect on other factors, but a significant interaction was obtained for 3 factors: freedom and independence; dating, courting, and etiquette; and drinking, swearing, and telling jokes. On these factors Caucasian females scored in the liberal direction and so did Chinese males. Caucasian males and Chinese females were consistently and significantly more conservative.

1436

Broderick, J. L. (1978). Psychological significance of the post-revolutionary Chinese family: A critical-emancipatory exploration. Dissertation Abstracts International, 38, *B4441.*

1437

Buhrich, N., & Haq, S. (1980). Profile of narcotic abuse in Peninsular Malaysia. American Journal of Drug & Alcohol Abuse, 7, *211-217.*

Demographic and drug abuse characteristics of 3,484 new drug abuse contacts presenting to the General Hospital, Kuala Lumpur, Malaysia are reported. The large majority were heroin inhalers. They were different from the traditional Eastern opium inhalers and similar to Western heroin injectors in that they were young, male, single, and frequently unemployed. These features and the relative underrepresentation of Chinese suggest that the Chinese of this study did not learn narcotic abuse from opium-smoking relatives.

1438

Bulatao, J. C. (1969). Mapping Manila society by photographs and factor analysis. Philippine Journal of Psychology, 2, *6-11.*

16 photographs of individuals taken in Manila were described through the use of 12 adjectives in a Q-technique and were intercorrelated. 20 male undergraduates served as Ss. The resulting matrix was factor analyzed and yielded 3 factors, which were interpreted as social classes, phenomenologically arrived at, i.e., (a) Westerner-Provinciano Filipino, (b) urban Filipino, and (c) Chinese.

1439

Bunzel, R. (1950). Explorations in Chinese culture. *Unpublished document, Columbia University Research in Contemporary Cultures, New York.*

1440

Bunzel, R., & Weakland, J. H. (1952). An anthropological approach to Chinese communism. *Unpublished document, Columbia University Research in Contemporary Cultures, New York.*

1441

Burch, B. B. (1979). Models as agents of change in China. In R. W. Wilson, A. A. Wilson, & S. L. Greenblatt (Eds.), Value change in Chinese society *(pp. 122-137). New York: Praeger.*

1442

Burrows, E. G. (1947). Hawaiian Americans: An account of the mingling of Japanese, Chinese, Polynesian and American cultures. *New Haven: Yale University Press.*

1443

Callan, V. J., & Kee, P. K. (1981). Sons or daughters? Cross-cultural comparisons of the sex preferences of Australian, Greek, Italian, Malay, Chinese and Indian parents in Australia and Malaysia. Population & Environment: Behavioral & Social Issues, 4, *97-108.*

Surveyed 1,239 parents and found son preference to be higher for Malaysian couples. Reasons centered on traditional values of old age support, continuation of the family name, and completion of male tasks in the home. The reasons for wanting a daughter indicate an even clearer breakdown of interests in the 2 countries over the traditional as compared to the more psychologically oriented benefits in having a girl. Results indicate a general decline in son preference from high- to low-fertility regimes and somewhat less concern with the traditional roles of children.

1444

Cameron, D. C. (1968). Youth and drugs: A world view. JAMA, 206, *1267-1271.*

Discusses government control, treatment and rehabilitation, international patterns (Iran, India, Thailand, Singapore, Hong Kong, Philippines, Sweden, and the United States), young people and drugs, and factors related to drug taking. Drug taking is likened to a communicable-disease model, and it is concluded that "it is not enough to try to clarify the origins of psychological readiness for escape, thrill seeking, rebellion, or some combination of these. We must also ask ourselves how it happens that drugs are used for the 'fulfillment' of these psychological needs."

1445

Cansdale, J. S. (1969). Cultural problems of Chinese students in a Western-type university. In I. C. Jarvie (Ed.), Hong Kong: A society in transition. *London: Routledge and Kegan Paul Limited.*

1446

Castell, P. J., & Goldstein, J. H. (1977). Social occasions for joking: A cross-cultural study. In A. J. Chapman & H. C. Foot (Eds.), It's a funny thing, humour *(pp. 193-197). Oxford: Pergamon Press. (Papers also presented in International Conference of Humor and Laughter, Temple University, Philadelphia, Quarters D, National Naval Medical Centre Bethesda, Md.)*

1447

Casterline, J. B. (1980). The determinants of rising female age at marriage: Taiwan, 1905-1976. Dissertation Abstracts International, 41, *A1226-1227.*

1448

Chan, D. W. O. (1985). Perception and judgment of facial expressions among the Chinese. International Journal of Psychology, 20, *681-692.*

1449

Chan, D. W. O., Chan-Ho, M. W., & Chan, T. S. C. (1984). Life event scaling: The Chinese experience. Social Science & Medicine, 18, *441-446.*

261 Chinese staff and student members (aged 18-60 yrs) in a university community rated 69 life events on a scale of "upsettingness" in order to (1) unidimen-

sionally scale Ss' perceptions of life events, (2) explore status-group differences in Ss' perceptions of life events, (3) examine status-group differences in Ss' perceptions of specific life events, and (4) uncover dimensions necessary to adequately characterize Ss' perceptions of life events. Results show that there was relatively great consensus in Ss' ratings as a group and relatively great consistency in their ratings across diverse status groups differing in age, sex, marital status, and staff-student membership. An examination of specific events, however, revealed subtle differences among groups. In general, perception of life events could be conceptualized in the following dimensions: personal loss and failure, gain and achievement, environmental and role change, personal catastrophe, minor interpersonal problems, and legal and court-related problems. It is suggested that adjustment, control, and desirability are event attributes that capture different aspects of perception of life events.

1450

Chan, J. (1976). Parent-child interaction and education: A cross-cultural comparative study. New Horizons, *No. 17, 69-81.*

Twelve parental factors (Father and Mother times Concerned, Restrictive, Democratic, Demanding, Rational, and Autocratic) were identified for Hong Kong and Singapore Chinese samples, using the Parent Image Differential. They were compared with those reported by Ginsburg et al. on American and Mexican samples. It was observed that the factor patterns were similar among the four cultural groups, indicating their cross-cultural stability. However, there were some interesting differences in the relative importance of factors among the four groups. It was hardly surprising that the factors were more similar in magnitude between Hong Kong and Singapore Chinese, and between Americans and Mexicans, than they were between the Asian and the American groups.

1451

Chan, K. H. (1984). A study of assimilation attitudes and behaviors of Chinese American registered voters in Santa Clara County, California. Dissertation Abstracts International, 45, *A1880.*

1452

Chan, L. M. (1970). Foot binding in Chinese women and its psycho-social implications. Canadian Psychiatric Association Journal, 15, *229-231.*

1453

Chan, W. T. (1966). The individual in Chinese religions. In C. A. Moore (Ed.), The Chinese mind. *Honolulu, HI: University of Hawaii Press.*

1454

Chan, Y. C. N. (1978). Educational needs in intergenerational conflict: A study of immigrant families in New York's Chinatown. Dissertation Abstracts International, 39, *A2010-2011.*

1455

Chandra, S. (1967). Stereotypes of university students toward different ethnic groups. Journal of Social Psychology, 71, *87-94.*

Attempted to determine the persistence and change in the stereotypes of university students toward Indians, Americans, Englishmen, Chinese, and Russians, in the context of Chinese aggression. Findings were: (1) Students have a positive attitude toward all ethnic groups except Chinese, (2) the pre-existing stereotypes show a tendency to persist, (3) stereotypes concerning the Chinese show an unfavorable attitude, and (4) self-image of Indians reflects an ambivalent picture.

1456

Chaney, D., & Podmore, D. (1973). Young adults in Hong Kong: Attitudes in a modernising society. *Hong Kong: University of Hong Kong, Centre of Asian Studies.*

1457

Chang, B. L., Chang, A. F., & Shen, Y. A. (1984). Attitudes toward aging in the United States and Taiwan. Journal of Comparative Family Studies, 15, *109-130.*

Compared attitudes toward aging and the needs of old people among 200 college students from Taiwan and 400 students of Chinese descent living in the US. Ss completed the Attitude Toward Old People Scale and the Needs of Old People Scale; they also indicated whether they lived in a household that included their grandparents, whether they would choose to live with their grandparents, and whether they had a religious affiliation. Results indicate that both groups had favorable attitudes toward aging and old people. However, Taiwanese held less stereotypical views of old people, while the Chinese-Americans held more positive views. Results are discussed in view of the role of increased urbanization and educational, societal, and family support for attitudes toward the aged.

1458

Chang, C. F. (1982). [Interpersonal relationships, self-concept, and attribution traits in college freshmen]. Journal of Education and Psychology, 5, *1-46. (In Chinese.)*

This study investigated the relationships between self-concept, attribution traits, and interpersonal relationships in 524 college freshmen. They were given the Tennessee Self Concept Scale, the Attribution Scale, and Social-Relations Questionnaires. The major findings of the study were. (1) There were significant correlations between interpersonal relations and personality traits; however, the size of correlations changed with kinds of situations. (2) Both boys and girls who scored higher in self-concept had better interpersonal relations in leisure and working situations. (3) In successful events, boys who had the stronger tendency to make ability or external (i.e. luck and fate) attribution had better interpersonal relations in leisure and working situations. (4) In failure events, girls who had the stronger tendency to make ability attribution had worse interpersonal relations in leisure and working situations. (5) The girls were significantly superior to the boys in interpersonal relations. (6) The girls living outside of campus were significantly superior to the girls living in school dormitory as far as interpersonal relations within academic situations were concerned.

1459

Chang, C. H. (1980). [Actual and perceived attitudes of adolescents and adults toward contemporary issues: A study of the "Generation Gap" in Chinese society]. Bulletin of Educational Psychology, 13, *1-12. (In Chinese.)*

The purpose of the study was to investigate the phenomenon of "generation gap" in modern Chinese society. A questionnaire of 50 statements concerning contemporary issues was administered to an adolescent group of 640 high school and college students and an adult group of 74 parents and high school teachers. The subjects were asked first to respond to each statement in terms of their own attitudes, and second to respond in terms of how they expected the other group would answer the same statement. The mean findings were: (1) Significant generational attitude differences were found in the samples on 5 out of 50 statements in terms of their own actual attitudes. (2) In respect of perceived attitudes, significant differences were found in the samples on 15 out of 50 statements. The results indicated that both the adults and adolescents tended to be traditionally oriented. The concept of "generation gap" has been overemphasized.

1460

Chang, C. H. (1986). [Parent-child relationship as related to educational success of school children]. Bulletin of Educational Psychology, 19, *1-20. (In Chinese.)*

This study tested the hypothesis that the parent-child relationship is related to educational success of school children in Chinese society. Two types of eighth and ninth grade students were selected; type I students were the 150 highest educational successes; type II students were the lowest 150 failures. A semi-structured interview questionnaire was administered on an individual basis to the students and his (or her) parents. The results indicated that: (1) The parents of type I students paid more attention to their children during time of homework; they visited the teachers more frequently, they knew more about school activities and understood better their children's abilities and interests. (2) The parent-child relationships of the type I students were better than those of the type II students. The implication of these results for parental education was discussed.

1461

Chang, H. B. (1973). Attitudes of Chinese students in the United States. Sociology & Social Research, 58, *66-77.*

Previous studies suggest that the most significant determinants of a foreign student's attitude toward the host country include the national status of his home country, the degree of his contact with Americans, the frustration he encounters during his sojourn, the length of time he has been in the U.S., and his authoritarianism. Results of a study of 250 students indicate that Chinese student attitudes toward the U.S. are positively associated with contact with Americans, but negatively associated with authoritarianism. A curve hypothesis concerning attitude changes through time was partially supported. No association was found between a Chinese student's attitude and the perceived national status of his home country, or his degree of frustration.

1462

Chang, K. K. (1973). [A study on family planning knowledge and attitude of twenty-year old single males in Taiwan]. Journal of the Formosan Medical Association, 72, *413-426. (In Chinese.)*

1463

Chang, L. L. (1980). Acculturation and emotional adjustment of Chinese women immigrants. Dissertation Abstracts International, 41, *A1809.*

1464

Chang, S. C. (1974). [A study of urban housewife's role in modern society]. Bulletin of the Institute of Ethnology *(Academia Sinica),* **37,** *39-84. (In Chinese.)*

1465

Chang, S. S. (1959). Value orientation of American and Chinese students. *Unpublished master's thesis, Ohio State University.*

1466

Chang, W. J. (1974). [The effects of cooperation and competition on interpersonal attraction, productivity, and aggression]. Bulletin of Research Institute of Education *(Taiwan Normal University),* **16,** *11-96. (In Chinese.)*

1467

Chang, W. J. (1976). [Interpersonal attraction as a function of opinion similarity and opinion presentation sequence]. Bulletin of Educational Psychology, 9, *73-84. (In Chinese.)*

This experiment was conducted to test two hypotheses: (a) Interpersonal attraction is a linear function of opinion similarity, and (b) a recency effect exists in a sequential presentation of similar and dissimilar opinions. In a 5 x 2 factorial design, five levels of opinion similarity (.10, .30, .50, .70, and .90), and two opinion sequences (similarity-dissimilarity and dissimilarity-similarity) were used. Each of the 100 subjects participating in this study interacted with a confederate in 1 of 10 experimental conditions. A significant effect on attraction was found only for the opinion similarity variable; no interaction between the opinion similarity and the presentation-sequence variables was noted. The implication of these findings to similarity-attraction theories is discussed and three explanations are suggested to account for the absence of the sequence effect.

1468

Chang, W. J. (1977). [Effects of opinion similarity and opinion social desirability on interpersonal attraction and interaction intention]. Bulletin of Educational Psychology, 10, *61-74. (In Chinese.)*

Eighty female subjects took part in a study of "impression formation," during which they evaluated a hypothetical stranger who was presented as either similar or dissimilar in opinions to themselves and as either having many socially desirable opinions or having many socially undesirable ones. The subjects were then asked to rate on the Interpersonal Judgment Scale the stranger's intelligence, knowledge of current events, morality, adjustment, attractiveness, and similarity in opinions to themselves, and to indicate their willingness to have the stranger as their intimate friend. It was found that both opinion similarity and opinion social desirability had a significant effect on interpersonal attraction. This finding seems to suggest that opinion similarity is a positively evaluated attribute or a reinforcing stimulus. It was also found that when the stranger was believed to have many socially desirable opinions, subjects tended to prefer the stranger similar in opinions as their intimate friend. On the other hand, when the stranger was perceived as having many socially undesirable opinions, subjects showed a nonsignificant preference to have the stranger dissimilar in opinions as their intimate friend. The nonsignificant difference was attributed to subjects' superficial involvement and the positively evaluated or the reinforcing nature of opinion similarity.

1469

Chang, W. J. (1980). [Affiliation tendency and sociometric status]. Bulletin of Educational Psychology, 13, *153-178. (In Chinese.)*

The present study examined the relationships between affiliation tendency and sociometric status. Subjects were 276 boys and 287 girls from two junior high schools in Taipei. It was found that: (1) Affiliation tendency was positively and linearly related to sociometric status and to perceived sociometric status, for boys but not for girls. (2) For both boys and girls, high affiliators had more contacts with peers than low affiliators. (3) For both boys and girls, affiliation tendency was linearly related to self-perceived sociometric status, self-evaluation, and loneliness. (4) Similarity in affiliation tendency made no significant contribution to the variance of attraction for both boys and girls. (5) Sensitivity to rejection was positively and linearly related to sociometric status for boys but not for girls. (6) For both boys and girls, the interaction between affiliation tendency and sensitivity to rejection had no effect on sociometric status. The findings implied that personality variables had differential effects upon boys and girls.

1470

Chang, W. J. (1985). [The prediction of sociometric status among junior high school students]. Bulletin of Educational Psychology, 18, *169-190. (In Chinese.)*

A two-year longitudinal study was conducted to investigate the relative importance of various factors as determinants of sociometric status. The subjects were 160 male and 353 female seventh graders from 12 junior high schools. In the second year of the study, a follow-up was conducted on 31 males and 64 females in 10 schools. Tests were given at the beginning of the first and second years, and again at the end of the second year. It was found that, at the early stage of acquaintance, personal trait desirability and subjective physical attractiveness were the most important determinants of sociometric status for both males and females. At the later stage, these two factors continued to be the most important determinants for males; for females, personal trait desirability, subjective physical attractiveness, intelligence, and affiliative tendency were the most important ones. Scholastic achievement increased prediction at the later stage for both males and females. The correlations between the sociometric status measured at the early stage and the late stage ranged from .42 to .62 when class membership was constant, and from .55 to .65 when class membership changed.

1471

Chang, Y. C. (1923). [One thousand Chinese superstitions]. Chinese Journal of Psychology, 2. *(In Chinese.)*

1472

Che, W. K. (1979). The modern Chinese family, 1959-1975. Dissertation Abstracts International, 39, *A4522.*

1473

Chen, C. F. (1975). [A study on child-bearing women's response to the promotion of family planning: Husbands and wives' motivation and decision regarding their ideal number of children]. *Unpublished master's thesis, Cheng-chi University, Taipei. (In Chinese.)*

1474

Chen, C. I. B. (1984). Chinese and American differences in group performance and strategies in problem solving groups. Journal of Education & Psychology, 7, *169-191.*

Under one of two drive-arousing conditions (luck or skill) manipulated within a laboratory setting, 12 American and 12 Chinese 3-male-student groups were compared in terms of group strategies and group performance outcomes in solving five jigsaw puzzles. Chinese students were assumed to be more group oriented and cohesive than American students because of their different cultural structures. Results showed that support for the hypotheses was found on measures of anticipated strategies used by Chinese versus American groups. Chinese groups, as compared to American groups, intended to use more group as opposed to individual orienting strategies. The hypotheses were not confirmed on the actual strategies used and the task outcome measures. Contrary to the hypothesis, groups performed better under the luck condition than the skill condition. Under the luck condition, American groups had better performance outputs than Chinese groups. Several factors that might account for this outcome were discussed.

1475

Chen, C. I., & Lam, S. P. (1984). [Effects of questionnaire length, salience, research authority and follow-up on response rates in a mail survey]. Chinese Journal of Psychology, 26, *77-84. (In Chinese.)*

This study examined the effects of questionnaire length, salience, researcher authority, and follow-up on the response rates of mailed questionnaires. A sample of 560 Taipei college students were sent questionnaires measuring attitudes toward missing classes. Results indicated that the response rate was 61.05%. The effect of researcher authority on response rate was statistically significant, but the effects of questionnaire length and salience were not. The effects of follow-ups on increasing response rates were statistically significant. The use of postcards increased the response rate from 61.05% to 73.01% and the use of replacement questionnaires increased the rate to 81.88%. The implications of these results are discussed.

1476

Chen, D., Denmark, F. L., & Adler, L. L. (1981). A study of political attitudes of Chinese and Puerto Rican women. International Journal of Group Tensions, 11, *59-80.*

Compared 30 foreign-born and 30 US-born females (aged 22-56 yrs) recruited from the Chinese and Puerto Rican population in New York City on their political attitudes and degree of political participation. Political participation was hypothesized to be positively correlated with the individual's sense of ethnic consciousness and degree of Americanization into the American culture. 15 foreign-born and 15 US-born of each ethnic group were matched with respect to age, education, and citizenship. The results show that the US-born group tended to participate in politically oriented organizations significantly more than the foreign-born group, while the voting pattern was similar between the groups. Length of residence in the US and view of the American political system were shown to be a good index of political participation.

1477

Chen, I. Y. (1978). [Political culture in college students in Taiwan: The effects of provincial origin, residential area, and college]. Bulletin of Chengchi University, 7. *(In Chinese.)*

1478

Chen, P. W. T. (1977). Chinese-Americans view their mental health. Dissertation Abstracts International, 37, *A6062-6063.*

1479

Chen, S. H., Wang, Y. T., & Foley, F. J. (1963). [Pattern of fertility in Taiwan] [Report of a survey made in "Attitude of women towards family size and birth control"]. Journal of Social Science ^ (College of Law, National Taiwan University), ***13*, 265-280.** (In Chinese.)

1480

Chen, S. M. (1974). [Interpersonal and intrapersonal inconsistent verbal instructions as related to children's resistance-to-temptation behavior]. *Bulletin of Educational Psychology*, *7*, **63-75.** (In Chinese.)

The purpose of this experiment was to examine the relationship between inconsistent verbal instructions and children's resistance to temptation. The subjects were 64 schoolchildren randomly drawn from the second grade of a primary school. They were divided into interpersonal- and intrapersonal-instruction groups, according to treatment conditions; each group was further divided into four subgroups: consistent-prohibitive, inconsistent (permissive first), inconsistent (prohibitive first), and consistent-permissive. The subject's toy-touching responses were analyzed in terms of latency, frequency, duration, and average duration scores. The results indicated that: (1) There were no significant group differences in manipulative responses between the interpersonal- and the intrapersonal-instruction groups. (2) The two subgroups of children who had received inconsistent instructions had significantly more toy-touching responses and shorter latencies than the consistent-prohibitive subgroup, but significantly less toy-touching responses and longer latencies than the consistent-permissive subgroup. (3) With regard to the means of latency, frequency, duration, and average duration scores, there were no significant differences between the two inconsistent subgroups.

1481

Chen, T. H. E. (1960). *Thought reform of the Chinese intellectuals.* **Hong Kong: Hong Kong University Press.**

1482

Chen, W. C. (1979). [*Political attitudes and their formation in secondary-school students in Taiwan*]. **Unpublished doctoral dissertation, National Cheng-chi University, Taipei.** (In Chinese.)

1483

Cheng, C. K. (1944). Familism: The foundation of Chinese social organization. *Social Forces*, *23*, **1.**

1484

Cheng, F. M., & Chen, M. C. (1972). [A quantitative study of cooperativeness of the students in junior middle schools]. *Psychological Testing*, *19*, **969-1019.** (In Chinese.)

1485

Cheng, F. M., & Yu, S. M. (1968). [A quantitative study of leadership among students in junior middle schools]. *Psychological Testing*, *15*, **464-498.** (In Chinese.)

1486

Cheng, M. C. E., Cheong, J., Khew, K. S., & Ratnam, S. S. (1977). Psychological sequelae of sterilization in women in Singapore. *International Journal of Gynaecology & Obstetrics*, *15*, **44-47.**

The Chinese in Singapore erroneously believe that there is an association between sterilization and castration. This belief has led to deep-seated fears that sterilization may result in obesity, physical weakness, and impairment of sexual functions. Beginning in 1969, the Singapore authorities introduced increasingly stronger social policies to reduce family size. Subsequently, there was a large increase in the number of tubal ligations. It was initially thought that this might result in a high incidence of psychological sequelae. A study of 150 women who had had culdoscopic ligations showed that 6.3% were dissatisfied at the end of 2 years. Women with fewer than four children or fewer than two sons tended to be more dissatisfied with sterilization.

1487

Cheng, W. Y., & Liao, L. L. (1985). [Response to pressure from family and career: A survey of career women in Taiwan]. *Chinese Journal of Mental Health*, *2*, **43-51.** (In Chinese.)

This study investigated the problem of women's adjustment to daily pressures from having both a family and a career. Data were gathered from 396 married career women in more than 10 white collar occupations. The results were: (1) Career women experienced conflicts between commitment to jobs and family life. Large individual differences were found as to how committed they were to their jobs. In most cases, career women gave priority to their family. This was interpreted as a result of their submission to male domination. (2) Some married career women felt that their work would have a negative impact on the work of their husbands. However, being a wife who earned additional income also had advantages. Career women felt that husbands should share housework. (3) Some career women held strong negative feelings toward "male chauvinistic" husbands, whereas others still held traditional attitudes. (4) Having an independent income sometimes improved the status of career women in the family. Many respondents felt that their income was for their own disposal.

1488

Cheng, Y. C. (1984). [The effects of life styles of married working women on their work and leisure relationships]. *Journal of Education & Psychology*, *7*, **200-201.** (In Chinese.)

1489

Cheong, S. C. (1970). Attitudes of Chinese parents and pupils towards studying in the Chinese type of high schools in Hong Kong. *Journal of Asian and African Studies*, *5*, **202-208.**

1490

Cheung, F., & Dobkin de Rios, M. F. (1982). Recent trends in the study of the mental health of Chinese immigrants to the United States. *Research in Race & Ethnic Relations*, *3*, **145-163.**

Examines some of the explanations offered by cultural psychologists on how migration affects mental health, with a focus on the Chinese who have migrated to the US in large numbers since the passage of the 1965 Immigration Act. The literature on Chinese-American (CA) mental health and migration is reviewed, and some of the important mental health problems (e.g., racism, underemployment/unemployment, maladjustment and stress, and culture shock) are discussed. A number of research issues on the complexity of the community from which the migrants originate, on the intricacies of the host communities, and on the vulnerability of the migrating population are clarified. Finally, the types of mental health services that are relevant for CAs are delineated.

1491

Cheung, F. M. (1981). [Mental health and recreational activities in a Chinese commune]. In R. P. L. Lee & S. K. Lau (Eds.), [*The people's commune and rural development*] (pp. 95-113). Hong Kong: Chinese University Press. (In Chinese.)

1492

Cheung, F. M. C., Lee, S. Y., & Chan, Y. Y. (1983). Variations in problem conceptualizations and intended solutions among Hong Kong students. *Culture, Medicine & Psychiatry, 7,* **263-278.**

Used a cognitive schema to explain health and illness behaviors among 78 19-26 yr old Chinese university students in Hong Kong. Ss were asked to attribute causes and suggest solutions to 5 health/mental health problems: weakness/fatigue, tension/anxiety, sleep difficulty, hollow/emptiness, and headache. The patterns of endorsement on the causal and solution categories used for the 5 problems were compared using a new asymptotic chi-squared test. The response patterns were found to be significantly different across the 5 problems. Each problem was attributed to multiple causes, including psychological, social, situational, somatic, and existential factors. The intended solutions were often related to the nature of the causal attributions especially when the problems were mild. In lay help-seeking, Ss would attempt a variety of self-help measures. However, for professional consultation, the medical doctor would be the primary care professional the Ss would turn to for most of the problems except in the case of hollow/emptiness.

1493

Chiao, C. (1984). Chinese strategic behavior: Some general principles. In R. Bolton (Ed.), *The content of culture: Constants and variants.* **New Haven: HRAF Press.**

1494

Chien, M. (1979). [*Chinese national character and Chinese culture: A historical perspective*]. Hong Kong: Chinese University of Hong Kong Press. (Also Taipei: Liang Ching.) (In Chinese.)

1495

Chien, M. F. (1977). [Factors related to peer interaction among school children in urban and rural areas]. *Psychology Testing, 24,* **32-40.** (In Chinese.)

1496

Chin, A. L. S. (1948). Some problems of Chinese youth in transition. *American Journal of Sociology, 54,* **1-9.**

1497

Chin, A. L. S. (1970). Family relations in modern Chinese fiction. In M. Freedman (Ed.), *Family and kinship in Chinese society* **(pp. 87-120). Stanford, CA: Stanford University Press.**

1498

Chin, A. S. (1964). The ideal local party secretary and the "model" man. *China Quarterly,* **No. 17, 229-240.**

1499

Chin, R., & Chin, A. L. (1963). [Comparative evaluations of aspects of contemporary Chinese culture by college students in Taiwan]. *Journal of Sociology* **(National Taiwan University), No. 1, 41-57.** (In Chinese.)

1500

Chinese Psychological Association. (1979). [*Attitudes towards the environment of life among college and university students in Taiwan*]. **Taipei: Chinese Psychological Association.** (In Chinese.)

1501

Chiu, H. Y. (1975). [A study of social change in Wanhua: Vol. 3. Changing social attitude in an urban community]. *Bulletin of the Institute of Ethnology* **(Academia Sinica), No. 39, 57-83.** (In Chinese.)

The author attempts to clarify the relation between social change and individual social attitude of an old and declined urban area of Taipei. Six scales for social attitudes were adopted, and a questionnaire was administered to obtain background data of the subjects. The following results were found: (1) When one of the social factors influences one kind of social attitudes, it also influences other social attitudes. (2) Different social attitudes are highly correlated, although each social attitude does have its own characteristics. (3) Individual attitudes are significantly influenced by factors such as educational level, religious behavior, family variables, political behavior, and age; but the relations are complicated.

1502

Chiu, H. Y. (1976). [Industrialization and social life in Yen village: Vol. 4. Social attitude]. *Bulletin of the Institute of Ethnology* **(Academia Sinica), No. 42, 97-118.** (In Chinese.)

According to recent studies, individual modernity has significant correlation with such social factors as individual education, parents' education, sex, age, religion, urban-rural experience, occupation, socioeconomic status, family pattern, exposure to mass media, travel experience, and political participation. In this empirical study, we find that the average educational level of family members, cognitive span, exposure to mass media, and religious affiliation have important effects on individual modernity. Expected number of children and aspiration about educational level of one's children are also significantly related to one's individual modernity. In addition, more perceived alienation is found among the people with higher modernity. Effects of the different programs of mass media and subcategories of folk religion on individual modernity are also analyzed in detail.

1503

Chiu, H. Y., & Wen, C. I. (1975). [Some determinants and correlates of attitude-value change: A comparative study in three different communities]. *Thought and Word, 12,* **1-14.** (In Chinese.)

1504

Chiu, H. Y., & Yuan, I. P. (1974). [Personality and stereotype in the revitalization process of a church]. *Bulletin of the Institute of Ethnology* **(Academia Sinica), No. 38, 115-150.** (In Chinese.)

1505

Chiu, L. H. (1972). A cross-cultural comparison of cognitive styles in Chinese and American children. *International Journal of Psychology, 7,* **235-242.**

221 rural Chinese male and female 4th and 5th graders from middle- or working-class families and 316 comparable American Ss took a 28-item cognitive style test adapted from I. Sigel. The hypotheses were tested that American Ss would be (a) superior in descriptive analytic style, (b) inferior in descriptive-whole style, (c) inferior in relational-contextual style, and (d) superior in inferential-categorical style. Results confirm all except hypothesis (b). The difference in the descriptive-whole responses was significant statistically for the 4th graders but in a direction opposite to that expected: Americans scored higher than Chinese. Chinese Ss preferred to categorize external stimuli on the basis of their interdependence or relationships while American Ss preferred to analyze and classify stimuli on the basis of inferences made about the stimuli grouped together. It is concluded that contrast in cognitive styles cannot be accounted for by child-rearing practices alone but must also consider cultural differences in attitudes, values, and ways of thinking.

1506

Chiu, W. C. (1967). [A study of the social values of Chinese university students]. *Psychological Testing, 14,* **377-382.** (In Chinese.)

1507

Chou, L. S. (1976). *[Psychological basis of democracy: A study of Chinese voters]*. **Unpublished master's thesis, College of Chinese Culture, Taipei.** (In Chinese.)

1508

Chow, C. S. (1984). Immigration and immigrant settlements: The Chinese in New York City. *Dissertation Abstracts International, 45,* **A1869.**

1509

Chow, L. P., Freedman, R., Potter, R. G. Jr., & Jain, A. K. (1968). Correlates of IUD termination in a mass family planning program: The first Taiwan IUD follow-up survey. *Milbank Memorial Fund Quarterly, 46,* **215-235.**

Discusses a follow-up study conducted in 1965 in Taiwan in which 2000 women wearing an intrauterine contraceptive device (IUD) were asked questions concerning: (1) circumstances of insertion, (2) complaints after insertion, (3) removal, (4) expulsion, (5) history after termination, (6) pregnancies after the initial insertion, (7) other questions related to the use of the IUD, and (8) questions concerning their social characteristics and reproductive behavior. Correlations were made between 3 reasons for terminating the use of the IUD for pregnancy, expulsion, or removal. Net and gross rates of termination were calculated according to length of time after the 1st insertion, the woman's age, parity, education, and type of doctor (male or female). These statistics were compared with those in Taichung, and the total termination rate was found to be significantly higher in Taiwan. General results indicate that (1) the woman's age and parity were closely related to each type of termination; (2) women with at least 1 induced abortion had significantly lower expulsion rates, and, therefore, lower termination rates than women who had never experienced abortion; (3) women of higher education had only slightly higher removal and termination rates than did those of lesser education; and (4) those women whose last birth was less than 6 mo. before insertion had very low pregnancy termination rates.

1510

Chow, N. W. (1983). The Chinese family and support of the elderly in Hong Kong. *Gerontologist, 23,* **584-588.**

Discusses how the elderly in Hong Kong should be supported in view of the tendency of more and more children to live away from their elderly parents when they start their own families. Government policies regarding the care of the elderly in Hong Kong support a community care approach in order to maintain the elderly as long as possible in their communities. It is argued that this policy has not been very successful because of its failure to ensure adequate services and to clearly define the relationship between the family and the provision of community support. Ways in which the family can continue to be a source of support are considered.

1511

Christensen, H. T. (1973). Attitudes toward marital infidelity: A nine-cultural sampling of university student opinion. *Journal of Comparative Family Studies, 4,* **197-214.**

Surveyed attitudes toward marital infidelity in 1968 among 1,543 male and 1,221 female college students at large state-supported universities in Sweden, Denmark, and Taiwan, a Catholic university in Belgium, 2 black colleges in the southern US, a large state university, a predominantly male Catholic college, a small Mennonite college in the midwestern US, and a Mormon university in the western US. Data were compared with a similar study by the author done in 1958. Extramarital coitus was totally rejected by more than half of all respondents, but proportions taking this position varied across cultures. Rejection (the conservative position) was disproportionately higher in Asian and in religious cultures, higher for females than males, higher with respondents who had not experienced premarital coitus, higher with each increase in competing commitments, and higher in 1958 than 1968. Generally, the rejection of marital infidelity and acceptance of the double standard were associated.

1512

Chu, C. P., & Ryback, D. (1973). Child-rearing practices in the Republic of China: A cross-cultural comparison. *Acta Psychologica Taiwanica, 15,* **6-9.**

To compare childrearing practices among some Asian countries, a 28-item questionnaire covering such areas as psychological security, feeding, weaning, toilet training, and socialization was administered to 167 Chinese students at National Taiwan University. Ss were asked to respond based on their general ideas about childrearing practices and the experiences of their own homes. A chi-square analysis of comparisons with data obtained previously from Ethiopian and Thai students indicated many significant differences among the 3 cultures (e.g., Chinese mothers were closest to their infants but least sensitive to their needs, whereas Ethiopian parents were most responsive to children's cries but least able to make them feel secure).

1513

Chu, G. (1972, May). Drinking patterns and attitudes of rooming-house Chinese in San Francisco. *Quarterly Journal of Studies on Alcohol,* **(Supp. 6), 58-68.**

Surveyed 41 52-85 yr old Chinese men concerning their drinking. 38 of these were born in China, lived alone, and had low annual incomes. 26 were abstainers, 2 were light-infrequent drinkers, 6 light-frequent, 2 moderate-infrequent, 2 moderate-frequent, and 3 heavy drinkers (1 or 2 drinks daily or 3 or 4 drinks on an occasion at least once a month). Drunkenness was proscribed by 83% and 24% disapproved of drinking. The recreational choices of the respondents included gambling, spending time in a park, and going to the movies. In surveys of the general population of San Francisco in 1962 and 1964, 11 of 36 Chinese respondents were abstainers, compared with 74 of 430 Caucasians; 7 Caucasians and 38 Chinese were light-infrequent drinkers; 5 and 62 light-frequent; 6 and 43 moderate-infrequent; 3 and 79 moderate-frequent; and 4 and 134 heavy drinkers. The low rate of alcoholism among Chinese in the U.S. is attributed to a nondrinking rather than a moderate-drinking pattern. Recreational gambling may serve as a functional equivalent of drinking among the Chinese.

1514

Chu, G. C. (1967). Prior familiarity, perceived bias, and one-sided versus two-sided communications. *Journal of Experimental Social Psychology, 3,* **243-254.**

The persuasive effects of 1-sided vs. 2-sided communications were retested in a non-western cultural setting. Perceived bias in the communication was hypothesized to account for the differential effects of the 2 styles of arguments. The impact of prior familiarity with the issue on the persuasive effects of the communication was examined. Ss were 273 high school students in Taiwan. Among the initially unfavorable, the 1-sided arguments were found more effective when the Ss were not familiar with the issue, while the 2-sided arguments were found more effective when the Ss were familiar. No such interaction appeared among the initially favorable. Regardless of the style of argument or initial attitudes, the effects of communication were an inverse function of detection of bias. When detection of bias was held constant, the interactive effects of the 1-sided and 2-sided communications all disappeared.

1515

Chu, H. M., Yeh, E. K., Klein, M. H., Alexander, A. A., & Miller, M. H. (1971). A study of Chinese students' adjustment in the U.S.A. *Acta Psychologica Taiwanica, 13,* **206-218.**

Studied the cross-cultural adjustment of 67 Taiwan-educated Chinese students at the University of Hawaii. 132 students who were about to depart for study abroad and 108 who were studying at home in Taiwan were selected as comparison groups. Ss' concept of the character of Chinese and Americans, their main reasons for coming to the United States, and their expected difficulties showed a very consistent pattern in the 3 groups. Their mental health was found to be related to their own American "character" and their Chinese "attitudes". A small number of significant changes in Ss' concepts after real exposure to cross-cultural life may be used to explain some mechanism of the paranoid formation in the Chinese students.

1516

Chu, J. L., & Yang, K. S. (1976). [The effects of relative performance and individual modernity on distributive behavior among Chinese college students]. *Bulletin of the Institute of Ethnology^ (Academia Sinica),* **41,** *79-95. (In Chinese.)*

There are reasons to believe that equity theory as developed by American social psychologists may not hold in Chinese society. To test this possibility, 64 high and 64 low scorers on a scale of Chinese individual modernity were selected as subjects. During the experimental session, the subject was made to believe that he was performing a task of copying French prose with a "partner" busy with the same task in another room, who actually never existed. After the task, the subject was informed of the actual number of letters copied by himself and a fictitious number of letters presumably copied by his "partner." The latter was either 7/3 or 3/7 times of the former, depending on the experimental condition (More-Than-Partner vs. Less-Than-Partner) to which he had been randomly assigned. The subject was then informed of the total amount of monetary reward earned by him and his "partner" as a team, and was asked to state his preferred way of allocating the reward. The effect of individual modernity was negligible, but relative performance turned out to be a powerful determinant of distributive behavior. Specifically, when informed of a poorer performance less than his "partner," the subject would prefer allocating the total reward according to their relative performance; but when informed of a better performance, the subject would prefer dividing the total reward equally between them. These results differ from those on Americans.

1517

Chu, K. et al. (1972). Population policy simulations performed with an econometric model of Taiwan. Simulation & Games, *3, 291-307.*

Describes a 24-equation econometric model of the economy of Taiwan. Factors delineated include consumption, investment, foreign trade, production, monetary sector, labor force, demographic sector, validation, and 4 policy experiments. It was shown that different program policies result in different per capita income.

1518

Chu, Y. H. (1979). Patterns of political participation in Taiwan. *Unpublished master's thesis, National Taiwan University, Taipei.*

1519

Chuang, Y. C. (1981). [The Chinese family in a changing society: Case analysis of five families in Nan-Ts'un]. Bulletin of the Institute of Ethnology *(Academia Sinica),* **52,** *1-31. (In Chinese.)*

1520

Chun, H. L. (1971). Jade Snow Wong and the fate of Chinese-American identity. Amerasia Journal, 1, *52-63. (Republished in S. Sue & N. N. Wagner (Eds.),* **Asian Americans: Psychological perspectives.** *Palo Alto, CA: Science Behavior Books, 1973.)*

1521

Chung, Y. C., & Hwang, K. K. (1981). [Attribution of performance and characteristics of learned helplessness in junior high school students]. Acta Psychologica Taiwanica, 23, *155-164. (In Chinese.)*

The present study investigated the relationships among causal attributions of performance, learning motivation, and learned helplessness. The subjects were 510 junior high school students. A canonical analysis indicated that one specific attribution style was strongly related to learned helplessness. Those students who tended not to attribute their success to ability and effort and to attribute their failures to lack of ability were lower in their performance expectation, persistence of study, self-esteem, sense of well-being, and academic achievement. The relationships between causal attribution variables and other variables (e.g., self-esteem) also corresponded to predictions derived from the attributional theory of motivation.

1522

Cline, R. J., & Puhl, C. A. (1984). Gender, culture, and geography: A comparison of seating arrangements in the United States and Taiwan. International Journal of Intercultural Relations, 8, *199-219.*

The investigators administered a 24-item questionnaire connected with seating arrangements at a library table to 100 female and 75 male U.S. undergraduates and to 54 female and 29 male Chinese technical and junior college teachers in Taiwan. The results showed that Chinese subjects were more likely than U.S. subjects to prefer side seating. It was suggested that the corner seating preferred by U.S. subjects for personal matters would be viewed as aggressive by Chinese subjects. In the U.S., seating preferences functioned to separate same-sex partners and to bring together males and females. The opposite functions were evident within the Chinese responses. In both cultures, the use of space functioned both physically and relationally to promote togetherness within sanctioned intimate relationships and to guarantee the separation of those for whom close interpersonal relationships were taboo.

1523

Columbia University Research in Contemporary Cultures: Chinese Series. *(1950). Unpublished documents, American Museum of Natural History, New York.*

1524

Coombs, L. C., & Chang, M. C. (1981). Do husbands and wives agree? Fertility attitudes and later behavior. Population & Environment: Behavioral & Social Issues, 4, *109-127.*

Analysis of the extent to which husbands and wives agree in their attitudes toward a number of key issues that may affect fertility behavior shows that although aggregate views of men and women are remarkably similar, marital couples are frequently in disagreement, particularly if measures discounting for chance agreement of responses are employed. In other words, one cannot accept either the husband or the wife as a surrogate respondent. These conclusions are based on data from cross-sectional surveys in Taiwan of 2,000 couples in which the wife was of childbearing age. The impact on fertility of such marital disagreement varied with the attitude in question. Follow-up birth data over a 4-yr period indicate that, when there was disagreement, it was the wife's attitude that had more influence on fertility, particularly if she had the stronger belief about the future security and status to be derived from a large family and from sons.

1525

Cooper, E. (1980). Colonialist fetishism: An answer to the Hong Kong apologists. Hong Kong Psychological Society Bulletin, *No. 4, 33-43.*

Briefly traces the extension of "fetishism" from an anthropological term meaning the veneration of objects believed to have magical powers in themselves to the concept of "fetishistic thought", which justifies the power positions of a ruling class by infusing those positions with a sacred character. This concept is applied to colonialism. When visiting members of the British Houses of Parliament expressed criticisms of the government of Hong Kong, defenders of the status quo either blamed the condition of the colonial system on the colonized or denied responsibility for the conditions. Seven of these "fetishistic propositions" are discussed and rebuttals offered. In extreme cases the colonized themselves may accept the colonizers' picture of them. It is felt that the concept of colonialist fetishism is widely applicable in the analysis of cross-cultural colonialism.

1526

Dai, B. (1944). Divided loyalty in war: A study of cooperation with the enemy. Psychiatry, *7, 327-340.*

1527

Daly, M. (1978). Gynecology: The metaethics of radical feminism. *Boston, MA: Beacon.*

edscusses women's "journey of becoming" from a radical feminist perspective. Topics include myths and deceptions embedded in language and patriarchal myths, goddess murder (e.g., Indian suttee, Chinese footbinding, African female genital mutilation, the massacre of witches, and gynocide practiced in American gynecology and psychotherapy), and the process of women's unfolding.

1528

Davreux, F. (1981). La minorite chinoise de San Francisco: De la societe du "ventre" a celle de "l'oeil" [The Chinese minority of San Francisco: Of the society of the "womb" to that of the "eye"]. Ethnopsychologie, 36, *53-68. (In other language.)*

The author analyzed the relationship of the Chinese minority in San Francisco to the White majority in terms of the suspicion and hostility with which both groups view each other, based on the writings of M. H. Kingston and J. S. Wong. The present author also considered the feeling of displacement experienced by American-Chinese individuals who find themselves in conflict, torn between two cultures and two countries.

1529

Dawson, J. L. (1972). Temne-Arunta hand-eye dominance and cognitive style. International Journal of Psychology, *7, 219-233.*

Gave 2 groups of Temne Ss from Sierra Leone and Australian aboriginals from Central Australian Arunta a variety of tests of intelligence, cognitive style, eye dominance, and handedness to determine the comparative effects of cultural pressures towards conformity upon incidence of left-handedness and the effects of mixed hand-eye dominance upon cognitive style. Results support the culture pressure hypothesis, since the conformist Temne culture sample revealed only 3.4% left-handed Ss while the more permissive Arunta sample showed 10.5% left-handed Ss. Data reported earlier on Chinese Hakka, Katanganese, and Temne agriculturalists (all "conforming" as gauged by the Asch Perceptual Conformity Test) revealed relatively little left-handedness among males and 1% incidence in females out of a total of 247 Ss, while the incidence of left-handedness was relatively high and not significant with respect to sex for Arunta and Eskimo Ss (low conforming). Mixed dominance (right-hand/left-eyed) Ss tended to show field-dependent cognitive style on all tests.

1530

Dawson, J. L., Law, H., Leung, A., & Whitney, R. E. (1971). Scaling Chinese traditional-modern attitudes and the GSR measurement of "important" versus "un-important" Chinese concepts. Journal of Cross-Cultural Psychology, 2, *1-27.*

The Traditional-Modern Attitude Theory states that individuals exposed to conflicting ideas either develop compromise attitudes or use alternate modes of inconsistency reduction. This paper presents theoretical and scaling problems involved in the Chinese Traditional-Modern Scale and a model of susceptibility to attitude change. In an accompanying GSR experiment it was found that more important concepts elicited a significantly higher level of arousal in response to attitude change in the direction of peer-group pressure. Such pressure resulted in important concepts changing in a traditional direction and unimportant concepts in a modern direction.

1531

Dawson, J. L., & Lonner, W. J. (1974). Readings in cross-cultural psychology. *Hong Kong: Hong Kong University Press.*

Presents the texts of lectures delivered at the inaugural meeting of the International Association for Cross-Cultural Psychology held in Hong Kong, August 1972. Topics covered include theoretical and methodological issues, learning and cognitive development, human ecology and behavior, perception, psychiatric and personality disorders, and roles and intergroup relations.

1532

Dawson, J. L. M. (1970). Attitude change and G.S.R. arousal among Hong Kong Chinese. *Oxford, UK: University of Oxford, Institute of Experimental Psychology.*

1533

Dawson, J. L. M. (1974). Ecology, cultural pressures toward conformity and left-handedness: A bio-social approach. In J. L. M. Dawson & W. J. Lonner (Eds.), Readings in cross-cultural psychology. *Hong Kong: Hong Kong University Press.*

1534

Dawson, J. L. M. (1975). Socio-economic differences in size-judgments of discs and coins by Chinese primary VI children in Hong Kong. Perceptual & Motor Skills, 41, *107-110.*

Conducted an experiment which provides some cross-cultural support for the hypothesis by J. S. Bruner and C. C. Goodman (1947) about perceptual accentuation. 20 Hong Kong Chinese 11-12 yr olds from a lower socioeconomic level overestimated valued coins more than 15 11-12 yr olds from a high socioeconomic level. The 2 samples used were matched for education, and both spoke the Cantonese dialect. There was also some evidence for H. Tajfel's (1957) "interserial" and "intraserial" effects more particularly for the lower socioeconomic Ss, although similar trends were apparent for the smaller group of higher socioeconomic Ss.

1535

Dawson, J. L. M. (1975). Theory and measurement in the study of individual modernity in Asia. In J. W. Berry & W. J. Lonner (Eds.), Applied cross-cultural psychology *(pp. 18-25). Amsterdam, Netherlands: Swets & Zeitlinger.*

1536

Dawson, J. L. M. (1976). Adjustment problems encountered by individuals in the process of modernization in the resolution of traditional-modern attitudinal conflict. In W. H. Lo (Ed.), Perspectives in mental health: Hong Kong, 1976 *(pp. 61-82). Hong Kong: Mental Health Association.*

1537

Dawson, J. L. M., & Ng, W. W. C. (1972). Effects of parental attitudes and modern exposure on Chinese traditional-modern attitude formation. Journal of Cross-Cultural Psychology, 3, *201-207.*

Following recent Traditional-Modern attitude change regarding research, additional evidence to support traditional-modern attitude change hypotheses is presented, and is concerned with the relative effects of parental socialization and other modernizing influences on attitude change among groups of Hong Kong Chinese. Younger Hakka village children were found, as expected, to have significantly more traditional attitudes than other children, while their traditional-modern attitudes also correlated more highly with those of their parents. Two matched adolescent Anglo-Chinese and Chinese Secondary samples were also chosen to examine the relative effects of parental socialization and mass media on attitude change. Both parental T-M attitudes and exposure to mass media were relevant to the development of student's T-M attitudes at the Anglo-Chinese school but for the Chinese Middle school only parental T-M attitudes were relevant, not exposure to mass media.

1538

Dawson, J. L. M., Whitney, R. E., & Lau, R. T. S. (1972). Attitude conflict, GSR, and traditional-modern attitude change among Hong Kong Chinese. Journal of Social Psychology, 88, *163-176.*

Tested predictions from J. L. Dawson's Traditional-Modern (T-M) Consistency Theory of attitude change in 2 experiments with a total of 44 Hong Kong Chinese college students. Ss were given a Chinese version of the Dawson T-M Scale as a premeasure of attitudes and attitude conflict on topics of traditional Chinese culture. This was followed by a discrepant communication which informed S of his peers' average opinion on these same topics. GSR was measured before and after Ss responded to the communication, following which Ss rated the importance of the topics. As predicted, belief importance was significantly related to the level of T-M attitude conflict. Attitude change which reduced the discrepancy between S and peers was significantly correlated with pre-GSR when attitude conflict and belief importance were high. When attitude conflict and belief importance were low, no such relationship emerged.

1539

DeFronzo, J. (1978). Nixon's visit to China and increased favorability toward communism. Psychological Reports, 42, *70.*

Exposure to TV coverage of Nixon's 1972 visit to the People's Republic of China and increased favorability toward communism were measured in 222 undergraduates. Results indicate that high levels of exposure were associated with increased favorability toward communism in China and communism in general.

1540

Demos, G. D., & O'Neill, W. F. (1984). "Groupthink": The study group in thought reform. ETC, 41, *187-205.*

Discusses the study-group procedure of thought reform that was most fully developed by the Chinese Communists. It is noted that, when an individual has been placed under sufficient stress and is significantly disoriented, it is possible with the study-group procedure to use a variety of methods to effect whatever ideological changes are desired. A study group ordinarily meets at least once a day for several hours, usually 6 days/week, typically for 6-12 mo. The study group operates to encourage and direct the course of self-criticism and serves as the basic instrument for more directive types of ideological re-education and for the consequent resocialization of the convert. The study group performs an essentially psychoanalytic function, in that it encourages self-examination, and employs group therapy techniques to promote ideological conversion. There are 4 types of group meetings that are used by the Chinese in study-group proceedings: accusation, study, criticism and self-criticism, and discussion meetings. Additional topics of discussion include the evolution of social identity, factors affecting group effectiveness, and coercive cooperation.

1541

Dingler, W. B. (Ed.) (1969). Youth and religion: A religious attitude study of Hong Kong secondary school students. *Hong Kong: Lutheran World Federation Broadcasting Service.*

1542

Doolittle, J. K. (1965). Social life of the Chinese. *New York: Harper & Bros.*

1543

Duane, M. (1979). The effect of maternal attitudes toward childrearing on social competence in preschool children. Dissertation Abstracts International, 39, *A6648.*

1544

Earle, M. J. (1967). Bilingual semantic merging and an aspect of acculturation. Journal of Personality & Social Psychology, 6, *304-312.*

Chinese-English bilingual students were classified according to the degree of assumed similarity between a sample of their own beliefs and those of representatives of the native-language community, and the 2nd-language community. Ss more similar to the 2nd-language community obtained significantly lower semantic differential d scores between Chinese and English translation-equivalent concepts than did Ss more similar to the native-language community. Students attending an English-language university obtained significantly lower d scores than students attending an English-language secondary school. Results are related to the Theory of Compound and Coordinate Bilingualism, and it is suggested that acceptance of beliefs of the 2nd-language community may result in a transformation from a coordinate to a compound bilingual system.

1545

Earle, M. J. (1969). A cross-cultural and cross-language comparison of dogmatism scores: A comparison of Hong Kong Chinese and British university students. Journal of Social Psychology, 79, *19-24.*

A cross-cultural comparison was made between Dogmatism (D) scores of British and Hong Kong Chinese students. The mean D score of Hong Kong Ss was significantly higher than the mean score of British Ss. It is suggested that Hong Kong Ss may be more closed-minded than British Ss, or they may be more acquiescent. For Chinese-English bilingual Ss the mean score on a Chinese translation of the D scale was significantly higher than the mean score on the English language scale. This last finding is considered to have important implications for cross-cultural measurement using verbal instruments, and it may also be relevant to studies in linguistic relativity.

1546

Eastman, L. E. (1973). Political conservatism in a revolutionary society: China. American Behavior Scientist, 17, *293-308.*

1547

Eber, I. (1974). The teaching of values in Chinese revolutionary fiction. China Notes, 13, *1-4.*

1548

Eberhard, W. (1967). Guilt and sin in traditional China. *Berkeley: University of California Press.*

1549

Eberhard, W. (1968 - 1969). Social interaction and social values in Chinese dreams. Journal of Sociology *(National Taiwan University), No. 4, 21-43; No. 5, 61-106.*

1550

Edwards, J. W. (1976). The concern for health in sexual matters in the "old society" and "new society" in China. Journal of Sex Research, 12, *88-103.*

Presents an array of issues relating to sex and health in Chinese culture. The lingering influence of "old society" sexual beliefs in China's "new society" based on scientific socialism can be traced in 2 related areas: (a) popularized concepts antagonistic to the antimysticism and public health campaigns, and (b) policies and attitudes propagated by the reformers themselves.

1551

Eisenbruch, M. (1984). Cross-cultural aspects of bereavement: Vol. 2. Ethnic and cultural variations in the development of bereavement practices. Culture, Medicine and Psychiatry, 8, *315-347.*

Noting that structures common to bereavement in a range of cultures can be identified by examining the social contexts in the transformations of Western bereavement practices, the present author compared the contemporary bereavement practices of several ethnic and cultural groups in North America. Consideration is given to the state of widowhood in different cultural systems. The impact of modernization among traditional societies demonstrates that, even though Western technologies are incorporated into the procedures followed by these modernizing societies, cultural codes remain intact. Five questions that require further clarification were identified. These concern whether bereavement is an illness, a rite of passage, or a normal life event; the usefulness of protective factors that facilitate successful resolution of grief; the effectiveness of mourning practices by various ethnic groups in preventing "bad grief"; the beneficial aspects of these practices if taken up by other ethnic groups; and ways in which Western health practitioners can determine whether a bereaved person from an unfamiliar culture is suffering "bad grief". Also addressed was the acceptability of Western grief counseling to non-Western clients.

1552

Eisner, V., & Tsuyemura, H. (1965). Interactions of juveniles with the law. Public Health Rep., 80, *681-691.*

1553

Endo, R. (1984). Use of informal social networks for service-related information. Psychological Reports, 54, *354.*

Administered a questionnaire on the use of informal social networks as the primary source of information about legal services to 4,214 individuals, including 399 Chinese Americans who used a federally funded legal program in a large western city in 1978. Three findings emerged from this research. First, the Chinese relied on informal social networks for information about legal services more than other groups including Whites, Blacks, Chicanos, other Hispanics, and Native Americans. Second, informal networks were also instructional in getting many Chinese to define their concerns within a legal framework and to seek legal action. Networks therefore played a crucial role in shaping personal problem-solving strategies. Third, there were differential patterns of use of informal networks. The most important variable in distinguishing between the Chinese who did (77%) and those who did not (23%) use networks was marital status. Chinese Ss who acquired information primarily from informal networks, compared to those who didn't, tended to be married and therefore to have access to additional family/relative social ties. The second most important variable was nativity. The Chinese who got information mainly from informal networks tended to be foreign-born. This finding is consistent with the greater underuse of formal services by the foreign-born. Ss who obtained information principally from informal networks tended to be female, to be older, and to have lower incomes and fewer years of schooling.

1554

Eng, M. (1983). Toward a general paradigm of majority-minority relationships: An exploratory analysis of the relationship of locus of control and individual-system blame attribution to personality characteristics, Chinese American ethnic identity, and psychological symptomatology. Dissertation Abstracts International, 43, *B3357.*

1555

Fan, C. Y. (1977). The Chinese language school of San Francisco in relation to family integration and cultural identity. Dissertation Abstracts International, 37, *A7414-7415.*

1556

Fei, H. T. (1946). Peasantry and gentry: An interpretation of Chinese social structure and its changes. American Journal of Sociology, 70, *1-17. (Reprinted in Y. A. Cohen (Ed.),* **Social structure and personality.***)*

1557

Fei, H. T. (1980). Ethnic identification in China. Social Sciences in China, 1, *94-107.*

1558

Feldman, D. L. (1985). Ideology and the manipulation of symbols: Leadership perceptions of science, education, and art in the People's Republic of China, 1961-1974. Political Psychology, 6, *441-460.*

Examined Mao Zedong's thoughts on science, education, and art and analyzed the content of one propaganda publication to study the impact of Mao's ideology on the Chinese leadership's perceptions of these activities between 1961 and 1974. It was concluded that the logical structure of Mao's thought has affected leadership perception of these activities. Various themes have been emphasized at different times, reflecting the shifting priorities of the elite and an assumption on the part of the leadership of the malleability of the human mind and the considerable power of propaganda to reinforce desirable perceptions.

1559

Folberg, J. (1983). A mediation overview: History and dimensions of practice. Mediation Quarterly, *No. 1, 3-13.*

Discusses the historical development of mediation in China, Africa, Japan, and in different religions. The most familiar model for mediation in the US comes from the dispute resolution procedures in labor-management relations. Divorce mediation is considered in terms of 4 distributional questions that must be decided: marital property, spousal support, child support, and child custody and visitation.

1560

Foley, L. A., & Kranz, P. L. (1981). Black stereotypes of other ethnic groups. Journal of Mind & Behavior, 2, *435-441.*

87 Black undergraduates attending a Black, religiously affiliated college indicated traits they felt were typical of each of 10 ethnic groups. The traits were selected from a list of 84 adjectives originally used by D. Katz and K. W. Braly (1933). Clear stereotypes emerged for 6 ethnic groups; all were relatively positive except the one for Whites, which was extremely negative. The most favorable stereotypes were of Chinese and Jews. The stereotypes of Blacks ranked third in favorableness, followed by those of Italians and Germans.

1561

Fong, S. L. (1973). Assimilation and changing social roles of Chinese Americans. Journal of Social Issues, 29, *115-127.*

Describes the effects of social change, primarily in the form of cultural and social assimilation, on adjustment and social roles in Chinese-Americans. Most affected have been traditional norms regarding the family and sex role stereotypes. It is reported that disparate life styles have led to subgrouping within the Chinese group.

1562

Fong, S. L. M. (1965). Cultural influences in the perception of people: The case of Chinese in America. British Journal of Social and Clinical Psychology, 4, *110-113.*

1563

Fong, S. L. M. (1965). Assimilation of Chinese in America: Changes in orientation and social perception. American Journal of Sociology, 71, *265-273.*

1564

Fong, S. L. M. (1970). Sex role in the modern fabric of China. In G. H. Seward & R. C. Williamson (Eds.), Sex roles in changing society. *New York: Random House.*

1565

Fong, S. L., & Peskin, H. (1969). Sex-role strain and personality adjustment of China-born students in America: A pilot study. Journal of Abnormal Psychology, 74, *563-567. (Republished in S. Sue & N. N. Wagner (Eds.),* **Asian-Americans: Psychological perspectives.** *Palo Alto, CA: Science & Behavior Books, 1973.)*

Since the role of student has been traditionally reserved for the male in Chinese society, hypothesized that China-born, female undergraduates would feel generally alienated from and in defiance of norms of the parent culture. Results on the CPI with 43 male and 43 female China-born undergraduates supported this view, with females scoring lower on Socialization and Good Impression. The Chinese model of the feminine role (reserve, patience, modesty, etc.) was most rejected by the subsample of females on student visas, and most accepted by the naturalized females (including permanent residents), as reflected on the CPI Femininity Scale. Regardless, of sex, naturalized and resident students clearly outranked visa students on important aspects of psychological health.

1566

Forgas, J. P., & Bond, M. H. (1985). Cultural influences on the perception of interaction episodes. Personality & Social Psychology Bulletin, 11, *75-88.*

Most human interactions take place within the framework of culture-specific social episodes, and the cognitive representations people have about such social encounters should thus reflect the salient characteristics of their surrounding culture. To investigate cultural influences on the perception of interaction episodes, 58 subjects 18-23 years old from Hong Kong and 80 subjects 17-24 years old from Australia provided judgments about their implicit representation of 27 social episodes common in both environments. The subjects' judgments were analyzed, using an individual-differences multidimensional scaling (INDSCAL) procedure. INDSCAL indicated significant differences in the cognitive representation of episodes, which were strongly related to the dominant features of the two cultures. Individual demographic, personality, and attitudinal variables were also related to episode perceptions in a culture-specific pattern. Findings were discussed in terms of the influence of culture on cognition.

1567

Foulks, E. F. (1969). On teaching child development and psychoanalytic theory: Views from nine cultures. Pennsylvania Psychiatric Quarterly, 9, *12-72.*

Introduces 9 studies on child development in India, Thailand, Korea, Taiwan, Iran, Mexico, Philippines, and 2 American minority groups.

1568

Fox, D. J., & Jordan, V. B. (1973). Racial preference and identification of black, American Chinese, and white children. Genetic Psychology Monographs, 88, *229-286.*

Studied the current validity of K. B. Clark and M. P. Clark's 1939 experiments which revealed negative racial identification among black children, and attempted to extend their research to American Chinese and white children. Using the Clarks' questions to test racial awareness, identification, and preference, 360 black and 360 white 5-7 yr olds chose between black and white dolls, and 360 Chinese and 294 white 5-7 yr olds chose between color photographs of Chinese and white children. Groups were matched on age, sex, and integrated vs segregated schooling. Findings reveal a significant positive shift in black racial identification from the original Clark data, to where majorities of black Ss expressed own-race preference. However, response patterns of Chinese Ss were often more negative than those of the black children studied by the Clarks. White Ss were nearly unanimous in preferring the white doll or photograph. Sex had no effect on racial awareness, identification or preference for any racial group, nor did age for white Ss. Although age had no effect on racial preference for black or Chinese Ss, larger proportions of older children in both groups were aware and identified with their own race. Integrated or segregated schooling had no effect on responses except that more integrated Chinese were aware of "white" and more integrated whites had positive perceptions of black children.

1569

Fraser, W. E. (1977). Population control: Part II. China. British Journal of Sexual Medicine, 4, *19-20.*

1570

Freedman, A., & Freedman, P. E. (1982). Mass line leadership: Another view of Mao's China. American Psychologist, 37, *103-105.*

Argues that in his analysis of mass leadership in China, J. Barlow presents a one-sided and highly misleading portrait of Mao's China. Barlow almost completely overlooks the fact that small study groups and other organs of participation in the People's Republic of China operate within a context of coercion and fear that conditions the individual's behavior. Mao's use of physical punishment and outright terror, and the power of his regime over the individual citizen are discussed.

1571

Fried, M. H. (1953). The fabric of Chinese society: A study of the social life of a Chinese country seat. *New York: Praeger.*

1572

Fried, M. H. (1976). Chinese culture, society, and personality in transition. In G. A. De Vos (Ed.), Response to change: Society, culture, and personality *(pp. 45-73). New York: van Nostrand.*

1573

Gabrenya, W. K., Latane, B., & Wang, Y. E. (1983). Social loafing in cross-cultural perspective: Chinese on Taiwan. Journal of Cross-Cultural Psychology, 14, *368-384.*

Hypothesized that members of cultures whose value emphases and social institutions have been characterized as group-oriented would tend to form more cohesive groups and be more likely to place group benefit over individual benefit than members of an individualistic US culture, hence evidencing less social loafing. Contrary to this expectation, 160 Chinese schoolchildren in Taiwan (in Grades 2-9), asked to produce sound by clapping and shouting alone and in pairs, evidenced levels of social loafing similar to those obtained in US research (K. Williams and K. Williams, 1981) employing this procedure. Several sources of this absence of a relationship between social loafing and cultural values are discussed, including the effects of the social restrictiveness of the sound production procedure on its ability to top cultural differences.

1574

Gallin, R. S. (1984). The entry of Chinese women into the rural labor force: A case study from Taiwan. Signs, 9, *383-398.*

Examined data, collected from 1957 to 1982, on women from a Taiwanese village that changed from an economic system based almost solely on agriculture to one founded predominantly on nonfarm employment. Although women moved from the domestic sphere to join men in the public sector, this has not been accompanied by a significant redefinition of their status. It is argued that these women's failure to achieve personal autonomy and authority on the basis of their productive labor derives from a system of patriarchal capitalism in which traditional ideology maintains and reinforces the subordination of women to the interests of the family, state, and international market economy.

1575

Galvin, J. E. (1985). Chinese immigrants and the experience of loneliness: An existential phenomenological investigation. Dissertation Abstracts International, 46, *A929.*

1576

Gardiner, H. W. (1969). A cross-cultural comparison of hostility in children's drawings. Journal of Social Psychology, 79, *261-263.*

Human figure drawings were collected from 2382 11-13 yr. old boys, comprising 26 cultural groups and scored for hostility on the basis of criteria established by Dennis and Gardiner. Results indicate notable variations in both the degree of hostility as well as the kind of hostile content portrayed. Hostility was highest in drawings from Thailand (35%) followed by such groups as Germany (26%), Taiwan (25 and 22%), Yugoslavia (17%), Algeria (15%), Mecca (6%), Syria (3%), Brooklyn nonorthodox Jews (1%), and Japanese (1%).

1577

Gardiner, H. W., & Lematawekul, D. (1970). Second-generation Chinese in Thailand: A study of ethnic identification. Journal of Cross-Cultural Psychology, 1, *333-344.*

176 adolescents were separated into those who used Chinese and those who used Thai family names; and those who did not attend Chinese schools. A number of standardized measures were used. 2nd-generation Chinese who used Chinese family names and/or attended Chinese schools had closer ethnic identification with the Chinese. Scores on various scales did not correlate with identification. Areas of possible future research are suggested.

1578

Gardner, R. C., Kirby, D. M., & Arboleda, A. (1973). Ethnic stereotypes: A cross-cultural replication of their unitary dimensionality. Journal of Social Psychology, 91, *189-195.*

Asked 250 Filipino college students to rate the concept "Chinese" (in the Philippines) along 40 stereotype differential scales and to indicate their degree of contact and feelings of social distance toward them. The stereotype about the Chinese was defined by the 10 attributes for which the stereotype differential ratings were most polarized. A factor analysis of all the variables yielded 3 factors, an Evaluative, Stereotype and Social distance dimension. Since the factors were orthogonal, results provide cross-cultural support for the independence of stereotypic and evaluative reactions previously noted in the North American context.

1579

Gardner, R. C., Kirby, D. M., Gorospe, F. H., & Willamin, A. C. (1972). Ethnic stereotypes: An alternative assessment technique, the Stereotype Differential. Journal of Social Psychology, 87, *259-267.*

Compares the stereotypes of 197 Filipino education students about 9 groups-Americans, Canadians, Chinese, Filipinos, Germans, Japanese, Jews, Russians and Spaniards-as assessed by the Katz and Braly technique and the Stereotype Differential (SD). It is concluded that the 2 techniques provide similar assessments but that the SD is more useful where an individual difference measure of stereotyping is required. A further analysis of the data from the SD indicates that Ss who stereotype 1 outgroup tend to stereotype others.

1580

Glenn, E. N. (1983). Split household, small producer and dual wage earner: An analysis of Chinese-American family strategies. Journal of Marriage & the Family, 45, *35-46.*

In contrast to the institutional approaches frequently used in studies of Black and Hispanic family life, research on the Chinese-American family has relied almost exclusively on cultural explanations. The latter perspective emphasizes the continuity of Chinese-American family patterns over time, portraying them as basically static. The present author, using an institutional framework, emphasizes the changing structure of Chinese-American families resulting from the interplay between shifting institutional constraints and the efforts of Chinese Americans to maintain family life in the face of these restrictions. Historical analysis revealed 3 distinct immigrant family types that emerged in different periods in response to particular political and economic conditions: split household, small producer, and dual-wage worker. The existence of these types suggests that characteristics often interpreted as products of Chinese culture actually represent strategies for dealing with conditions of life in the US.

1581

Glenn, N. D. (1974). Recent trends in white-nonwhite attitudinal differences. Public Opinion Quarterly, 38, *596-604.*

Examines the evidence against the "assimilationist" hypothesis that as racial differences in income, education, occupation, and regional distribution become smaller, racial differences in attitudes and behavior will also diminish. A comparison of responses of 1,375 whites and 125 nonwhites to 15 attitudinal questions revealed increased white-nonwhite dissent rather than consensus between the 1950s and the 1960s. Maximum dissent was found on the issues of capital punishment, religious involvement in social issues, family size, political conservatism vs liberalism, and prohibition. Increased consensus was found on issues favoring admission of Red China to the United Nations, a Jewish President, and less isolationism in US foreign policy.

1582

Godbill, B. M. (1983). Power relations, homosexuality and the family: A review of the literature, including cross-cultural studies (homosexuality and the family in the Mohave, Chinese and Iraqi cultures). Journal of Comparative Family Studies, 14, *315-331.*

The author reviews the literature on family dynamics and the etiology of homosexuality, the socioeconomic aspects of the family and homosexuality, the acceptance or rejection of gender roles by the parents of homosexuals, and the aspirations of homosexuals. Psychoanalytic studies of homosexuality are critiqued, and researchers' awareness of the sociocultural and temporal definitions of homosexuality is questioned. An examination of cross-cultural studies shows an acceptance of alternative sex roles for both men and women in Mohave culture. In China, the conflicts of the Oedipal period and puberty are mitigated by clearly defined social roles for each generation and sex. When homosexuality does appear, it tends to be somaticized. In Iraq, homosexuality was traditionally practiced as a "normal" phase in masculine development. It is concluded that the biases of psychoanalysis have blinded it to factors important to the solution of intimate human problems.

1583

Gordon, L. V. (1967). Q-typing of Oriental and American youth: Initial and clarifying studies. Journal of Social Psychology, 71, *185-195.*

Intercorrelations among 19 student samples tested in Hong Kong and Taiwan, India, Japan, Samoa, the Philippine Islands, and the United States, based on mean scores on a survey of interpersonal values, were factor analyzed followed by varimax rotation. Three resultant factors clearly distinguished among the cultures. When marker variables from a previous American analysis were added to the student samples, four readily interpretable factors emerged. Also, relationships between specific groups were interpretable at the correlational level. The methodology, termed q-typing, appears to have utility for clustering groups on the basis of similarity of interpersonal value orientations and relating individuals, groups or types to one another. Applicability of the methodology in cross-cultural research is discussed.

1584

Graham, M. A. (1983). Acculturative stress among Polynesian, Asian and American students on the Brigham Young University--Hawaii Campus. International Journal of Intercultural Relations, 7, *79-103.*

Conducted a 5-yr study of the acculturation effects on college freshmen attending the Hawaiian campus of the Brigham Young University. Although all Ss belonged to the same religious denomination (i.e., the Church of Jesus Christ of Latter-day Saints), 9 cultural groups were studied: Hawaiian, Samoan, Tongan, New Zealand Maori, Fijian, Chinese, Japanese, Filipino, and US mainland White Ss. 109 US military personnel (17-20 yrs old) who were White, Hispanic, and Black were also studied for comparison. Ss were administered a battery of measures, including the Bell Adjustment Inventory and the IPAT. There were significant differences among Ss in assimilation patterns, affective contingencies, points of conflict, and cultural stereotyping. Findings also show the following: (1) Acculturative stress was significantly greater among Samoan Ss. (2) Chinese Ss were academically the most successfully adaptive cultural group. (3) English language usage imposed the greatest discriminatory barrier to all non-American cultures. Cultural configurations relative to Samoan Ss and recommendations to minimize acculturative stress are discussed.

1585

Grant, P. R., & Holmes, J. G. (1981). The integration of implicit personality theory schemas and stereotype images. Social Psychology Quarterly, 44, *107-115.*

Asked 89 female undergraduates to form an impression of either an Irish or a Chinese stimulus person described by 2 traits. These traits were either part of the stereotype image of the stimulus person's ethnic group or were unrelated to this image. Results show that the Irish stereotype traits were used to characterize the Irish stimulus persons and Chinese stereotype traits were used to characterize the Chinese stimulus person, whatever their trait descriptions. In addition, when Ss characterized an individual described by traits unrelated to the individual's ethnic group stereotype, they included these traits in their impressions of that person. Thus, Ss' impressions of such a person included all the stereotype traits associated with the person's ethnic group and these unrelated traits. Results suggest that stereotypes play an important role in social perception. Specifically, they support the notion that stereotypes are overgeneralizations that are applied to any ethnic group member regardless of his or her individual characteristics. They also suggest that stereotypes do not act to minimize perceived individual differences between ethnic group members along dimensions independent of the stereotype image.

1586

Gregory, R. J. (1977). Drug abuse in China: II. Contemporary and implications. Drug Forum, 6, *299-314.*

Examines the abuse of opiates in China in historical perspective. Political, economic, and social changes in China which have affected drug abuse patterns are discussed to clarify reasons for the elimination of opiate use. Further, why the contemporary use of opiates is continued elsewhere is discussed, and some of the social and cultural influences in the American drug scene are presented. It is suggested that to deal effectively with the abuse of drugs in the US, lessons can be learned from cross-cultural evidence.

1587

Gregory, R. J. (1977). The Chinese drug scene: I. History. Drug Forum, 6, *235-247.*

Examines the widespread abuse of opiates in China from a historical viewpoint. Political, economic, and social changes in China have affected drug abuse patterns and accordingly provide insight on reasons for the elimination of opiate use. Light is shed on why the contemporary use of opiates is continued elsewhere, and on some of the social and cultural influences on the American drug scene. It is argued that to deal effectively with the abuse of drugs in the US, lessons can be learned from cross-cultural evidence.

1588

Grichting, W. L. (1971). Occupation prestige structure in Taiwan. Journal of Sociology *(National Taiwan University), 7, 67-80.*

1589

Gui, C. L. S. (1985). A cross-cultural study of the relation between degree of American acculturation and androgyny. Dissertation Abstracts International, 45, *A3097.*

1590

Gulick, R. H. V. (1961). Sexual life in ancient China. *Leiden: E.J. Brill.*

1591

Guskin, A. E. (1969). Changing identity: The assimilation of Chinese in Thailand. Dissertation Abstracts International, 30, *A4415-416.*

1592

Hahn, C. C. (1928). Psycho-social effects of the Chinese family systems. Society and Social Research, 12.

1593

Hale, R. W., & Char, D. F. B. (1982). Sexual and contraceptive behavior on a college campus: A five-year follow-up. Contraception, 25, *125-134.*

1594

Haque, A. (1969). National stereotypes of college students in Hyberabad (Pakistan) during the Indo-Pakistan war. Pakistan Journal of Psychology, 2, *21-38.*

200 undergraduate female Pakistani Ss were given 80 adjectives and assigned the 5 most appropriate to each of 14 national groups which had been classified into 5 groups on the basis of their relationship to Pakistan. It was found that groups classified as ingroup (Pakistani) and friendly outgroup (Chinese, Indonesians, Iranians, Saudi Arabs, and Turks) received 100% favorable traits, as did 1 member of the neutral (Japanese) outgroup. The enemy group (Indians) and 1 member of the unfriendly outgroup (Malaysians) received 100% unfavorable traits. An "index of uniformity" of responses made it possible to differentiate between groups undistinguishable on the basis of attitude scores. Results "were explained in terms of the functional relations between Pakistan and other countries . . . . ". It is concluded that the nature of acceptable and unacceptable categories is different, attitude scores are a weak measure of stereotype, and the "degree of uniformity is positively related to the degree of favourable or unfavourable attitudes . . . .".

1595

Harding, C. (1980). East meets West: A conflict of values. Hong Kong Psychological Society Bulletin, *No. 5, 35-43.*

Contrasts in terms of personal construct theory the cultural values and hence the core roles taught to Chinese and to Western children. Where the Chinese emphasize social responsibilities, especially toward the family, Western children are socialized to value independence and individualism. The usefulness of the repertory grid technique in understanding the sociopsychological processes that take place in forming and changing core role constructs is illustrated by the case of a 25-yr-old woman whose original Chinese values were coming into conflict with Western values.

1596

Hare-Mustin, R. T. (1982). China's Marriage Law: A model for family responsibilities and relationships. Family Process, 21, *477-481.*

Discusses China's Marriage Law of 1981, which encompasses the responsibilities of spouses, parents, children, grandparents, and siblings to one another. The new law is contrasted with the 1950 Marriage Law, which prohibited such feudal practices of former times as arranged marriages and child betrothals. The 1981 law is concerned with equality and the lawful needs of women, children, and the aged. It encourages family planning, makes divorces easier to obtain and provides for adoptees and stepchildren. The law provides a legislative model for personal relationships.

1597

Harkness, E. G. (1973). Culture and role of Chinese health professionals with multi-ethnic clients. Dissertation Abstracts International, 34, *B2428.*

1598

Harrell, S. (1980). Normal & deviant drinking in rural Taiwan. In A. Kleinman & T. Y. Lin (Eds.), Normal and Abnormal Behavior in Chinese Culture *(pp. 49-59). Dordrecht, Netherlands: D. Reidel.*

1599

Harvey, C. B. (1985). Child care in China: Recent developments. Journal of Child Care, 2, *25-30.*

The author provided a descriptive overview of child- and healthcare in China from the philosophical bases established during the cultural revolution (post 1949) to the present. Efforts to modernize education, which have centered on making families, kindergarten, schools, and society an integrated environment for the fostering of socialist morality and cultural harmony, were discussed. It was reported that preschool education presently centers on the enhancement of innate abilities, the encouragement of high levels of knowledge acquisition, and the instruction of specific technical skills. Primary school education was described as focusing on the encouragement of love of motherhood, labor, and science; the creation of good study habits; the provision of basic knowledge of nature and society; and the instruction of basic skills in reading, writing, and arithmetic. Recent trends in special and after-school education were briefly described along with advances in child healthcare. It was suggested that the children, as the center of Chinese family life, are the focus of central government attention and that changes in the childcare situation in China reflect the changes in the overall dynamics of the country's politicocultural situation.

1600

Headland, I. T. (Ed.). (1914). Home life in China. *London: Methuen.*

1601

Heiligman, A. C. (1978 - 1979). Racism in United States: Drug legislation and the trade-off behind it. Drug Forum, 7, *19-26.*

1602

Hepburn, C., & Locksley, A. (1983). Subjective awareness of stereotyping: Do we know when our judgments are prejudiced? Social Psychology Quarterly, 46, *311-318.*

272 undergraduates rated the likelihood of criterial traits among diverse social groups and also rated individual targets from those groups on commensurate scales to investigate whether Ss could accurately assess the influence of their own stereotypes on relevant judgments of individuals. Six stereotypic beliefs were involved: that males are more assertive than females, Blacks are more athletic than Whites, Chinese are more modest than Americans, nocturnal people are more rebellious than diurnal people, physically attractive people are more sociable than unattractive people, and overweight people are more impulsive than normal-weight people. After each target judgment, Ss indicated the extent to which their judgment was influenced by their own stereotypic beliefs, permitting construction of a subjective index of stereotypic effects. An objective index of stereotypic effects was constructed by subtracting the posterior difference between judgments of individuals from contrasted social groups from the prior difference between stereotypic judgments of the groups. Results show that no correlation was found between subjective and objective indices of stereotypic effects on judgment, suggesting that Ss did not have direct introspective awareness of the impact of their own stereotypes on their judgments of individuals. Data indicate that Ss relied on several different inferential strategies to infer stereotypic effects. The cumulative effect of these strategies was to inflate Ss' estimates of the actual impact of stereotypes on judgment.

1603

Hermalin, A. I., & Chow, L. P. (1971). Motivational factors in IUD termination: Data from the second Taiwan IUD follow-up survey. Journal of Biosocial Science, 3, *351-375.*

1604

Hewstone, M., Bond, M. H., & Wan, K. C. (1983). Social facts and social attributions: The explanation of intergroup differences in Hong Kong. Social Cognition, 2, *142-157.*

56 male undergraduates of 2 Hong Kong universities were asked to explain 8 generally accepted facts distinguishing the 2 groups to an experimenter and a future audience from one or the other group. Four of the 8 facts favored each of the universities. Results show Ss of both universities made group-serving attributions, this bias being more marked on the ex-

planations made by the lower-status group. The favorability of the facts to one's own group and the group identity of the experimenter/audience had no impact on the attributions made. Results are discussed in terms of H. Tajfel's (1978) social identity theory, which proposes that this positive ingroup image is achieved by favoring the ingroup over the outgroup on positively valued dimensions. Findings support the theory's applicability in a collectivist culture emphasizing harmony.

1605

Hewstone, M., & Ward, C. (1985). Ethnocentrism and causal attribution in Southeast Asia. Journal of Personality & Social Psychology, 48, *614-623.*

The present study tested the hypothesis of ethnocentric attribution. In Experiment I, 34 Malay and 34 Chinese male Malaysian university students were asked to ascribe to internal or external causes the behavior of ingroup and outgroup members performing socially desirable or undesirable acts. The hypothesis was supported only for the Malays, whereas the Chinese favored the outgroup. These results were consistent with a limited analysis of auto- and heterostereotypes. Experiment II, with 60 Singaporean male university students, again revealed ingroup favoritism for the Malays, although the Chinese no longer favored the outgroup. These less extreme results mapped onto the stereotypes and mirrored the more multicultural environment in Singapore. Differences between the studies were discussed in terms of wider sociostructural and cultural influences that indicate that ethnocentric attribution is not a universal tendency.

1606

Heyer, V. (1953). Relations between men and women in Chinese stories. In M. Mead & R. Metraux (Eds.), The study of culture at a distance *(pp. 221-234). Chicago, IL: University of Chicago Press.*

1607

Hicks, J. M., Goldman, M., & Kang, J. (1968). Attitudes toward Negroes and stereotypes about Americans among Chinese students in Taiwan and the United States. Journal of Social Psychology, 76, *139-141.*

Cross-cultural comparisons were made with respect to attitudes and stereotypes of Chinese in Taiwan, Chinese in the United States, and Americans. Each group was presented a questionnaire consisting of a direct measure of attitudes toward Negroes and a list of trait adjectives. Degree of prior contact with Negroes was also indicated by each respondent. Attitudes of Chinese in the United States were found to measure significantly more in the direction of American attitudes than attitudes of Chinese in Taiwan. Analysis of stereotypes of Americans pointed in the same direction as the above finding. Chinese in Taiwan and long-term Chinese in the United States (4-8.1 yr.) expressed the most favorable attitudes, with Chinese of intermediate length of stay in the United States expressing less favorable attitudes toward Negroes.

1608

Hill, A. M. (1985). A preliminary perspective on kinship and ethnicity among Chinese in Thailand [Special Issue: Family, kinship and ethnic identity among the Overseas Chinese]. Journal of Comparative Family Studies, 16, *143-159.*

The influence of kinship on individual choices of ethnicity among overseas Chinese and Yunnanese Chinese in Thailand were examined. It was contended that kinship is relevant to the acquisition of social skills and cultural knowledge, factors that are related to ethnic identity. Reasons for allying with or denying Chinese heritage and kinsmen were discussed, and it was suggested that Chinese women are instrumental in providing the foundation of ethnic identity through their familial roles as wives and mothers.

1609

Hines, R. H. (1968). Social distance components in integration attitudes of Negro college students. Journal Of Negro Education, 37, *23-30.*

Using a ranking technique, the social distance attitudes and preferences of Negro students toward whites, Jews, American Indians, Mexicans, and Chinese were measured for 9 social situations ranging from very general to intimate interaction. Results indicate a general preference for whites due to their role as the dominant element of power in American culture. Self-identification and commitment to other Negroes showed a decrease in ambivalence, preference for whites decreased, and preference for other minority groups increased, as the nature of the social example became more intimate. The effect of the disadvantaged status of the Negro on his social distance attitudes is discussed.

1610

Hiniker, P. J. (1965). Chinese attitudinal reactions to forced compliance. *(Monograph No. c/65-18, pp. 1-63). (Summary of "Socialization in the Confucian patterns"). Cambridge, MA: Massachusetts Institute of Technology, Center for International Studies.*

1611

Hiniker, P. J. (1969). Chinese reactions to forced compliance: Dissonance reduction or national character. Journal of Social Psychology, 77, *157-176.*

Constitutes an experimental test of forced compliance dissonance reduction tendencies against the predictions of a characterological theory of Chinese reactions to forced compliance. The experiment was concluded in Hong Kong in 1964 with 50 refugees from Mainland China. The experimental situation involved the delivering of counterattitudinal statements regarding the changing level of rice rations on Mainland China under variable levels of inducement. The results generally support the characterological predictions as against those of dissonance reduction due to forced compliance. Of particular importance in the characterological explanation of the results was the tendency of Chinese as compared to Americans to maintain a separation between overt formalism and covert feelings.

1612

Hirschman, C., & Rindfuss, R. (1982). The sequence and timing of family formation events in Asia. American Sociological Review, 47, *660-680.*

Examined the sequence and time interval between age at 1st marriage and birth of 1st child in 7,759 30-44 yr old married women in South Korea, Taiwan, Peninsular Malaysia, and Thailand. A general conceptual framework for the study of the determinants of early family formation is presented. Within this framework, the effects of educational attainment and urban-rural origins on the timing of 1st marriage and 1st birth were examined. Some common patterns of family formation that modestly support W. Goode's (1963) convergence thesis were found, but there were also significant unexplained interpopulation differences.

1613

Hirschman, E. C. (1982). Ethnic variation in hedonic consumption. Journal of Social Psychology, 118, *225-234.*

Explored variation in hedonic consumption patterns among members of religion- and nationality-based ethnic groups. It was assumed that observed differences in types and levels of hedonic consumption would increase understanding of the hedonic aspects of ethnicity and the effects of ethnic socialization upon consumption. Religious groupings of the college students and their social contacts were Catholic (n = 167), Jewish (n = 228), and Protestant (n = 55). Nationality groupings were Chinese (n = 29), Greek (n = 23), Irish (n = 20), Italian (n = 68), Jewish (n = 200), and English (n = 49). Ss were administered a questionnaire that assessed hedonic consumption, including projective behavior, imagery, favorite physical activities, enthusiasm, and motives. It was found that significant ethnic differences were present in projective behavior, imagery, behavioral motives, and preferred leisure activities, thus supporting the utility of further investigating the hedonic behavior-ethnicity linkage.

1614

Ho, D. Y. (1985). Psychological aspects of slavery and colonialism. Bulletin of the Hong Kong Psychological Society, *No. 15, 37-42.*

The author described the evolution of the master-slave relationship and compared colonialism with slavery, arguing that both result in a loss of the sense of self-sovereignty and of personal dignity, manifested in self-doubt, self-rejection, and possibly self-hatred. The roles of prejudice and racism in colonialism and slavery were discussed. It was asserted that healthy interethnic relations are more likely when: (1) equality exists between the ethnic groups, (2) neither group perceives the other to be a threat to its security or interests, and (3) adequate channels of communication are present.

1615

Ho, D. Y. F. (1972). The affectional function in contemporary Chinese families. In Proceedings of the 24th Annual Meeting of the World Federation for Mental Health *(pp. 131-137). Hong Kong: Mental Association of Hong Kong.*

1616

Ho, D. Y. F. (1973). Changing interpersonal relations in Chinese families. In H. E. White (Ed.), An anthology of Seminar papers: The changing family, East and West *(pp. 103-118). Hong Kong: Baptist College.*

1617

Ho, D. Y. F. (1974). Face, social expectations, and conflict avoidance. In J. L. M. Dawson & W. J. Lonner (Eds.), Readings in cross-cultural psychology *(pp. 240-251). Hong Kong: Hong Kong University Press.*

It is argued that different sets of criteria for judging face are definable in terms of social expectations or requirements, which are, in turn, functions of social positions (statuses and roles). The requirements for conduct in general, however, are invariant with respect to social positions. Accordingly, questions of face may involve various facets of social functioning: status maintenance, role performance, and conduct in general. Furthermore, they may arise not only from an individual's own direct actions but also from how he or she is treated by others, since expectations in interpersonal relations are reciprocal in nature. To give face to others is no less important than to save one's own face. The traditional Chinese mode of dealing with conflicts allow for mutual face saving, but this has the disadvantage of leading to confrontation avoidance without a genuine resolution of the underlying conflicts.

1618

Ho, D. Y. F. (1976). On the concept of face. American Journal of Sociology, 81, *867-884.*

The concept of face is clarified and distinguished from other closely related constructs: authority, standards of behavior, personality, status, dignity, honor, and prestige. The claim to face may rest on the basis of status, whether ascribed or achieved, and on personal or nonpersonal factors; it may also vary according to the group with which a person is interacting. Basic differences are found between the processes involved in gaining versus losing face. While it is not a necessity for one to strive to gain face, losing face is a serious matter which will, in varying degrees, affect one's ability to function effectively in society. Face is lost when the individual, either through his action or that of people closely related to him, fails to meet essential requirements placed upon him by virtue of the social position he occupies. In contrast to the ideology of individualism, the question of face frequently arises beyond the realm of individual responsibility and subjective volition. Reciprocity is inherent in face behavior, wherein a mutually restrictive, even coercive, power is exerted upon each member of the social network. It is argued that face behavior is universal and that face should be utilized as a construct of central importance in the social sciences.

1619

Ho, D. Y. F. (1978). Self-knowledge or the lack of it--a psychocultural view. Hong Kong Psychological Society Bulletin, *No. 1, 12-14.*

1620

Ho, D. Y. F. (1978). Face and stereotyped notions about Chinese face behavior. In M. Akita (Ed.), Proceedings of the 1st Planning Committee for a Pan-Asian Conference of Psychology *(pp. 7-25), Kyoto, Japan. (Republished in* **Philippine Journal of Psychology,** *1980,* **13,** *20-33.)*

The present paper examines both Chinese and Western views on face. It is an attempt to answer two questions: (1) Is face behavior universal, or is it unique to or distinctive of the Chinese and other peoples who have been influenced by them? (2) What are the factors which have contributed to the formation of the stereotype that Chinese attach an overriding importance to face? Several conclusions were reached after a critical review of the literature: (a) Serious conceptual and methodological difficulties (specifically ethnocentric bias) are often present which render research conclusions ambiguous and suspect; (b) there is a consensus of opinion that the rituals of face behavior operate to avoid confrontation and to conserve the traditional Chinese sociopolitical structure characterized by the dominance of vertical authority relationships; and (c) observers are unanimously agreed that Chinese attach great importance to face, although there is disagreement on whether or not this is unique to them. A more accurate formulation would be that Chinese are more conscious of the significance of face in social processes than are other peoples. This greater consciousness may be partly traced to the Chinese language, which has rich symbolic representations of face behavior since early history. It may be more meaningful to study variations in face behavior in different cultural contexts, rather than to investigate which ethnic groups attach more importance to face.

1621

Ho, D. Y. F. (1979). Psychosocial implications of collectivism: With special reference to the Chinese case and Maoist dialectics. In L. H. Eckensberger, W. J. Lonner, & Y. H. Poortinga (Eds.), Cross-cultural contributions to psychology *(pp. 143-150). Lisse, Netherlands: Swets & Zeitlinger.*

1622

Ho, D. Y. F. (1985). Prejudice, colonialism, and interethnic relations: A East-West dialogue. Journal of Asian and African Studies, 20, *218-231.*

A dialogue between two psychologists, Dr. East and Dr. West, discussed: (a) ethnocentric bias and the social consequences, stereotyping in particular, of ethnicity and cross-cultural research; (b) the responsibility Asian psychologists should assume for their lack of organization and research efforts, while recognizing that they may be subject to severe sociopolitical constraints; (c) prejudice and ideology: East and West; (d) colonialism and its psychological consequences; (e) Asian collective identity; and (f) social change as a precondition for desirable psychological changes to occur.

1623

Ho, D. Y. F. (1986). A dialogue on pornography and censorship. Hong Kong Journal of Mental Health, 15, *65-71.*

This dialogue was an attempt to clarify some of the major issues involved in the debate on pornography between moralists and libertarians. The discussion encompassed semantic clarification, criteria for making judgments about pornographic materials, an examination of the evidence for alleged harmful effects of pornography and the methodological issues involved in research, the dilemmas of censorship, and the Hong Kong situation.

1624

Ho, E. H. (1979). A study of the implications of the Piagetian theory of moral development for Seventh-Day Adventist schools: Based on a comparison of selected schools in Hong Kong, Michigan and Indiana. Dissertation Abstracts International, 39, *A7300.*

1625

Ho, F. (1979). Political attitudes toward democracy in university students. In K. S. Yang & C. C. Yeh (Eds.), Contemporary social problems in Taiwan. *Taipei: Chu-Liu Publishing Co.*

1626

Ho, Y. C. (1981). [The relationship between sex role and self-concept in college students]. Bulletin of Educational Psychology, 14, *221-230. (In Chinese.)*

The relations of sex role to self-concept and locus of control were examined in this study. The Sex Role Inventory, Tennessee Self Concept Scale and Rotter's Internal-External (I-E) Scale were completed by 208 college students. The data were analyzed by 2 (sex) x 4 (sex role) MANOVA and ANOVA. The data indicated that: (1) There were no significant differences in I-E Scale scores between the sexes and among four sex-role identities (androgynous, masculine, feminine, and undifferentiated). (2) Androgynous subjects had the highest self-esteem scores, and undifferentiated subjects had the lowest; masculine and feminine subjects' scores were close to those of androgynous subjects. Differences in self-esteem in terms of traditional sex-role identities (masculine men, feminine women) and cross-sex-role identities (feminine men, masculine women) were discussed. Implications for counseling and further research were suggested.

1627

Ho, Y. C. (1986). [The student subculture and its correlates: A study of university students in Taiwan]. Bulletin of Educational Psychology, 19, *105-147. (In Chinese.)*

Research on 3,220 students from 25 colleges and universities showed: (1) The students placed a greater emphasis on social and spiritual values than on individual and material values; on family life and social welfare than on social status and material life. They placed a greater emphasis on effort and ability than on luck, family background and human relations. (2) Contemporary students placed a greater emphasis on economic and political values than on social and religious values. (3) Contemporary students tended to be more politically involved and have more liberal attitudes toward sex and fashions. (4) Some negative characteristics of the Chinese student subculture were revealed: a greater emphasis on competence than on moral values; opportunistic, self-centered, with little academic motivation; and pleasure-oriented. (5) The student subculture could be categorized as male-female, science-humanities, self-social orientation, and opportunistic-idealistic. Some recommendations were offered to universities and educational authorities.

1628

Ho, Y. T. (1972). A first study of local attitudes and problems in providing sex education in Hong Kong secondary schools. *Unpublished master's thesis, University of Hong Kong.*

1629

Hoadley, J. S. (1970). "Hong Kong is the lifeboat": Notes on political culture and socialization. Journal of Oriental Studies, 8, *206-218.*

1630

Hofstede, G. (1977). Cultural elements in the exercise of power. In Y. H. Poortinga (Ed.), Basic problems in cross-cultural psychology. *Amsterdam, Netherlands: Swets & Zeitlinger.*

1631

Hofstede, G. (1979). Value systems in forty countries: Interpretation, validation and consequences for theory. In L. Eckensberger, W. J. Lonner, & Y. H. Poortinga (Eds.), Contributions to cross-cultural psychology. *Lisse, Netherlands: Swets & Zeitlinger.*

1632

Hofstede, G. (1980). Culture's consequences: International differences in work-related values *(abr. ed.). Beverly Hills and London: Sage.*

1633

Hofstede, G. (1983). Dimensions of national cultures in fifty countries and three regions. In J. B. Deregowski, S. Dziurawiec, & R. C. Annis (Eds.), Expectations in cross-cultural psychology *(pp. 335-355). Lisse, Netherlands: Swets & Zeitlinger.*

1634

Hofstede, G., & Bond, M. H. (1984). An independent validation of Hofstede's cultural dimensions using Rokeach's value survey. Journal of Cross-Cultural Psychology, 15, *417-433.*

1635

Hong Kong Council of Social Service, Working Group on Alcoholism Study. (1983). Exploratory study on alcohol abuse in Hong Kong. *Hong Kong: Author.*

1636

Hong Kong Young Women's Christian Association & Hong Kong Shue Yan College. (1982). Report on working mothers in family functioning. *Hong Kong: Author.*

1637

Hong, L. K. (1976). The role of women in the People's Republic of China: Legacy and change. Social Problems, 23, *545-557.*

Interviewed 10 female Chinese emigrants and 8 Hong Kong Chinese who had recently visited relatives on China's mainland. The data show that after 25 years of communist rule, women in China have made significant progress toward emancipation; however, some aspects of traditional sex role differentiation still persist in the family. Furthermore, in work outside the home, women still experience discrimination in pay and important jobs. In the political area, women are still discriminated against on the national level. Most of the important government positions are held by men. It is concluded that, although the magnitude of sex inequality in the past can explain some of these legacies, a more complete explanation must take into account the survival of the patrilineal kinship system, the ancestral cult in China, and the inadequacy of the socialist revolution.

1638

Hong, L. K. (1978). Risky shift and cautious shift: Some direct evidence on the culture-value theory. Social Psychology Quarterly, 41, *342-346.*

Reports evidence in support of the culture-value explanation of risky and cautious shifts. By comparing 75 Chinese students from Taiwan and 75 American students, it was found that Chinese were more cautious than Americans in making solitary decisions; cautious shifts occurred among the Chinese when they made the decisions as a group; and risky shifts occurred among the Americans. This difference in choice-shifts between the 2 samples could be attributed to the Chinese Confucian ethic and Chung Yung (or Doctrine of the Mean). Attention is also called to the need for studying the relationship between cultures and types of decision in explaining risky and cautious shifts.

1639

Honig, A. S. (1978). Comparison of childrearing practices in Japan and in the People's Republic of China: A personal view. International Journal of Group Tensions, 8, *6-32.*

Describes childrearing in China and Japan, as observed during a 1976 summer tour. Topics covered include the importance of children, fathering, child care facilities, early education curriculum, moral development, discipline and the treatment of behavior problems, physical fitness, the importance of work chores, aesthetics, politics, and religion. It is concluded that in both countries children are imbued with a sense of beauty, pride in cultural heritage, moral development, hard work habits, and positive sociability.

1640

Hsieh, P. Y. (1943). The autobiography of a Chinese girl. *(C. Tsui, Trans.). London: Allen & Unwin.*

1641

Hsieh, T. T., Shybut, J., & Lotsof, E. J. (1969). Internal versus external control and ethnic group membership: A cross-cultural comparison. Journal of Consulting & Clinical Psychology, 33, *122-124.*

To investigate a relationship between internal vs. external control and ethnic group membership, 3 groups of high school Ss (Chinese, American-born Chinese, and Anglo-American) were compared in their responses to the Internal-External Control Scale. A hypothesis that a belief in internal vs. external control is significantly related to ethnic group membership was confirmed.

1642

Hsien, C. H. (1944). The Chinese concept of face. American Anthropologist, 46, *45-64.*

1643

Hsiung, H. L. (1967). [Ethnic attitude and prejudice]. The National Chengchi University Journal *(Taipei),* **15,** *501-562. (In Chinese.)*

1644

Hsu, F. L. (1971). The challenge of the American dream: The Chinese in the United States. *Belmont, CA: Wadsworth. (Reviewed by L. D. Boreman, in* **American Anthropologist, 75,** *1007-1008.)*

1645

Hsu, F. L. K. (1940). The problem of incest tabu in a North China village. American Anthropologist, 42, *122-135.*

1646

Hsu, F. L. K. (1948). Under the ancestors' shadow: Chinese culture and personality. *New York: Columbia University Press. (Republished London: Routledge & Kegan Paul, 1949.)*

The characteristic patterns of behavior in a small semi-rural community in southwest China are described, with particular attention to patterns of family and religious life. Analysis of the culture of the community reveals the two most important influences upon the basic personality type to be authority and competition, the former deriving from ancestral tradition and operating through the father-son tie, and the latter carried on within a framework determined by such authority. The most important status personality configuration difference occurs between the rich or highly placed and the poor or lowly placed. The end results of authority and competition applied to both these groups are radically different, and are offered as the explanation of the cycles of the rise and fall of families and dynasties.

1647

Hsu, F. L. K. (1949). Suppression versus repression: A limited psychological interpretation of four cultures. Psychiatry, 12, *223-242. (Also in R. C. Teevan & R. C. Birney (Eds.),* **Readings for Introductory Psychology.** *New York: Harcourt, Brace & World, 1965.)*

1648

Hsu, F. L. K. (1951). The Chinese of Hawaii: Their role in American culture. Transactions of the New York Academy of Sciences, 13, *243-250.*

1649

Hsu, F. L. K. (1953). Americans and Chinese: Two ways of life. *New York: Abelard-Schuman. (Republished London: Cresset Press, 1955.)*

1650

Hsu, F. L. K. (1961). Kinship and ways of life: An exploration. In F. L. K. Hsu (Ed.), Psychological anthropology: Approaches to culture and personality *(pp. 509-567). Homewood, IL: Dorsey Press.*

1651

Hsu, F. L. K. (1963). Clan, caste, and club: A comparative study of Chinese, Hindu, and American ways of life. *New York: van Nostrand.*

It is argued that differences in the family system lie at the root of three worlds: the Chinese situation-centered world, the Hindu supernatural-centered world, and the American individual-centered world. The Chinese family system is characterized by the dominance of the father-son relationship, in contrast to the dominance of the mother-son relationship in the Hindu system and the dominance of the husband-wife relationship in the American system. Father-son dominance sets the stage for the situation-centered orientation characterized by a strong tendency to seek mutual dependence.

1652

Hsu, F. L. K. (1964). Americans and Chinese: The beginnings of contrast. In M. McGiggert (Ed.), The character of Americans. *Homewood, IL: Dorsey.*

1653

Hsu, F. L. K. (1967). Under the ancestors' shadow: Kinship, personality, and social mobility in village China *(rev. and exp. ed.). New York: Doubleday. (Revised edition of* **Under the ancestors' shadow,** *1948. New York: Columbia University Press.)*

1654

Hsu, F. L. K. (1968). Chinese kinship and Chinese behavior. In P. T. Ho & T. Tang (Eds.), China in crisis: Vol. 1. China's heritage and the Communist political system. *Chicago: University of Chicago Press.*

1655

Hsu, F. L. K. (1970). Americans and Chinese: Purpose and fulfillment in great civilizations. *New York: Doubleday/Natural History Press.*

1656

Hsu, F. L. K. (1971). Psychosocial homeostasis and jen: Conceptual tools for advancing psychological anthropology. American Anthropologist, 73, *23-44.*

Considers that the basic importance accorded personality in psychological anthropology has obscured the understanding of how Western man lives in Western society and culture, or how any man lives in any society and culture. What is missing is the central ingredient in the human mode of existence: man's relationship with his fellow men. The concepts of psychosocial homeostasis and jen are designed to extricate psychological anthropology from this intellectual prison. The 1st describes the process whereby every human individual tends to seek certain kinds of affective involvement with some of his fellow humans. The 2nd refers to the internal and external limits of the individual's affective involvement. With the aid of 5 major hypotheses based on these concepts, a review is made of familiar facts drawn from China, the United States, and Japan.

1657

Hsu, F. L. K. (1971). Filial piety in Japan and China: Borrowing, variation and significance. Journal of Comparative Family Studies, 2, *67-74.*

1658

Hsu, J. (1972). [Chinese parent-child relationships as revealed in popular stories for children]. In Y. Y. Li & K. S. Yang (Eds.), [Symposium on the character of the Chinese: An interdisciplinary approach] *(Monograph Series B, No. 4, pp. 201-218). Taipei: Academia Sinica, Institute of Ethnology. (In Chinese.)*

1659

Hsu, J., & Tseng, W. S. (1974). Family relations in classic Chinese opera. International Journal of Social Psychiatry, 20, *159-172.*

Categorizes the stories of 111 classic Chinese operas according to the familial relations of the principal actors. Descriptions of repeated themes for each relationship form the basis for a description of traditional Chinese family culture. Implications for cultural modernization are drawn.

1660

Hsu, M. (1973). Cultural and sexual differences on the judgment of criminal offenses: A replication study of the measurement of delinquency. Journal of Criminal Law & Criminology, 64, *348-353.*

In stating their 2 hypotheses, Sellin and Wolfgang have cautioned that the scale values in quite different cultures might not conform to their expectations. The present study shows that this indeed is the case. The difference between Chinese male and female raters indicates that sex also plays an important role in forming an individual's value judgment. The question is posed that if sex does made a difference in value judgment, what could this mean to the presently male-dominated judicial system.

1661

Hsu, V. (1983). Maxine Hong Kingston as psycho-autobiographer and ethnographer. International Journal of Women's Studies, 6, *429-442.*

The Woman Warrior can be considered as a psychoautobiography, in that it relates the author's psychic experiences, and as ethnography, in that these psychic experiences interface with the objective concrete experiences common to Chinese-Americans. The idiosyncratic characteristics of Kingston's personality and her childhood circumstances and the broader cultural experiences represented in the book are discussed.

1662

Hu, C. T. (1960). China: Its people, its society, its culture. *New Haven: Human Relations Area Files Press.*

1663

Hu, F. (1982). [Yu-Chuan and Wu-chuan: A conceptual and empirical analysis of political value orientation]. In K. S. Yang & C. I. Wen (Eds.), [The Sinicization of social science research] *(pp. 381-416). Taipei: Academia Sinica, Institute of Ethnology. (In Chinese.)*

1664

Hu, H. C. (1944). The Chinese concepts of face. American Anthropologist, 46, *45-64. (Reprinted in D. G. Haring (Ed.),* **Personal character and cultural milieu.** *Syracuse: Syracuse University Press, 1956).*

1665

Hu, H. C. (1949). Emotions, real and assumed, in Chinese society^ (CH-668). Unpublished manuscript, Columbia University Research in Contemporary Cultures, New York.

1666

Hu, H. C. (1951). *Sex experiences of children.* **Unpublished document (RCC-CH-PR4), Columbia University Research in Contemporary Cultures, New York.**

1667

Huang, K., & Pilisuk, M. (1977). At the threshold of the Golden Gate: Special problems of a neglected minority. *American Journal of Orthopsychiatry, 47,* **701-713.**

Notes that the residents of San Francisco's Chinatown demonstrate the consequences of economic and social ills deriving from the history of Chinese-Americans and the orientation of American society towards them. Changes in the immigration laws have presented particularly stressful circumstances for the traditional Chinese-American family. The relationship of such social stresses to the incidence and form of psychopathology--including an unusually high incidence of suicide--is noted.

1668

Huang, L. (1956). Dating and courtship innovations of Chinese students in America. *Marriage and Family Living, 18,* **25-29.**

1669

Huang, L. C. (1974). A cross-cultural study of conformity in Americans and Chinese. *Dissertation Abstracts International, 34,* **B5714. (Also available on University Microfilms 74-11, 788.) New Mexico, 1973.**

1670

Huang, L. C., & Harris, M. B. (1973). Conformity in Chinese and Americans: A field experiment. *Journal of Cross-Cultural Psychology, 4,* **427-434.**

Conducted a cross-cultural field experiment to determine the effects of a model's social status and specific task competence on imitation or conformity. Ss were 2 groups of 80 adults in Taiwan and the US. Results indicate that Chinese were more conforming than Americans and that, in both countries, the model's status had a significant effect and competence a negligible effect on conformity. A Status * Competence interaction effect for Americans and for both groups combined indicated that a high-status model was imitated slightly more if low in competence, but a low-status model was imitated only if he was highly competent.

1671

Huang, L. C., & Harris, M. B. (1974). Altruism and imitation in Chinese and Americans: A cross-cultural experiment. *Journal of Social Psychology, 93,* **193-195.**

Conducted a field experiment with 130 Chinese in Taipei, Taiwan, and 115 Americans in Albuquerque, New Mexico, to determine the effects of observing a model on accepting and actually mailing a letter. It was predicted that Chinese, being more conformist, would help less than more "materialistic" Americans in the refusing model and helpful rewarded model conditions, and more in the no model and helpful unrewarded model conditions. However, the only statistically significant difference found was that a higher percentage of letters accepted by Chinese Ss were actually received.

1672

Huang, L. J. (1976). The family and the communes in People's Republic of China: Retrospect and prospect. *Journal of Comparative Family Studies, 7,* **97-109.**

The author examines the role of the commune in the economic patterns of the People's Republic of China. This commune system, with three levels of production, is primarily the social innovation of the communist regime of the People's Republic. Research indicates that the system seems to be enjoying relative success, and this is attributed partly to its origin. That is, instead of the spontaneous inception of the many varieties of the American communes by members themselves, the Chinese communes were organized and planned by political leaders with the masses participating on different levels of production. The author maintains that the Chinese commune system, with its trials and errors, has been successful in raising the economic standards of the country through large-scale participation of the masses.

1673

Huang, L. J. (1982). Planned fertility of one-couple/one-child policy in the People's Republic of China. *Journal of Marriage & the Family, 44,* **775-784.**

The People's Republic of China, with the population reaching 1 billion in 1981, is the 1st country to institute a 1-couple/1-child planned fertility policy. The target is to achieve zero population by the year 2000. Major rationales and measures for implementing this policy are discussed. Also addressed is the resistance among the masses that arises from the conflict between the birth-planning policy and centuries-old Chinese cultural values.

1674

Huang, L. L., & Hwang, K. K. (1979). [Influence of authoritarian and dogmatic personality upon the perception of the U.S. recognition of the Republic of China]. *Bulletin of the Institute of Ethnology^ (Academia Sinica), No. 48, 155-196. (In Chinese.)*

The purpose of this research was to study the psychological responses of the Chinese in Taiwan to the normalization of diplomatic relation between the United States and the People's Republic of China. The questionnaires included Chinese versions of the F-scale, D-scale, and three sets of Semantic Differential scales for evaluating the American people, the American government, and the event of normalization. The subjects consisted of students from high schools and colleges, as well as some people working in enterprise organizations. The results showed that: (1) The subjects' attitudes toward the American people tended to be positive, whereas those toward the American government tended to be negative. (2) The dimensions of semantic differential scales for evaluating the American people, the American government, and the event of normalization were 4, 3, and 3 respectively. (3) The factorial structure of the F-scale included seven factors, and that of D-scale included three. (4) The personality pattern of Dogmatism, non-Cynicism and Traditionalism had a high canonical correlation with a set of attitudes toward the American people, the American government, and the event of normalization that were similar to that advocated in the mass media at the time.

1675

Huang, L. T., Phares, R., & Hollender, M. H. (1976). The wish to be held: A transcultural study. Archives of General Psychiatry, 33, *41-43.*

M. H. Hollender et al noted that "a strong desire to be held or cuddled correlated with a general leaning toward openness in emotional expression". The present study assessed the influence of cultural attitudes on the wish to be held. Questionnaires were given to 5 groups of Asian women living in Kuala Lumpur, Malaysia. Ss, most of them in their twenties or thirties, totaled 190. The most striking differences found were between 2 groups of Chinese, one Chinese-educated, and the other English-educated. The Chinese-educated group inhibited the expression of sensual needs. An English education overturned the traditional mode of response; Ss in this group scored highest in their wish to be held and lowest in their inclination to keep their body-contact desires secret. It is concluded that cultural as well as psychological forces exert a profound influence on the wish to be held.

1676

Huang, M. S., & Singer, A. E. (1984). Ethnic group stereotyping by police and university students in New Zealand. Journal of Psychology, 116, *89-93.*

42 university students, 41 police recruits, and 37 senior policemen completed a 12-item semantic differential to rate 4 of the New Zealand ethnic groups: Maori, Samoan, Chinese, and English. Results indicate no overall attitudinal differences among the 3 samples. However, a differential pattern of attitude stereotyping for the 4 ethnic groups was observed. Maoris were considered as law-breaking and generous; Samoans as

humble, ignorant, and generous; Chinese as patient, clever, hard-working, and law-abiding; and English as impatient, talkative, and clever.

1677

Huang, S. C. (1963). A comparison of selected values among Formosan and American adolescents (Doctoral dissertation, Ohio State University, 1962). Dissertation Abstracts International, 24, *381.*

1678

Huang, W. Y. (1977). [A study of students' interpersonal relationships in a junior high school in Taipei]. Research in Education & Psychology, 1, *117-141. (In Chinese.)*

This study adopted the sociometric techniques of Moreno to investigate the social behavior of 270 junior high school students in Taipei. Factors such as age, height, weight, birth order were evaluated as to their effects on interpersonal relations and group-forming processes.

1679

Huang, X. T., Shi, K., & Wang, X. S. (1984). [A psychological study of interpersonal relations in college classes]. Acta Psychologica Sinica, 16, *455-465. (In Chinese.)*

This is a study of interpersonal relations among freshmen, sophomores, and seniors in 21 college classes treated as separate collectives. Data from interviews, observation, and sociometric techiques were collected. Certain features in the informal inner structure of college classes were revealed. Significant personality traits were identified in two extreme types in a class, the most popular and the most unpopular. It was found that the basic criteria used by college students in choosing friends were moral character and psychological similarity. The college students expected their class leaders to possess certain mental traits as basic requirements. There was a close connection between a college student's self-concept and his or her interpersonal relations with classmates.

1680

Huang, Y. H. (1974). [Popularity as related to the amount of reinforcement given to the statement of others]. Bulletin of Educational Psychology, 7, *23-32. (In Chinese.)*

It was hypothesized that the more popular a person is, the more reinforcement he or she will give to the statements of others in an interpersonal situation. Popularity was measured by a sociometreic technique, and the amount of reinforcement was counted from the agreement, nodding or uh-hum responses made while listening to a recording of statements spoken by males and females. The results confirmed the hypothesis.

1681

Hughes, S. P. (1982). Cultural and ethnic patterns of alcohol consumption in a university environment. Dissertation Abstracts International, 43, *A280.*

1682

Humana, C., & Wu, W. (1972). Ying-Yang: The Chinese way of love. Sexual Behavior, 2, *20-25.*

Presents passages from Confucian and Taoist writings to illustrate traditional Chinese sexual practices and beliefs. Major topics include the relationship between mind and body and the role of women.

1683

Hummel, A. W. (1960). The art of social relations in China. Philosophy East and West, 10, *13-22.*

1684

Hung, N. S. (1973). Attitudes of Chinese in Hong Kong towards Japan. *Unpublished master's thesis, Hong Kong University.*

1685

Hwang, C. H. (1974). [Attitudes of Chinese university students toward dating and mate selection]. Bulletin of Educational Psychology, 7, *1-14. (In Chinese.)*

Administered a questionnaire concerning attitudes toward dating and mate selection to 128 college students in 1959 and to 321 college students in 1974. Results show that the attitudes of the young people in Taiwan today toward dating and mate selection are more practical and less restrictive than they were 15 yrs ago. However, the relative importance of personal criteria for mate selection remains unchanged. Likewise, their unfavorable attitude towards premarital (80%) and extramarital sex behavior (90%) showed little change during this period.

1686

Hwang, C. H. (1974). A comparative study on social attitudes of adolescents in Glasgow and in Taipei. *Taipei: Orient Cultural Service.*

1687

Hwang, C. H. (1974). [The use of a semantic differential in studying social attitudes of Chinese and Scottish adolescents]. Psychological Testing, 21, *39-46. (In Chinese.)*

1688

Hwang, C. H. (1975). A follow-up study on social attitudes of Chinese and Scottish adolescents. Bulletin of Educational Psychology, 8, *95-106.*

42 Scottish and 40 Chinese junior high school pupils from a 1974 study were retested 2 yrs later using a

selected set of TAT cards. Several differences between Scottish and Chinese adolescents found in the previous study were confirmed.

1689

Hwang, C. H. (1977). [Filial piety from a psychological point of view]. Bulletin of Educational Psychology, 10, *11-20. (In Chinese.)*

Used an anonymous questionnaire to survey the opinions of 687 junior high school, 311 high school, and 198 university students on the role of filial piety in modern Chinese society. Most respondents indicated that filial piety is still necessary. The practice of filial conduct was not considered to be difficult. Results also indicate several differences between current and traditional ideas of what constitutes filial piety, thus reflecting changing attitudes characteristic of modern society.

1690

Hwang, C. H. (1981). [A preliminary study of time perception and pace of life in Chinese university students]. Bulletin of Educational Psychology, 14, *1-14. (In Chinese.)*

The time perception of Chinese university students was studied. A questionnaire was used to determine: (a) the frequency of being late in social engagements; (b) their feelings of being late; (c) their perceptions of being early and late; (d) the attributions they would make in case of being late; and (e) their evaluation of the personality of people who were punctual, occasionally late, or chronically late. When the results were compared with those on American and Brazilian college students reported by Levine et al., Chinese students seemed to have a stricter sense of punctuality. Although they made a greater allowance for people arriving early in social gatherings, they showed less tolerance than Westerners for latecomers; and they themselves would always try to be present ahead of the scheduled time. The accuracy of public clocks and personal watches was checked at 15 localities in Taiwan. There was no systematic difference in accuracy between big cities and small towns.

1691

Hwang, C. H. (1986). [An analysis of the responses of junior high students in Taipei to a sentence completion test]. Bulletin of Educational Psychology, 19, *21-36. (In Chinese.)*

The Revised Sentence Completion Test developed by the present author was administered to students in eight junior high schools in Taipei City. The responses of 480 randomly selected subjects were investigated by content analysis through categorization. The results were compared with those collected by this author in 1974 with similar method. Suggestions in regard to parent-child relationship and school education were made based on the findings.

1692

Hwang, K. K. (1977). The patterns of coping strategies in a Chinese society. Acta Psychologica Taiwanica, 19, *61-73.*

Investigated the coping strategies of 180 married Chinese men living in Taipei and having at least 1 child. Ss were first asked to report their frequently used strategies for dealing with daily problems; they then completed a questionnaire which assessed their coping styles. Analysis of Ss' responses on the questionnaire resulted in a classification system consisting of 4 broad categories. Factor analysis of the quantitative data resulted in 6 patterns of coping. Each of the 6 patterns is discussed in terms of the classification system and Formosan culture.

1693

Hwang, K. K. (1978). The dynamic processes of coping with interpersonal conflicts in a Chinese society. Proceedings of the National Science Council, R.O.C., 2, *198-208. Taipei: National Science Council.*

1694

Hwang, K. K. (1978). [The adjustment to urban life and individual's modernization]. In Y. M. Tsai & W. H. Kuo (Eds.), [Modern urban society: A collection of essays] *(pp. 53-66). Taipei: Chu Liu Book Co. (In Chinese.)*

1695

Hwang, K. K. (1979). Coping with residential crowding in a Chinese urban society: The interplay of high-density dwelling and interpersonal values. Acta Psychologica Taiwanica, 21, *117-133.*

Studied various patterns of coping with different kinds of life stress and the accompanying psychopathological reactions of 180 30-60 yr old Chinese men residing in a Chinese urban community. Ss were administered the Life Stress Scale, the Views of Life Scale, and the Comprehensive Problem Behavior and Feeling Checklist. Findings indicate that Ss of low socioeconomic status not only reside in a dwelling where each resident has a small average living space but also frequently experience life stress from various domains of life (e.g., work, economic state, marriage, and housing conditions). Their coping strategies are characterized by a lack of self-confidence, and they tend to suffer from a depression syndrome, including withdrawal from social interaction, feelings of loneliness, and somatic disturbances. It is concluded that an individual, living in a residence with many others, who sets a high value on the traditional cultural norm of interpersonal cooperation and getting along with others on friendly terms will experience no interpersonal conflicts and psychopathological disturbances. However, one who values the individualistic values of self-assertion and enhancing one's achievement will suffer from interpersonal hostility and suspiciousness, and is likely to be disturbed by psychosomatic disorders and agitated depression.

1696

Hwang, K. K. (1984). [The organization pattern of family business in Taiwan]. In C. T. Wei & H. H. Lee (Eds.), [Tides of thought] *(pp. 327-371). Taipei: Linking Publishing. (In Chinese.)*

1697

Hwang, K. K., & Yang, K. S. (1971). [The relationship of individual modernity to social orientation among Chinese university students]. Bulletin of the Institute of Ethnology *(Academia Sinica), No. 32, 245-278. (In Chinese.)*

1698

Hwang, K. Y. (1982). [An exploratory study of sex knowledge, attitude and behavior of social youth]. Journal of Education and Psychology, 5, *115-176. (In Chinese.)*

This study investigated the sex behavior of social youths, and analyzed the learning style of sex knowledge and attitude of social youths. A questionnaire on sex knowledge, attitude and behavior was administered to 160 boys and 105 girls. The results were: (1) The level of sex knowledge was moderate. (2) The sources of sex knowledge were newspaper and journal, classmates, school curriculum and teacher. (3) Sex knowledge was influenced by sex difference and the level of education, and not by parental occupation and education, the area of residence, or age. (4) Most subjects admitted their sex knowledge was inadequate. (5) There was a significant sex difference in attitude to premarital sex, boys being more liberal than girls; if premarital sex occurred, the girls felt more regret and disgust against their lovers. (6) Most of the subjects agreed that abortion should be legalized. (7) The percentages of reported masturbation, nocturnal emission and homosexuality of the subjects were lower than those of other countries.

1699

Hwang, M. C. (1967). [A sociometric study of elementary school children]. Psychological Testing, 14, *393-402. (In Chinese.)*

1700

Hwang, W. C. (1980). [America as perceived by Chinese high school students]. *Taipei: Dai-yen Publishing Co. (In Chinese.)*

1701

Ikels, C. (1983). The process of caretaker selection. Research on Aging, 5, *491-509.*

Describes the findings of a survey conducted among families of Chinese and Irish ancestry (N = 242 Ss aged 60 + yrs) to assess the relative value of certain factors in predicting patterns of family support for the elderly. These factors included values and attitudes of parents and adult children toward caretaking; the presence, absence, and degree of proximity of these kin to an older person; and neighborhood characteristics. The utility of the genealogy in helping to understand the meaning of kinship resources to the elderly is discussed.

1702

Issacs, H. (1958). Scratches on our mind: The images of Indians and Chinese held by Americans. *New York: John Day.*

1703

Iu, C. R. (1982). Ethnic and economic correlates of marital satisfaction and attitude towards divorce of Chinese American women. Dissertation Abstracts International, 43, *A1293.*

1704

Iwawaki, S., Williams, J. E., & Wu, J. J. (1979). Sex-trait stereotypes in Japan and Taiwan. *Paper presented at the First Asian Regional Conference of the International Association for Cross-Cultural Psychology, Hong Kong.*

1705

Jackson, J. P. (1968). The management of projected aggression by South Vietnamese people: A study of acculturation. Dissertation Abstracts International, 29, *B1834-1835.*

1706

Jahoda, G., Deregowski, J. B., & Sinha, D. (1974). Topological and Euclidean spatial features noted by children: A cross-cultural study. International Journal of Psychology, 9, *159-172.*

415 4-12 yr olds from Hong Kong, Glasgow, Allahabad (India), and Lusaka (Zambia), ranging from low to high in socioeconomic background and industrialization of their society, designated the odd figures in each set of 3 regular or irregular shapes, presented in a manner that controlled order effects. 2 shapes shared a Euclidian property (e.g., round), 2 shared a topological property (e.g., solid), and 1 showed both topological and Euclidean features. Only a small number of Ss consistently chose Euclidean or topological figures as the odd member. Although only 1 age difference and no sex differences appeared, regular forms elicited significantly fewer topological responses for each sample than irregular ones. The assumption that topological responses decline with age received no support. Instead, choice of figures marked by both topological and Euclidean features appeared to reflect spatial ability.

1707

Jain, U. (1967). A study of stereotypes of college students and teachers toward themselves and seven other national groups. Indian Psychological Review, 3, *134-139.*

A questionnaire containing 60 attributes (positive and negative balanced) was administered to 50 Ss of each sex, students and teachers in 3:2 ratio, to obtain the 10 most appropriate characteristics for their own and 7 other nationalities (African, American, British, Chinese, French, Pakistani, and Russian). A high degree of agreement, ranging from 70-90%, was found between the 2 groups of Ss. The findings are relatively parallel to earlier studies. American, British, and Russian nationalities are seen mostly positively, while the French are observed ambivalently. Africans are attributed with mostly impersonal, derogatory traits, while the Chinese and Pakistanis are seen in emotionally loaded, derogatory and negative posture. Indians see themselves, for instance, as superstitious, tradition loving, and easily satisfied.

1708

Jen, S. M. (1974). Cybernetic analysis of Chinese cultural evolution. Dissertation Abstracts International, 35, *B2405-2406.*

1709

Joesting, J., Ogus, A., & Joesting, R. (1973). Consistencies in views of deviants by college students. Psychological Reports, 33, *138.*

Administered a questionnaire to 134 college students in a southern state university relating to their views of deviants. Germans were the most favored deviants, followed by intellectuals, Jews, Mexicans, Chinese, Negroes, marijuana smokers, women's liberation, etc. All product-moment correlations were significant (p .01), showing that Ss who discriminated against 1 group of deviates tended to generalize this discrimination to all other deviants.

1710

Johnson, R. C. et al. (1985). A cross-ethnic comparison of reasons given for using alcohol, not using alcohol or ceasing to use alcohol. Journal of Studies on Alcohol, 46, *283-288.*

The author assessed the reasons given by drinkers for drinking, abstainers for not drinking, and former drinkers for ceasing to drink in 674 Caucasian, 656 Chinese, 654 Filipino, 645 Japanese, 640 Hawaiian/part Hawaiian, and 443 mixed Oriental and Caucasian descendants in Hawaii. Results of questionnaires indicated that although there were group differences in frequencies of endorsement of reasons given for drinking, for not drinking, or for ceasing to drink, the findings of similarity were most impressive. Drinkers, abstainers, and former drinkers were similar across racial-ethnic groups in their proportions of endorsement of reasons for drinking, abstaining, or ceasing to use alcohol. Although reasons for drinking varied across racial-ethnic groups, they varied much more across groups that differed in alcohol consumption independent of ethnicity, with all reasons for drinking being more often endorsed as consumption increased. In addition, the citation of more pathological reasons for drinking was associated with a greater number of drinking problems. It was suggested that differences among ethnic groups in a number of problem drinkers may have to do with different ethnic norms for alcohol use.

1711

Jones, S. E. (1971). A comparative proxemics analysis of dyadic interaction in selected subcultures of New York City. Journal of Social Psychology, 84, *35-44.*

2 studies investigated subcultural and sex differences in spatial orientation behavior. 2-person groups of adults in 4 separate poverty subcultures (Negro, Puerto Rican, Italian, and Chinese) were observed engaging in social interaction on the public streets of New York City. Trained judges made estimates of the interpersonal distance and mutual shoulder orientation of each dyad. Regardless of subcultural group membership, women were found to be more direct in shoulder orientation than men, an outcome which appears to parallel the findings of previous studies of eye-contact behavior. There was some evidence, as informants had predicted, that black males were less direct than males in other minority groups, although this result did not approach statistical significance. Finally, interaction distance was strikingly similar in all of the subcultures studied, contrary to expectations, suggesting the inference that poverty groups are rather homogeneous in the structuring of interpersonal distance.

1712

Jordan, D. K. (1982). Taiwanese poe divination: Statistical awareness and religious belief. Journal for the Scientific Study of Religion, 21, *114-118.*

Explores the statistical properties of "poe" as they are used by Hokkien speakers in Taiwan and suggests that these qualities are known and deliberately manipulated by Taiwanese when they use poe, even though they simultaneously believe the fall of the poe to be governed by divine will. Poe divination is akin to multiple coin-flipping in form and is the most common Taiwanese divination. The usual procedure is for the petitioner to pose a question, phrase an answer, and then throw the poe for confirmation or disconfirmation. Most revelations must be reformulated several times before they are confirmed. The religious believer using poe must rely on sleight-of-hand and individual or collective self-deception concerning control of the response.

1713

Joshi, B. L. (1969). [Review of The spirit of Chinese politics: A psychoculture study of the authority crisis in political development]. *Contemporary Psychology, 14,* **213-215.**

1714

Jung, C. G. (1958). Psychological commentary on the Tibetan Book of the Great Liberation. In H. Read, M. Fordham, & G. Adler (Eds.), *The collected works of C. G. Jung* **(Vol. 11). London: Routledge & Kegan Paul.**

1715

Jung, C. G. (1958). Psychological commentary on the Tibetan Book of the Dead. In H. Read, M. Fordham, & G. Adler (Eds.). *The collected works of C. G. Jung* **(Vol. 11). London: Routledge & Kegan Paul.**

1716

Kagitcibasi, C. (1982). Old age security value of children and development: Cross-national evidence. *Journal of Comparative Family Studies, 13,* **133-142.**

Conducted a 9-country survey on motivations for childbearing. 2,000-3,000 married respondents each from Indonesia, the Republic of Korea, the Philippines, Thailand, Singapore, Taiwan, Turkey, the Federal Republic of Germany, and the US completed a 103-item questionnaire. Results show that the value placed on children in old age decreased as a society or country became more developed. This fact contributes to the lower fertility in Westernized societies. The economic value for old-age security of children was positively related to the number of children.

1717

Kalish, R. A., & Yuen, S. (1971). Americans of East Asian ancestry: Aging and the aged. *The Gerontologist, 11,* **36-47. (Republished in S. Sue & N. N. Wagner (Eds.),** *Asian-Americans: Psychological Perspectives.* **Palo Alto, CA: Science & Behavior Books, 1973.)**

1718

Kang, T. K., & Ng, K. T. (1986). Children from single-parent families: prevalence in the school setting. *Hong Kong Journal of Mental Health, 15,* **45-50.**

A total of 3,544 primary and secondary school children from nine schools were screened for parental absence, using a two-phase screening procedure. Home background information was gathered using a screening questionnaire (Phase 1), and confirmed with an in-depth child questionnaire (Phase 2) for those suspected with parental absence. Six percent of the sample was identified as children from single-parent families. There were more children affected by father-absence resulting from death. Children living without a father or a mother were about equal in single-parent homes resulting from marital disruption. Findings were compared with demographic data on overseas single-parent families. The utility of the screening for future use and the potential of using schools for study of children from single-parent families were discussed.

1719

Kang, T. S. (1972). Name and group identification. *Journal of Social Psychology, 86,* **159-160.**

Hypothesized that change of name is a symbolic representation of identity change. This shift of social identity implies a restructuring of group identification, relation to the culture, and patterns of interpersonal interaction. 118 questionnaires from Chinese university students were analyzed. Results indicate that those Ss who changed their names displayed significantly more outgroup oriented attitudes and behaviors than those who did not change their names.

1720

Karlins, M., Coffman, T. L., & Walters, G. (1969). On the fading of social stereotypes: Studies in three generations of college students. *Journal of Personality and Social Psychology, 13,* **1-16.**

1721

Katz, D., & Braly, K. W. (1933). Racial stereotypes of one hundred college students. *Journal of Abnormal and Social Psychology, 28,* **280-290.**

1722

Katz, D., & Braly, K. W. (1933). Verbal stereotypes and racial prejudice. In E. E. Maccoby, T. M. Newcomb & E. L. Hartley (Eds.), *Readings in social psychology* **(3rd ed.). London: Methuen.**

1723

Kee, D. W., & Rohwer, W. D. (1973). Noun-pair learning in four ethnic groups: Conditions of presentation and response. *Journal of Educational Psychology, 65,* **226-232.**

Assessed noun-pair learning efficiency within 4 low socioeconomic status ethnic groups (black, Chinese-American, Spanish-American, and white) as a function of presentation conditions and method of measurement (verbal recall vs pictorial recognition). A mixed-list paired-associate task was administered individually to 40 2nd-grade children from each group. Results reveal substantial effects for presentation conditions but not for ethnic groups. In addition, similar patterns of condition effects emerged across response modes for all ethnic groups. Results are taken as evidence of the generality of presentation condition effects in noun-pair learning and as an empirical demonstration of parity in learning ability for children from different ethnic backgrounds.

1724

Keil, T. J. (1978). Sex role variations and women's drinking: Results from a household survey in Pennsylvania. *Journal of Studies on Alcohol, 39,* **859-868.**

Data on 876 21-65 yr old women were analyzed by means of the Automatic Interaction Detection algorithm developed to ascertain the effects of a variety of predictors on the dichotomous dependent variable, abstinence-drinking. Drinkers were more likely to belong to religious groups that do not have proscriptions against drinking or else are ineffective in enforcing such proscriptions; attend religious services less than once/wk; have mothers who drink; have European, Black, Puerto Rican, or Chinese backgrounds; be 21-32 yrs old; have 10-17 yrs of education; associate with peers who drink; work full time, attend school or, if homemakers, be retired from work outside the home or attend school in addition to being a homemaker.

1725

Kennedy, W. B. (1975). Education for liberation and community. *Religious Education, 70,* **5-44.**

Reviews materials prepared for the education section of the Fifth Assembly of the World Council of Churches. Excerpts and analyses represent statements from Africa, Asia, Europe, Latin America, and North America, with passing reference to China and the general problem of literacy. The papers generally call for radical education reforms to correct social injustices in both developed and developing nations. The "deschooling" of I. Illich and the writings of P. Freire are prominent influences. The role of the church in education varies greatly among nations, including church schools and seminaries and also broader catalytic functions related to national public education systems.

1726

Khor, D. (1985). Alienated allies: Fetters of feminism [Special Issue: Psychology and Women]. *Hong Kong Psychological Society Bulletin,* **No. 14, 47-58.**

Based on personal experience, research conducted in Hong Kong, and surveys of the British and American literature, the present author discusses the role of public support on the score of the women's movement. Feminism is seen as a recognition of women's oppression in society--an antisexist stance aimed at securing legitimate rights of women and liberating both men and women from stereotypical gender roles. Reasons for not supporting the women's movement are distinguished: lack of knowledge, misconceptions, or rational disagreements with its premises. The depiction of women and feminism by the media is discussed, and its impact on attitudes toward feminism is examined. Reasons for the lack of support from men, who would be expected to be somewhat sympathetic to some of the movement's aims (e.g. sex-role liberation), are also considered, along with unintentional ways that women themselves may hurt the cause of feminism. Suggestions for correcting these problems are included.

1727

King, A. Y. C. (1981). An analysis of "Jen-ching" in inter-personal relationships: A preliminary inquiry. *Proceedings of the International Conference on Sinology,* **held in Taipei, August 1980. Taipei: Academia Sinica.**

1728

King, A. Y. C., & Lee, R. P. L. (Eds.). (1981). *Social life and development in Hong Kong.* **Hong Kong: The Chinese University Press.**

1729

King, A. Y. C., & Myers, J. T. (1977). *Shame as an incomplete conception of Chinese culture: A study of face* **(Working paper No. A63-18-1-1). Hong Kong: Chinese University of Hong Kong, Social Research Center.**

1730

Kinloch, G. C. (1973). Race, socio-economic status, and social distance in Hawaii. *Sociology & Social Research, 57,* **156-167.**

Tested a typology of race groups to explain social distance in Hawaii using 2 factors, a group's position in the society's social economic strúcture and its level of cultural viability, to form the axis. 1,346 undergraduates at the University of Hawaii were administered the Bogardus Social Distance Scale as part of a larger questionnaire. Results indicate that the higher a race is on both dimensions, the more likely its members will reject individuals of other race groups. Thus, Chinese, Japanese, and Korean students showed higher levels of prejudice than Filipinos, Negroes, and Caucasians. Variations in the data suggest the relevance of political factors and kinds of racial admixture. Overall results suggest that race relations as measured by the concepts of social distance are structured by cultural and economic variables.

1731

Kinloch, G. C., & Borders, J. A. (1972). Racial stereotypes and social distance among elementary school children in Hawaii. *Sociology & Social Research, 56,* **368-377.**

Studied 293 elementary school students with regard to racial stereotypes and social distance patterns among Japanese, Chinese, and racially mixed children in Hawaii. Both stereotyping and a high degree of social distance were found. Some stereotypes were accepted while others were related to racial origin. Social distance patterns revealed low rejection of Japanese, Chinese, and Hawaiians in contrast to Caucasians, Filipinos, Negroes, and Samoans. Age, sex, and family size were associated with both stereotyping and social distance. It is concluded that racial attitudes in Hawaii in elementary school students show a clear socioeconomic hierarchy and are affected by demographic data and the setting in which they occur.

1732

Kirkpatrick, J. (1972). Some unexamined aspects of childhood association and sexual attraction in the Chinese minor marriage. *American Anthropologist, 74,* **783-784.**

1733

Kitano, H. H., & Sue, S. (1973). The model minorities. *Journal of Social Issues, 29,* **1-9.**

Presents an overview of model Asian minorities in the U.S. -- the Chinese and Japanese. Despite the increased educational, economic, and occupational opportunities for all minorities, and despite the more obvious dissatisfactions of the more vocal and less culturally conforming Blacks and Chicanos, it is considered questionable that the Asian minorities are more satisfied or more successful. Prejudice still exists in more subtle form and expectations are much higher.

1734

Kitano, H. H., & Yeung, W. T. (1982). Chinese interracial marriage. *Marriage & Family Review, 5,* **35-48.**

Examined data on the inmarriage and outmarriage patterns of the Chinese in Los Angeles County for 1975, 1977, and 1979. Outmarriage rates for these 3 yrs were 44, 49.6, and 41%, respectively. The rise from under 10% in the 1950's to over 40% in the 1970's reflects (1) internal changes in the ethnic community, most often brought about by cultural contact and acculturation, and (2) external changes, primarily a decrease in the barriers set up by other groups (e.g., prejudice and discrimination).

1735

Kitano, H. H., Yeung, W. T., Chai, L., & Hatanaka, H. (1984). Asian-American interracial marriage. *Journal of Marriage & the Family, 46,* **179-190.**

Presents data on the rates of in- and outmarriage for Chinese, Japanese, and Koreans in Los Angeles and Hawaii. Data were obtained from marriage licenses with Asian surnames. In 1979 in Los Angeles, the Japanese rates of outmarriages were the highest (60.6%), followed by the Chinese (41.2%), and the Korean (27.6%). The figures were reversed for Hawaii in 1980, with the Korean rates of outmarriage the highest (83%), followed by the Chinese (76%), then the Japanese (59%). Females of all 3 groups outmarried at a higher rate than males. A social-psychological model based on the ethnic group and its interaction with the dominant community was developed. Variables considered included historical factors, the family, the community, personal factor, and the receptivity of the dominant community. Generation was found to be the most important variable related to outmarriage, with the 3rd generation outmarrying at a higher rate than the 1st.

1736

Klatsky, A. L., Siegelaub, A. B., Landy, C., & Friedman, G. D. (1983). Racial patterns of alcoholic beverage use. *Alcoholism: Clinical & Experimental Research, 7,* **372-377.**

Reports data showing that among 59,766 persons who had routine health examinations from 1978 to 1980 at a California medical care program, the proportions of patients reporting drinking in self-classified racial groups were the following: White, 89.5%; Latin, 84.8%; Japanese, 81.9%; Black, 79.8%; Chinese, 68.1%; and Filipino, 63.9%. Men of all races reported more drinking than women. Specific data on types of alcohol consumed by sex and associations with cigarette smoking are reported.

1737

Klein, M. H., Miller, M. H., & Alexander, A. A. (1974). When young people go out in the world. In W. P. Lebra (Ed), *Mental health research in Asia and the Pacific: III. Youth, socialization, and mental health.* **Honolulu, HI: University Press of Hawaii.**

Discusses the effects of working, traveling, or studying beyond one's national or cultural boundaries, using data from studies of US and Taiwanese students. Comparisons of American and Taiwanese "ways of going out," the expectations and the actual incidence of friendship among the different students, and the causes and consequences of "not making it" in a foreign country are examined.

1738

Klein, M. H., Miller, M. H., & Alexander, A. A. (1981). The American experience of the Chinese student: On being normal in an abnormal world. In A. Kleinman & T. Y. Lin (Eds.), *Normal and abnormal behavior in Chinese culture* **(pp. 311-330). Dordrecht, Netherlands: D. Reidel.**

1739

Klein, T. W., & DeFries, J. C. (1973). Racial and cultural differences in sensitivity to flickering light. *Social Biology, 20,* **212-217.**

Examined (a) the extent of individual differences in the ability to detect flicker in a sinusoidally modulated stimulus at each of 5 frequencies and for critical flicker frequency and (b) whether population differences might account for a significant proportion of the observed variability. Ss were 12 male and 12 female undergraduates from each of 4 racial groups (Caucasian, Chinese, Japanese, and part-Hawaiian). Comparisons on 3 measures of sensitivity to flickering light suggested the possibility of genetic involvement in observed differences. Evidence consistent with a hypothesis that sensitivity at high and at low frequencies is under the control of independent mechanisms was also found.

1740

Kleinman, A., Kunstadter, P., Alexander, E. R., & Gate, J. L. (1978). *Culture and healing in Asian societies: Anthropological, psychiatric and public health studies.* **Cambridge, MA: Schenkman.**

Includes chapters on traditional and modern psychiatric care in Taiwan and problems and prospects in comparative cross-cultural medical and psychiatric studies.

1741

Kleinman, A., & Sung, L. H. (1979). Why do indigenous practitioners successfully heal? *Social Science & Medicine, 13B,* **7-26.**

In a follow-up of 12 consecutive patients of a shaman in Taiwan, 10 Ss rated themselves at least partially cured. Only the 2 cases of severe, acute somatic and psychological diseases led to negative evaluations of treatment by patients and families. The 10 improved Ss had suffered from chronic, self-limited, and masked minor psychological disorders, and behavioral or social gains were responsible for the positive evaluations. It is concluded that in most cases indigenous practitioners must heal because the treatment of disease plays a small role in the care of the disorders that are usually treated successfully. The possibility of a placebo effect in the shaman's treatment of severe, acute, and life-threatening chronic diseases is discussed.

1742

Klineherg, O. (1938). Emotional expression in Chinese literature. *Journal of Abnormal and Social Psychology, 32,* **517-520. (Reprinted in B. H. Stoodley (Ed.),** *Society and self.* **New York: Free Press of Glencoe, 1962.)**

1743

Klinger, M. R. B. (1962). Moral values across cultures. *Personnel & Guidance Journal, 41,* **139-143.**

1744

Ko, L. H. (1970). [*Value system and behavior pattern of Chinese adults in Taiwan*]. **Taipei, Taiwan: Ministry of Education, Cultural-affairs Bureau.** (In Chinese.)

1745

Koh, Y. Y. (1958, Oct.). Study of the intelligence of juvenile delinquents in Taiwan. *Democratic Review.*

1746

Koo, L. C. (1985). The (non)status of women in Chinese society [Selected papers from the 1984 Annual Conference]. *Hong Kong Psychological Society Bulletin,* **No. 14, 64-70.**

Reviews historical sources to illustrate the role of women in traditional Chinese society. The inferior and subordinate position of women was reinforced by cultural and social expectations, Confucian principles, and attitudes. The extent to which this legacy of cultural and institutionalized subordination still exists in Hong Kong is considered.

1747

Krader, L. (1968). Person and collectivity: A problem in the dialectic of anthropology. *Transactions of the New York Academy of Sciences, 30,* **856-862.**

Traces the philosophical, legal, and historical roots of the concept of person. Some peoples, such as the Eskimo and the Chukchi have neither a concept of person nor of society. Concepts of person and collectivity, as abstractions, are potentially discoverable in any society. In our culture, the externalized form of the individual has become the person, although this may not be the case in China. Legal practice tends to reify the concept of person.

1748

Kramer, J. C. (1979). Speculations on the nature and pattern of opium smoking. *Journal of Drug Issues, 9,* **247-255.**

1749

Kramers, R. P. (1963). On being polite in Chinese. *Bible Translator, 14,* **165-173.**

1750

Kriger, S. F., & Kroes, W. H. (1972). Childrearing attitudes of Chinese, Jewish, and Protestant mothers. *Journal of Social Psychology, 86,* **205-210.**

Administered the Parental Attitude Research Instrument (PARI) to 105 Jewish, Chinese, and Protestant mothers. Chinese Ss scored significantly higher than both Jewish and Protestant Ss on the PARI Control scale; no significant differences were found between Jewish and Protestant Ss' scores on Control. Contrary to predictions, no significant differences were found among the 3 groups on the PARI Rejection scale. Results are interpreted in light of cultural differences in assimilation, family structure, and childrearing attitudes.

1751

Kuchner, J. F. (1981). Chinese-American and European-American: A cross-cultural study of infant and mother. *Dissertation Abstracts International, 42,* **B1151.**

1752

Kung, L. (1976). Factory work and women in Taiwan: Changes in self-image and status. *Signs, 2,* **35-58.**

Discusses findings of informal interviews with 82 unmarried female factory workers in Taiwan. Increased participation in the labor force by young Chinese females has not resulted in a clear sense of elevated social status among them. The reasons adduced for this apparently puzzling situation center primarily on the low prestige value of factory work and the hardships of manual labor in a society that prizes educational attainment and white-collar occupations. For many young women the transition from life in their small villages to the industrialized centers is painful and demoralizing. In addition, the economic import of their labor has not increased women's influence in the family. Individual interpretation of the meaning of social change is seen as a critical factor in the understanding of that change.

1753

Kung, S. S. (1955). *Personal and professional problems of Chinese students and former students in the New York metropolitan area.* **Unpublished doctoral dissertation, Columbia University.**

1754

Kuo, C. L. (1982). Perceptions of assimilation among the Chinese in the United States. *Research in Race & Ethnic Relations, 3,* **127-143.**

Discusses the perceptions that Chinese in the US have held of their position there, traces the ways those perceptions have changed over time, and analyzes the factors that have influenced them. Three phases are distinguished in the historical development of Chinese attitudes toward their assimilation (AS) into the larger society: the period prior to World War II, from World War II to the mid-1960's, and from the mid-1960's to the present. The perceptions of 3 modern Chinese organizations--2 clubs that originated on Long Island (New York) and the Organization of Chinese Americans--are examined to illustrate the changes in Chinese attitudes that occurred in the mid-1960's and to show the role these organizations have played in the AS of their members. It is suggested that (1) AS is more than a behavioral phenomenon in that it includes an attitudinal dimension, (2) cultural AS need not precede structural AS, and (3) AS often depends on forces outside of the host nation itself.

1755

Kuo, W. (1976). Theories of migration and mental health: An empirical testing on Chinese-Americans. *Social Science & Medicine, 10,* **297-306.**

This investigation tested the applicability of four migratory theories in specifying the most stressful life changes among immigrants and the impact of these stresses on their mental health. The four theoretical notions, social isolation, cultural shock, goal striving stress, and cultural change, were explicated and tested against a data set on Chinese immigrants. The empirical evidence showed that the four theories accounted for less than a quarter of the variance of the mental impairment scores. These theories differed in explanatory utility and in some instances predicted contradictory directions for relationships between mental illness and immigration experience. The results of the study suggest the need for further cross cultural and comparative investigations dealing with the applicability of the existing migratory theories to mental illness.

1756

Kuo, Y. Y. (1971). Family constellation in the Chinese language. *Journal of Individual Psychology, 27,* **181-184.**

Although there is no word in the Chinese language which corresponds simply to "brother" or "sister", linguistic provisions are made for expressing birth-order position. Available information suggests that observations regarding the psychological significance of birth order in Western culture may be applied also to the Chinese.

1757

Kuo, Z. Y., & Lam, Y. H. (1968). Chinese religious behavior and the deification of Mao Tse-Tung. *Psychological Record, 18,* **455-468.**

Presents a survey of the development of Chinese religion and of its status immediately prior to the ascension of the communist regime to power. The manner in which Mao Tse-Tung utilized the preexisting religious base to deify himself is described. Failure of the process of deification is ascribed to the nature of Chinese religious behavior and the reactions of the masses to the failures of certain of the communist programs.

1758

Kurokawa, M. (1968). Acculturation and childhood accidents among Chinese- and Japanese-Americans. *Dissertation Abstracts International, 28,* **A4726.**

1759

Kurokawa, M. (1969). Acculturation and childhood accidents among Chinese and Japanese Americans. *Genetic Psychology Monographs, 79,* **89-159.**

Based on the previous study which indicated higher accident rates among Caucasian than among Oriental children, it was hypothesized that acculturated Oriental children are more likely to have accidents than the nonacculturated. It was also hypothesized that children who suffer from acculturation conflict are likely to incur accidents. From members of the Kaiser Hospital Prepaid Medical Plan in California, 151 Chinese and Japanese American children were selected to compose high-, medium-, and low-accident groups. Mailed questionnaires and interviews with mothers of these children provided data in support of the above hypotheses.

1760

Kwan, K. M. (1958). *Assimilation of the Chinese in the United States.* **Doctoral dissertation, University of California, Berkeley.**

1761

Lai, E. J. (1973). [*A study of decision making in Taiwan's rural families*]. **Unpublished master's thesis, National Taiwan University, Taipei.** (In Chinese.)

1762

Lam, M. P. (1980). The problems of Chinese students at the University of Illinois at Urbana-Champaign. *Dissertation Abstracts International, 40,* **A5323.**

1763

Lang, O. (1946). *Chinese family and society.* **New Haven, CT: Yale University Press.**

1764

Lao, R. C., Chuang, C. J., & Warren Lee, B. (1983). Reactions of students in Taiwan to severance of U.S. relations. *Journal of Social Psychology, 119,* **17-20.**

Surveyed the psychological reactions of 299 female and 207 male Taiwanese undergraduates concerning the abrupt 1978 move by the US to sever diplomatic relations with the Republic of China (ROC). A 14-item political attitude questionnaire was administered to Ss shortly after President Carter's announcement that he would sever relations with the ROC and establish them with the People's Republic of China. It was found that at the emotional level, Ss felt angry and depressed about this political move. At the cognitive level, however, they felt that it would lead to no substantive harm for the ROC and that some positive aspects might occur as a consequence of the new US policy. These psychological reactions were examined in relation to how much control the people believed they had over their own lives. In general, a higher sense of internal control and a lower sense of control by others were associated with a more optimistic and positive perspective. An unusual sex effect was also revealed: females and males were similar emotionally but differed cognitively in that females were more precise and analytical. Females split the issues into domestic and international concerns, whereas the males had a more general and global perspective.

1765

Lau, M. P. (1967). *An epidemiological study of narcotic addiction in Hong Kong.* **Hong Kong: Hong Kong Government Press.**

1766

Lau, S. (1982). The effect of smiling on person perception. *Journal of Social Psychology, 117,* **63-67.**

The effect of smiling on interpersonal attraction and perception was examined in a 2 (sex of perceiver) by 2 (sex of stimulus person) by 2 (facial expression) experiment. 133 Chinese college students were presented a photograph of a stimulus person either smiling or not smiling. As predicted, Ss liked a smiling person more and evaluated him/her more positively than a nonsmiling person. Ss regarded a smiling person to be more intelligent than a nonsmiling person and experienced a warmer feeling as well.

1767

Lau, S. K. (1981). Chinese familism in an urban-industrial setting: The case of Hong Kong. *Journal of Marriage & the Family, 43,* **977-992.**

Depicts the content of familism in the Chinese society in the urban-industrial setting of Hong Kong. Chinese familism has taken the form of utilitarianistic familism. This new type is characterized by (1) primacy of familial interests, (2) perception of the social-political context as the arena for the pursuit of familial interests, (3) utilitarianistic considerations in the structuring of intrafamilial relationships, (4) the nonsignificance of the social status of the familial group, (5) utilitarianistic recruitment of familial members and the resultant vagueness of the boundary of the familial group, and (6) the dilution of authority relationships between familial members. To account for the emergence of utilitarianistic familism, 3 structural factors--Chinese immigration, institutional inadequacy, and socioeconomic development-- are singled out and their relationship to utilitarianistic familism discussed. The theoretical relevance of utilitarianistic familism is elaborated by putting it into a comparative perspective.

1768

Law Reform Commission of Hong Kong. (1983). *Report on laws governing homosexual conduct* **(Topic 2). Hong Kong: Hong Kong Government Printer.**

1769

Law, S. K. (1979). Child molestation: A comparison of Hong Kong and Western findings. *Medicine, Science, & the Law, 19,* **55-60.**

A retrospective study of all defendants referred for psychiatric evaluation by the courts over a 10-year period for sexually molesting children was carried out. Offenders were more often of a young age, assaulting children in places accessible to the public and tending to resort to violent means if their demands were not met. Middle-aged and elderly offenders usually suffered from social isolation and sexual frustration and inclined to approach neighbouring children in a non-violent manner. Cases of severe disorder were few, but a significant number were labelled schizoid or of psychopathic personality. The characteristics of the victims closely resembled those described in Western series. Fondling was the commonest offending act, but intercrural and attempted vaginal intercourses were also frequent.

1770

Law, T. T. (1974). **Differential childrearing attitudes and practices of Chinese-American mothers.** *Dissertation Abstracts International, 34,* **A4406.**

1771

Lazure, D. (1962). **The family and youth in New China: Psychiatric observations.** *Canadian Medical Association Journal, 86,* **179-183.**

1772

Lebra, T. S. (1973). **Compensative justice and moral investment among Japanese, Chinese, and Koreans.** *Journal of Nervous and Mental Disease, 157,* **278-291.**

1773

Lee, C. (1981). **Values and conflict: A deontic assertion analysis as applied to Chinese leadership, 1956-1965.** *Dissertation Abstracts International, 42,* **A2282.**

1774

Lee, C. C. (1985). **Acculturation and value change: Chinese immigrant women.** *Dissertation Abstracts International, 45,* **A3586-3587.**

1775

Lee, J. (1977). **Patterns of mental ability in Chinese children reared in the United States and in the Republic of China.** *Dissertation Abstracts International, 38,* **A2667.**

1776

Lee, M. C. (1977). **The effect of just and unjust punishment on the imitation of aggression.** *National Chengchi University Journal^ (Taipei), 36, 93-105.*

1777

Lee, P. H. (1986). **[Changes in stereotypes toward other ethnic or national groups among students at National Taiwan University during eighteen years]. In H. Y. Chiu & Y. H. Chang (Eds.), [Social and cultural change in Taiwan]** *(Monograph Series B, No. 16, Vol. 2, pp. 513-554). Taipei: Academia Sinica, Institute of Ethnology. (In Chinese.)*

1778

Lee, R. (1952). **Acculturation of Chinese Americans. Sociology and Social Research, 36,** *319-321.*

This paper is a discussion about three groups into which most Americans of Chinese descent and non-American Chinese living in America can be placed. Various degrees of acculturation are shown among them. It is concluded that, while most of them have become Americanized, only a slow and painful process will tell whether they can ever become Americans.

1779

Lee, R. H. (1960). **The Chinese in the United States of America.** *Hong Kong: Hong Kong University Press.*

1780

Lee, R. P. L. (1985). **Social stress and coping behavior in Hong Kong. In W. S. Tseng & D. Y. H. Wu (Eds.), Chinese culture and mental health** *(pp. 193-214). Orlando, FL: Academic Press.*

1781

Lehman, P. E. (1972). **Some comments on witches, heresy, and the "dope fiend" mythology. Drug Forum, 1,** *177-185.*

Traces the development of the term "dope fiend" to the Christian missionaries in China during the 1800's. The relationship between the dope fiend concepts, witchcraft, and social heresy is examined. Antinarcotic legislation is considered as symbolic rather than instrumental in purpose.

1782

Lei, T., & Yang, K. S. (1986). **[Changes in values among university students: Twenty years later]. In H. Y. Chiu & Y. H. Chang (Eds.), [Social and cultural change in Taiwan]** *(Monograph Series B, No. 16, Vol. 2, pp. 479-511). Taipei: Academia Sinica, Institute of Ethnology. (In Chinese.)*

1783

Leifer, A. (1972). **Ethnic patterns in cognitive tasks. Dissertation Abstracts International, 33,** *B1270-1271.*

This thesis compared Chinese, Italian, Negro and Puerto Rican disadvantaged 4 yr. old Head Start students on tests of constructional ability, ability to copy geometric forms, verbal ideational fluency and understanding of parts of the body.

1784

Leon, J. J. (1975). Sex-ethnic marriage in Hawaii: A nonmetric multidimensional analysis. Journal of Marriage & the Family, 37, *775-781.*

High ethnic intermarriage rates have long been characteristic of Hawaii. These rates have often been pointed to as another indicator of assimilation in these islands. This analysis explores the dimensions of ethnic in- and intermarriage for 2 time periods: 1948-1953 (N=33,798) and 1965-1969 (N=38,120). The common elements that predispose males and females to marry in and out of their ethnic groups were examined. Utilizing a mapping sentence and nonmetric multidimensional analysis, sex and ethnicity of the marriage partners were mapped into the same structural space for each time period. Findings, depicted spatially, show 2 general clusters. One cluster consists of Japanese, Chinese, and Korean males and females (East); the other consists of Caucasian, part-Hawaiian, Hawaiian, Filipino, and Puerto Rican (West) males and females. Findings suggest that the East cluster ethnic groups, regardless of sex, prefer other East cluster ethnic groups and vice versa. In general, this interpretation lends support to the idea of social homogamy on a broader level than ethnicity.

1785

Leonetti, D. L. (1978). The biocultural pattern of Japanese-American fertility. Social Biology, 25, *38-51.*

A comparison of age-specific fertility data on 2nd-generation Japanese-American women with published data on modern and premodern women in Japan and with data on modern US White women shows the persistence of a fertility pattern among all Japanese groups. This pattern was significantly different from that of US Whites. It appears that continuity in certain family and kinship elements has played a central role in the persistence of this pattern. In addition, it is suggested that the introduction of modern contraceptive techniques may have the consequence of merely intensifying a cultural pattern of fertility, rather than changing its basic outlines.

1786

Leong, F. T., Tseng, W. S., & Wu, D. Y. (1985). Cross-cultural variations in stressful life events: A preliminary study [Special Issue: Attitudes toward counseling and mental health in non-Western societies]. American Mental Health Counselors Association Journal, 7, *72-77.*

Using qualitative responses from five psychiatrists and one psychologist from Japan, Korea, Indonesia, Thailand, Shanghai, and Mainland China, cross-cultural variations in stressful life events were assessed. The most stressful life events for the subjects from the different countries were, respectively, interpersonal problems in one's company, conflicts with family members, marital problems caused by the caste system, divorce or infidelity, housing shortages, and death of a close family member. The cross-cultural variations in life events perceived as stressful illustrate the need for the empirical study of the influence of culture on the experience of stress.

1787

Leong, J. H. K. (1974 Oct-Dec). Cross cultural influences on ideas about drugs. Bulletin on Narcotics, 26, *1-7.*

1788

Leung, E. (1985). Family support and postnatal emotional adjustment. Bulletin of the Hong Kong Psychological Society, *No. 14, 32-46.*

The author questioned the general view that postnatal emotional changes are mental illnesses rather than adjustments made by women to motherhood. Clinicians and researchers generally view the absence of negative reactions as a sign of good adjustment. The present study emphasized the role of family and social support in helping the woman cope with motherhood. A study of 35 new mothers' reactions to motherhood was carried out in which interviews with the women and their ratings of the social support given by various significant others were conducted. Results indicated that family support was important in postnatal adjustment. Women who received support from their families were likely to be less anxious and depressed than women who did not receive such support. Husbands were the most important source of assistance and emotional empathic understanding. Lack of marital support was correlated with depressed mood. The support network per se was critical; new mothers were emotionally upset by the knowledge that they were not receiving support. The role of family support as both a stressor and a buffer in postnatal experience was discussed.

1789

Leung, K., & Bond, M. H. (1982). How Chinese and Americans reward task-related contributions: A preliminary study. Psychologia: An International Journal of Psychology in the Orient, 25, *32-39.*

In light of G. Hofstede's (1980) dimension of individualism-collectivism, it was predicted that Chinese would be more moderate in their overt responses than Americans. 60 Chinese and American male undergraduates were presented with a scenario in which the target person (TP) either facilitated or hindered his group's completion of a class project. In their overt reactions to the TP, both cultural groups were rewarding to the helpful TP and punitive toward the unhelpful one. As predicted, the Chinese were less rewarding to the helpful TP and less punitive toward the unhelpful TP than were American Ss. It is suggested that this tendency toward moderation in the overt Chinese reaction supports group harmony and integrity. Future studies varying socioemotional as well as task inputs are discussed in relation to a pan-cultural model of equity in social exchange.

1790

Leung, K., & Bond, M. H. (1984). The impact of cultural collectivism on reward allocation. Journal of Personality & Social Psychology, 47, *793-804.*

It is argued that the collectivism of a culture leads to different styles of reward allocation with in-group and out-group members. Two studies using Chinese and American subjects examined this issue. In the first study an out-group situation was used, in which subjects were led to believe that they worked with a partner whom they would not meet, to obtain a group reward. The collectivistic Chinese subjects were found to follow the equity norm more closely in dividing the group reward than the individualistic American subjects when pressure of social evaluation was removed. In the second study Chinese and American subjects read a scenario in which an allocator who divided the group reward equally with an in-group member more and regarded such an allocation as fairer. When subjects were asked to assume that they were the allocator and to hypothetically divide the reward, Chinese subjects followed the equity norm more closely than did American subjects when the recipient was an out-group member or when the subjects' input was low. However, when the subjects' input was high and the recipient was an in-group member, Chinese subjects followed the equality norm more than did American subjects. These findings are discussed in terms of the desire for maintaining group solidarity in a collectivist culture.

1791

Leung, K., & Lind, E. A. (1986). Procedural justice and culture: Effects of culture, gender, and investigator status on procedural preferences. Journal of Personality & Social Psychology, 50, *1134-1140.*

Sixty Chinese and 66 American undergraduates were asked to indicate their preferences for using adversary and nonadversary procedures of dispute resolution. Subjects read a dispute scenario and description of the two procedures, rated the preference for each procedure, gave reasons for their rating, and completed rating scales assessing their perceptions of each procedure on several dimensions. Two additional factors included in the design were: the status of the investigator in the dispute resolution procedure and the gender of the subject. Results showed that American subjects in general preferred the adversary procedure, and the Chinese subjects were in general indifferent about the two procedures. Status of investigator and gender of subject interacted in their effects of American subjects' preferences, but did not affect Chinese subjects' preferences. Results suggested that the Chinese subjects might have perceived the process control afforded them by the adversary procedure to be desirable, but that the confrontation and competitiveness inherent in this procedure might have mitigated their preference for it.

1792

Lew, W. J. F. (1979). A Chinese woman intellectual: Family, education, and personality. Education Journal *(Hong Kong), 7, 166-197.*

1793

Lewis, M. (1982). Aging in the People's Republic of China. International Journal of Aging & Human Development, 15, *79-105.*

Examines the treatment of the elderly in China, particularly under the Communist regime. The 1949 Revolution in China brought major changes for the elderly including (1) an ideal of greater egalitarianism among generations, (2) growing economic security for the elderly, and (3) changes in family structure as areas were communalized and families dispersed. One function of the elderly in China is the promoted practice of lecturing on the hardships of the old (prerevolutionary) days. Another change has been the liberation of women from bondage to men. The government is attempting to provide retirement security for workers, promote community life, run homes for family-less retired persons, establish an inexpensive medical care system, promote physical fitness, and treat senility on an outpatient basis and as a physiological disorder--all changes that would benefit their rapidly growing number of elderly.

1794

Li, F. C. (1955). A study of the heterosexual social life of a single male Chinese college student in New York City. *Unpublished doctoral dissertation, Columbia University, New York.*

1795

Li, M. C. (1981). [The construction of Sex Trait Inventory and the comparisons of four sex trait categories on achievement motive and attitudes toward marriage, career and sex]. Acta Psychologica Taiwanica, 23, *23-37. (In Chinese.)*

On the basis of 191 male and female college students' judgments, and testing of reliability and validity, the Li Sex Trait Inventory (LSTI) was constructed. In LSTI there are 20 masculine items of instrumental characteristics and 20 feminine items of expressive characteristics. All of these items are of positive social desirability. 502 male and female college students were tested with LSTI, Family Orientation and Working Orientation Scale and Marriage, Sex Attitude Scale. It was found that students with high masculine traits had high mastery motivation in spite of his or her sex. Generally speaking, males were highly competitive, but androgynous female students were as competitive as most male students. Male and female students with undifferentiated sex traits were less likely to work and lack competition. There was no significant difference on "fear of success" between male and female students and among students of four sex trait categories. Females were more conservative than males on attitudes toward virginity and sexuality, but were more liberal than males on attitudes toward a woman's independent status in the family and marriage relationship.

1796

Li, M. C. (1983). [Like, love and premarital sexual permissiveness between both sexes]. Acta Psychologica Taiwanica, 25, *121-135. (In Chinese.)*

The first part of this study was an investigation of characteristics that were important for attracting members of the opposite sex. Both male and female college subjects showed traditional sex stereotyping; characteristics important for females to possess were more consistent than those important for males to possess. Females' expectations of males were higher than males' expectations of themselves. It was found in the second part of this study that factors of love and like were different from each other. Male and female subjects with intimate opposite-sex friends gave higher scores on the love factor for these friends than for their ordinary opposite-sex friends. There was a significant difference between the scores on the like factor for intimate and ordinary opposite-sex friends as judged by the female, but not male, subjects. The third part of the study showed that the degree of premarital sex permissiveness was higher for male subjects than for female subjects, and higher for female subjects with intimate boy friends than for those without intimate boy friends. The premarital sex permissiveness of male seniors was higher than that of lower-grade college students.

1797

Li, W. L., & Liu, S. S. (1975). Ethnocentrism among American and Chinese youth. Journal of Social Psychology, 95, *277-278.*

Simultaneously administered questionnaires requiring ratings of 33 adjectives describing a national character to 296 American and 265 Chinese (Taiwanese) undergraduates. American Ss perceived the Chinese much more favorably than their own group, but a reciprocal pattern was not observed among the Chinese Ss.

1798

Li, W. L., & Yu, L. (1974). Interpersonal contact and racial prejudice: A comparative study of American and Chinese students. Sociological Quarterly, 15, *559-566.*

Data from 298 US and 261 Taiwanese undergraduates indicated that: (a) Family socioeconomic status was significantly related to cross-national contact among both the Americans and Chinese, (b) increased contact did not linearly reduce prejudice for both the Americans and Chinese, and (c) family socioeconomic status was more important than interpersonal contact in its relation to prejudice.

1799

Li, Y. Y. (1966). [Comparative evaluations of Chinese culture by overseas Chinese students in Taiwan]. Bulletin of the Institute of Ethnology *(Academia Sinica),* **21,** *215-231. (In Chinese.)*

1800

Li, Y. Y., Yang, K. S., & Wen, C. I. (Eds.). (1985). [Collected essays on modernization and sinicization]. *Taipei: Kuei Kuan. (In Chinese.)*

1801

Lieh-Mak, F., Luk, S. L., & Chung, S. Y. (1985). Child abuse: A review. Journal of the Hong Kong Psychiatric Association, 5, *18-19, 22-25.*

1802

Lieh-Mak, F., O'Hoy, K. M., & Luk, S. L. (1983). Lesbianism in the Chinese of Hong Kong. Archives of Sexual Behavior, 12, *21-30.*

Discusses some historical and literary background regarding lesbianism in China. Data on demographic information, family background, and behavioral characteristics of 15 Chinese lesbians (aged 19-61 yrs) were collected by means of semi-structured interviews and compared with a matched group of married women. It was found that more lesbians were adopted, reported unhappy childhoods and hostile family atmospheres, had parents who preferred them to be boys, and attended sexually segregated schools. Ss differed from their Western counterparts in having a closer relationship with their mothers and in the absence of oral sexual practice.

1803

Lieh-Mak, F., & Tam, W. Y. K. (1981). Hong Kong married abortion applicants: A comparison with married women who elect to complete their pregnancy. Journal of Biosocial Science, 13, *71-80.*

1804

Lifton, R. J. (1956). Thought reform of Chinese intellectuals: A psychiatric evaluation. Journal of Asian Studies, 16, *75-88. (Republished in* **Journal of Social Issues,** *1957,* **13,** *5-20.)*

1805

Lifton, R. J. (1961). Thought reform and the psychology of totalism: A study of "brain washing" in China. *New York: Norton. (Also published by Harmondsworth: Penguin.)*

Research in Hong Kong, 1954-55, is the basis for case studies of Western and Chinese subjects from Communist China. Varying degrees of response to thought control techniques are described. Attitude-change "according to an imposed ideological myth" is contrasted with "open" personal change, "a commitment made autonomously and in the face of alternatives." The menace of thought control is stressed. The appendix contains the confession obtained from a Chinese intellectual.

1806

Lifton, R. J. (1976). Revolutionary immortality: Mao Tse-tung and the Chinese Cultural Revolution. *New York: W. W. Norton.*

Discusses revolution in general, and the Cultural Revolution in Communist China in particular, from a psychological and psychohistorical viewpoint. The thesis of the 1st edition (1968) is reaffirmed: The concept of revolutionary immortality is an ongoing sense of continuing evolution and revolution in culture and thought processes which connects the individual and the culture to man's general past and future. It is a "shared sense of participating in permanent revolutionary fermentation and of transcending individual death by living on indefinitely within the continuing revolution".

1807

Lin, C. C. (1979). [Political attitudes and participation behavior in college students in Taiwan]. *Unpublished master's thesis, National Taiwan University, Taipei. (In Chinese.)*

1808

Lin, H. T. (1976). [Familial correlates of vocational choice attitudes of junior high school students]. Journal of the Taiwan Provincial College of Education, 1, *79-108. (In Chinese.)*

1809

Lin, I. M. (1977). [Multidimensional self-attribution attitude scale]. Psychological Testing, 24, *46-51. (In Chinese.)*

1810

Lin, M. J. (1982). [Teachers' and psychologists' attitudes toward the behavior problems of children]. Journal of Education and Psychology, 5, *281-307. (In Chinese.)*

The Wickman's questionnaire was administered to 34 psychologists and 560 junior high school teachers. The results were: (1) There were significant differences between teachers' and psychologists' attitudes toward both the behavior problems of children and the general types of behavior problems. (2) Although the similarity between the general attitudes of male and female teachers toward the behavior problems of children was high, male teachers considered some behaviors as more serious problems than did female teachers. (3) The general attitudes of different age groups of teachers and different teaching experiences toward the behavior problems of children were similar; there were some differences in terms of which behaviors presented more serious problems. (4) The general attitudes of various positions of teachers toward the behavior problems of children were similar.

1811

Lin, M. J. (1983). [An investigation of college students of social distance of the exceptional children]. Journal of Education & Psychology, 6, *55-73. (In Chinese.)*

This study investigated the social distance of the exceptional college student. The Jones' paired comparisons questionnaire was administered to 493 college students. The results were: (1) The average and the gifted comprised the most acceptable groups in most situations. The severely mentally retarded and the delinquent comprised the unacceptable end of the psychological continuum in most interpersonal situations. The mild incapacitations were generally higher on the acceptance continuum. (2) As the level of intimacy increased to a willingness to marry, most college students would accept the average and the gifted. (3) There was no significant difference between the students who had taken psychology courses dealing with exceptional children and those who had not taken these courses.

1812

Lin, N., Ensel, W. M, Simeone, R. S., & Kuo, W. (1979). Social support, stressful life events, and illness: A model and an empirical test. Journal of Health & Social Behavior, 20, *108-119.*

The effects of social support and stressors (stressful life events) on illness (psychiatric symptoms) are examined in a model with data from a representative sample of the Chinese-American adult population in Washington, D.C. The analysis shows that, as expected, stressors are positively related to the incidence of psychiatric symptoms, and social support is negatively related to psychiatric symptoms. Further, the contribution of social support to predicting symptoms is greater in magnitude than that of stressful life events. When marital status and occupational prestige are incorporated into the model, the significant (negative) contribution of social support to symptoms is not reduced. Implications for the theoretical development of a sociomedical theory of illness are discussed.

1813

Lin, P. C. (1979). [Relationship between attribution and adjustment in junior high school students]. Acta Psychologica Taiwanica, 21, *61-73. (In Chinese.)*

The purpose of this study was to investigate the relationship between the attribution and the personal and social adjustment of junior high school students. The subjects were 280 second graders (146 boys and 134 girls) from two Taipei junior high schools. Hung-Yang's Attribution Scale and the California Test of Personality were used as research instruments. The data obtained were statistically treated by principal component analysis and step-wise multiple regression. The main findings of the study were: (1) There were two common factors in the eight attribution variables. Interaction effects among kinds of attribution, sex, and the nature of events were found. (2) Internal attribution for positive events was positively correlated with personal and social adjustment, but internal attribution for negative events was negatively correlated with adjustment. (3) External attributions for positive events and for negative events have negative correlations with personal and social adjustment. (4) The practices of combining different attribution scores into subtotals may reduce the relationship between these scores and adjustment.

1814

Lin, P. C. (1981). [The relationship of sex typing to self defensiveness, life adjustment, and cognitive measures]. Acta Psychologica Taiwanica, 23, *107-129. (In Chinese.)*

Data on seven variables were obtained from 486 students in junior high schools in Taipei city: positive and negative masculinity and femininity, personal adjustment, social adjustment, self-defensiveness, dogmatism, creativity, and Piagetian formal operational thought and concrete operational thought. Analysis of variance and canonical correlation analysis were used to analyze relations between sex typing and the above variables. The main findings were: (1) Among four positive sex-role types, the androgynous person had better life adjustment than the undifferentiated person, but the differences between the androgynous and the masculine or the feminine individuals were small. (2) Among four negative sex-role types, the androgynous person had worse life adjustment than the undifferentiated person, and the differences among the androgynous, the masculine, and the feminine individuals were very small. (3) Measures of sex-role inventory were significantly correlated with self-defensiveness. The positive androgynous and the negative undifferentiated individuals made more untrue responses than the other sex-role types. The implications of these findings to theories of androgyny were discussed.

1815

Lin, R. K. (1983). Parent-child relationships among the Chinese in San Francisco. Dissertation Abstracts International, 43, *A3532.*

1816

Lin, R. M. (1983). Differences in meanings of cultural values between the Nationalist Revolution and the Communist Revolution in contemporary China. Dissertation Abstracts International, 43, *B3411.*

1817

Lin, T. H. (1978). [A study on the Changhwa country residents attitudes toward physical education]. Journal of the Taiwan Provincial College of Education, 3, *205-240. (In Chinese.)*

1818

Lin, T. Y., & Lin, M. C. (1981). Love, denial, and rejection: Responses of Chinese family to mental illness. In A. Kleinman & T. Y. Lin (Eds.), Normal and abnormal behavior in Chinese culture *(pp. 387-401). Dordrecht, Netherlands: Reidel.*

1819

Lin, W. T. (1966). Chinese value orientation in Hong Kong. Sociological Analysis, 27, *53-66.*

1820

Lind, A. W. (1958). Adjustment patterns among the Jamaican Chinese. Social & Economic Studies, 7, *144-164.*

1821

Lindgren, H. C., & Yu, R. (1975). Cross-cultural insight and empathy among Chinese immigrants to the United States. Journal of Social Psychology, 96, *305-306.*

Identified correlates of cross-cultural sensitivity, insight, or empathy that 91 17-66 yr old Chinese immigrants living in San Francisco develop with respect to their host culture. Results show that cultural understanding is likely to be enhanced by increased exposure to a host culture, and that education in the homeland is positively correlated with social sophistication and a sharpened awareness of social behavior patterns.

1822

Li-Repac, D. C. (1983). The impact of acculturation on the child-rearing attitudes and practices of Chinese-American families: Consequences for the attachment process. Dissertation Abstracts International, 43, *B2695.*

1823

Liu, A. P. (1980). The ideology and personality of the radical left in the People's Republic of China. Political Psychology, 2, *3-21.*

Analyzed the context, ideology, and personality of 4 Chinese Communist leftists (Mao Tse-tung, Chiang Ch'ing, Chang Ch'ung-ch'iao, and Yao Wen-yuan). Three contextual factors that gave rise to the leftists are (1) alienation of Mao from the Communist Party, (2) anxiety of a group of middle-level propagandists about the post-Mao era, and (3) disaffection of the public. The ideology of the leftists warns about the danger of "bourgeois restoration" and calls on China to return to the spirit of the revolutionary time before 1949. The radicalism of Mao, Chiang, Chang, and Yao is seen as a combination of personal need and "social molding".

1824

Liu, C. Y., & Yang, K. S. (1976). [A comparative test of four mathematical models of birth intention]. Acta Psychologica Taiwanica, 18, *149-168. (In Chinese.)*

132 suburban Chinese housewives participated in a study that tested four mathematical models of birth intention. The reliability of one model over the other three is demonstrated.

1825

Liu, I. M., & Huang, H. J. (1979). [Cognitive structure and a change in attitude toward the goal of taking a job]. Acta Psychologica Taiwanica, 21, *35-39. (In Chinese.)*

A group of subjects were surveyed for their goals in taking jobs (Study 1). Another group of subjects rank ordered eight main goals in taking jobs and were tested for the attitude strength of their three main goals. It was found that the rank ordering of their goals was consistent with the strength of their attitude (Study 2). Two months later, the same group of subjects in Study 2 read a story describing a botanist's achievement through years of hard work, and rank-ordered the main goals from the botanist's standpoint as well as from their own (Study 3). It was found that subjects' attitude toward the goal of taking a job was similar to the attitude of the botanist in the story, possibly due to vicarious reinforcement.

1826

Liu, W. (1964, January). Values and social relations in China: A reappraisal. *Paper presented at the seminar Personality and Motivation in Chinese Society, Bermuda.*

1827

Liu, W. (1964, January). Family interactions and values: A study of refugees and non-refugee families in Hong Kong by the R.D. method. *Paper presented at the seminar Personality and Motivation in Chinese Society, Bermuda.*

1828

Liu, W. T. (1966). Chinese value orientations in Hong Kong. Sociological Analysis, 27, *53-66.*

1829

Liu, W. T. (1966). Family interactions among local and refugee Chinese families in Hong Kong. Journal of Marriage and the Family, 28, *314-323.*

1830

Liu, W. T., & Yu, E. S. H. (1977). Variations in women's roles and family life under the socialist regime in China. Journal of Comparative Family Studies, 8, *201-215.*

Beyond the simple dichotomy of urban and rural China there are other significant factors which could be expected to have an impact on fertility behavior but which have not been adequately or sufficiently analyzed. Some of these factors are: the genuine desire of the Chinese to push for sex-role equality and to equalize opportunities, the possible emergence of a new form of conjugal relations in the family, the reported increase in labor participation of married women, commune organization, and the structure of urban neighborhoods, among others. The authors concern themselves with the ways in which these factors are articulated with the family system, the economic structure, and the sociopolitical context in China. They wish to examine the economic motivation of women's participation in the labor force and some of the factors that are conducive to women's ascendance to political leadership roles. They look at the requisites of the kinship structure, housing conditions, coresidence patterns and other factors external to the family and assess their implications on women's roles, fertility behavior, and family life in China.

1831

Lo, C. F. (1942). Moral judgments of Chinese students. Journal of Abnormal and Social Psychology, 37, *264-269.*

1832

Locksley, A., Hepburn, C., & Ortiz, V. (1982). On the effects of social stereotypes on judgments of individuals: A comment on Grant and Holmes's "The integration of implicit personality theory schemas and stereotypic images". Social Psychology Quarterly, 45, *270-273.*

P. R. Grant and J. G. Holmes investigated the effects of stereotypic beliefs about Chinese and Irishmen on judgments of individuals. They concluded that social stereotypes strongly influence judgments even when case information is available. This conclusion runs counter to the results of experiments by the 1st author et al, which demonstrate that the presence of case information significantly and substantially reduces effects of stereotypes on judgments of individuals. The present authors contend that this apparent difference in results is not real. It is established that the design of Grant and Holmes's study does not permit evaluation of the argument advanced by Locksley et al, thus precluding comparisons between the 2 sets of data. Moreover, reanalyses of the Grant and Holmes data demonstrate that their Ss relied more heavily on case information than on social category information to make target judgments and did not adjust the weight they assigned to case information as a function of social category information.

1833

London, I. D. (1974). The revenge of heaven: A brief methodological account. Psychological Reports, 34, *1023-1030.*

Presents a chronological account of the psychopolitical research that lead to The Revenge of Heaven: Journal of a Young Chinese, K. Ling's idiographic study of China's Cultural Revolution. The underlying methodological rationale of using literary techniques and conceptions in group-dependent, as a way of reconstituting perceived reality from the data is discussed.

1834

London, I. D., & Lee, T. L. (1977). Socio/psycholinguistics of the cultural revolution: An empirical study. Psychological Reports, 40, *343-356.*

Sample analyses are provided to show how political terms in vogue during China's Cultural Revolution developed colloquial meanings at variance with the official "dictionary". Responses to these terms made by 56 respondents, most of whom were under 30 yrs of age and were at that time in Kwangtung and Fukien Provinces, constitute the empirical data. A methodology with anthropological overtones is developed to meet the exigencies of handling such data.

1835

London, I. D., & London, M. B. (1975). Rumor as a footnote to Chinese national character. Psychological Reports, 37, *343-349.*

Details a case study of an odd rumor, widely current in China after Nixon's visit. Based on interviews of respondents from Kwangtung and Fukien Provinces, an examination of the stabler aspects of this rumor not only points to its probable source, but also reveals 2 traditional components of Chinese national character.

1836

Long, F. Y., & Lee, M. M. (1974). Some psychosocial characteristics of sexual reassignment requestors in Singapore: A report on 23 cases. Medical Journal of Malaysia, 28, *208-212.*

1837

Loo, C., & Mar, D. (1982). Desired residential mobility in a low income ethnic community: A case study of Chinatown. Journal of Social Issues, 38, *95-106.*

Interviewed 108 Chinese Americans about desired residential mobility in Chinatown to investigate social theories of urban location regarding ethnic settlement and neighborhood homogeneity. Results underscore the importance of social and environmental contributors to the desire to move: age, class, perceptions of crowding, and attitudes toward ethnic homogeneity. Neighborhood homogeneity occurred along these lines as well. Both class and ethnicity were determinants of residential location.

1838

Loveridge, D. (1982). Communication between people. Hong Kong Psychological Society Bulletin, *No. 9, 19-26.*

In this paper presented at the 1982 Annual Conference of the Hong Kong Psychological Society, the author discusses client-therapist communication and cross-cultural work on familial communication. Western familial communication is compared to that of Chinese, Vietnamese, and Thai communication. Work with Vietnamese refugees is briefly presented.

1839

Lu, L. G. et al. (1986). [A study of the mental state of 100 recipients of oviductligation for sterilization]. Chinese Journal of Neurology and Psychiatry, 19, *329-331. (In Chinese.)*

This is a study of 100 recipients of oviductligation for sterilization, with special reference to their mental state before, during, and after the operation, and to the relation between their personality characteristics and the emergence of psychosomatic complications. It was found that 68 of the patients were willing to receive the operation; 96% felt nervous and fearful. The recipients with weak characters developed psychosomatic complications more easily.

1840

Lu, Y. H. (1972). [A study of farmers' learning aspiration in Taiwan]. Bulletin of the Institute of Ethnology *(Academia Sinica), No. 34, 99-118. (In Chinese.)*

1841

Lu, Y. H. (1980). [Women's attitudes toward career role and family role in Taiwan's social change]. Bulletin of the Institute of Ethnology *(Academia Sinica), No. 50, 25-66. (In Chinese.)*

The present study was an attempt to explore women's attitudes to changing roles as a result of social changes. A sample of 293 women from 20 to 60 years old in Taiwan were studied in an islandwide survey. The results indicated that most women took a multiple-role perspective. The family role and the career role were regarded as equally important. It was found that education was more important in contributing to different attitudes to the career role than to the family role, whereas social-environmental factors were more significant to attitudes toward the family role. It appears that women's attitudes toward the two different roles are independent of each other. In addition, the data on attitudes toward employment suggests that most of the women aspire to be employed. As a compromise to the inherent role conflict, most of them suggested an interrupted career plan according to their family life cycle.

1842

Luce, T. S. (1974). The role of experience in inter-racial recognition. Personality & Social Psychology Bulletin, 1, *39-41.*

75 Black and 72 White undergraduates, all of whom attended a university, had lived all their lives in the Southwest, and had no previous interactions with Chinese or Japanese persons, and 65 Chinese and 60 Japanese undergraduates, all of whom attended school and lived in a multi-ethnic setting, studied photographs of members of these 4 racial groups and then were given a recognition test on them. All 4 groups of Ss displayed the "own-race" phenomenon (i.e., they performed best on own-race photos), and there were no other significant findings.

1843

Luce, T. S. (1974). Blacks, whites and yellows: They all look alike to me. Psychology Today, 8, *105-108.*

Compared black, white, Chinese, and Japanese college students in terms of their ability to select photographs of faces already seen from photographs not previously seen. The photographs were of individuals from the same 4 racial/ethnic groups as the Ss. Blacks could recognize blacks, whites, and, to a lesser extent, Orientals. Orientals could recognize fellow Orientals and, to a lesser extent, blacks. Experience with members of other races does not explain the pattern of these findings, since neither the blacks nor the whites had had experience with Orientals, but the Oriental Ss had had experience with both blacks and whites.

1844

Lynn, R. (1977). The intelligence of the Chinese and Malays in Singapore. Mankind Quarterly, 18, *125-128.*

Presents data for the Raven Progressive Matrices for samples of 13-yr-old Chinese and Malay schoolboys. In relation to British norms, Chinese Ss obtained a mean IQ of 110, Malay Ss of 96. Implications of these means and of the Chinese-Malay differences are discussed.

1845

Ma, M. C. (1986). [Application of a fuzzy statistic approach to the evaluation of the seriousness of offenses]. Information on Psychological Sciences, *No. 4, 10-16. (In Chinese.)*

The Multistage Evaluation Method based on a fuzzy model of category judgment was used to explore the relationship between the amount stolen and seriousness of offense, as estimated by law enforcement officials, students, and criminals. It has been shown consistently that the logarithmic function is applicable to the description of this relationship. However, in the present study there was a statistically significant difference between criminals and law enforcement officials in the speed of increase of the function, whereas there was no significant difference between law enforcement officials and students in this respect.

1846

Mading, K. (1968). Research on family values and culture change in Hong Kong's modern Chinese novels. Journal of the Hong Kong Branch of the Royal Asiatic Society, 8, *154-156*

1847

Mahdihassan, S. (1980). Chinese origin of the word alcohol. American Journal of Chinese Medicine, 8, *239-244.*

1848

Mandel, D. E. (1982). Aspects of the adaptive process in migration: The Chinese in Canada. Dissertation Abstracts International, 43, *B509.*

1849

Marquette, J. F. (1981). A logistic diffusion model of political mobilization. Political Behavior, 3, *7-30.*

Previous studies have argued that a predisposition toward political mobilization is based on a high level of individual identity anxiety. The present study suggests a simplification of the theory of political mobilization that treats the ideology of a mobilizing agent as an innovation. The process of political mobilization is then treated as a process of innovation diffusion. The theory is tested using extended time series for 7 societies: the US, Britain, USSR, Sweden,

Nazi Germany, Fascist Italy, and the People's Republic of China.

1850

Marsella, A. J., DeVos, G., & Hsu, F. L. K. (Eds.). (1985). Culture and self: Asian and Western perspectives. *New York: Tavistock.*

1851

Marsella, A. J., Murray, M. D., & Godlen, C. (1974). Ethnic variations in the phenomenology of emotions: I. Shame. Journal of Cross-Cultural Psychology, 5, *312-328.*

Investigated ethnic variations in the connotative meaning of emotions, using as Ss 324 American college students of Japanese, Chinese, and European ancestry. Ss were administered a 20-scale semantic differential for various emotions including shame. Results were factor analyzed and yielded the following dimensions: Evaluative, Dynamism, Synesthesia, Awareness, Arousal, and Intensity. Results show ethnic group differences in the endorsement pattern of the different scales and in the factorial structures. The concept of "shame" is discussed and related to the cultural traditions of the ethnic groups studied. Implications for ethnopsychiatry are noted.

1852

Marsh, R. M. (1971). The explanation of occupational prestige hierarchies. Social Forces, 50, *214-222.*

The ranking of occupational prestige in Taiwan is highly similar to that in the United States and the numerous other societies both modernized and relatively nonmodernized in which such studies have been conducted. Previous explanations of this important cross-societal invariant, occupational prestige evaluation, have emphasized common structural features of any complex society, whether industrialized or not. It is not clear how this proposition can be empirically falsified. A more satisfactory explanation is sought in terms of specific properties of occupational roles in any society, i.e., education, responsibility (or authority), and income. The relationship of each of these variables to prestige is analyzed, using data from Taiwan, Denmark, and the United States.

1853

Matejko, A. (1970). Task versus status: The contradiction of modernization. Revue Internationale de Sociologie, 6, *329-354.*

Based on social systems theory, equilibrium between task and status orientations is described as critical to social change. Elitist and egalitarian models are presented for both task and status orientations, e.g., American capitalist democracy is described as a combined model, task-oriented elitist and status-oriented egalitarian. Modernization is furthered by a task orientation bolstered by the development of education and mass media and retarded by a rigid status orientation. The model is applied to underdeveloped nations including Ethiopia, China, Africa, and Cuba.

1854

Maykovich, M. (1971). White-yellow stereotypes: An empirical study. Pacific Sociological Review, 14, *447-467.*

1855

Maykovich, M. (1972). Reciprocity in racial stereotypes: White, black and yellow. American Journal of Sociology, 77, *867-897.*

1856

McCauley, C. (1982). More about thought reform. American Psychologist, 37, *102-103.*

Criticizes J. A. Barlow's contention that although mass-line leadership is manipulative, it is not simply authoritarian or dictatorial and may even have an advantage for the followers not often achieved in political democracies. It is argued that Barlow's comparison of mass leadership with Lewinian democratic leadership suggests that Chinese leaders guide group discussion and decision in much the same way that democratic leaders in the K. Lewin et al (1939) study guided their 10-yr-old Ss. Treating citizens like children may be mass leadership, but it is hardly Lewinian or democratic. Barlow minimizes the importance of force and the threat of force in maintaining mass leadership. Other criticisms include a significant omission in Barlow's description of the Red Army and its success in converting captured Nationalist troops during the Chinese civil war and his lack of distinction between brainwashing and thought reform.

1857

McClelland, D. C. (1963). Motivational patterns in Southeast Asia with special reference to the Chinese case. Journal of Social Issues, 19, *6-19.*

Three sets of Chinese stories used to teach children in public schools were compared: one from Republic China (1920-9), one from Taiwan (1950-9), and one from mainland China (1950-9). The stories were objectively scored for need for achievement, need for affiliation, and need for power. The results showed that the pattern of scores for Republican China corresponded to that found very frequently in static, tradition-oriented societies governed by an authoritarian regime--low need for achievement, very low need for affiliation, and very high need for power. Both Taiwan and mainland China showed an increase in the need for achievement and in the need for affiliation, but the increases were much higher in the mainland than in Taiwan.

1858

McCoy, M. (1979). Culture-shocked marriages in Hong Kong. Hong Kong Psychological Society Bulletin, *No. 2, 9-16.*

Discusses "culture-shocked marriages" -- couples consisting of Hong Kong Chinese males and Western females who met and married elsewhere, but who now reside in Hong Kong -- in terms of the husband's experience, the wife's experience, and the interaction of these experiences on the marriage. Although the author was unable to isolate any one of the above factors, the wife's experience in moving to Hong Kong as an expatriate is the primary focus. A culture shock model is proposed as a view of the transitional experience precipitated by exposure to a 2nd culture. The model has 5 stages, each associated with a typical behavior and affect: (1) contact, (2) disintegration, (3) reintegration, (4) autonomy, and (5) independence. Data were collected from 20 expatriate wives, using the case study method. The benefits of using such an approach are discussed.

1859

McCoy, M. (1980). Further explorations of the culture-shocked marriage hypothesis: The exceptions. Hong Kong Psychological Society Bulletin, *No. 5, 17-28.*

Following the author's (1979) paper that described "culture-shock marriages" in Hong Kong--i.e, marriages between a Chinese male returned from overseas and a Western female, and the problems faced by such a couple--3 successful intercultural marriages are described in terms of P. S. Adler's (1975) 5-stage model of cultural shock. As the husbands were inaccessible for cultural reasons, only the wives were interviewed, using personal construct theory and the repertory grid technique. The factors in each of the 3 exceptional cases that influenced the marriage favorably are pointed out.

1860

Mead, M., & Metraux, R. (Eds.). (1953). The study of culture at a distance. *Chicago: University of Chicago Press.*

1861

Meade, R. D. (1970). Leadership studies of Chinese and Chinese-Americans. Journal of Cross-Cultural Psychology, 1, *325-332.*

Chinese and Chinese-American college students ranked 9 issues of importance, discussed them under conditions of authoritarian, democratic, or laissez-faire leadership atmospheres, arrived at a group ranking, and then ranked them individually again. With Chinese Ss, authoritarian leadership and male leadership produced greater group cohesiveness. With Chinese-Americans, both authoritarian and democratic produced group cohesiveness as did male leaders. Emergent leaders appeared only in laissez-faire groups of Chinese with female leaders. Differences may be due to the Chinese being familiar with the authoritarian form of leadership only.

1862

Meade, R. D., & Barnard, W. A. (1973). Conformity and anti-conformity among Americans and Chinese. Journal of Social Psychology, 89, *15-24.*

Asked 2 groups of 60 male college students in the United States and Hong Kong to state their private opinions about a series of controversial issues. 5 peer-group confederates then individually stated opinions which were opposite from those of the S. All Ss and confederates than gave reasons for their opinions and were allowed to change their opinions if they wished. Hesitancy in answering, revision of original opinions, and amount of revision were the dependent variables. There was a greater hesitancy and number of opinion changes among Chinese than among Americans. Americans had greater amounts of opinion changes. Both Americans and Chinese had shorter hesitancies and fewer opinion changes in the presence of female confederates than in the presence of males. Results are interpreted in terms of F. Hsu's anthropological theory and contemporary motivational theory.

1863

Meade, R. D., & Barnard, W. A. (1975). Group pressure effects on American and Chinese females. Journal of Social Psychology, 96, *137-138.*

Females in both cultural groups responded to group pressure effects both similarly and differently from males studied previously by the authors. Chinese females exhibited greater latency and greater tendency to shift opinion than American females, and they shifted more often. The degree of these effects in the presence of male confederates appeared to be greater than for male Ss.

1864

Meade, R. D., & Whittaker, J. O. (1967). A cross-cultural study of authoritarianism. Journal of Social Psychology, 72, *3-7.*

The California f scale was administered to college students in India, Hong Kong, Rhodesia, Arabia, Brazil and the United States. Within each cultural group there were no sex differences in authoritarianism. American students scored significantly lower than all other groups while Rhodesians and Indians together scored highest. Arabians and Chinese did not differ and scored 2nd highest. Brazilians scored lower than all groups except Americans. Results are interpreted in terms of social and leadership research.

1865

Mendelson, J. H., & Mello, N. K. (1975). Plasma testosterone levels during chronic heroin use and protracted abstinence: A study of Hong Kong addicts. Clinical Pharmacology & Therapeutics, 17, *529-533.*

The effects of heroin use and subsequent prolonged abstinence on plasma testosterone levels were examined in 31 male heroin addicts. Heroin (alone and in combination with methadone) significantly suppressed plasma testosterone levels. However, drug induced testosterone suppression does not appear to be permanent in adult addicts. Recovery of testosterone levels to normal occurred after about one month of heroin abstinence.

1866

Mendes, H. A. (1976). Single fatherhood. Social Work, 21, *308-312.*

Presented interview data from 15 Black, 14 White, 2 Mexican-American, and 1 Chinese-American single fathers who were characterized as either seekers or assenters according to whether they had actually chosen to be single parents. Findings indicate that seekers were generally more successful in the single parent role and that this group had less diversity in sociological and psychological make-up than assenters.

1867

Meredith, G. M. (1969). Sex temperament among Japanese-American college students in Hawaii. Journal of Social Psychology, 77, *149-156.*

With the rapid acculturation of Oriental minorities to American middle-class life, there are corresponding changes in culture-linked definitions of masculinity and femininity. The Terman-Miles M-F Test was administered to 65 Caucasian, 98 Japanese-American, and 40 Chinese-American undergraduates. Few differences were found between male groups. The differences between Caucasians and female Oriental groups were statistically significant. The findings are discussed with reference to exploitative and accommodative sex-role strategies. Attention was devoted to the local distinction between Meiji-type and Haole-type among the Japanese-Americans.

1868

Merry, J. (1975). A social history of heroin addiction. British Journal of Addiction, 70, *307-310.*

1869

Metzger, T. A. (1981). Selfhood and authority in neo-Confucian political culture. In A. Kleinman & T. Y. Lin (Eds.), Normal and abnormal behavior in Chinese culture *(pp. 7-27). Dordrecht, Netherlands: D. Reidel.*

1870

Mickolus, E. F. (1980). The double standard in nation perception: Artifact versus main effect. International Journal of Group Tensions, 10, *38-60.*

Attempted to replicate S. Oskamp's findings of a double standard in the perception of different nations. A revised form of Oskamp's Index of Mirror Images and Double Standards, with items referring to identical actions taken by the US, USSR, and China, was administered to 53 US college students and 52 foreign citizens who attended a program at Yale University in 1974. The effects of 2-sided, impartial presentation of these actions were assessed. The study replicated the findings of divergent attribution patterns of the US and USSR and extended them to the US and China pair. Artifacts in previous research were isolated and assessed, including problems involved in scale distortion and factor analysis generalization. Bivariate and multiple regression analysis were used to assess the interaction of demographic characteristics with international attitudes. Women showed less of a double standard than men, as did Ss with more information, those who had traveled to more places, and Ss exposed to a religion oriented toward the individual.

1871

Minkowski, L. (1969). [Children in Communist China and North Vietnam during the preschool period: Communication with a film and photos]. Annales Medico-Psychologiques, 1, *818. (In other language.)*

Early apprenticeship in adult behavior, life experiences and responsibilities begin in nursery school and this is believed to be an important educational factor contributing toward the "heroic resistance" and self-reliance of the North Vietnamese. Other personal observations indicate that their highly developed preventive medicine and family planning programs are achieved through explanation, teaching, and "a system of individual persuasion without coercion". The formation of "a new type of man does not appear to hinder the free development of personality", despite the prevalence of propaganda, sexual taboos, and the collectivity over individualism.

1872

Mitchell, R. E. (Ed.). (1972). Family life in urban Hong Kong. *Taipei: Oriental Cultural Service.*

1873

Mitchell, R. E. (1972). Levels of emotional strain in Southeast Asian cities: A study of individual responses to the stresses of urbanization and industrialization. *Taipei: Oriental Cultural Service.*

1874

Mitchell, R. E. (1972). Husband-wife relations and family-planning practices in urban Hong Kong. Journal of Marriage and the Family, 34, *139-146.*

1875

Mitchell, R. E., & Lo, I. (1968). Implications of changes in family authority relations for the development of independence and assertiveness in Hong Kong children. Asian Survey, 8, *309-322.*

1876

Money, J. (1977). Peking: The sexual revolution. In J. Money, (Ed.), Handbook of sexology *(chapter 39, pp. 543-550). North Holland: Bio-medical Press, Elsevier.*

1877

Montgomery, R. L. (1977). Rural-to-urban migrants on Taiwan: Variations in informal and formal groups based on ethnic, marital, and religious differences. Dissertation Abstracts International, 37, *A7990-7991.*

1878

Moore, C. A. (1966). The Chinese mind. *Honolulu: University of Hawaii Press.*

1879

Morland, J. K. (1969). Race awareness among American and Hong Kong Chinese children. American Journal of Sociology, 75, *360-374.*

1880

Morland, J. K. (1972). Race awareness among American and Hong Kong Chinese children. In S. S. Guterman (Ed.), Black psyche: The modal personality patterns of black Americans. *Berkeley, CA: Glendessary.*

Results of a cross-cultural comparison show significant differences between 4-7 yr. old Hong Kong Chinese, Caucasian Americans, and Negro Americans on racial preference and racial self-identity. Findings support the normative theory of racial prejudice.

1881

Morris, C. W. (1956). Varieties of human value. *Chicago: University of Chicago Press.*

1882

Moser, M. J. (1975). Death in Chinese: A two-dimensional analysis. Journal of Thanatology, 3, *169-185.*

Discusses traditional Chinese behavior as an aspect of Chinese social relationships. The way in which the deceased is projected into a number of functionally different relationships with the living members of the community is described. Seen from this perspective, the loss of one of society's members is not construed as a total severance from the world of the living, but as the starting point for a series of continuing social interactions which continually cross the boundary between life and death.

1883

Munro, D. J. (1975). The Chinese view of modeling. Human Development, 18, *333-352.*

Points out that while interest in imitation and observation by Western students of learning processes has only recently been activated, writers in Confucian and Communist China have long given it central focus. The Chinese stress the role of models in moral education; peer respect is advocated as the primary reward available to the exemplar and vicariously to the learner. Among other things, the use of this reward, viewed as preferable to money, sets the Chinese position apart from the one reflected in Soviet theory and practice. Model selection and presentation is formalized in accordance with principles derived from Soviet socialist emulation campaigns, from a rationalization of practical experiences encountered during the guerrilla period, and from Confucianism. In conclusion the Chinese theory is critically evaluated; emphasis is placed on implications for motivation and creativity.

1884

Murphy, G. J. (1978). The family in later life: A cross-ethnic study in marital and sexual satisfaction. Dissertation Abstracts International, 39, *A2553.*

1885

Murphy, H. B. M. (1974). Mass youth protest movements in Asia and the West: Their common characteristics and psychiatric significance. In W. P. Lebra (Ed.), Mental health research in Asia and the Pacific: Vol. 3. Youth, socialization, and mental health. *Honolulu, HI: The University Press Hawaii.*

1886

Murphy, N. C. (1983). Homosexuality, Hong Kong, and hubris: A study of deceit. *Hong Kong: Author.*

1887

Nakanishi, N. (1969). Symbol perception of the Kahn Test of Symbol Arrangement among four cultures. International Journal of Symbology, 1, *20-24.*

Presents a cross-cultural study of enculturation and acculturation processes as they are reflected in the learning of visual symbols. Popular responses of naming to the Kahn Test of Symbol Arrangement showed enculturation differences between the Christian country of America, the Buddhist country of Japan, the Taoist-Buddhist country of China (Formosa), and the Islamic country of East Pakistan as the people drew in their learning from very different cultural sources.

1888

Newman, R. G., & Whitehill, W. B. (1979). Double-blind comparison of methadone and placebo maintenance treatments of narcotic addicts in Hong Kong. Lancet, 2, *485-488.*

In a double-blind study carried out between 1972 and 1975 in Hong Kong, 100 heroin addict volunteers were initially admitted to hospital for 2 weeks for stabilization on 60 mg of methadone before being assigned at random to two groups: one group received methadone (range 30-130 mg, average 97 mg/day); those in the other group had their dose of methadone reduced at the rate of 1 mg/day and were maintained on placebo. All subjects were provided with a broad range of supportive services. After 32 weeks 10% of the controls were still on treatment, compared with 76% of those receiving methadone. At the end of the 3-year project, only 1 of the original 50 placebo subjects still turned up for treatment (2%), whereas the retention-rate (proportion still on treatment) for methadone subjects was 56%. Subjects who had dropped out of the study and were readmitted for methadone treatment under known conditions had the same retention rate as the original treatment group.

1889

Ng, K. M. (1980). Mathematical cognitive structure: An exploratory study of Hong Kong Chinese, Chinese American, and Euro-American junior high school students. Dissertation Abstracts International, 40, *A5770.*

This thesis examines the cognitive structure, particularly with respect to mathematics achievement, in Hong Kong Chinese, Chinese American and Euro-American 7th and 8th graders.

1890

Ng, S. H. (1984). Equity and social categorization effects on intergroup allocation of rewards. British Journal of Social Psychology, 23, *165-172.*

Examined the effects of equity and social categorization on reward allocation by inserting a veridical input factor into the minimal categorization paradigm unconfounded by any need for inequity prevention. Forty-seven Hong Kong Chinese students divided a monetary reward between two recipients who had contributed unequally to the reward. The more productive recipient was either an in-group or out-group member, or there was no group distinction between them (noncategorization). Significant main effects of equity (favoritism to the more productive recipient) and social categorization (in-group bias) were found on intergroup allocation, as was the main effect of equity on interpersonal allocation. When the forces of social categorization and equity were in harmony, equity effect was accentuated and nearly all the subjects behaved equitably, when in conflict, equity effect was neutralized and subjects were evenly split into equitable and inequitable allocators. The need for integrating equity and social categorization was highlighted.

1891

Ng, S. H., Akhtar Hossain, A. B. M., Ball, P., Bond, M. H., Hayashi, K., Lim, S. P., O'Driscoll, P. M., Sinha, D., & Yang, K. S. (1982). Human values in nine countries. In P. Rath, H. S. Asthana, D. Sinha & J. B. P. Sinha (Eds.), Diversity and unity in cross-cultural psychology *(pp. 196-205). Lisse, Netherlands: Zeit Unger.*

1892

Niu, P. K. (1976). A proposed Christian psychological guidance program for Catholic college and university students in Taiwan. Dissertation Abstracts International, 37, *A1995.*

1893

Ochsner, M. A. (1969). Chinese communist attitudes toward the Soviet Union, 1949-1965: A content analysis of official documents. Dissertation Abstracts, 29, *A4080.*

1894

O'Hara, A. R. (1968). [Comparative responses to interpersonal conflict by university students in Mexico, United States, and Taiwan]. (C. H. Chang, Trans.). Journal of Sociology *(National Taiwan University), 4, 13-20. (In Chinese.)*

1895

O'Hara, A. R. (1972). [Social & culture change among Chinese university students]. (K. C. Hong, Trans.). Journal of Sociology^ (National Taiwan University), *8,* **19-26.** (In Chinese.)

1896

O'Neill, W. F., & Demos, G. D. (1977). The semantics of thought reform. *ETC, 34,* **413-430.**

Examines the nature and effectiveness of Communist thought reform practices (brainwashing) and relates them to education and psychotherapy. Chinese Communist practices are distinctive, especially the use of language as a tool for ideological conversion. Four phases are noted: resistance; noncognitive reform (behavioral counterconditioning); ideological action; and ritualization of ideology. Aspects of thought reform include (a) formulation of a new ego-identity in which selfhood disappears by altering values and vocabulary; (b) instrumental conditioning of identity and behavior; (c) the use of language to direct and sustain behavior; (d) self-reinforcing ideology; (e) symbolic reconditioning; (f) similarities to religious faith; (g) establishment of correct semantics and syntax; and (h) the formulation of automatic reactions.

1897

O'Neill, W. F., & Demos, G. D. (1983). The Yeshov method. *ETC, 40,* **422-432.**

Describes the Yeshov method of thought reform used by both the Soviet and Chinese communists to bring about significant modifications in personal identity. The Yeshov method, as originally conceived, was a method of interrogation developed during the era of the Soviet purge-trials of the 1930's. It was largely abandoned in the USSR and has since been adapted by the Chinese. It can be broken down into 3 major phases: an accusation, a confession, and a "reconstructed confession". The method commences when the prisoner is charged with being guilty of some offense against the state. At the same time, he/she is subjected to intense physical and psychological pressures to confess and repent. In effect, the prisoner is subjected to extreme duress for failing to confess to what are often purely imaginary or, at the very least, unrecognized acts. If such stress continues for a sufficient period of time, 2 results ordinarily occur: The prisoner develops a need to be guilty and also develops a corresponding need to discover some appropriate sort of crime that can serve as an effective explanation (or justification) for such guilt. The advantages of the Yeshov method from the viewpoint of the thought reformers are noted, including that the method results in a self-sustaining dedication to a continuous process of ideological self-psychoanalysis. The individual undergoes the "subjectification of truth", because in the total institution, truth exists only in context; reality is situational.

1898

Osgood, C. (1975). *The Chinese: A study of a Hong Kong community^ (Vols. 1-3). Tucson, AZ: University of Arizona Press.*

1899

Osgood, C. E. (1964). Semantic differential technique in the comparative study of cultures. American Anthropologist *(Special Publication),* **66** *Part 2, 171-200.*

1900

Pak, A. W., Dion, K. L., & Dion, K. K. (1985). Correlates of self-confidence with English among Chinese students in Toronto. Canadian Journal of Behavioural Science, 17, *369-378.*

Examined the relation between 174 Chinese undergraduates' self-ratings of confidence with English and indicators of assimilation and psychological adjustment. Measures included adaptations of the Social Readjustment Rating Scale, the Rosenberg Self-Esteem Scale, and Rotter's Internal-External Locus of Control Scale. Factor analysis revealed that confidence with English was positively associated with linguistic assimilation into English-Canadian society and with several components of psychological adjustment (e.g. sense of personal control, self-esteem). Indicators of cultural assimilation (e.g., social distance toward anglophone groups) and involvement in the Chinese community were not, however, related to confidence with English. Findings suggested that for some ethnolinguistic minorities in Canada, self-rated confidence with the language of the majority group is not necessarily indicative of the loss of ethno-cultural identity by its members.

1901

Palinkas, L. A. (1982). Ethnicity, identity and mental health: The use of rhetoric in an immigrant Chinese church. Journal of Psychoanalytic Anthropology, 5, *235-258.*

Studied the impact of church membership in 2 Mandarin-speaking Christian churches in San Diego. Ethnicity in these churches was tied to (1) members' sociocultural adjustment to their new environment and the psychological stress engendered by the adjustment; (2) the juxtaposition of the Chinese and Western cultural traditions; and (3) the role of religious discourse in anxiety reduction and identity resolution. The church was supportive to many Chinese because it offered a healing-redemptive fellowship concerned with spiritual and mental health; it also served as a substitute for the Chinese kinship network and acted as an arena for sociocultural change. Three strategies helped form a Chinese-Christian identity: the combining of the Chinese and Christian worlds, the promotion of a united church, and the minimization of personal conflicts. Rhetoric also tied together group and individual perspectives. Three brief sketches are presented of 22- and 24-yr-old males and a 62-yr-old female whose depression, anxiety, and loneliness were alleviated through their church membership.

1902

Pan, M. T. (1973). The attitudes of Taiwan businessmen toward the entertaining girls of the city of Taipei. Dissertation Abstracts International, 34, *B2432-2433.*

1903

Parameshvara Deva, M. (1978). A seven year study of opiate dependence in Malaysia. Medical Journal of Malaysia, 32, *249-254.*

1904

Parish, W. L. (1981). Family and community in the People's Republic. In A. Kleinman & T. Y. Lin (Eds.), Normal and abnormal behavior in Chinese culture *(pp. 203-212). Dordrecht, Netherlands: Reidel.*

1905

Parish, W. L., & Whyte, M. K. (1978). Village and family in contemporary China. *Chicago: University of Chicago Press.*

1906

Park, J. Y. et al. (1984). The flushing response to alcohol use among Koreans and Taiwanese. Journal of Studies on Alcohol, *45, 481-485.*

Investigated alcohol use and the existence of and amount of alcohol required to evoke a flushing response to alcohol in 87 homeland Korean and 101 Taiwan Chinese families. Results indicated that while both groups reported similar incidences of flushing, Koreans drank more. Comparisons with five ethnic groups in Hawaii revealed that fast flushing (after one drink or less) but not slow flushing (after two or more drinks) led to decreased alcohol use in all seven groups.

1907

Peabody, D. (1968). Group judgments in the Philippines: Evaluative and descriptive aspects. Journal of Personality & Social Psychology, 10, *290-300.*

Judgments about Chinese living in the Philippines, and about Filipinos, Americans, and Japanese were made by members of the 1st 2 groups using 14 pairs of scales designed to separate evaluative and descriptive aspects. Results showed major effects for both aspects: the groups tended to (1) disagree about their evaluations of each other, but (2) agree about the descriptive characteristics of each group. The Chinese were judged tight in impulse control and unassertive; the Japanese tight and assertive; the Filipinos more loose in impulse expression and unassertive; and the Americans a mixture of tight and loose characteristics and assertive.

1908

Pearson, V. (1986). Mental health legislation in Hong Kong: Some thoughts on recent developments. The Hong Kong Journal of Social Work, 20, *34-39.*

1909

Pedersen, P. B. (1970). Youth in Asia: A report on research among 451 Chinese and English speaking youth responding to a 400 item survey in English and Chinese. *Kuala Lumpur: Lutheran Church in Malaysia.*

1910

Peng, D. L., Yang, M., & Yang, L. Z. (1985). [Role of situational and facial clues in expression judgment]. Information on Psychological Sciences, *No. 2, 26-32. (In Chinese.)*

1911

Peng, R. X., Sun, X. R., Lin, Z. X., & Zhao, M. (1980). [Preferred Chinese skin color in TV reproduction]. Acta Psychologica Sinica, 12, *189-194. (In Chinese.)*

Ss viewed 24 photographs of a young Chinese woman's face, with various chromaticities of the skin. The category-judgment method was employed for subjective evaluation of the quality of the reproduced skin color on the TV monitor. In comparing the chromaticity of preferred TV skin color with that obtained for real skin color, the dominant wavelength remained unchanged, but the purity of the preferred skin color was much higher than that for real skin.

1912

Pierson, H., Postiglione, G., & Hu, S. (1982). Toward a theory of cultural conflict in Hong Kong. New Horizons, *No. 23, 75-81.*

1913

Plattner, S. (1975). Rural market networks. Scientific American, 232, *66-79.*

Describes Christaller's central-place theory, which has stimulated important conceptual developments in economic geography. Field research in a Chinese province has shown geographical distributions of markets to match Christaller's models closely. "Socialization" of rural trade disrupted trade and the traditional rural market system was re-established. Research on market systems in Guatemala and other former colonial possessions demonstrates limitations on the ability of central-place theory to duplicate all the subtleties of real-world situations.

1914

Podmore, D., & Chaney, D. (1972). Attitudes towards marriage and the family among young people in Hong Kong, and comparisons with the United States and Taiwan. Journal of Comparative Family Studies, 3, *228-238.*

1915

Podmore, D., & Chaney, D. (1974). Educational experience as an influence on "modern" and "traditional" attitudes: Some evidence from Hong Kong. Journal of Social Psychology, 94, *139-140.*

On 11 attitude statements, it was hypothesized that young people in Hong Kong with (a) some secondary education would be relatively "modern" compared with those without secondary education, (b) some higher education would be relatively "modern" compared with those without higher education, and (c) an education exclusively in Anglo-Chinese schools would be relatively "modern" compared with those with an education exclusively in Chinese schools. Results confirm hypotheses.

1916

Podmore, D., & Chaney, D. (1974). Family norms in a rapidly industrializing society: Hong Kong. Journal of Marriage & the Family, 36, *400-407.*

A sample of 1123 young people in Hong Kong were interviewed and responded to a number of statements concerning family norms. The data suggest that with regard to relationships between husband and wife, and parents and children, views are more consonant with the norms of the Western conjugal family than the traditional Chinese family. A pattern consonant with traditional norms is found concerning relationships with the older generation and a substantial minority support the notion of extended family living. It is argued that the coexistence of some traditional family norms and some norms typical of the conjugal family is functional in thc Hong Kong context.

1917

Podmore, D., Chaney, D., & Golder, P. (1975). "Don't know" responses among young adults in Hong Kong. Journal of Social Psychology, 96, *307-308.*

Investigated a previous finding of a relatively large number of "don't know" responses given by Hong Kong residents to questions about attitudes toward police, government, and the political future of Hong Kong. Data from 1,123 interviews with 15-29 yr olds living in urban areas show that the percentage of "don't knows" was significantly greater for politically sensitive than for politically neutral statements.

1918

Podmore, D., Chaney, D., & Golder, P. (1975). Third parties in the interview situation: Evidence from Hong Kong. Journal of Social Psychology, 95, *227-231.*

Studied the effect of the presence or absence of parents during interviews with 1,123 15-19 yr olds in Hong Kong. Parental presence significantly affected responses to 2 of 11 statements presented during the interviews concerning respondents' attitudes toward the family and family relationships. Results are interpreted in terms of the differential sensitivity of the 11 statements (i.e., whether they related to specific family events or wider social issues).

1919

Prachuabmoh, V., Knodel, J., & Alers, J. O. (1974). Preference for sons, desire for additional children, and family planning in Thailand. Journal of Marriage & the Family, 36, *601-614.*

The extent of son preference in Thailand and its effect on desire for additional children and practice of family planning is examined using data from a national social-demographic sample survey and a follow-up survey of family planning acceptors. The data suggest that there is some preference for sons although generally couples prefer to have children of both sexes. Among the urban ethnic Chinese, however, son preference was more pronounced. With the exception of this group the preference for sons does not seem to have much effect on desire for additional children or family planning practice. The number of children a couple has appears to be a much more important determinant of desire for additional children and use of contraception than is the particular sex composition of the offspring. The general lack of a strong son preference is interpreted in terms of broader social and cultural patterns characteristic of Thai families.

1920

Pruitt, I. (1945). A daughter of Han: The autobiography of a Chinese working woman. *New Haven, NT: Yale University Press. (Republished Stanford, CA: Stanford University Press, 1967.)*

1921

Pye, L. W. (1968). The spirit of Chinese politics: A psychocultural study of the authority crisis in political development. *Cambridge, MA: MIT Press.*

1922

Rabushka, A. (1970). Affective, cognitive, and behavioral consistency of Chinese-Malay interracial attitudes. Journal of Social Psychology, 82, *35-41.*

Analysis of a random sample of Chinese and Malay residents in George Town (Penang), Malaysia, provided an opportunity to estimate empirically the relationships between the major components of attitudes affective, cognitive, and behavioral. Data reveal that affect and behavior are positively correlated, but that behavior and cognition along with affect and cognition do not appear in a consistent arrangement. These findings vary from the results of recent experimental inquiries which have shown that attitude components appear in a consistent arrangement. The difference in results may be explained by use of survey research techniques among a relatively uneducated mass of urban residents in an underdeveloped country, rather than relying on college students as experimental Ss.

1923

Raddock, D. M. (1974). Growing up in New China: A twist in the circle of filial piety. History of Childhood Quarterly: The Journal of Psychohistory, 2, *201-220.*

Carried out an "intensive interviewing project" in Hong Kong with 35 male emigres from China using a quasi-psychoanalytic format. Formerly, affection for parents and reverence for authority figures were inseparable. The revolutionary process gradually removed the ethos and gnawed away at the devices for maintaining rigid stratification within the family. For the Communist intellectuals, liberation of the country was preceded by liberation of the individual. Increased stature of the new generation is changing the standards of behavior within the family.

1924

Rajah, K. S. (1979). Drug problems in adolescence. Journal of Singapore Paediatrics Society, 21, *Suppl., 87-97.*

1925

Raschke, V. (1976). Premarital sexual permissiveness of college students in Hong Kong. Journal of Comparative Family Studies, 7, *65-74.*

Compared the premarital sexual permissiveness of 264 American college students in the midwest, 26 students from Hong Kong who were studying in the US, and 153 students attending colleges and universities in Hong Kong. Results show that (a) I. L. Reiss's (1965) Premarital Sexual Permissiveness Scales worked as Guttman scales for the Chinese students, (b) Chinese students in Hong Kong were less permissive and less active concerning premarital sex, and (c) the majority of determinants of premarital sexual permissiveness found by Reiss and others to hold for Americans also held as determinants of permissiveness for Chinese students. Results also show that Chinese students who were studying in America tended to adopt American standards of premarital sexual attitudes and behaviors.

1926

Record, J. C., & Record, W. (1976). Totalist and pluralist views of women's liberation: Some reflections on the Chinese and American settings. Social Problems, 23, *402-414.*

Views women's movements in the US and China in light of ideological differences which are described as pluralist-totalist. The interests of individuals and intermediate groups such as the feminists have independent value in the pluralist state, while the interests of the collectivity have overriding importance in the totalist state. The crux of the issue is whether feminists' interests are best served by the aggressive assertion of individuals and private groups or by the subordination to a larger revolutionary movement whose explicit goals include ultimate liberation and equality for all. Although conflicts (e.g., land reform and birth control) between women's interests and revolutionary goals in the totalist Chinese society clearly exist, Chinese women leaders defer their own feminist interests to socialist production and other revolutionary purposes. The conflict between totalist and pluralist positions is discussed in reference to goals defined by collective and particular interests. The means by which feminist goals should be pursued is considered with respect to the role of the state in (a) intervening to reshape sex roles and (b) assuming initiative in providing new opportunities for women.

1927

Reddy, U. V. (1981). Some psychological factors in the perception of national groups by Indians. Managerial Psychology, 2, *79-83.*

Administered a questionnaire including an open-mindedness measure to 300 Indian college students and professionals. Profiles of the images the Ss held of 6 national groups (US, USSR, UK, Arab countries, China, and West Germany) were compared with Ss' own self-images. Although findings indicate that certain demographic factors and personal qualities affected Ss' perception of national groups, it is concluded that generalizations about perceptions and the social and psychological bases of these perceptions are not feasible. Since foreign countries are not similar, images are not associated with general independent factors.

1928

Reed, T. E., Kalant, H., Gibbins, R. J. et al. (1976). Alcohol and acetaldehyde metabolism in Caucasians, Chinese and Americans. Canadian Medical Association Journal, 115, *851-855.*

Ethanol (0.4 to 0.8 g/kg in 30 minutes) was given by mouth to 102 healthy young volunteers (37 Caucasian men, 21 Caucasian women, 20 Chinese men and 24 Ojibwa men). Venous blood concentrations of ethanol and acetaldehyde 60, 90, 120 and 150 minutes after the end of drinking were measured by gas chromatography. The calculated rates of ethanol metabolism in the Caucasian men and women did not differ, but the overall group means for subgroups of Caucasians (103.6 mg/kg.h), Chinese (136.6 mg/kg.h) and Ojibwa (182.7 mg/kg.h) with decreasing postabsorption values differed significantly from each other. Mean acetaldehyde values paralleled the rates of ethanol metabolism: Ojibwa, 14.6 mug/ml; Chinese, 10.0 mug/ml; and Caucasians, 9.4 mug/ml. The high rate of ethanol metabolism in American subjects differs from previous findings. Habitual level of alcohol consumption, proportion of body fat and genetic factors appear to account for most of the group differences.

1929

Reid, F. T. Jr. (1979). Psychosocial structure in China. Arizona Medicine, 36, *679-681.*

1930

Richardson, R. A. (1971). The cross-cultural validity of Freudian sexual symbolism. International Journal of Symbology, 2, *1-7.*

Studied samples obtained from Sweden and China, from a Negro and a Caucasian population, and one which represented a potpourri of cultural backgrounds. Ss were asked to identify a variety of sexual symbols as male or female. Identification of the symbols varied significantly from culture to culture thereby questioning Freud's position concerning the cross-cultural generality of sexual symbolism. Such variability reflects a cultural influence on sexual symbolism unrecognized by Freud, which necessitates a reformulation of Freud's position to accommodate the cultural conditioning.

1931

Ridley, C. P., Godwin, P. H. B., & Doolin, D. G. (1971). The making of a model citizen in Communist China. *Stanford, CA: Hoover Institution.*

1932

Rin, H., Cheng, L. T., & Chen, T. (1974). [Some trends found among suicides reported on a newspaper]. Acta Psychologica Taiwanica, 16, *7-23. (In Chinese.)*

In this study, a total of 364 suicides reported in a popular newspaper in Taipei during the years 1969-71 were analyzed. The first part dealt with socio-psychological variables; trends found in the distribution of cases as to age, sex, given reasons, methods, and immediate result of suicide. Heightened rates of suicide were seen among young females and middle-aged males. Women were more afflicted by the difficulty encountered in love making, marital life and family relationship, and men were frequently disturbed by legal problems and social maladaptation. Men who killed themselves after murdering others in situations involving conflict with their marriage partners specifically drew public attention. In the second part, newspaper writers' reactions toward suicide were analyzed by examining the printed title size and number of letters written in reporting suicide. Reporters tended to react dramatically to matters related to criminal acts, mental derangement, social conflict, and especially to theatrical behavior. Articles on homicide-suicide victims were the longest and had the largest titles. Exaggerated newspaper reports on suicide might influence other susceptible persons and thus increase the rate of suicide.

1933

Rindfuss, R. R., & Hirschman, C. (1984). The timing of family formation: Structural and societal factors in the Asian context. Journal of Marriage & the Family, 46, *205-214.*

Examined the timing of family formation in 4 Asian countries: Taiwan, South Korea, Thailand, and Malaysia. Since the focus was explicitly comparative, data from the 4 countries were merged. Data were from 5,457 married Malaysian women, 1,883 married Korean women, 5,588 married Taiwanese women, and 1,921 never-married Thai women. The extent to which various social-structural variables operated the same way in these societies was tested by comparing the determinants of age at first birth. Factors affecting age at first birth included background, adolescent and early adulthood, and biological and societal factors. Results of fertility surveys indicate that education and rural/urban origins had the same effect on the timing of family formation in each of these countries. Once such social-structural variables were controlled, country or ethnicity remained an important predictor of the timing of family formation. Three Confucian heritage groups--Taiwanese, Koreans, and the Malaysian Chinese--were essentially identical with respect to the timing of family formation, suggesting the importance of a shared heritage. Factors accounting for this influence are discussed.

1934

Rohlen, T. P. (1971). Father-son dominance: Tikopia and China. In F. L. K. Hsu (Ed.), Kinship and culture. *Chicago, IL: Aldine.*

1935

Rohrlich-Leavitt, R. (1975). Women cross-culturally: Change and challenge. *Hague, Netherlands: Mouton.*

Presents a group of papers describing the status, roles, experiences, and outlook of women in various cultures of Islam, Africa, Latin America, and in the US, the USSR, China, and Israel. The status of women in the profession of anthropology is particularly considered.

1936

Romalis, C., & Romalis, S. (1983). Sexism, racism, and technological change: Two cases of minority protest. International Journal of Women's Studies, 6, *270-287.*

Describes 2 cases of technological change in which mechanical improvements introduced into preindustrial societies caused social and economic disadvantage to specific groups. Beginning in the 1930's, the Igbo women of southeastern Nigeria found their social and financial statuses sharply diminished by the new mills introduced to produce palm oil; their protests against these innovations are seen not only as resistance to technological change but also as feminist rebellion against the sexist attitudes of European colonials operating the palm oil industry. In California of the 1880's, Chinese operators of hand laundries were disadvantaged by the development of expensive steam laundry machinery. These 2 structurally comparable cases are discussed in terms of the responses of the aggrieved minorities to the curtailment of their economic power and the larger societies' perception of the minorities' protests. Conclusions are drawn about the historical visibility of racism and sexism and the legitimacy they have been accorded as bases for grievances.

1937

Rootman, I., & Hughes, P. H. (1980). Drug-abuse reporting systems. WHO [World Health Organization] Offset Publication, *No. 55, 98.*

1938

Rosen, S. (1978). Sibling and in-law relationships in Hong Kong: The emergent role of Chinese wives. Journal of Marriage & the Family, 40, *621-628.*

Using data from a case study of young families in an affluent Hong King housing complex, the author (1976) contends that role reorganization within the nuclear family and, specifically, the changing role of Chinese wives, has created a new family structure which reinforces rather than rejects traditional norms of shared residence and reciprocal aid among kin. Four new variants of the traditional pattern--life-cycle variation, inclusion of uxorial relatives, emergence of "extended family households" encompassing several separate residences, and strengthening of intragenerational ties--are cited, along with attitudinal changes which have also contributed to the new style of extended-family interaction.

1939

Rosenbaum, L. L., & Rosenbaum, W. B. (1975). Persuasive impact of a communicator where groups differ in apparent co-orientation. Journal of Psychology, 89, *189-194.*

To test the hypothesis that the extent of attitude change in the advocated direction would be related to the degree of co-orientation between a communicator and different groups, the chapter president of a college sorority attempted to influence the attitudes toward the admission of mainland China to the United Nations of 94 undergraduate females (chapter pledgees, chapter actives, actives of a nearby chapter, and actives of a comparable sorority at a nearby university). Attitudes were measured by asking the Ss to respond to 8, 7-point Likert-type items. The pledgees manifested a significantly greater attitude change in the advocated direction than did each of the remaining 3 groups. It is suggested that variables more important than co-orientation between communicator and receiver were operating. The pledgees probably experienced greater need for social approval and valued membership in the group more than the actives of the other groups and, therefore, perceived greater reward in changing their attitude in the direction advocated by the sorority president.

1940

Rosenberg, R. R. (1970). The apathetic majority: Political socialization of university students in Nationalist China. Youth and Society, 2.

1941

Rosenfeld, P., Giacalone, R. A., Tedeschi, J. T., & Bond, M. H. (1983). The cross-cultural efficacy of entitlements in American and Hong Kong Chinese students. In J. B. Deregowski, S. Dziurawiek & R. C. Annis (Eds.), Expiscations in cross-cultural psychology *(pp. 266-269). Lisse, Netherlands: Swets & Zeitlinger.*

1942

Ross, E. A. Q. (1911). The changing Chinese: The conflict of oriental and western cultures in China. *New York: The Centary.*

1943

Rump, E. E. (1972). Comparing Australia and New Zealand on color prejudice. International Journal of Psychology, 7, *39-45.*

Assessed racial prejudice by having comparable university subsamples, consisting of 149 male and 145 female Australian, and of 69 male and 66 female New Zealand beginning psychology students, rate person descriptions (using Canadian, Maori, Aborigine, and Chinese concepts as stimuli) with corresponding behavioral statements. Australian Ss showed significantly more prejudice than New Zealand Ss, especially for Maori and Chinese concepts. Mean prejudice scores, with 2-tail t-tests applied to determine significance of deviations from zero, revealed that both Australian and New Zealand groups showed prejudice for the 3 "colored" concepts but not for the control Canadian concept. While sex differences were small, the largest component appeared for the Chinese concept on the Marital Rejection scale, with females showing relatively higher prejudice. Pronounced results common to both groups were their significant prejudice scores, manifesting rejection of the Chinese concept, and in their particularly high prejudice scores on the Marital Rejection scale.

1944

Russell, R. D. (1983). "Old" ideas still valuable: A review of cross-cultural case studies. Journal of School Health, 53, *112-115.*

Discusses a book, Health, Culture, and Community, written by B. Paul (1955) of 16 case studies of public reactions to medical and health programs that were instituted in places such as Chile, Natal, China, and Yap. The book's relevance for developing a multicultural, ecological perspective on health is also discussed.

1945

Ryback, D. (1976). Childrearing and child-care practices among Israeli students. Psychological Reports, 38, *922.*

Results from a comparison of data obtained from 150 Israeli university students with previously published data from Thai, Ethiopian, and Chinese students suggest that some childrearing practices in Israel are very similar to those in other cultures. However, more Israeli than Ethiopian, Thai, or Chinese (a) saw children as being made to feel loved, (b) saw parents as being sensitive to children's needs, and (c) expected their children to become quickly independent of the family.

1946

Ryback, D., Sanders, A. L., Lorentz, J., & Koestenblatt, M. (1980). Childrearing practices reported by students in six cultures. Journal of Social Psychology, 110, *153-162.*

A questionnaire exploring childrearing aspects of psychological security, feeding and weaning, toilet training, and socialization was administered to respondents of 6 cultures: a total of 1,187 undergraduates from Ethiopia, the Republic of China, Thailand, Israel, India, and the US. Ss responded to the questionnaire on the basis of their general ideas about childrearing practices in their own culture and their own home experience. Significant differences across all cultures within each item were found. For example, Ethiopian, followed by Indian mothers were seen as most likely to suckle a crying infant. Israelis were thought to be most likely to feed a child on a schedule convenient to the mother and most likely to wean by sudden withdrawal rather than by gradual stages.

1947

Sargent, M. J. (1971). A cross-cultural study of attitudes and behaviour towards alcohol and drugs. British Journal of Sociology, 22, *83-96.*

Cultural groups were chosen to reflect Bale's 4 setting attitudes toward drinking: abstinence (Chinese), ritual usage (Jewish), convivial usage (Japanese), and utilitarian (Australian). The Chinese subgroup (n = 207), Jewish subgroup (n = 112), and Australian-born subgroup (n = 1,594) were selected from a larger group of undergraduate students at 3 Australian universities; Japanese (n = 278) Ss were drawn from 4 universities in northern Japan. Ss' drinking behavior was assessed by the Knupfer Frequency Quantity Index and the Park Problem Drinking Scale; questions about attitudes and drug usage were also included. In addition, several unstructured discussion groups were organized and transcribed to verify some of the underlying attitudes assumed. 3 of the 8 predictions that Australian men would have higher representation of heavy drinkers, that the Chinese would have the highest representation of abstainers, that there would be a greater proportion of abstainers among Australians than among Jews or Japanese were confirmed. Substitution of drugs for alcohol was higher among Australian women and Jewish people, for whom alcoholic intoxication is proscribed. The data were interpreted as support for Bales's Theory that alcoholism is related to cultural attitudes.

1948

Schafer, B. (1973). [Measurement of ethnic differences on a semantic differential]. Archiv fur Psychologie, 125, *29-38. (In other language.)*

Attempted to evaluate the measurement of ethnic differences on the popular "judging people" basis on a semantic level. The instrument used represents 2 empirically derived factorial concepts with 5 scales each. The dimensions are characterized as social and economic status and temperament. 71 Ss responded to a list of 66 bipolar adjectives describing ethnic groups (e.g., Anglo-Americans, Chinese, or French) in order to determine various semantic constellations for each nation. 4 factors were used, (2 in addition to those mentioned above), resulting in 284 concept judgments.

1949

Schmeidler, G., & Windholz, G. (1976). Sex roles and the subjective: A cross-cultural test. Signs, 2, *207-212.*

Explored differences and similarities in line drawings produced by over 1,000 college students from Korea, Japan, Okinawa, Taiwan, Thailand, and New York. Using M. Scheerer and J. Lyons's study as a model, Ss drew lines in response to 10 words: "father", "mother", "husband", "wife", "love", and 5 of the abstract words used by Scheerer and Lyons. Each drawing was scored for pressure, size, openness, direction, pattern, shape, and regularity. Results established that despite dissimilarities of language, the attributes of the drawings by the various groups showed strong similarities. Cross-comparison of drawings denoting sex-role words showed that words were paired by sex (i.e., "father" and "husband") rather than by status (i.e., "husband" and "wife"), and that the lines for female roles were less similar than those for male roles. Comparisons of abstract and sex-role words showed associations of the female sex roles with happiness and love, and the male sex roles with pride and strength. Differences in the drawings by the 2 sexes were also investigated. Implications of the results center around cross-cultural variability and modifiability of attitudes with regard to sex roles as expressed in line drawings.

1950

Schneider, M. J. (1980). Cross-cultural communication and the acquisition of communicative competence. Dissertation Abstracts International, 40, *A6071.*

1951

Schwartz, L. L., & Isser, N. (1979). Psychohistorical perceptions of involuntary conversion. Adolescence, 14, *351-360.*

Discusses 2 19th-century cases of forced conversion of Jewish children to Catholicism and their effects on the people involved. Comparison is made with modern "cult" conversions and with thought reform techniques used by the Chinese in the Korean War. Numerous parallels in techniques are cited, and aid for returning Vietnam veterans, cult converts, and their families is recommended.

1952

Schwertfeger, M. M. (1982). Interethnic marriage and divorce in Hawaii: A panel study of 1968 first marriages. Marriage & Family Review, 5, *49-59.*

Findings from a 9-yr longitudinal study of 3,405 1st marriages of Hawaiian residents in 1968 support previously reported (e.g., A. Lind, 1964), slightly lower divorce rates for Japanese and Chinese marriages. The data underscore the remarkable stability of Chinese in marriages in comparison to those of other ethnic groups. The overall divorce rates were higher for inter- rather than intraethnic marriages, reflecting sex and ethnicity interaction effects between interethnic partners.

1953

Shiang, J. (1984). The significance of transactions: Reciprocity between Chinese elderly and their adult children living in Boston and its suburbs. Dissertation Abstracts International, 45, *A1157.*

1954

Shih, L. (1971). [Conflicts among the Paiwanese families: Some cases from Su-Paiwan Village]. Bulletin of the Institute of Ethnology *(Academia Sinica), No. 32, 311-324. (In Chinese.)*

1955

Shih, L. S., Nelson, D. L., & Duncombe, L. W. (1984). Mood and affect following success and failure in two cultural groups. Occupational Therapy Journal of Research, 4, *213-230.*

It was hypothesized that a success experience and a failure experience would elicit different moods and affects in participants and that cultural background would affect responses to success and failure. The subjects were 20 Chinese graduate students currently enrolled in US graduate schools and 20 U.S. graduate students. The semantic differential technique and the bipolar form of the Profile of Mood States (POMS) were used as dependent variables. The independent variables were success-failure, nationality, and gender. Results revealed that across the nationalities and across the sexes, the success experience resulted in significantly more positive moods and affects than the failure experience. The only significant interaction between nationality and success-failure occurred on the composed-anxious factor of the POMS; the Chinese group felt especially composed after the success activity in comparison with the American group. Females' moods were generally lower than males' on preactivity, postsuccess, and postfailure measurements.

1956

Shu, T. (1985). Attitudes toward one's own ethnic language: The Chinese in Houston. Dissertation Abstracts International, 46, *A413-414.*

1957

Shyi, C. W., & Li, M. C. (1982). [The relationships among locus of control, modernity and political attitude]. Journal of Education and Psychology, 5, *251-262. (In Chinese.)*

Ninety-six male and 115 female college students were tested with Internal-External (I-E) Locus of Control Scale, Individual Modernity Scale and Political Attitude Scale. The I-E Scale and Individual Modernity Scale were each divided into four factors and Political Attitude Scale was divided into three factors. It was found that subjects with higher internal control had higher scores on the factors of political autonomy and modernity, while subjects with higher external control had lower scores on the factors of political autonomy and changing social condition. Modernity was negatively related to conservative political attitude and positively related to attitudes of political autonomy and changing social condition. The relationship pattern between I-E and political attitude was the same as found for American black college students, but different from findings for American white college students. The reasons for this different result were discussed.

1958

Sidel, R., & Sidel, V. W. (1975). Education in the People's Republic of China: How many wheelbarrows of nightsoil do the Red Guards collect to serve the people of the commune? Teachers College Record, 76, *605-616.*

Examines the educational process in China as a major tool for providing a basis for putting governmental authority into the hands of the people and improving life for those who formerly had least authority. Both physical and intellectual labor are regarded as productive and each as necessary for the other. Persons are expected to participate and become competent in both general spheres. Students thus learn the varied roles of citizens and the fact that they themselves are important to the proper functioning of their society. Education as such occurs throughout life, with the individual acting as student or teacher, depending on the needs of the situation.

1959

Singer, K. (1975). The prognosis of narcotic addiction. *London: Butterworths.*

1960

Singer, K. (1975). Depressive disorders from a transcultural perspective. Social Science & Medicine, 9, *289-301.*

1961

Sinha, A. K. P., & Upadhyaya, O. P. (1960). Stereotypes of male and female university students in India toward different ethnic groups. Journal of Social Psychology, 51, *93-102.*

1962

Sinha, A. K. P., & Upadhyaya, O. P. (1962). Eleven ethnic groups on a social distance scale. Journal of Social Psychology, 57, *49-54.*

1963

Sinha, G. S., & Sinha, S. P. (1966). A study of national stereotypes. Indian Journal of Social Work, 27, *163-173.*

100 graduate and undergraduate students of Patna University were asked to select 3 characteristics for each of 10 national groups (American, Burmese, Ceylonese, Chinese, English, French, Indian, Nepali, Pakistani, and Russian). They were also asked to judge the 100 checklist characteristics in terms of desirability. Findings include: (1) The 2 student groups differed significantly in the assignment of desirability traits to Ceylonese, Chinese, Indian, and Pakistani (the undergraduates were more favorably disposed); (2) the stereotype of the Chinese has changed considerably since the Sino-Indian War as compared to previous studies; (3) considerable agreement (range 90-40% for American and French, respectively) was found between the groups concerning the 10 most frequently assigned traits; and (4) Ss see Asian nations as more similar to each other than to European nations.

1964

Smith, A. H. (1894). Chinese characteristics. *New York: Fleming H. Revell. (Reprinted London: Oliphont, Amderson & Ferrier, 1972.)*

1965

Smith, A. (Ed.). (1890). The natural history of the Chinese boy and the Chinese girl: A study in sociology. *Shanghai: North China Herald Office.*

1966

Smith, M. W. (1952). Different cultural concepts of past, present, and the future: A study of ego extension. Psychiatry, 15, *395-400.*

1967

Smith, N. V. O., & Vinacke, W. E. (1951). Reactions to humorous stimuli of different generations of Japanese, Chinese, and Caucasians in Hawaii. Journal of Social Psychology, 34, *69-96.*

1968

Smith, W. C. (1970). Americans in process: A study of our citizens of Oriental ancestry. *New York: Arno Press. (Original work published 1937)*

1969

Solomon, R. (1978). The evolution of opiate use in China: The origins of the illicit international trade. Journal of Psychedelic Drugs, 10, *43-49.*

1970

Solomon, R. H. (1969). Mao's effort to reintegrate the Chinese polity: Problems of authority and conflict in Chinese social processes. In A. D. Barnett (Ed.), Chinese Communist politics in action *(pp. 271-361). Seattle: University of Washington Press.*

1971

Solomon, R. H. (1971). Mao's revolution and the Chinese political culture. *Berkeley, CA: University of California Press.*

1972

Spradley, J. P., & Phillips, M. (1972). Culture and stress: A quantitative analysis. American Anthropologist, 74, *518-529.*

Although anthropologists often employ the concept of stress to account for behavior, they have seldom studied differences in the way stressful situations are appraised. A method for quantifying the perceived magnitudes of events leading to culture shock is described. The resultant Cultural Readjustment Rating Questionnaire was administered to 83 returned Peace Corps volunteers, 34 Chinese foreign students, and 42 United States students with no intercultural experience. Results suggest that there are universal stressors, encountered by those who experience culture shock, as well as culture-related differences in the definition of stress. Other applications of the method which may increase the rigor of comparative studies are discussed.

1973

Stein, D. J. (1974). The phenomenology of resettlement: An exploration into the experiences of Chinese immigrants in San Francisco. Dissertation Abstracts International, 34, *B3477.*

1974

Stoessinger, J. G. (1970). China and America: The burden of the past. American Journal of Psychotherapy, 24, *579-596.*

Traces America's involvement in Chinese affairs through recent centuries, and the accompanying misinterpretations by both sides regarding the nature of the other's intent. Contends modern attitudes have seeds in specific historical events.

1975

Stoodley, B. H. (1967). Normative family orientations of Chinese college students in Hong Kong. Journal of Marriage & the Family, 29, *773-782.*

Chinese college students were interviewed with reference to family norms. The data suggest that the younger generation, while adopting the western norm of individual choice in marriage, observes proprieties of parental respect and Confucian tradition while only partially accepting western norms of dating and romantic love. This movement toward an extended family type may be functional in the urban context.

1976

Stover, L. (1962). "Face" and verbal analogues of interaction in Chinese culture: A theory of formalized social behavior based upon participant-observation of an upper-class Chinese household, together with a biographical study of primary informant. *Doctoral dissertation, Columbia University, Ann Arbor. (University Microfilms No. 62-5199, 184-197).*

1977

Stover, L. E. (1974). The ecology of Chinese civilization. *New York: New American Library.*

1978

Stover, L. E., & Stover, T. K. (1976). China: An anthropological perspective. *Pacific Palisades, CA: Goodyear.*

1979

Stratton, G. M., & Henry, F. M. (1943). Emotion in Chinese, Japanese and Whites: Racial and national differences and likeness in physiological reactions to an emotional stimulus. American Journal of Psychology, 56, *161-180.*

1980

Streufert, S., & Sandler, S. I. (1971). A laboratory test of the mirror image hypothesis. Journal of Applied Social Psychology, 1, *378-397.*

Chinese and American nationals participated in an experimental inter-nation simulation as a test of Bronfenbrenner's Mirror Image hypotheses. Perceptions of own and opposing nations were measured for (a) a rebel movement, and (b) a large power fighting a rebel movement in a foreign nation. The effects of information availability (relevance) and of increasing threat from a 3rd power were also investigated. It was found that evaluative mirror image perceptions of the opposing nation as "bad" and one's own as "good" were easily established. Mirror image perceptions of "they are the aggressors" were found for Chinese but not for Americans. Information relevance had only limited effects. Threat from a 3rd power produced, in general, decreased mirror image perceptions for Ss representing the large power, but did not affect Ss representing the rebel movement.

1981

Streufert, S., & Sandler, S. I. (1973). Perceived success and competence of the opponent, or the Laboratory Dien Bien Phu. Journal of Applied Social Psychology, 3, *84-93.*

Studied the effect of information relevance and information availability on perceptual differences between Chinese and American nationals. 24 U.S. citizens and 24 nationals of Hong Kong or Taiwan participated as same-national pairs in the Tactical and Negotiations Game. Participants' perceptions of success, failure, and competence levels for their own team (under conditions where judgments could be based on varying levels of relevant information) and for a supposed opposing team (under conditions where perceptions had to be inferred in the absence of information) were obtained. It was found that Americans and Chinese did not differ in ratings of their own team. Chinese, as opposed to Americans, perceived the opposing team as having more success, less failure, and more competence. The perceptual errors of the French and Viet Minh which led to the defeat of the French at Dien Bien Phu were replicated in the laboratory for Americans and Chinese. Areas in which such potential cultural differences (oriental vs occidental) might be important are mentioned.

1982

Su, C. W. (1968). [The child's perception of parent's role]. Psychology and Education *(Taiwan Normal University),* **2,** *87-109. (In Chinese.)*

The main purpose of this investigation was to obtain information on parental roles through the child's perception. The subjects were 708 children in the fourth, fifth, and sixth grades in Taiwan. A questionnaire with 47 items concerning child-training attitudes and practices was used. The data showed that either parent could function as the main disciplinarian. There was no appreciable difference between parents in the frequency of giving punishments, even though in most cases it was the mother who spent more time in disciplining the child. In a majority of cases, the father was perceived to be the harsher disciplinarian and the authority figure in the home, and was the parent of whom the child was more afraid. In contrast, the mother was more likely than the father to be perceived as the more forgiving parent and to be better liked by the child.

1983

Su, C. Y., Lin, S. H., Wang, Y. T. et al. (1978). Effects of beta-endorphin on narcotic abstinence syndrome in man. Journal of Formosan Medical Association, *77, 133-141.*

Eight adult Chinese male addict volunteers with long histories of high-dosage narcotic addiction were studied under strict surveillance. Human beta-endorphin was administered intravenously to 4 patients who exhibited a severe withdrawal syndrome from heroin. The intensity of the abstinence syndrome experienced by each patient was scored by the Kolb-Himmelsbach system with minor modification. Thirty minutes after the injection of 80 mug/kg of beta-endorphin, the improvement of the abstinence syndrome was very impressive and dramatic in 2 patients who were previously in a very severe withdrawal condition. The results suggest that beta-endorphin may have practical importance in the treatment of narcotic addiction, and implicate the possibility that endogenous beta-endorphin may play some role in the mechanism of narcotic tolerance and dependence.

1984

Sue, D., Ino, S., & Sue, D. M. (1983). Nonassertiveness of Asian Americans: An inaccurate assumption? Journal of Counseling Psychology, 30, *581-588.*

Tested the view that Asian Americans are nonassertive and the possibility that they display differential assertiveness depending on situational variables. To determine if race of the individual with whom they are interacting is an influencing variable on assertion in Asian Americans, 51 Chinese-American and 25 Caucasian undergraduate males were randomly assigned to 1 of 2 conditions: role playing a series of 13 situations requiring assertion with an Asian experimenter or role playing the same situations with a Caucasian experimenter. Ss also completed the Social Avoidance and Distress Scale, Fear of Negative Evaluation Questionnaire, and Rathus Assertiveness Schedule. Results indicate that Chinese-Americans were as assertive as Caucasians on all behavioral measures and that the race of experimenter was not an important variable in the performance of Asians. Consistent with previous studies, significant differences on self-report measures were obtained. Chinese-Americans were more likely to report anxiety in social situations, greater apprehension in evaluative situations, and lower assertiveness than Caucasians.

1985

Sue, D. W., & Frank, A. C. (1973). A typological approach to the psychological study of Chinese and Japanese American college males. Journal of Social Issues, 29, *129-148.*

Applied a typology formed from scores on the School and College Ability Test, SVIB, and Omnibus Personality Inventory to 104 Chinese- and 50 Japanese-American males to identify certain homogeneous subgroups and their resultant psychological characteristics. Chinese- and Japanese-American males tended to concentrate in certain groups and exhibit unique characteristics that seem explicable in terms of their cultural background and historical experience in America. Results suggest that Asian-Americans are experiencing more stress than their Caucasian counterparts.

1986

Sue, S., & Kitano, H. H. (1973). Stereotypes as a measure of success. Journal of Social Issues, 29, *83-98.*

Discusses the fact that Chinese and Japanese stereotypes have undergone dramatic changes. Early stereotypes were uniformly negative, reflecting the social, economic, and political climate in America. After passage of discriminatory laws and the entrance of other minorities, Asians were considered less dangerous and the favorability of stereotypes increased. World War II revived negative stereotypes against the Japanese. Today Asian Americans are viewed as successful, model minorities. The question is raised whether these positive stereotypes and views are accurate. It is suggested that methodological and conceptual problems in the study of stereotypes have hindered a clear analysis of this question. The partial truth and potential negative consequences of favorable stereotypes are also discussed.

1987

Sue, S., & Nakamura, C. Y. (1984). An integrative model of physiological and social/psychological factors in alcohol consumption among Chinese and Japanese Americans. Journal of Drug Issues, 14, *349-364.*

This is a review of the physiological and social-cultural factors contributing to the low rate of alcohol consumption among Chinese and Japanese Americans. It is contended that while drinking, particularly at social functions, is permissible, excess drinking is discouraged and tightly regulated by family and community attitudes and values. It is also suggested that Chinese and Japanese exhibit different physiological responses in alcohol metabolism and cardiovascular sensitivity from those of Caucasians. A reciprocity model is proposed to conceptualize and integrate these factors and to explain the problems faced by Asian American adolescents. It is argued that the progressive assimilation of Asian Americans to American values is likely to increase alcohol consumption and that Asian Americans confronted with alcohol must also contend with the different influences of their parents' Asian culture and that of the larger American society. Implications for future research that simultaneously consider physiological and social-cultural influences are discussed.

1988

Sue, S., Sue, D. W., & Sue, D. W. (1975). Asian Americans as a minority group. American Psychologist, 30, *906-910.*

Based on the 1970 US Census and available studies, the status of Chinese, Filipinos, and Japanese is examined. 2 views are presented: Asian Americans as a successful minority group and as an oppressed minority group. It is suggested that (a) statistics regarding income, education, interracial marriage, and mental health need to be critically examined because of prevailing myths and stereotypes and (b) an accurate assessment of the needs and experiences of Asian Americans is necessary in order to provide adequate psychological services.

1989

Sue, S., & Wagner, M. (Eds.) (1973). Asian-Americans: Psychological perspectives. *Palo Alto, CA: Science & Behavior Books.*

1990

Sue, S., Zane, N., & Ito, J. (1979). Alcohol drinking patterns among Asian and Caucasian Americans. Journal of Cross-Cultural Psychology, 10, *41-56.*

Results of a study of 47 Asian- and 77 Caucasian-American university students suggest the importance of the cultural factor hypothesis in drinking patterns, rather than the genetic hypothesis, which assumes racial physiological differences in alcohol reactions.

1991

Suedfeld, P., Epstein, Y. M., Buchanan, E., & Landon, P. B. (1971). Effects of set on the "effects of mere exposure". Journal of Personality & Social Psychology, 17, *121-123.*

Replicated 1 of R. B. Zajonc's studies on the attitudinal effects of differential exposure, using 6 "Chinese characters" at exposure frequencies of 0, 1, 2, 5, 10, and 25. Each of 72 undergraduates saw 1 stimulus at each frequency. 1/2 of the Ss were given a favorable set toward the stimuli, the other 1/2, an unfavorable set. The 1st group's ratings were similar to those reported by Zajonc. The other group's ratings were a curvilinear function of exposure, with the most negative ratings at 0 and 25 exposures. Set apparently determines evaluation after the stimulus becomes moderately familiar.

1992

Sun, L. K. (1983). [The "deep structure" of Chinese culture]. *Hong Kong: Ji Xian. (In Chinese.)*

1993

Tan, M. G. (1969). Social mobility and assimilation: The Chinese in the United States. Dissertation Abstracts International, 30, *A416-417.*

1994

Tanaka, Y. (1972). Values in the subjective culture: A social psychological view. Journal of Cross-Cultural Psychology, 3, *57-69.*

Using POLDI (a variation of the semantic differential method) as a measuring instrument, Japanese and German subjects judged a set of nation concepts. The results indicated a subtle but real cultural uniqueness of evaluative criteria despite the over-all consistency in the semantic frame of reference. Next, Evaluative Atlases of several critical concepts were constructed on the basis of data collected in 15 language/culture communities by means of multi-lingual semantic differentials, and comparisons were made among the 15 communities. Finally, a plan of intercultural cooperation was proposed, stressing the responsibility of social and behavioral scientists for both devising and executing plans for the engineering of such intercultural cooperation.

1995

Tao, L. K. (1934). Some Chinese characteristics in the light of the Chinese family. In E. E. Evans-Pritchard et al. (Eds.), Essays presented to C. G. Selingman. *London: Kegan Paul, Trench, & Trubner.*

1996

Tarwater, J. W. (1966). Chinese and American students' interpersonal values: A cross-cultural comparison. Journal of College Student Personnel, *7, 351-354.*

1997

Tavris, C. (1974, May). The speak-bitterness revolution, everybody is a psychologist, and field report: Women in China. Psychology Today, 7, *43-49, 92-93, 97-98.*

1998

Thakerar, J. N., & Iwawaki, S. (1979). Cross-cultural comparisons in interpersonal attraction of females toward males. Journal of Social Psychology, 108, *121-122.*

Tested the hypotheses that (a) females from different cultures would judge 10 photographs of modern Greek males similarly as to physical attractiveness and (b) the 2 groups of females would attach different levels of importance to the physical and psychological traits of attraction. Results with 17 English and 17 Eastern (10 Chinese and 7 Indian) Ss (mean age 21.7 yrs) support the hypotheses.

1999

The Asian American Elderly. (1972). Whitehouse Conference on aging, 1971. *Washington, DC: U.S. Government Printing Office.*

2000

Tong, B. (1974). A living death defended as the legacy of a superior culture. *Working papers by the University of California, Los Angeles, Asian-American Studies Center. (Reprinted in Amerasia Journal.)*

2001

Tong, B. R. (1971). **The ghetto of the mind: Notes on the historical psychology of Chinese America. Amerasia Journal, 1,** *1-31.*

2002

Topley, M. (1966). **Some basic conceptions and their traditional relationships to society. In M. Topley (Ed.), Some traditional Chinese ideas and conceptions in the Hong Kong social life today.** *Hong Kong: Hong Kong Branch of Royal Asiatic Society.*

2003

Triandis, H. C. et al. (1984). **Individual models of social behavior. Journal of Personality & Social Psychology, 46,** *1389-1404.*

Presents a technique that extracts individual models of social behavior. Such models reflect each individual's ideas about what social behaviors are interrelated, and what aspects of social situations are linked to different levels of probability that particular patterns of social behavior will occur. The method was used in 2 studies, one with bicultural Ss (1 American, 6 Latin Americans, 2 Hong Kong Chinese, and 1 Greek) and the other with 22 monocultural Mexican and Chinese Ss and 8 of the bilinguals from the 1st study. For each S, factor analysis of the judgments concerning the probability of occurrence of specific social behaviors in specific social situations provided information of how the S linked social behaviors. ANOVA on the factor scores provided information about the S's beliefs concerning how attributes of social situations are linked to social behaviors. Inspection of the individual models of social behavior indicated that some common elements across models are probably linked to culture. The technique has wide applicability for social and personality psychology because it permits idiographic comparison of models of social behavior across individuals who share some attribute.

2004

Triandis, H. C., McGuire, H., Saral, T. G., Yang, K. S., Loh, W., & Vassiliou, V. (1972). **A cross-cultural study of role perceptions. In. H. G. Triandis et al. (Eds.), The analysis of subjective culture.** *New York: Wiley-interscience.*

2005

Tsai, W. H. (1966). **[A study of interpersonal relationships in the family of Taiwan]. Thought and Word, 4,** *28-33. (In Chinese.)*

2006

Tsai, W. H. (1968). **[A study of social interactions in college students' daily life]. Journal of Sociology** *(National Taiwan University),* **4,** *156-167. (In Chinese.)*

2007

Tsai, W. H. (1973). **[The freedom of love in the changing Chinese society]. Thought and Word, 10,** *41-51. (In Chinese.)*

2008

Tsao, K. H. (1981). **[Generation gap among Taipei high school students]. Acta Psychologica Taiwanica, 23,** *9-16. (In Chinese.)*

Generation gap is defined as differences between two generations in values, interests, and attitudes. In this study, perceived agreements with parents and with peers on 15 moral and value issues were compared. The subjects were 2,557 students, 1,439 males, and 1,118 females, from nine Taipei high schools. The main findings were: (1) Attitudes toward religion were similar to perceived parental attitudes; attitudes toward homework, choice of friends, choice of clothing, hair style, TV programs, music were similar to perceived peer attitudes. (2) Attitudes toward spending money, smoking cigarettes, drinking alcohol, premarital sex, discipline, and view of life interacted with attitudes toward parents; subjects favorable toward parents held attitudes which were more similar to perceived parental attitudes, whereas subjects unfavourable toward parents held attitudes more similar to perceived peer attitudes. (3) Sex differences were evident in attitudes toward smoking cigarettes, drinking alcohol, and premarital sex. (4) Attitudes toward parents were positively related to interaction with parents.

2009

Tseng, W. S., & Hsu, J. (1969). **Chinese culture, personality formation and mental illness. International Journal of Social Psychiatry, 16,** *5-14.*

Elements of Chinese culture, especially childrearing practices, may influence the frequency and types of mental illness observed in China. Depression, homosexuality, and alcoholism are examples of disorders diagnosed less frequently in China than in the United States. These differences are explained by such Chinese cultural factors as the use of shame in conscience-formation, the presence of an extended family participating in infant care, and an aversion to the public expression of strong emotions. In comparison to United States culture, Chinese culture places less emphasis on emotional adjustment and greater stress on physical well-being. As a result, Chinese patients present a higher proportion of neurasthenic, hypochondriacal, and psychosomatic symptoms than American psychiatric patients.

2010

Tseng, W. S., & Hsu, J. (1972). **The Chinese attitude toward parental authority as expressed in Chinese children's stories. Archives of General Psychiatry, 26,** *28-34.*

The classic Twenty-Four Stories of Filial Piety, which has been influential in Chinese child rearing, is presented to illustrate the relationship between generations. Other well-known children's stories are also presented and are arranged according to stages of human development: (a) transition from omnipotent fantasy to reality orientation; (b) triangular conflict between the child and parents; and (c) interference with the alliance of a young couple by authority. In Chinese children's stories, defiance of parental authority results in the admonition, punishment, or death of the transgressor. If he survives, however, he is given opportunity for training and atonement. In conflicts between generations, the elders always triumph.

2011

Tsien-Lee, M. (1974). [Attitudes toward past, present, and future among Chinese subjects]. Psychologica Belgica, 14, *297-312. (In other language.)*

Administered semantic differential scales measuring attitudes toward past, present, and future to 724 Chinese of both sexes, 16-68 yrs old, from different social strata and different regions, including native Taiwanese and continental Chinese. Results show that Ss' attitude toward the future was the most positive one. Female Ss' attitudes toward the past were more positive, and their attitudes toward the present and future were less positive, than those of male Ss. Young people had a more positive attitude toward the future and a less positive attitude toward the past than older Ss. Attitudes toward the future were less positive among continental Chinese than among Taiwanese but this difference was smaller among younger Ss. Discussion includes critical examination of methodology employed, with suggestions for improvement.

2012

Tsung, S. K. F. (1978). Moms, nuns and hookers: Extrafamilial alternatives for village women in Taiwan. Dissertation Abstracts International, 39, *A2390.*

2013

Tucker, G. R., Taylor, D. M., & Reyes, E. (1971). Ethnic group interaction in a multiethnic society. International Journal of Psychology, 6, *217-222.*

120 male Manilan Ss (average age, 11.5), who said their native language was Tagalog and identified themselves as members of the Tagalog regional group, watched a videotape skit of the same scene repeated 4 times with different combinations of Tagalog and Chinese boys. The skit portrayed a discussion about how to spend a free afternoon. 2 boys (actors) consistently overruled a 3rd who suggested a game of table tennis in preference to swimming. In the mixed ethnic-group conditions, the actor different in ethnic affiliation was also the one overruled in the skit. Before watching the skit, Ss rated on a 7-point scale how well they anticipated the actors would "get along" and were asked to select the language they expected them to use in the dialogue. 12 test sessions corresponded to each of the experimental conditions. Results reveal that Ss perceived that members of homogeneously composed groups would get along better than heterogeneous groups, especially for all-Chinese groups. While Ss unanimously correctly identified the language spoken, they showed much less accuracy in deciding which actors were Tagalog and which Chinese. This technique may be appropriate to study changes in ethnic group relations due to changes in language policy.

2014

Tung, M. P. (1980). Symbolic meaning of the body in Chinese culture: A psycholinguistic inquiry. Dissertation Abstracts International, 40, *B3427.*

2015

Tyagi, A. K. (1975). A comparative study of some techniques of psychological interrogation of the prisoners of war. Journal of Psychological Researches, 20, *49-55.*

Studied the manner in which prisoners of war (POWs) were interrogated by the Chinese and Pakistanis during a series of border disputes in 1962 and the techniques used to indoctrinate the Indian soldiers to obtain information and convert POWs to their captors' political ideologies. 178 ex-POWs of China and Pakistan were interviewed. It was found that, while the Chinese had adopted scientific methods of indoctrination to get strategic information and to impress the POWs with their ideologies, the Pakistanis interrogators did not use any sophisticated techniques of indoctrination and were interested only in tactical information of immediate utility.

2016

Ullman, L. P., Freedland, K. E., & Warmsun, C. H. (1978). Sex and ethnic group effects on attitudes toward women. Bulletin of the Psychonomic Society, 11, *179-180.*

Two popular measures of attitudes toward women, the short version of the Attitudes Toward Women Scale (AWS) and the Feminism (FEM) Scale were administered to 208 women and 106 men who identified themselves as Caucasian, American of Japanese ancestry, Chinese, Hawaiian and part Hawaiian, and other. The 2 scales correlated highly with each other. The sex and ethnic identity main effects were statistically significant on both scales, and the AWS yielded a significant Sex by Ethnic Identity interaction, while the FEM did not.

2017

Upmanyu, V. V., & Vasudeva, P. N. (1981). A study of attitude towards Chinese, Pakistanese and Russians in relation to socio-economic status. Journal of Psychological Researches, 25, *5-14.*

Administered a modified version of L. L. Thurstone's (1929) attitude scale to 500 male and 500 female 18-38 yr old Indian college students. Independent of socioeconomic status, Ss held favorable attitudes toward Russians and unfavorable attitudes toward Pakistanis. Attitudes toward the Chinese were influenced by socioeconomic status, with those Ss whose fathers had had more education having less unfavorable attitudes than Ss whose fathers only had a high school education.

2018

Van den Berghe, P. L. (1983). Human inbreeding avoidance: Culture in nature. Behavioral & Brain Sciences, 6, *91-123.*

Much clinical and ethnographic evidence suggests that humans, like many other organisms, are selected to avoid close inbreeding because of the fitness costs of inbreeding depression. The proximate mechanism of human inbreeding avoidance seems to be precultural and to involve the interaction of genetic predispositions and environmental conditions. As first suggested by E. Westermarck (1891) and supported by evidence from Israeli kibbutzim, Chinese sim-pua marriage, and convergent ethnographic and clinical evidence, humans negatively imprint on intimate associates during a critical period of early childhood (between 2 and 6 yrs of age). There is also much evidence that humans, like other social animals, do not seek to maximize outbreeding, but rather to maintain an optimal balance between outbreeding and inbreeding. Close inbreeding reduces fitness through inbreeding depression, but some inbreeding brings the benefits of nepotism. For simple, stateless, horticultural societies, the optimal balance seems to be achieved by a combination of precultural inbreeding avoidance of relatives and cultural rules of preferential marriage. Adjustment of the coefficient of inbreeding to other ecological settings seems to be largely cultural. An interactive model of "culture in nature" is presented in which culture is seen as co-evolving with genes to produce the maximization of individual inclusive fitness. Commentaries on the article and the author's response are included.

2019

Van Gulik, R. H. (1961). Sexual life in ancient China. *Zeiden: E. J. Brill.*

2020

Vandenberg, S. G. (1967). The primary mental abilities of south American students: A second comparative study of the generality of a cognitive factor structure. Multivariate Behavioral Research, 2, *175-198.*

In an earlier study, the primary mental abilities (PMA) of Chinese students studying in American universities was compared with those of American college students. In the present study, the PMAs of South American college students are compared with the Chinese students. 31 Tests (20 with English instructions and 11 with Spanish) were administered to 92 South American students who were participating in the English language institute of the University of Michigan. After treating the South American data by Ahmavaara's Transformation Analysis, 7 factors were matched between the south American and Chinese studies; the congruence indices for the 2 sets of factors ranged between .953 And .780.

2021

Vernon, P. (1980). Chinese immigrants and citizens in Canada. New Horizons, *No. 21, 12-25.*

2022

Vinacke, W. E., & Fong, R. W. (1955). The judgment of facial expressions by three national-racial groups in Hawaii: II. Oriental faces. Journal of Social Psychology, 41, *185-195.*

2023

Vinake, W. E. (1949). Stereotyping among national-racial groups in Hawaii: A study in ethnocentrism. Journal of Social Psychology, 30, *265-291.*

2024

Vogel, E. (1965). From friendship to comradeship: The change in personal relations in Communist China. China Quarterly, 21, *46-60.*

2025

Vogel, E. F. (1969). A preliminary view of family and mental health in urban Communist China. In W. A. Caudill & T. Y. Lin (Eds.), Mental health research in Asia and the Pacific *(pp. 393-404). Honolulu: East-West Center Press.*

2026

Wan, K. C., & Bond, M. H. (1982). Chinese attributions for success and failure under public and anonymous conditions of rating. Acta Psychologica Taiwanica, 24, *23-31.*

The self-serving or egocentric bias is a well-documented effect whereby subjects attribute their success more to internal factors and less to external factors than they do their failure. The present study adopted the methodology of Snyder, Stephan, and Rosenfield to explore this phenomenon in Chinese culture. Attributions for successful and unsuccessful performance on a competitive matrix game were collected under both anonymous and public conditions of responding. Under both conditions of responding, a self-serving bias was found for the subjects' attributions of ability and effort. For attributions to luck, however, conditions of responding interacted with competition outcome so that the egocentric bias was found under anonymous conditions, but a self-effecting bias was found under public conditions. Discussion focussed on the universality of the self-serving bias in private attributions and the impact of culture on the size and direction of the self-serving bias in public explanations. The construct of luck may play an important role in moderating private egocentrism during social interaction.

2027

Wang, F. K. (1958). [A study of social attitudes]. Psychological Testing, 6, *398-401. (In Chinese.)*

2028

Wang, G., & McKillip, J. (1978). Ethnic identification and judgements of an accident. Personality & Social Psychology Bulletin, 4, *296-299.*

Examined the effect of ethnic identity on judgments of an accident made by samples of Chinese students studying in the US, of American college students, and of American small town residents. 90 Ss read 3 versions of an automobile accident: (1) a Chinese driver hit an American victim, (2) an American driver hit a Chinese victim, and (3) no ethnic identification included in the scenario. Results reveal that ethnic identity mediated assessments of fine and judgments of personality characteristics for Chinese students and town residents, but not for American students. Ethnic identity plays a significant role in determining attributions for intergroup interaction, but only for those for whom the particular ethnic categorization is important. The implication is that where group identity is weak, bias in perception and attribution will also be weak.

2029

Wang, J. F. (1981). Education and fertility behavior: A case study in Taipei, Taiwan. Dissertation Abstracts International, 41, *A4895.*

2030

Wang, P. S. (1973). Father-son relationship problems over three generations. Journal of Sociology *(National Taiwan University), 9, 30-90.*

2031

Wang, S. G. (1982). [Sociology and the population problem]. Shehui Kexue Zhanxian [Social Science Front], 5, *98-103. (In Chinese.)*

2032

Wang, V. L. (1975). Motivating the masses for family planning in the People's Republic of China. Bulletin of the Pan American Health Organization, 9, *95-111.*

China's family planning program has been praised by some for being among the most rational and extensive in the developing world. This paper focuses on Chinese attitudes, knowledge, and behavior in this area, and describes the network of supportive services and motivational efforts undertaken to promote birth control in the People's Republic.

2033

Wang, Y. C. (1950). Columbia University Research in Contemporary Cultures *(CH-179). Unpublished document, American Museum of Natural History, New York.*

2034

Ward, B. E. (1985). Through other eyes: Essays in understanding "conscious models"--mostly in Hong Kong. *Hong Kong: Chinese University Press.*

This is a collection of papers of anthropological, sociological, and psychological interest. The papers are mainly preliminary studies of the boat-people of Hong Kong and China, socioeconomic topics in South-East Asia, the socialization of children, and the position of women in Asia. Papers attempt to answer not only questions of "What is meant by being Chinese?" but those relating to the reasons Chinese people give for keeping to, and passing on, traditional behaviors (the "conscious model"). Two papers on child development lean on the author's observations of temper tantrums and self- and parental-control within a small Hong Kong fishing village, and introduce some simple concepts as a basis for description of the integration of children into the social world of this village.

2035

War-on-Rape Committee. (1978). [Manual on rape victims counselling]. *Hong Kong: Author.*

2036

Watrous, B., & Hsu, F. L. (1972). An experiment with TAT. In F. L. Hsu (Ed.), Psychological anthropology *(new ed.). Cambridge, MA: Schenkman.*

Administered the TAT to 300 Chinese, Hindu, and American undergraduates to explore the possibility of using some form of projective test on a large cross-cultural scale to aid anthropological field work. Results indicate that the use of the full TAT may be an impediment rather than an advantage in understanding intergroup differences; the use of a few cards, however, may prove to be a better aid for understanding personality in its group than individual perspective.

2037

Weakland, J. H. (1950). The organization of action in Chinese culture. Psychiatry, 13, *361-370.*

2038

Weakland, J. H. (1953). An analysis of seven Cantonese films. In M. Mead & R. Metraux (Eds.), The study of culture at a distance. *Chicago, IL: University of Chicago Press.*

2039

Weakland, J. H. (1953). Chinese family images in international affairs. In M. Mead & R. Metraux (Eds.), The study of culture at a distance. *Chicago, IL: University of Chicago Press.*

2040

Weakland, J. H. (1956). Orality in Chinese conceptions of male genital sexuality. Psychiatry, 19, *237-247.*

2041

Weakland, J. H. (1958). Family imagery in a passage by Mao Tse-tung: An essay in psychocultural method. World Politics, 10, *340-387.*

2042

Weeks, J. R., & Cuellar, J. B. (1983). Isolation of older persons: The influence of immigration and length of residence. Research on Aging, 5, *369-388.*

Current theories suggest that migration tends to exacerbate isolation of older people, although such isolation should be mitigated by length of residence. Propositions derived from these theories were tested using data collected in San Diego from 1,139 people (aged 55 + yrs) representing 10 ethnic groups (Black, Hispanic, Filipino, Guamanian, Samoan, Japanese, Chinese, Korean, American Indian, and nonminority). Findings suggest that recent older immigrants are more isolated than elders in other migration/residence statuses. However, immigration seems to exert an overall low level of influence on isolation, whereas ethnicity independently appears to exert a greater influence.

2043

Wei, Z. (1983). Chinese family problems: Research and trends. Journal of Marriage & the Family, 45, *943-948.*

Since the enactment of the marriage laws of 1950 and 1980, family life in the People's Republic of China has undergone several dramatic changes including, more recently, a raising of the legal marriage age, less restrictions on divorce, and official promotion of family planning and reduced fertility throughout the country. Because these policies and practices conflict with Chinese traditions, inevitable problems have arisen. Economic and social problems, such as inflation and juvenile delinquency, are also addressed; and efforts toward improvement are described.

2044

Weisman, S., Snadowsky, A., & Gannon, M. (1972). Chinese college students perceive their cultural identity. Education, 92, *116-118.*

Assessed several factors of cultural heritage and identification in a sample of Chinese college students attending a large urban college. The majority of the Asian born Ss indicated a greater identification with Eastern culture, whereas the American born Ss were more inclined toward Western culture. Although a majority felt that the Chinese suffered discrimination in the United States, they also expressed confidence in the American democratic process. This apparent inconsistency is related to the finding that a majority chose their major in engineering or natural sciences, skills at the core of the American technological system. Other aspects of the Chinese Ss' educational experience and differences in responses between men and women also are considered.

2045

Weiss, M. S. (1970). Selective acculturation and the dating process: The patterning of Chinese-Caucasian interracial dating. Journal of Marriage and the Family, 32, *273-278. (Also in S. Sue & N. N. Wagner, Eds.,* **Asian-Americans: Psychological perspective.** *Palo Alto, CA: Science & Behavior Books, 1973.)*

The recent increase in Chinese-Caucasian dating may reflect a growing Chinese-American female preference for Caucasian courtship behavior. Chinese-American girls have internalized the dominant dating values of the Caucasian teenager to a greater extent than Chinese-American boys. Because many Chinese boys seem unable to master the American dating game, they often cannot meet the girls' expectations prompting the girls to seek romance, companionship and adventure in Caucasian arms. Divergent expectations and/or dating behavior between Chinese-American boys and girls may be related to: (1) the pervasive influence of American racial stereotyping; (2) Chinese-American interpersonal relationships in American society; (3) sex-linked psychological profiles and socialization practices; and (4) the closed nature and efficient information exchange system in the Chinese community.

2046

Weisskopf-Joelson, E. (1970). On surrender. Journal of Psychology, 76, *57-66.*

While modern alienated man longs to surrender to an entity which transcends his self, Western culture views such surrender as undesirable and, thus, blocks important avenues to mental health. Oriental acceptance of self-renunciation is compared with Occidental individualism. Suggestions made by a Chinese-American are quoted, stressing the importance of turning down our excessive self-reliance in favor of mutual dependency.

2047

Weller, R. P. (1985). Bandits, beggars, and ghosts: The failure of state control over religious interpretation in Taiwan. American Ethnologist, 12, *46-61.*

The author explored one way in which popular religion provides a sphere of resistance to state institutions and ideologies. Throughout the past century, both popular interpretation and official manipulation of ghosts were reworked and renewed as they interacted with each other (especially with regard to the Universal Salvation Festival) and as material conditions changed in Taiwan. The symbolic background of the ghost cult ceremony, the history of popular performances of it, and state manipulations of ghosts were examined.

2048

Welsh, C., & Wu, E. C. (1985). [Cognition of household roles, disturbance in marital relationships and husband's extra-marital affairs]. Chinese Journal of Mental Health, 2, *105-118. (In Chinese.)*

This study examined extramarital affairs in which the husband was the unfaithful partner. The subjects included a "main group" of 409 wives seeking help for marriages troubled by their husbands' unfaithfulness. Two control groups consisted of: a "problem group" of 55 wives seeking help for a variety of problems other than an extramarital affair, and a "normal group" of 139 wives from normal marriages. Data was collected through structured interviews. The results indicated degree of marital satisfaction had a considerable effect on extramarital behavior. Affective changes had a dual impact on both marital satisfaction and extramarital behavior. The long term deterioration in affective relationship was strongest in the main group, slightly less in the problem group, and virtually nonexistent in the normal group. Path analysis indicated that the effect of the cognitive difference between husband and wife concerning household roles on the extramarital behavior of the husband was mediated by four marital variables: marital satisfaction, long term change in affective relationship, communication between husband and wife, and daily life problems.

2049

Wen, C. I. (1972). [Stability and change of Chinese traditional values]. Bulletin of the Institute of Ethnology *(Academia Sinica), No. 33, 287-301. (In Chinese.)*

2050

Wen, C. I. (1979). [Community differences in values: A comparison of four Chinese communities]. In [Collection of Papers for the Celebration of Professor H. S. Tao's 80th Birthday Anniversary*]. Taipei: Shih Huo. (In Chinese.)*

2051

Westermeyer, J. (1976). The pro-heroin effects of anti-opium laws in Asia. Archives of General Psychiatry, 33, *1135-1139.*

Over a period of 25 yrs anti-opium laws were enacted by 3 Asian governments in countries (Hong Kong, Thailand, and Laos) where opium use was traditional. Within months, heroin use suddenly appeared; and within a decade, heroin addiction surpassed opium addiction. The laws led to (a) increased price of narcotic drugs, (b) a heroin "industry", (c) corruption of the law enforcement system, and (d) major health problems involving parental drug use. The Asian experience indicates that antinarcotic laws can be effective only with careful preparations, such as changing society's attitude toward the traditional drug from ambivalence to opposition, mobilizing resources to treat and rehabilitate all addicts within a short period of time, developing the social will to incarcerate all "recidivist" addicts for a prolonged period, and preventing narcotic production or importation.

2052

White, G. M., & Prachuabmoh, C. (1983). The cognitive organization of ethnic images. Ethos, 11, *2-32.*

Hypothesized that the attribution of behavioral characteristics to categories of persons is likely to be constrained by implicit models of personality and social behavior. Evidence for this type of conceptual influence was found in an analysis of ethnic images associated with 3 types of ethnic identity in southern Thailand among Thai- and Malay-speaking Thai Muslims educated at national or Islamic schools. Factor analysis of trait attributions made by each of the 3 samples produced a model of 2 orthogonal factors interpreted as Solidarity/Conflict and Dominance/Submission. These factors were used to examine similarities and differences within each ethnic group. Results indicate that ethnic images are not monolithic cognitive constructions distributed uniformly throughout ethnic populations. Comparison of 2 samples of Thai Muslims differing in type of education indicated distinct differences in Ss' images of Thai and Thai-Muslim identities. Ss educated in national schools showed greater evidence of identification with

Thai national culture and greater facility with language and culture than Islamic-educated Ss. The ethnic images held by Ss educated at national schools mediated those that contrasted the 2 populations. This type of conceptual process portrays ethnic images as dynamic cognitive constructions that are susceptible to both situational variation and social, historical change.

2053

Whitney, R. E. (1971). **Agreement and positivity in pleasantness ratings of balanced and unbalanced social situations: A cross-cultural study. Journal of Personality & Social Psychology, 17,** *11-14.*

A 2 * 2 factorial experiment tested the relative importance of interpersonal agreement, positivity, and balance in determining a judge's pleasantness ratings of various social situations. Positivity refers to both positive interpersonal relations, as in "P and O are friends", and positive orientations toward objects and events, as in "P likes X". Chinese undergraduates read about and rated the pleasantness of 8 different social situations constructed from balance theory propositions. Results indicate that the main determinants of pleasantness are interpersonal agreement and positivity. The Agreement * Positivity interaction was not significant, indicating that balance did not affect the subject's pleasantness ratings.

2054

Whittaker, J. O. (1967). Attitudes toward civil liberties: A cross-cultural study. Journal of Psychology, 65, *145-152.*

A Likert-type Attitude Scale was administered to college students in the United States, Hong Kong, Lebanon, Brazil, India, and Rhodesia. Overall scores on this scale revealed the most democratic attitudes to be found among American students, although every group of Ss scored on the "democratic" side of the scale. Significant differences were found among the various groups in responses to specific items, and possible reasons for such differences are discussed.

2055

Whittaker, J. O., & Meade, R. D. (1967). Sex and age as variables in persuasibility. Journal Of Social Psychology, 73, *47-52.*

Attempted to determine if sex differences in persuasibility reflect unique features of a specific culture or if the differences are universal. A test of persuasibility was administered to college students in Rhodesia, Lebanon, Brazil, Peru, and Hong Kong. Only the difference between males and females in Hong Kong was significant. Another purpose was to determine if sex differences in persuasibility occur in Ss of ages different from those utilized in previous studies. Differences were found only among adolescent Ss in the United States. Finally, the relationship between persuasibility and ca was explored. Older Ss, regardless of sex, appear less persuasible than younger Ss.

2056

Whittaker, J. O., & Meade, R. D. (1967). Social pressure in the modification and distortion of judgment: a cross-cultural study. International Journal Of Psychology, 2, *109-113.*

Cross-cultural replication of Asch's experimental study of the effects of social pressures upon conformity shows that Brazilian, Arab, and Chinese college Ss perform like Americans while Rhodesian Ss show considerably greater conformity than is true in the other groups. Regardless of cultural background, Ss yield to group influence more as stimulus ambiguity increases. Because of the nature of the laboratory task and because all Ss were volunteers, the origins of similarities and differences in compliance deserve more careful scrutiny.

2057

Whittaker, J. O., & Meade, R. D. (1967). Sex of the communicator as a variable in source credibility. Journal of Social Psychology, 72, *27-34.*

This paper compares the credibility of male and female sources of information in communication, for both oral and written presentations. It examines this issue in a cross-cultural comparison of subjects from Brazil, Hong Kong, India, Rhodesia and Jordan.

2058

Whittaker, J. O., & Meade, R. D. (1968). Retention of opinion change as a function of differential source credibility: A cross-cultural study. International Journal of Psychology, 3, *103-108.*

College Ss from Brazil, Hong Kong, Lebanon, Rhodesia, and India showed greater opinion change toward high rather than low credibility sources, though both sources produced positive change that declined over time. Perceived credibility bore some relationship to the issues involved, yet certain sources tended to have higher credibility regardless of issue. Highest ranking groups included professors, physicians, and engineers. Lowest ranking groups included majority opinion, businessmen, and priests and other clergymen.

2059

Whyte, P. (1979). Cross-cultural marriage: An overview. Hong Kong Psychological Society Bulletin, *No. 2, 5-8.*

Provides statistics on interethnic marriages in various cultures such as England, the US, and China, and discusses personality types (e.g., the demoralized or promiscuous person) of people who may decide to enter cross-cultural marriages. Psychological tensions experienced by the couple as well as by significant others are also discussed.

2060

Wible, D. S., & Hui, C. C. H. (1985). Perceived language proficiency and person perception. Journal of Cross-Cultural Psychology, 16, *206-222.*

The influence of language proficiency on listeners' perceptions of second-language speakers was examined. Twenty native Mandarin Chinese speakers listened to tapes of six American females speaking in Chinese as their second language and evaluated each speaker on a set of 22 traits. Another group of nine native Chinese speakers listened to the same tapes and evaluated the six speakers on areas of Chinese language proficiency. The trait evaluations were then correlated with the language evaluations. Evaluations of 8 of the 22 traits showed significant correlations with evaluations in every language area. The results indicated two distinct groups of traits. One group was traits that the judges somehow associated with language proficiency. In evaluating these traits, the judges depended on cues of language proficiency. The other group was traits that apparently the judges evaluated independently of spoken language proficiency.

2061

Williams, J. E. (1965). Connotations of racial concepts and color names. Journal of Personality and Social Psychology, 3, *531-540.*

2062

Williams, J. E., Morland, J. K., & Underwood, W. L. (1970). Connotations of color names in the United States, Europe, and Asia. Journal of Social Psychology, 82, *3-14.*

Explored the hypothesis of cross-cultural generality in the connotative meanings of common color names via semantic differential ratings by 6 groups of college students: American Caucasians, American Negroes, Germans, Danes, Hong Kong Chinese, and Asiatic Indians. The hypothesis was supported by the finding of general agreement in the rank-order placement of the 10 color names along the evaluation, potency, and activity dimensions. On evaluation, "white" was rated most positively by all 6 groups, while "black", "brown", and "gray" were rated most negatively. Some possible explanations of these cross-cultural meanings are discussed.

2063

Wilson, A. A., Auerbacher, A., Greenblatt, S. L., & Wilson, R. W. (Eds.). (1977). Deviance and social control in Chinese society. *New York: Praeger.*

2064

Wilson, R. W. (1973). Shame and behavior in Chinese society. Asian Profile, 1, *431-447.*

2065

Wilson, R. W. (1974). The moral state: A study of the political socialization of Chinese and American children. *New York: Free Press.*

2066

Wilson, R. W. (1977). Perceptions of group structure and leadership position as an aspect of deviance and social control. In A. A. Wilson, A. Auerbacher, S. L. Greenblatt, & R. W. Wilson (Eds.), Deviance and social control in Chinese society *(pp. 52-66). New York: Praeger.*

2067

Wilson, R. W. (1981). Moral behavior in Chinese society: A theoretical perspective. In R. W. Wilson, S. L. Greenblatt, & A. A. Wilson (Eds.), Moral behavior in Chinese society *(pp. 1-37). New York: Praeger.*

2068

Wilson, R. W., Wilson, A. A., & Greenblatt, S. L. (Eds.). (1979). Value and change in Chinese society. *New York: Praeger.*

2069

Windholz, G. (1978). B. F. Skinner's design of culture: A lesson, its pitfalls, and hopes. International Journal of Group Tensions, 8, *5-17.*

Skinner has proposed that the behavior of society members should be systematically controlled if humankind is to survive. In a historical precedent the application of reward and punishment to change the behavior of the Chinese people toward the goals of the Ch'in dynasty (221-206 BC) ended in aggressive behavior of the controllees against the controllers. Skinner's approach to modification of behavior differs from that of the Ch'in by disavowing punishment in favor of nonreinforcement of prevalent socially undesirable behavior. However, the experimental analysis of behavior shows that the outcome of punishment is similar to that of nonreinforcement; both eliminate the undesirable behavior but also elicit aggression.

2070

Wolf, A. P. (1964). Aggression in a Hokkien village: A preliminary description. *Paper presented at a seminar on Personality and Motivation in Chinese Society, Burmuda. New York: SSRC.*

2071

Wolf, A. P. (1970). Childhood association and sexual attraction: A further test of the Westermarck hypothesis. American Anthropologist, 72, *503-515.*

Studied E. Westermarck's contention that intimate childhood association promotes sexual aversion. A preliminary study of household registration records from Taiwan covering the period of 1900-1925 and information from informants support Westermarck's conclusion. Women who were forced to marry a childhood associate (a) bore fewer children, (b) were more likely to leave or divorce their husbands, and (c) were more likely to commit adultery. Evidence suggests that the incest taboo does not prohibit what men's feelings incline them to do, but is instead an expression of these feelings, socially unnecessary but psychologically inevitable.

2072

Wolf, M. (Ed.). (1968). The house of Lim: A study of a Chinese farm family. *Englewood Cliffs, NJ: Prentice-Hall.*

2073

Wolf, M. (1972). Women and the family in rural Taiwan. *Stanford, CA: Stanford University Press.*

2074

Wolff, P. H. (1972). Ethnic differences in alcohol sensitivity. Science, 175, *449-450.*

Studied the effects of alcohol in 34 Caucasoid, 38 Japanese, 24 Taiwanese, and 20 Korean 25-35 yr. olds. Mongoloid Ss showed marked facial flushing and mild to moderate symptoms of intoxication after drinking amounts of alcohol that had no detectable effect on Caucasoids. Group differences were also found in a study of 55 infants. Results present are related to probable variations in autonomic reactivity.

2075

Wong, A. K. (1970). Political apathy and the political system in Hong Kong. United College Journal, 8, *1-20.*

2076

Wong, B. (1985). Family, kinship, and ethnic identity of the Chinese in New York City, with comparative remarks on the Chinese in Lima, Peru and Manila, Philippines. Special Issue: Family, kinship and ethnic identity among the Overseas Chinese. Journal of Comparative Family Studies, 16, *231-254.*

Data compiled from fieldwork and several research reports were used as a basis for discussing how U.S. immigration policies and economic adaptation of the Chinese affect and modify the Chinese-American family system. Also discussed was the development of several types of Chinese-American families who differ not only in size but also in intrafamilial relationships and cultural identity. Similarities between the family types with regard to the family system and the incorporation of friends into the family network were also discussed, and data were compared with comparative findings from Peru and the Philippines.

2077

Wong, C. K. J. (1981). The changing Chinese family pattern in Taiwan. Dissertation Abstracts International, 41, *A3745.*

2078

Wong, F. M. (1975). Industrialization and family structure in Hong Kong. Journal of Marriage & the Family, 37, *985-1000.*

This study examines the relationship between industrialization and the family structure in Hong Kong. Data are collected from several related studies as well as a representative sample study of 2,270 families, analyzed and interpreted from a historical-functional perspective. The results show that, as the development of industrialization moves along a pre-early-advanced continuum, there have been corresponding changes in the structure of the family which evolves from a temporary, broken extended form, to a settled stem one, and currently toward a small nuclear one. Correlational analyses have also confirmed the associations of such industrialization correlates as native township, education, occupation and religion, with the family structure.

2079

Wong, J. S. (1950). Fifth Chinese daughter. *New York: Harper & Row. (Republished London: Hurst & Blackett, 1952.)*

2080

Wong, S. L. (1965). [Adjustment problems between 2 generations arising from the change of social values in Hong Kong]. Chung Chi Journal, 5, *31-39. (In Chinese.)*

2081

Wong, S. L. (1970). Social change and parent-child relations in Hong Kong. In R. Hill & R. Kong (Eds.), Families in East and West. *Mouton: Hague.*

2082

Wong, S. L. (1984). Consequences of China's new population policy. China Quarterly, *No. 98, 220-240.*

2083

Wong, S. L. (1986). Modernization and Chinese culture in Hong Kong. China Quarterly, *No. 106, 306-325.*

2084

Wong, S. Y. (1984). [The values and life style of college students in northern Taiwan]. Journal of Education & Psychology, 7, *95-117. (In Chinese.)*

Data on Life Style Survey (LSS) and Rokeach Value Scale (RVS) from 248 college students revealed that: (1) Both male and female college students emphasized more on internal values than external values. (2) In terms of value orientation, male subjects emphasized achievement more than the female subjects did. (3) Female subjects thought their life style more faddish than the male subjects; male subjects thought they were more confident and competent, more traditional-sex-role-oriented, and more social. (4) The business students perceived themselves as more faddish than the law, agricultural and medical students, and the law students perceived themselves as more confident and competent than literature students. (5) The lower the family income was, the more the subjects emphasized self-respect and intelligence. (6) There were sex differences in the correlations between the RVS scores and LSS scores.

2085

Wong, T. (1982). Aggression, personality, and political culture. Hong Kong Psychological Society Bulletin, *No. 9, 5-17.*

Responds to an article on aggressive behavior in Chinese society by M. Bond and S. H. Wang (1982) and proposes that the introduction of the concept of political culture helps in analyzing aggression and personality. Bond and Wang found that researchers disagree on the nature of the socialization practices of Chinese parents and the extent of aggressiveness in Chinese children. It is noted that Solomon related aggression and hostility to particular relations of authority via the mechanisms and anxiety created through childrearing and socialization practices and sanctioned by the Confucian ideology of societal hierarchy and interrelatedness. Also reviewed is the work of R. W. Wilson (1974) who wrote that the learning environment of Chinese children is characterized by a socialization that emphasizes love-withdrawal and shaming techniques as methods of control. The present author concludes that any study of aggressive behavior in Chinese society must take into account the cultural standards of conformity and accommodation to group sanction and to the psychological accommodations of shaming and anxiety.

2086

Wongswadiwat, J. (1974). The psychological assimilation of Chinese university students in Thailand. Dissertation Abstracts International, 34, *A7602-7603.*

2087

Woodson, R. H., & da Costa-Woodson, E. M. (1984). Social organization, physical environment, and infant-caretaker interaction. Developmental Psychology, 20, *473-476.*

Examined the relationships of the infant-caretaker interaction with the home's social organization and physical environment in rural Malay and Chinese families living in Malaysia. 12 families in each group were observed every 4-6 wks until the target infant's 1st birthday. Most infant-caretaker interaction in the nuclear Malay family occurred in areas physically separate from work and cooking facilities, which were compatible with infant crawling and exploration. The extended family in the Chinese home interacted with the infant in a large room that contained cooking, storage, and work areas. These differences in the social and the physical environments paralleled differences in infant-caretaker interaction between Malays and Chinese, including the role of alternate caretakers in the management of infant crying, the distribution and context of physical contact, and the proximity regulation between infant and mother. Findings are discussed in terms of the integration of behavioral characteristics, patterns of social organization, and arrangement of the physical environment that constitutes a culture's caretaking practices.

2088

Wright, B. R. (1964). Social aspects of change in the Chinese family pattern in Hong Kong. Journal of Social Psychology, 63, *31-39.*

2089

Wright, G. N., Phillips, L. D., Whally, P. C., Choo, G. T., Ng, K. O., Tan, I., & Wisudha, A. (1978). Cultural differences in probabilistic thinking. Journal of Cross-Cultural Psychology, 9, *285-299.*

Studied cultural differences in 3 aspects of "probabilistic thinking", Ss were university students--43 from Britain, 53 from Hong Kong, 101 from Indonesia, and 96 from Malaysia--who completed several questionnaires. The largest cultural difference was found between Asian and British groups. The British adopted a more finely differentiated view of uncertainty, both verbally and numerically, than the Asians in response to uncertain situations. These differences are predictable neither on the basis of the relative abundance of probability expressions in the Indonesian language nor by the Malay Ss' ability to discriminate English probability words on a meaningful probability discrimination dimension. For numerical probabilities assigned to almanac questions, the British were less extreme and better calibrated than the Asians. Potential cultural influences that could account for the cultural differences were examined, and the possibility that Asian ways of dealing with uncertainty do not involve the verbal or numeric response modes studied is presented.

2090

Wright, G. O. (1954). Projection and displacement: A cross-cultural study of folktale aggression. Journal of Abnormal and Social Psychology, 49, *523-528.*

2091

Wu, D. L. (1980). Beyond the Bamboo Door: A psychosocial study of women and organizations in Metropolitan China, 1978-1979. Dissertation Abstracts International, 40, *B5876.*

2092

Wu, H. I. (1983). Conflict and cooperation of Sino-American relations in the great-power triangle: The approaches of cybernetics, social psychology, and social field theory. Dissertation Abstracts International, 43, *A2785.*

2093

Wu, T. H. (1982). [The relationship between moral judgment and attribution for male and female adolescents]. Bulletin of Educational Psychology, 15, *149-166. (In Chinese.)*

The purpose of this study was investigate relations among attribution, moral judgment, grade level, and sex. The subjects were 324 first-year junior high school and 357 first-year senior high school students; there were 335 males and 346 females. The results indicated that: (1) About 80% to 90% of the subjects were internally controlled. (2) About successful events, senior high students were more internally controlled than junior high students. (3) About failure events, junior high females and senior high males had higher internal scores than senior high females. (4) Among the internal group, females tended to attribute success to effort more than males did; there was an interaction between sex and grade for failure events. (5) Senior high students had higher moral judgment scores than junior high students. (6) There was no significant relation between attribution and moral judgment.

2094

Yamamoto, K., Davis, O. L., & McEachron-Hirsch, G. (1983). International perceptions across the sea: Patterns in Japanese young adults. International Journal of Intercultural Relations, 7, *69-78.*

Examined the international perceptions of 172 Japanese college students. Ss classified 30 nations according to their current and future affinity to Japan. Little difference was detected in the Q-sorts between institutions and sexes, while the current and future sorts correlated .96 with each other. In cluster analyses, many 2-nation units (e.g., Czechoslovakia-Yugoslavia) were the building blocks for the overall pattern. The total configuration consisted of 3 broad groups: mostly Western European nations, problematic nations (e.g., China, Russia, Israel, and Egypt), and remote and neutral nations. Structurally, the results are similar to another study by the 1st and 3rd authors of US undergraduates, but the contents are different. Findings tentatively support the notion of cultural metastereotypes.

2095

Yamanaka, K., Chang, H. C., & Lorenz, F. O. (1982). Modernity and fertility preference in Taiwan. Sociological Quarterly, 23, *539-551.*

Data from interviews with 973 14-44 yr old Taiwanese women having at least 1 child and living with their husbands were used to study the effects of modernity (with respect to nonfatal attitudes, activity orientation, planning values, and kinship orientation) and social status (SS) on fertility preferences (FPs). Analysis showed that the modernity attitude contributed significantly to the explanation of FPs, independent of SS variables. SS variables also contributed directly to the explanation of FPs. There was little evidence to support theories that modernity acts as an intervening variable between SS and FP. Results seem to indicate that both SS and modern attitudes work directly to inhibit fertility, with the bulk of the direct effect coming from Ss' education and modern values. Data reinforce the belief that what one believes and perceives, or the attitudes one holds, will eventually be manifested in preferences and perhaps in action.

2096

Yang, C. F. (1982). [Change of value orientation and its influences on Chinese gift-giving behavior]. Hong Kong Journal of Business. *(In Chinese.)*

2097

Yang, H. H. (1981). [A survey of sexual knowledge, attitude, and behavior among university and college students in Taiwan]. Journal of Education & Psychology, 4, *99-100. (In Chinese.)*

2098

Yang, H. J. (1978). Communicative competence in Formosan sociable events: A participant observation study. Dissertation Abstracts International, *39, A2622-2623.*

2099

Yang, K. S. (1975). An analysis of direct questioning and pictorial thematic interviewing as two methods of measuring ideal family size and son preference. Acta Psychologica Taiwanica, 17, *85-103.*

Evaluated the effects of differences in wording among various direct questions on the respondent's fertility-related responses and examined the differences between preferences in the number and sex of children obtained by the direct-questioning method and those by the pictorial thematic interviewing. 161 native Chinese husband/wife pairs were individually interviewed. The major findings were: (a) While the direct question worded with a respondent-directed referent gave a greater mean of ideal family size than did the direct questions with an other(s)-directed referent, the latter type of questions tended to give comparable ideal numbers of children whether the referent was specified as an individual or a group, whether a reference to some point of time was made, or whether the referent had a close relationship with the respondent. (b) There was a tendency for the 2 sets of measures of ideal family size and son preference obtained by direct questioning and thematic interviewing to positively correlate with each other. (c) The means of ideal family size obtained by the direct questions phrased with an other(s)-directed referent were comparable to those obtained by the corresponding thematic questions.

2100

Yang, K. S. (1976). Psychological correlates of family size, son preference, and birth control in Taiwan. Acta Psychologica Taiwanica, 18, *67-94.*

Interviewed 322 native Chinese (161 husbands and 161 wives) to investigate the relationships between several psychological variables, chosen on the basis of their theoretical relevance, and a number of fertility-related measures. Findings show the following: (a) Individual modernity was negatively correlated with actual and ideal family size and son preference and positively with contraceptive behavior. (b) Internal-external control tended to correlate positively with ideal family size and son preference and negatively with contraceptive behavior. (c) Authoritarianism had a positive correlation with ideal family size and a negative one with contraceptive behavior. (d) Need for affiliation correlated positively only with ideal family size among wives. (e) Need to raise and maintain status through having a child showed a positive correlation with ideal family size and a negative one with contraceptive behavior. (f) Husband's tendency to withdraw affection for his wife and wife's fear of loss of her husband's affection, due to sonlessness, correlated positively with actual and ideal family size and negatively with contraceptive behavior. Implications for the work of the family planning fieldworker are discussed.

2101

Yang, K. S. (1982). [Yuan and its functions in modern Chinese life]. In Proceedings of the Conference on Traditional Culture and Modern Life *(pp. 103-128). Taipei: Committee on the Renaissance of Chinese Culture. (In Chinese.)*

2102

Yang, K. S. (1986). [The new filial piety in modern society]. Chinese Cultural Renaissance Monthly, 19, *51-67. (In Chinese.)*

2103

Yang, K. S., & Bond, M. H. (1980). Ethnic affirmation by Chinese bilinguals. Journal of Cross-Cultural Psychology, 11, *411-425.*

Examined the effect on the response of bilinguals when they were presented with a questionnaire in their 1st or 2nd languages. 121 university students whose 1st language was Chinese completed a survey on their identification with Chinese or Western practices. The questionnaire was written in Chinese or English and administered in small groups by 1 of 4 investigators--2 Chinese and 2 Western. Results show higher levels of Chinese identification in response to the English version of the attitude survey. It is proposed that this ethnic affirmation depends on the respondent's level of identification with the 1st culture and the availability of behaviors to affirm or deny that culture. The phenomenon of ethnic affirmation extends beyond questionnaire responding and would seem applicable to any situation where one's ethnic salience is heightened. Cross-cultural interaction, particularly in a research context, is a prime example.

2104

Yang, K. S., & Huang, L. L. (1986). [Changes in philosophy of life among university students: Twenty years later]. In H. Y. Chiu & Y. H. Chang (Eds.), [Social and Cultural change in Taiwan] *(Monograph Series B, No. 16, Vol. 2, pp. 443-447). Taipei: Academia Sinica, Institute of Ethnology. (In Chinese.)*

2105

Yang, K. S., Lee, P. H., & Yu, C. F. (1963). The social distance attitudes of Chinese students towards twenty-five national and ethnic groups. Acta Psychologica Taiwanica, *No. 5, 37-51.*

2106

Yang, L. S. (1957). The concept of pao as a basis for social relations in China. In J. K. Fairbank (Ed.), Chinese thought and institutions *(pp. 291-309). Chicago: University of Chicago Press.*

2107

Yang-Lee, P. H., & Yang, K. S. (1970). [National-ethnic stereotypes of 240 Chinese students at the National Taiwan University]. Acta Psychologica Taiwanica, 12, *7-23. (In Chinese.)*

2108

Yang-Lee, P. H., & Yang, K. S. (1972). [Change in the stereotypes of National Taiwan University students towards different national and ethnic groups from 1962 to 1971]. Acta Psychologica Taiwanica, 14, *137-156. (In Chinese.)*

Compared the social stereotypes of Taiwanese university students toward 10 national and ethnic groups (Americans, Arabs, Chinese, English, French, Germans, Indians, Japanese, Negroes, and Russians) at the end of 1971 with those in a 1962 study. Change was found in both trait content and percentage for almost all of the groups, indicating a general decline in ethnic stereotyping among Chinese students in Taiwan during the last decade. In addition to this general "fading effect", there were marked differences in the degree of change among different groups. The Japanese and Americans were the 2 groups toward which Taiwan students' stereotypes had been modified most. The change was apparently in the unfavorable direction and is viewed as the result of a series of unusual international events during 1971 in which China, Japan, and the U.S. were actively involved.

2109

Yang, M. C. (1945). A Chinese village. *New York: Columbia University Press.*

2110

Yang, M. J., & Hwang, K. K. (1980). [The Vedge Model of self-disclosure and its correlates]. Acta Psychologica Taiwanica, 22, *51-70. (In Chinese.)*

This research is aimed at studying some problems related to the Vedge Model of Self-Disclosure. The subjects were 194 male and 234 female junior high school students. A self-disclosure scale was used to measure their willingness to disclose themselves while interacting with father, mother, best friend, and friend in general; and a parent's childrearing practice scale was used to measure their parents' attitude toward them. The results showed that the topics of conversation with others could be classified into three categories; sex, family, and general affairs. Male and female subjects were different in their willingness to disclose particular topics to different social targets. The most preferred target of self-disclosure was mother, followed by best friend, father, and friend in general. Compared with males, females tended to be more willing to disclose themselves to others. The perceived parents' disciplinary attitudes toward subjects were composed of three factors: authoritarian control, love and acceptance, and high expectation of academic achievement. Father's and mother's disciplinary attitudes were highly correlated on each of these factors. The disciplinary attitudes of authoritarian control and rejection were negatively correlated with children's willingness to disclose themselves to their parent on topics of general affairs but not those related to sex and family.

2111

Yao, E. L. (1979). The assimilation of contemporary Chinese immigrants. The Journal of Psychology, 101, *107-113.*

Studied the assimilation patterns of the Chinese who immigrated to the US after World War II by selecting 133 first-generation Chinese Americans in metropolitan areas. Their assimilation in terms of extrinsic and intrinsic cultural traits was measured by 2 attitude inventories. Comparison between the intrinsic and extrinsic cultural traits showed that the former had a lower degree of assimilation than the latter. The inconsistent patterns of assimilation demonstrated by the sample are coherent with the theoretical schemes proposed by M. M. Gordon (1964), C. W. Kiefer (1974), and W. M. Newman (1973).

2112

Yaung, C. L. (1980). Development strategy, relative deprivation and fertility behavior in Taiwan. Dissertation Abstracts International, 40, *B4755.*

2113

Yee, A. H. (1973). Myopic perceptions and textbooks: Chinese Americans' search for identity. Journal of Social Issues, 29, *99-113.*

2114

Yee, A. H. (1974). Spirit and values of the Chinese people: Reflections for Americans. School Psychology Digest, 3, *25-35.*

Describes the opportunity for cultural and spiritual exchange between China and America due to the recent opening up of the Peoples Republic of China. It is suggested that the average Chinese views China more as a reformed country than as a convert to world communism. The self-sacrificial spirit, collective interest, and state loyalty of the Chinese are contrasted with the individualistic spirit of the West. An understanding of current Chinese cultural pride is offered for the Western reader.

2115

Yee, D. H., & Yang, K. S. (1977). [Differences in attributional and coping responses between the actor and the observer under cheating situations]. Acta Psychologica Taiwanica, 19, *111-124. (In Chinese.)*

Based on justice theory, attribution theory, and appraisal and coping theory, two experiments were conducted to investigate the differences in attributional and coping responses between the actor and the observer under different cheating situations. The hypotheses were: (1) The actor would attribute his cheating behavior to some external causes as a way of self-defense, whereas the observer would attribute it to some internal causes as a way of restoring justice. (2) The more unjust the cheating situations, the larger the differences in attribution between the actor and the observer. (3) The actor would tend to adopt palliative responses to relieve his psychological stress, whereas the observer would tend to adopt active responses to restore his feeling of justice. In Experiment 1, 121 college students were instructed to role play as either actor or observer under five different cheating situations. The results confirmed the first hypothesis mentioned above and this finding was interpreted as evidence supportive of the justice theory. In Experiment 2, two cheating situations each with an actor and an observer, where the actor was punished in one but not the other, were presented through videotape to 88 college students and the subjects were asked to infer the causes of the actor's cheating behavior and his coping responses. The major findings were: (1) The actor's tendency of external attribution was higher than the observer's. (2) Under the punishment situation, the actor tended to be perceived as more self-derogatory and the observer as more forgiving; under the nonpunishment situation, the actor was perceived as tending to defend himself by denial and self-preservational responses and the observer as tending to punish the actor by criticism and derogatory remarks. These findings were interpreted as partial support for the justice theory.

2116

Yee, T. N. (1980). Chinese American conceptualization of physical and mental well-being. Dissertation Abstracts International, 41, *B706.*

2117

Yeh, E. K. (1972). The Chinese mind and human freedom. International Journal of Social Psychiatry, 18, *132-136.*

Discusses the concept of freedom in Chinese culture. Freedom for Western man is considered to be the lack of external pressures and the ability to make political and economic decisions for himself. This meaning of freedom is seldom found in Chinese thought. Instead, mutual interdependence and subordination to group welfare are stressed. Diversity of behavior results not from individual freedom but from the changing demands of diverse specific social situations.

2118

Yeh, E. K., & Chu, H. M. (1974). The images of Chinese and American character: Cross-cultural adaptation by Chinese students. In W. P. Lebra (Ed.), Mental Health Research in Asia and the Pacific: III. Youth, socialization, and mental health *(pp. 200-216). Honolulu, HI: University Press of Hawaii.*

2119

Yeh, M. D. (1985). Student movements in the People's Republic of China, 1957-79. Dissertation Abstracts International, 46, *A786.*

2120

Yenko, R. M. (1970). The affective component of racial stereotypes and its relation to attitudes of social distance. Philippine Journal of Psychology, 3, *45-61.*

Conducted a study with 49 male Filipino undergraduates to investigate the relationship between Ss' attitudes of social distance (ASD) toward Americans, Chinese, Japanese, and Spanish mestizos and the presence or absence of affect in the stereotypes of these 4 groups. Stereotypes were measured by an Adjective Check List (ACL) composed of semantic-differential sets of traits that described the same behavior but connoted opposing social desirability valences, e.g., thrifty vs. stingy. ASD was measured by a modified version of the Bogardus Social Distance scale and a paired-comparisons scale. A few affectless stereotypes were found for Americans and Chinese only. A noncongruent relationship was obtained between the affective component found in American, Chinese, and Japanese stereotypes and the ASD toward these groups. It is hypothesized that the relationship between the ACS and the ASD was affected by Ss' contact with members of these 4 groups and by the lack of control of image factors that may have been associated with the groups concerned.

2121

Ying, Y. W. (1983). Chinese-Americans view the quality of their lives: An exploratory study in San Francisco. Dissertation Abstracts International, 43, *B2699.*

2122

Young, K. P. H. (1985). A report on single parent families in Hong Kong *(Department of Social Work Resource Paper, Series No. 9). Hong Kong: University of Hong Kong.*

2123

Young, N. F. (1972). Independence training from a cross-cultural perspective. American Anthropologist, 74, *629-638.*

Studies relating age of independence training with achievement motivation and achievement have resulted in contradictory findings. The responses of 52 Chinese mothers in Hawaii to Winterbottom's Independence Training Questionnaire were analyzed in conjunction with (a) ethnographic observations of Ss' childrearing practices, and (b) their 9-12 yr. old sons' school grades, ratings by teachers, and scores on the TAT. The lack of significant relationships between independence training and sons' achievement motivation and achievement behaviors was explained by the failure of the questionnaire to tap the mother's underlying motives for stating particular ages. The Chinese ethnographic data reveal that cultural factors, e.g., values, strongly affected the mothers' responses.

2124

Young, N. F. (1972). Changes in values and strategies among Chinese in Hawaii. Sociology & Social Research, 56, *228-241.*

Studied 48 Hawaiian born and 32 immigrant Chinese families with preadolescent boys in terms of their assimilation in Hawaii. Data indicate that while cultural changes are occurring, there is much persistence of values and strategies of traditional China. Values related to success, hypothetical expenditures, family systems, and interethnic relations were investigated. Results suggest some of the problems of unilateral assimilation and raises questions on the direction to be taken by the Chinese in Hawaii.

2125

Yu, L. C. (1981). Filial piety, generational conflict, acculturation and stress among Chinese Americans. Dissertation Abstracts International, 42, *B2609.*

Five-hundred and ten Chinese Americans were divided into four age groups and four acculturation groups to see (1) how age and acculturation affect their filial belief and behavior towards their parents, and (2) how acculturation of generations affects the stress levels of respondents. It was found that age did not significantly affect belief and behavior. Acculturation had no significant effect on psychological stress symptoms; it decreased the number of negative life events, decreased life dissatisfaction, but it did not have a significant effect on the respondents' discomfort levels. It was also found that of the four acculturation groups, the totally acculturated group, those who were born and grew up in this country, had a higher stress level than the immigrant groups.

2126

Yu, L. C. (1984). Acculturation and stress within Chinese American families. Journal of Comparative Family Studies, 15, *77-94.*

Explored the effects of acculturation on stress levels of 277 male and 233 female Chinese-Americans living in the US midwest. Ss completed a bilingual questionnaire with acculturation as the independent variable and stress as the dependent variable. Acculturation was assessed by grouping Ss by the number of years they had been in the US. Stress was measured by 4 stress indicators: number of psychological stress symptoms, number of negative life events, life dissatisfaction, and discomfort levels. Three major components of filial piety were chosen for exploration: concern for parental health, financial support of parents, and housing needs of parents. Results indicate that for males, the number of psychological stress symptoms and life dissatisfaction decreased as the level of acculturation increased. Results were similar, but not significant, for females. Females belonging to the least and the most acculturated groups reported the highest level of discomfort regarding financial support to aged parents.

2127

Yu, L. C., & Harburg, E. (1980). Acculturation and stress among Chinese Americans in a university town. International Journal of Group Tensions, 10, *99-119.*

Studied the effects of filial responsibility on adult Chinese Americans. 510 Chinese Americans in a midwestern university town completed a bilingual questionnaire used to measure 4 levels of acculturation with 4 stress indicators (psychological stress symptoms, negative life events, life dissatisfaction and discomfort levels in taking care of aged parents' health, in giving financial support to parents, and in meeting aged parents' housing needs). An ANOVA was computed using acculturation as the independent variable and stress as dependent variable. Results show that the most acculturated group reported the lowest number of psychological stress symptoms and the lowest level of discomfort regarding their filial responsibility to their aged parents; the US-born reported more psychological stress symptoms than the most-acculturated group; the least-acculturated group reported the highest negative life events among the 4 acculturation groups; the totally acculturated group reported the lowest level of life dissatisfaction. Within immigrant groups, acculturation decreased the number of negative life events and decreased the discomfort of Ss when they did not fulfill their filial responsibility. Findings imply that the US-born Chinese are more susceptible to stress because they lack subculture support.

2128

Yu, L. C., & Harburg, E. (1981). Filial responsibility to aged parent: Stress of Chinese Americans. International Journal of Group Tensions, 11, *47-58.*

Examined the effects of increasing age and acculturation on stress levels resulting from the filial responsibilities toward aged parents of 510 Chinese-American Ss (aged 18 yrs and older). Ss were administered a bilingual, self-administered questionnaire. ANOCOVA was computed using 4 acculturation levels (least, more, most, totally) as independent variables, 4 stress indicators (psychological stress symptoms, negative life events, life dissatisfaction, and discomfort levels) as dependent variables, and age as the covariate. Acculturation significantly affected the number of psychological stress symptoms reported while increasing age did not. Those who were born in the US reported more psychological stress symptoms than immigrants who had lived in the country for 16 yrs or longer. Within immigrant groups, higher level of acculturation decreased the number of negative life events. Higher level of acculturation also decreased life dissatisfaction, and age, not acculturation, affected the discomfort level resulting from filial responsibility toward their parents.

2129

Yu, L. C., & Wu, S. C. (1985). Unemployment and family dynamics in meeting the needs of Chinese elderly in the United States. Gerontologist, 25, *472-476.*

The authors studied the effects of unemployment on the discomfort level of providing financial support and housing among the Midwestern Chinese-American elderly. A survey of 510 first-generation immigrants, aged 18 to 90 years, showed that married, employed females were more likely to give money to their parents and in-laws than single, unemployed subjects. Employment decreased the discomfort level of subjects who were meeting the needs of elderly relatives. The data also showed that one spouse's discomfort in meeting such needs affected the discomfort of the other spouse.

2130

Zeiner, A. R., Paredes, A., & Christensen, H. D. (1979). The role of acetaldehyde in mediating reactivity to an acute dose of ethanol among different racial groups. Alcoholism: Clinical & Experimental Research, 3, *11-18.*

Physiologic changes after the ingestion of alcohol were monitored in Chinese and white volunteers. Absorption rate, acetaldehyde concentration, facial flushing, and heart rate increases were correlated.

The following references are also relevant to this chapter:

4, 11, 53, 54, 85, 154, 160, 238, 263, 290, 297, 299, 320, 323, 328, 330, 393, 418, 538, 542, 563, 575, 598, 631, 636, 658, 660, 680, 681, 684, 691, 697, 703, 744, 758, 762, 772, 783, 784, 806, 810, 812, 817, 824, 850, 869, 879, 922, 987, 989, 991, 1022, 1029, 1035, 1072, 1079, 1081, 1083, 1086, 1089, 1111, 1121, 1169, 1205, 1230, 1250, 1266, 1267, 1273, 1285, 1292, 1302, 1305, 1334, 1350, 1352, 1362, 1378, 2131, 2139, 2142, 2144, 2162, 2229, 2280, 2286, 2299, 2300, 2313, 2317, 2415, 2419, 2422, 2494, 2495, 2518, 2522, 2542, 2562, 2596, 2598, 2681, 2697, 2766, 2827, 2838, 2854, 2872, 2886, 2887, 2949, 2993, 3019, 3029, 3109, 3114, 3197, 3212, 3224, 3231, 3285, 3325, 3327, 3364, 3366, 3390, 3446, 3449, 3451, 3513, 3520, 3536.

EDUCATIONAL PSYCHOLOGY 10

Frequency data on citations in this chapter, in terms of content classification subcategories, are presented in Table 9.

Table 9: *Number of Citations by Content Classification, Language, and Geographical Area*

Content classification	Total	CL	EL	OL	PRC	T	HK	US
Educational psychology	59	12	45	2	12	6	14	0
Educational administration, personnel, and training	18	8	10	0	3	12	1	0
Curriculum, programs, and teaching methods	48	28	19	1	30	10	2	1
Academic learning and achievement	89	54	35	0	22	35	11	1
Classroom dynamics, student adjustment and attitudes	64	33	31	0	3	40	5	3
Special and remedial education	19	6	11	2	5	6	1	0
Counseling and measurement	64	37	27	0	2	41	6	3
Total		361	178	178	5	77	150	408

Note: CL = Chinese language; EL = English language; OL = other languages. PRC = People's Republic of China; T = Taiwan; HK = Hong Kong; US = United States (Chinese Americans--according to the frequency of the subject term Asian Americans).

Subject terms used for indexing citations related to educational psychology are grouped according to geographical area, subject population, and topic. These are presented below, in a descending order of frequency. (The frequency of single-word subject terms includes those of compound terms in which the single word appears. Subjects terms used for indexing citations from other chapters may have been included. Terms with a frequency of less than 10 are not shown.)

Geographical area

167	Taiwan
139	Asia
91	Peoples Republic of China
46	Hong Kong
12	United States

Subject population

203	students
96	children
69	college students
64	school age children
43	high school students
42	junior high school students
39	adolescents
29	adults
28	elementary school students
26	teachers
17	Asians
12	Asian Americans
12	foreign students
10	preschool age children

Topic

108	achievement
94	education
62	academic achievement
47	attitudes
42	teaching
40	learning
39	ability
38	development
38	sex
36	curriculum
35	mathematics
34	language
32	cross cultural differences
32	personality
32	reading
29	teaching methods
28	adulthood
26	curriculum development
26	motivation
25	counseling
20	adjustment
19	intelligence
19	mathematics education
17	achievement motivation
17	personality traits
17	teacher attitudes
16	ethnic groups
14	cognitive processes
14	psychology
14	student attitudes
13	teacher characteristics
12	behavior
12	cognitive development
12	educational psychology
12	health

12	human sex differences
12	test validity
11	foreign language learning
11	schools
11	sociocultural factors
10	age differences
10	comprehension
10	concepts
10	special education

Table 10 shows that studies of academic learning and achievement are the most numerous (24.7%). As to geographical area, Taiwan predominates, but has given little attention to special and remedial education. Research in the PRC is deficient in the following subcategories: educational administration, personnel, and training; classroom dynamics, student adjustment and attitudes; special and remedial education; and counseling and measurement.

Not surprisingly, the subject term *achievement* ranks first in frequency; *academic achievement* ranks third. Again, a reflection of the preoccupation with achievement, academic achievement in particular, in Chinese education--a preoccupation apparently not matched by sufficient concern for students who need special or remedial education. Significantly, *creativity* is absent.

2131

Ahmad, H. B. (1980). Achievement, social environment and background characteristics in lower secondary schools: Peninsular Malaysia. *Dissertation Abstracts International, 40,* **A4991.**

2132

Ai, J. W. (1953). [A preliminary report on the Chinese language test for middle schools]. *Psychological Testing, 1,* **35-38.** (In Chinese.)

2133

Ai, J. W. (1954). [A comparative study of reading abilities of high school pupils in Taiwan, Hupeh, Kweichow and Szechuan]. *Psychological Testing, 2,* **135-139.** (In Chinese.)

2134

Amada, G. (1983). Mental health consultation on the college campus. *Journal of American College Health, 31,* **222-223.**

Describes the City College of San Francisco Mental Health Program designed to offer short-term, crisis-oriented psychological services to students. Since its inception in 1970, over 6,000 students have been provided with approximately 15,000 hrs of individual and group psychotherapy. Specific activities of the program have included consultation with police science students, consultation for interviewing applicants for the Radiologic Technology Department, lectures to engineering students on the psychology of corporate organizations, bilingual therapy for Chinese-American students, a workshop for clerical and janitorial personnel, and the provision of psychological services for an on-campus childcare facility.

2135

Anon, A. (1978). Special education in the Republic of China. *Australian Journal of Mental Retardation, 5,* **6-9.**

Describes the types of special education programs and services available in Taiwan, the training of special education teachers, and existing problems and future trends in the areas of special education in the Republic of China.

2136

Armfield, A. (1985). A comparison of high-ability and low-ability pupil scores on Raven's Standard Progressive Matrices at the Primary School attached to South China Normal University and the Guangzhou School for the Deaf/Mute, Guangzhou, People's Republic of China. *School Psychology International, 6,* **24-29.**

The Raven Standard Progressive Matrices were administered to 1,000 students in Grades 1-5 at a school attached to South China Normal University and 280 8-yr-olds at the Guangzhou School for the Deaf/Mute. Subjects perceived to receive the highest and the lowest grades and subjects perceived to be the most or the least clever were designated for comparison purposes. Results showed that earning high marks and being considered clever by teachers was associated with a high ability to make observations and reason in the visual mode.

2137

Atkinson, D. R., Maruyama, M., & Matsui, S. (1978). Effects of counselor race and counseling approach on Asian Americans' perceptions of counselor credibility and utility. *Journal of Counseling Psychology, 25,* **76-83.**

Conducted 2 studies in which Asian Americans rated a counselor's performance in a simulated counseling session with an Asian American student. Two tape recordings of a contrived counseling session were prepared in which the client responses were identical but the counselor responses differed, 1 depicting a "directive" counseling approach and 1 a "nondirective" approach. Each tape recording was paired with 2 different introductions, 1 in which the counselor was identified as Asian American and 1 in which the counselor was described as Caucasian American. In the 1st study, 52 Asian American university students were randomly assigned to 1 of the 4 introduction-approach combinations. In the 2nd study, 48 Japanese Americans who were members of the Young Buddhist Association were randomly assigned to the 4 introduction-approach combinations. In both studies, the counselor was rated as more credible and approachable when employing the directive counseling approach than when using the nondirective counseling approach. Evidence was found that Asian American university students see Asian American counselors as more credible and approachable than Caucasian American counselors, while the association members viewed them as equally credible and approachable.

2138

Attaprechakul, D. (1985). Learning scientific information through reading in a first or second language. *Dissertation Abstracts International, 46,* **A366.**

2139

Barclay, J. R., & Wu, W. T. (1980). Classroom climates in Taiwanese and American elementary schools: A cross-cultural study. *Contemporary Educational Psychology, 5,* **65-82.**

The responses of 438 Taiwanese and 513 American children to the Barclay Classroom Climate Inventory were analyzed by sex, grade, socioeconomic status, and achievement. Results strongly suggest that multidimensional cross-cultural studies provide a key to the specific support systems that provide socialization through formal and informal education.

2140

Beasley, S. R. (1972). The use of biographical data as a predictor of academic success for minority students at the University of Colorado. *Dissertation Abstracts International, 32,* **A6753.**

This thesis used biographical data, including vocational and academic plans and needs, extra-curricular plans, need for financial assistance, and notable high-school accomplishments to predict academic success at the University of Colorado. The students studied were all from minority groups -- American-Indian, Asian-American and black students.

2141

Blumenthal, E. P. (1977). Models in Chinese moral education: Perspectives from children's books. *Dissertation Abstracts International, 37,* **A6357A-6358.**

The author analysed a set of 252 children's stories published since the Cultural Revolution in the People's Republic of China. It was found that achievement appeared as the central behavior in half the stories. The next most frequent behavior was altruism, and the third was social and personal responsibility. Since achievement was almost always for the group, rather than personal goals, the three behaviors together indicate a strong emphasis on actions which further the interests of society as a whole. Regarding techniques of control and discipline, a content analysis of 30 stories revealed that physical punishment was the most common, though social disapproval and rejection also ranked high. Social rewards were the most frequent kind of reward. The main characters in the stories were consistently and immediately rewarded for socially desirable acts, and negative characters were punished for evil deeds.

2142

Boakari, F. M. (1984). The nationality group in cross-cultural adjustment: The case of Koreans and Taiwanese at the University of Iowa. *Dissertation Abstracts International, 44,* **A3605-3606.**

2143

Bochner, S., McLeod, B. M., & Lin, A. (1977). Friendship patterns of overseas students: A functional model. *International Journal of Psychology, 12,* **277-294.**

Studied 30 foreign students at the University of Hawaii (6 each from Japan, Korea, the Philippines, Taiwan, and Thailand) and 6 host national (American) students, balanced for sex. Ss identified their 5 best friends, and the 5 people with whom they spend most of their time. Ss were then presented with a list of 15 activities and identified a preferred companion for each of the situations. The data were used to test a functional model of the academic sojourn, which predicts that foreign students will belong to 3 social networks, in descending order of salience: (a) a conational network whose function is to affirm and express the culture of origin; (b) a network with host nationals, whose function is the instrumental facilitation of academic and professional aspirations; and (c) a multinational network whose main function is recreational. Results confirm the existence, predicted differential function, and salience hierarchy of these 3 social networks and reconcile previous conflicting reports regarding the social relations of foreign students.

2144

Bourne, P. G. (1975). The Chinese student: Acculturation and mental illness. *Psychiatry, 38,* **269-277.**

Reviews the history of the Chinese student in America and examines the conflicts created by the special role of the Chinese on campus. The types of problems manifested by Chinese students, who sought help from a university student health program, as a result of the stresses caused by currently changing attitudes toward assimilation are examined. The problems of male and female students are considered separately, and 6 brief case examples are presented.

2145

Brimer, M. A., & Griffin, P. (1985). *Mathematics achievement in Hong Kong secondary schools -- A report on the conduct in Hong Kong of the second international mathematics study: Within the International Association for the Evaluation of Educational Achievement* **(Occasional Papers and Monographs No. 65). Hong Kong: University of Hong Kong, Centre of Asian Studies.**

2146

Brownstein, M. A. (1986). A study of the adaptation and application of Bloom's Taxonomy of educational objectives: Cognitive domain, to science education in the People's Republic of China. *Dissertation Abstracts International, 46,* **A2647.**

2147

Cen, G. Z., & Li, B. S. (1982). [The effects of training on moral judgments among children]. *Acta Psychologica Sinica, 14,* **432-440.** (In Chinese.)

This investigation tested the effects of two different training procedures on moral judgments in young children. A total of 125 kindergartens and primary school children aged 5-11 years were involved. The results indicated that a brief training programme could immediately change the orientation of children's moral judgment, but this might be somewhat restricted by maturation variables. The results also demonstrated that the principle-explanation type of training was more effective than the verbal-approval type of training.

2148

Chan, J. (1974). Intelligence and intelligence tests in Hong Kong. *New Horizons*, **No. 15, 82-88.**

2149

Chan, J. (1977). Parent-child interaction variables as predictors of academic attainment. *New Horizons*, **No. 18, 60-67.**

2150

Chan, J. (1980). Certain factors affecting academic success of secondary students in Hong Kong: An empirical investigation. *New Horizons*, **No. 21, 65-79.**

2151

Chan, J. W. C. (1970). *The construction and validation of a scholastic aptitude test for Hong Kong sixth form Chinese science students aged 17 to 22.* **Unpublished master's thesis, University of London.**

2152

Chan, K. M. (1970, May). The culturally deprived child in Hong Kong: His educational and psychological needs. *Mental Health Association of Hong Kong Newsletter*, **2-8.**

2153

Chang, C. H. (1975). [Effects of the discovery approach of science instruction on elementary school children's logical thinking development]. *Bulletin of Educational Psychology*, *8*, **11-24.** (In Chinese.)

This study was designed to test the following hypotheses: (1) Children trained by the discovery method will subsequently have an improved ability to solve scientific reasoning problems, compared with those trained by the traditional didactic method. (2) The relative effectiveness of the discovery method is related to variables such as grade, sex, intelligence, and personality traits. The subjects were 100 fourth graders (50 boys and 50 girls) and 80 sixth graders (40 boys and 40 girls) from experimental classes of discovery instruction. A matched group of children was drawn from classes instructed by the traditional didactic method. The Raven's Progressive Matrices and the Chinese form of the children's Manifest Anxiety Scale were used to assess the children's intellectual and personality traits respectively. The results indicated that: (1) There were no significant differences between the groups given different types of instruction in terms of retention and transfer of principles. (2) No significant sex difference was found among fourth graders, but among sixth graders boys were significantly superior to girls in terms of reasoning performance. (3) The hypothesized negative relationship between anxiety level and reasoning performance was not confirmed.

2154

Chang, C. H. (1976). [Sex differences of children in school learning as related to sex differences of teachers: An analytical study of the effect of the availability of sex-role identification models on children's school learning]. *Bulletin of Educational Psychology*, *9*, **1-20.** (In Chinese.)

Studied achievement motivation, scores on achievement tests, and attitudes toward learning experiences in 284 4th-, 5th-, and 6th-grade boys and girls, half of whom were taught by men and half by women. In addition, 32 women and 31 men teachers were surveyed on their attitudes toward students of either sex. Results indicate no difference in intellectual abilities of students taught by men and women (measured by Raven's Progressive Matrices). However, 4th and 5th graders taught by women scored higher on classroom Chinese and mathematics examinations than those taught by men. 6th graders taught by men had higher scores in classroom examinations and standardized achievement tests (in Chinese and mathematics), but had lower achievement motivation (measured by a modified Achievement Motivation Scale) than their counterparts taught by women. Fifth-grade boys, and 6th graders of both sexes, who were taught by women rated their learning experiences higher. On a forced-choice survey of teacher opinions, teachers believed that their own behavior influenced students of the same sex the most. Teachers identified boys as classroom troublemakers more often than girls, and attributed less favorable characters to them. They expected boys to achieve more than girls, and were more disappointed when boys failed than when girls did.

2155

Chang, C. H. (1981). [Relationships between academic achievement and the discrepancies between students' perception of parental expectations and perception of their own performance]. *Bulletin of Educational Psychology*, *14*, **31-40.** (In Chinese.)

This study examined relations between high school students' academic achievement and discrepancies between their perceptions of parental expectations and perceptions of school performance. The subjects were 150 twelfth grade students from 15 classes, in which the top five students were selected as high achievers and the bottom five students were selected as low achievers. A questionnaire of 30 statements concerning school work was administered. The subjects were asked to respond to each statement first in terms of their perceptions of parental expectations, and second in terms of perceptions of their own performance. It was found that discrepancies between perceptions of parental expectations and of their own performance were smaller for the high-achievement group than for the low-achievement group. On 8 of the 30 statements there was a significant discrepancy between the two groups. The educational implications for parental expectations were discussed.

2156

Chang, C. H. (1982). [Ego identity status in Chinese university students: A test of the validity of Marcia's categorization of ego identity]. *Bulletin of Educational Psychology, 15,* **31-46.** (In Chinese.)

Tested the validity of J. E. Marcia's categorization system for ego identity in university students. An identity status questionnaire on occupational- and self-certainty was administered to 578 male and 539 female students (273 freshmen, 280 sophomores, 278 juniors, and 286 seniors) at 2 universities in Taipei. Results indicate that (1) 26.3% of Ss were classified as identity achievers; (2) there was a significant increase in the achievement identity status as Ss advanced from freshmen to seniors; (3) there were more identity achievers among Ss who had work experience; (4) Ss with higher academic status tended to be identity achievers; and (5) Ss who participated in student organizations also tended to be identity achievers.

2157

Chang, C. H. (1985). [Analytical studies of the attitudes of junior high school students toward ability grouping]. *Bulletin of Educational Psychology, 18,* **17-38.** (In Chinese.)

These studies investigated the attitudes of junior high school students toward the issues of ability grouping of students based on different criteria in instructional programs. A questionnaire with 20 questions was administered to a sample of 5,000 students, divided into one group of eighth graders and one group of ninth graders. The major findings were: (1) There was no significant difference between the two groups concerning their educational goals; most students wanted to go to senior high school after graduation. (2) Eighth graders showed more positive reactions toward school than ninth graders. (3) Eighth graders had better relations with their teachers; they felt they were more liked by their teachers than the ninth graders did. The problems concerning ability grouping were discussed.

2158

Chang, C. H., & Chen, L. C. (1977). [Sex differences in elementary school achievement as related to sex differences of teachers]. *Bulletin of Educational Psychology, 10,* **21-33.** (In Chinese.)

Compared the effect of male vs female teachers on achievements in Chinese and arithmetic of 141 boys and 124 girls in Grades 1-6. Female teachers tended to have superior female students, and male teachers to have superior male students. A questionnaire administered to 141 male and 124 female teachers indicated that teachers of both sexes showed a more favorable attitude toward female students.

2159

Chang, C. H., & Chien, M. F. (1969). [The effect of knowledge of results of intelligence and personality tests on the academic achievement of university students: An experimental test of Atkinson's theory of achievement motivation]. *Psychology and Education, 3,* **89-99.** (In Chinese.)

The relationship between academic achievement and knowledge of performance on intelligence and personality tests was examined. The subjects were 78 freshmen enrolled in an introductory psychology course at Taiwan Normal University. They were divided into two matched groups: subjects in the experimental group who were informed of their test scores, and subjects in the control group who were not informed. The main finding were: (1) There were no significant differences in academic achievement between the two groups. (2) In both groups, there were more overachievers among subjects in the middle range of intellectual ability. (3) There was no correlation between measures of academic achievement and personality traits. These results were discussed with reference to Atkinson's theory of achievement motivation.

2160

Chang, F. Y. (1981). [Academic cheating in high school students: The contribution of sex, moral judgment, and situational variable]. *Journal of Education & Psychology, 4,* **91-93.** (In Chinese.)

2161

Chang, H. T. (1960). [A psychological analysis of the process of mastering scientific concepts in school children]. *Acta Psychologica Sinica,* **No. 3, 172-181.** (In Chinese.)

Concepts are the basic components and also the results of the thinking process. According to the way they are mastered, concepts can be divided into two kinds: the pre-scientific concept and the scientific concept. One of the most important tasks in teaching is to make the pupils master the scientific concept quickly and correctly. In this article, the author sums up the teaching experiences gained from several courses in primary and middle schools, analyzes them from a psychological point of view, and finally puts forward the following points to be considered by the teacher: (1) providing abundant sensory material by stimulating relevant memories and using class demonstrations; (2) selecting adequate and using correct sensory material; (3) promoting active thinking of the pupils, paying attention to the relationship between previously and newly acquired knowledge, using the method of contrast and eventually fixing the meaning to a certain definition; and 4) using the concept in practice, in which it can be consolidated and developed.

2162

Chang, K. Y. (1980). A comparison of the personal development of American and Chinese college students within an Eriksonian framework. *Dissertation Abstracts International, 40,* **A6196.**

2163

Chang, L. S. Y. (1984). Values, attitudes and modernization: Values and attitudes of Chinese graduate students studying in Pittsburgh. *Dissertation Abstracts International, 45,* **A564-565.**

2164

Chang, T. M. (1978). [The effects of locus of control and arrangement of item difficulty on school achievement]. *Research in Education & Psychology, 2,* **245-246.** (In Chinese.)

2165

Chao, C. C. (1975). A study of conceptual elements involved in two physics terms for students of different cultural backgrounds. *Dissertation Abstracts International, 35,* **A5146-5147.**

2166

Chao, K. Y. (1958). [Full report on Learning Ability Test results from Hsinchu Middle School]. *Psychological Testing, 6,* **444-449.** (In Chinese.)

2167

Chao, L. J., & Tsao, J. C. (1963). [Studies on the methods of memorization used by junior middle school pupils: Vol. 1. Methods for memorizing four-word sentences]. *Acta Psychologica Sinica,* **No. 4, 312-320.** (In Chinese.)

A list of 20 four-word sentences was memorized by 40 first grade junior middle school pupils. The results showed: (1) The methods of memorization used by the pupils were: grouping the materials by meaning, grouping into quantitatively equal portions, using the first word of a sentence as a hint, grouping by rhyming the materials. (2) The efficiency of different methods of memorization was conditioned by the nature of the materials and the learning task. If all parts of the material were learned to approximately the same degree, the materials were better retained. (3) The method of memorization adopted by the pupils was dependent upon their understanding of the materials. Those who understood the materials equally well could, however, use different methods for memorization. (4) The different methods of memorization revealed to a certain degree the different processes of memorizing the materials.

2168

Chen, J., & Goon, S. W. (1976). Recognition of the gifted from among disadvantaged Asian children. *Gifted Child Quarterly, 20,* **157-164.**

Using the 6th grade of New York City schools with more than 10% enrollment of Chinese pupils and a criterion of giftedness 2 yrs above grade level in reading and 1.5 yrs above in the Metropolitan Achievement Test mathematics section, a median incidence of giftedness was found of about 19% compared with normal expectation of 4.75% for these criteria.

2169

Chen, L. C. (1978). [Sexes of teachers and students in relation to students' achievement in mathematics, motivation, and their perceptions of teachers' leadership patterns]. *Bulletin of Educational Psychology, 11,* **131-140.** (In Chinese.)

The purpose of this study was to investigate relationships among the sex of teachers and students and achievement in mathematics, achievement motivation, and perceptions of teachers' leadership patterns. The subjects were 212 junior high school students who took mathematics, divided into four groups: 53 boys taught by male teachers, 53 girls taught by male teachers, 53 boys taught by female teachers, and 53 girls taught by female teachers. The instruments used were an achievement test in mathematics, a questionnaire on achievement motivation, and a questionnaire on the perceived leadership of teachers. The results were: (1) Boys taught by male teachers did better in mathematics than girls taught by male teachers, whereas girls taught by female teachers did better in mathematics than boys taught by female teachers. (2) Boys' and girls' scores in achievement motivation were not related to sex of teachers; girls obtained higher achievement motivation scores than boys did. (3) Concerning teacher leadership, boys were more inconsistent in their perceptions of female than of male teachers, whereas girls were more inconsistent in their perceptions of male than of female teachers.

2170

Chen, L. C. (1980). [Relationship between teachers' preference and pupils' social status, achievement motivation and internal-external control construct]. *Bulletin of Educational Psychology, 13,* **187-194.** (In Chinese.)

This study explored relations among teachers' preference and students' social status, achievement motivation, and internal-external locus of control. The subjects were 305 fifth and sixth grade elementary school students (153 boys and 152 girls). They were given the Internal-External Control Scale, tests and questionnaires to measure teachers' preference, pupils' social status, and achievement motivation. The main results were: (1) There were positive correlations among teachers' preference and students' social status, achievement motivation, and locus of control.

(2) Well-liked and high-status students had stronger achievement motivation and a stronger belief in internal control than less well-liked and low-status students. (3) Girls were generally better liked by teachers than were boys; they also had stronger achievement motivation than boys did.

2171

Chen, M. (1986). [On the socio-psychological structure of communication between teachers and students]. *Acta Psychologica Sinica, 18,* **238-247.** (In Chinese.)

The problems concerning communication between teachers and students is discussed from the angle of social psychology, emphasizing that the structure of communication between teachers and students is composed of three principal aspects--interaction, exchange of information, and mutual recognition, and of three principal levels--personality, role, and community. The author proposed a communication pattern called "triangular prism of three aspects and three levels." Each of the three aspects in this pattern consists of several factors, and each factor plays a role in the communication between teachers and students at every level. Various problems may occur in every aspect and at every level which would affect the process of education. A preliminary analysis of these problems was made and some general solutions to them were suggested.

2172

Chen, P. L., & Mao, Y. Y. (1965). [On the processes of mastering typical verbal arithmetic problems in school children]. *Acta Psychologica Sinica, 32,* **215-222.** (In Chinese.)

The aim of this research was to analyze the processes of different stages in the understanding and mastery of typical verbal arithmetical problems in primary school children. The indices used were the amounts of correct classifying, solving and composing typical problems. Experiments were carried out individually on 30 fifth grade children. The results were as follows: (1) There were positive correlations among the achievements in classifying, solving and composing problems. (2) Six levels of understanding and mastery could be identified which might be used as a scale to test the children's mastery of verbal problems.

2173

Chen, S. F. (1984). The attitudes of faculty members and department chairpersons toward student evaluation of instruction in a selected university in the Republic of China. *Dissertation Abstracts International, 45,* **A1652-1653.**

2174

Chen, S. M. (1970). [A study of the preschool children's response in a seriation test]. *Psychology and Education, 4,* **47-63.** (In Chinese.)

This study deals with the children's response in a seriation test. Subjects were 192 kindergarten children, 96 drawn from lower social class and another 96 selected from upper-middle class, matched in sex and age. The material used was the Learning Readiness System Seriation Test, developed by R. Scott. Analysis of variance yielded statistically significant differences between two social classes, among four age groups, and insignificant differences between two sexes. The seriation score of each child may be used to determine the general grouping and the guidelines for experiences which will facilitate the overall learning readiness growth of preschool children. Educational implications are discussed in terms of the possible importance of integrating perceptual and language activities into compensatory programs for disadvantaged children.

2175

Chen, S. M. (1980). [A study of sociometric status of Chinese school children]. *Bulletin of Educational Psychology, 13,* **119-132.** (In Chinese.)

Investigated the sociometric status of 746 2nd-, 5th-, and 7th graders, using a sociometric questionnaire, Raven's Intelligence Test, Tennessee Self-Concept Scale, Children's Internal-External Control Scale, and ratings of 8 traits by teachers. Sociometric status was positively related to intelligence, academic achievement, internality, and self-acceptance. Sociometric status was positively correlated with teacher ratings of academic achievement, health, happiness, leadership, and popularity; and was negatively correlated with aggression, dependency, and problem behavior. There were no significant differences between sociometric status of boys and girls.

2176

Chen, W. K. C. (1936). Variations of the same students through a series of tests and scholarship records. *Chinese Journal of Psychology, 1,* **130-139.**

2177

Chen, W. S. (1977). The job satisfaction of school teachers in the Republic of China as related to personal and organizational characteristics. *Dissertation Abstracts International, 38,* **A3167.**

2178

Chen, Y. H. (1975). [What can the University-College Joint Entrance Examination predict]? *Psychological Testing, 22,* **95-98.** (In Chinese.)

2179

Chen, Y. H. (1982). [The efficacy of special class placement for the mentally retarded students in junior high schools in Taipei city]. *Bulletin of Educational Psychology*, *15*, **47-66.** (In Chinese.)

Conducted 2 studies to (1) compare the views of special class placement by special class teachers of 21 junior high schools in Taipei city; (2) investigate the variables of sex, age, teaching experience, and professional training background of special class teachers in rating the achievement of mentally retarded (MR) students; and (3) compare the academic achievement and social adaptive behavior of 2 groups of MR students in special classes and in regular classes. In Study 1, the academic achievement and personal adjustment of MR students were measured by 176 special class teachers using rating scales. A pretest-posttest control group design was used in Study 2 to compare the efficacy of special class placement. The experimental group consisted of 30 students who had been placed in MR class for the 1st time during the 1981-1982 school year. The 30 control students were eligible for MR placement, but were retained in regular classes during the entire school year. Results show that (1) there were significant differences among the teachers regarding their attitude toward special class placement; (2) among the teachers, no rating differences were found in terms of age, sex, and teaching experience; and (3) over 6 mo, the special class MR students had significantly greater gains in arithmetic, but not in reading or social adaptive behavior.

2180

Chen, Y. H., Lu, C. M., Hung, Y. Y., & Chen, L. C. (1980). [A survey on the opinions about corporal punishment of teachers, students and parents]. *Bulletin of Educational Psychology*, *13*, **57-74.** (In Chinese.)

The purposes of this study were to study views on corporal punishment of teachers, students, and parents in Taiwan, to investigate the forms and frequency of corporal punishment given by teachers, and to compare these views and practices with those in Western countries. The subjects included 1,073 teachers, 1,111 parents, and 4,582 elementary and secondary students. Three questionnaires were used, for teachers, parents, and students respectively. The major results were: (1) Most teachers, parents, and students thought that, as long as no injury was inflicted, proper corporal punishment was permissible. (2) Most parents and teachers admitted that they had been forced to practice corporal punishment, primarily for misbehaviors, though it was not a usual practice. (3) Most teachers, parents, and students regarded exhortation as a better way to correct students' misbehaviors. (4) The most pervasive forms of corporal punishment supported by teachers, parents, and students were "palm swatting," "standing," and "extra homework."

2181

Cheng, F. (1965). [An achievement test of nature study]. *Psychological Testing*, *12*, **225-234.** (In Chinese.)

2182

Cheng, F. M. (1959). [A new method for the evaluation of compositions]. *Psychological Testing*, *7*, **494-502.** (In Chinese.)

2183

Cheng, H. H., & Fan, C. M. (1976). [Comparisons of directive and non-directive counseling methods in vocational counseling]. In H. H. Cheng (Ed.), [*Counseling studies in the Republic of China*] **(pp. 129-163). Taipei: Young Lion.** (In Chinese.)

2184

Cheng, H. H., & Lui, S. E. (1976). [Effectiveness of nondirective counseling techniques among high school students]. In H. H. Cheng (Ed.), [*Counseling studies in the Republic of China*] **(pp. 59-78). Taipei: Young Lion.** (In Chinese.)

2185

Cheng, H. H., & Wu, E. C. (1977). [Effectiveness of counseling in terms of method and frequency with high school students]. *Mental Health Bulletin*, *21*, **35-46.** (In Chinese.)

2186

Cheng, H. L., & Yang, K. S. (1977). [The effects of attributional process on achievement motivation and scholastic achievement]. *Bulletin of the Institute of Ethnology (Academia Sinica)*, *43*, **85-127.** (In Chinese.)

This study investigated the main and moderating effects of causal attribution on achievement motivation and scholastic achievement. The subjects were 491 Chinese students drawn from two junior high schools in Taipei. The major findings were: (1) The causal attribution of scholastic achievement had no significant relationship with general intelligence. (2) Achievement motivation tended to be positively correlated with internal attribution (effort and ability) and negatively correlated with external attribution (luck and task). (3) Causal attribution had a moderating effect on the relationship of achievement motivation to scholastic achievement; that is, the correlation between the two achievement-related variables tended to be higher both for subjects with a stronger tendency to attribute to either effort or ability and for those with a weaker tendency to attribute to either luck or task. (4) Causal attribution had no significant main effect on scholastic achievement.

2187

Cheng, K. M. (1986). Traditional values and Western ideas: Hong Kong's dilemma in education. *Asian Journal of Public Administration, 8,* **195-213.**

2188

Cheng, W. J. (1971). [Adjustment of evening class students at high school level-problems analysis and guidance principles]. *Bulletin of Research Institute of Education Normal University, 13,* **485-593.** (In Chinese.)

2189

Chern, C. C. (1977). [Effects of image instructions on phrase learning in children of different language abilities]. *Research in Education & Psychology, 1,* **214-217.** (In Chinese.)

2190

Cheung, C. P. (1982). Student perceptions of parental practices and effort: A comparison of Chinese, Anglo, and Hispanic students. *Dissertation Abstracts International, 43,* **A1811-1812.**

2191

Cheung, F. (1982). A network of counselling services for college students. *New Horizons,* **No. 23, 92-98.**

2192

Cheung, F. M. C., & Lee, P. L. M. (1984). Anxiety among secondary school students in Hong Kong and its relationship with academic performance. *Chinese University Education Journal, 12,* **56-63.**

2193

Chia, C. S., Cheng, T. H., Wang, H. T., Liu, S. J., & Kuan, S. W. (1960). [An experimental study on the teaching of counting to children in the kindergarten]. *Acta Psychologica Sinica,* **No. 4, 245-253.** (In Chinese.)

2194

Chia, F. M. (1970). [Student ranking of desirable teacher characteristics]. *Psychological Testing, 17,* **790-794.** (In Chinese.)

2195

Chiang, C. F. (1977). [Effects of counselor's reputation and client's personality on the willingness of accepting counseling]. *Research in Education & Psychology, 1,* **203-204.** (In Chinese.)

2196

Chiang, D. M. (1986). Evaluation of a microcomputer CAI program to teach percentiles in Taiwan, the Republic of China: The effects of English comprehension ability and graphics on student achievement and attitudes. *Dissertation Abstracts International, 46,* **B2723-2724.**

2197

Chien, M. F. (1974). [A comparative study of adjustment problems among Chinese and American college students]. *Bulletin of Educational Psychology, 7,* **77-87. (Also** *Dissertation Abstracts International, 34,* **A2380-2381.)** (In Chinese.)

Investigated college students' adjustment problems in the light of different cultural backgrounds, with variables of sex, class, and college major. Ss were 720 undergraduates drawn by stratified sampling from 1 university in Taiwan and 1 university in the US. The Mooney Problem Check List (college form) and a supplementary questionnaire devised by the author were used. Results show that (a) cultural backgrounds were significantly correlated with the number of problems, (b) in both universities lower classmen reported more problems than did upper classmen, and (c) "curriculum and teaching procedure" is a major problem area for Chinese students but not for Americans.

2198

Chien, M. F. (1975). [A review of studies on college students' adjustment problems]. *Bulletin of Research Institute of Education Taiwan Normal University, 17,* **1-18.** (In Chinese.)

2199

Chien, M. F. (1975). [Science aptitude of the gifted students in junior high schools]. *Psychological Testing, 22,* **52-58.** (In Chinese.)

2200

Chien, M. F. (1984). [The effect of teacher leadership style on adjustment of elementary school children]. *Bulletin of Educational Psychology, 17,* **99-120.** (In Chinese.)

The purpose of this study was to investigate the relationship between the perceived teacher's instructional attitudes, and elementary school children's locus of control and adjustment. Subjects were 256 sixth graders from one elementary school in Taipei City. The Teacher's Instructional Leadership Description Questionnaire, the Revised Form of Nowicki-Strickland Locus of Control for Children, and the Chinese Revision of California Test of Personality were administered to the subjects in regular classroom settings. The data were statistically treated by analysis of variance, Scheffe' method of multiple comparisons, and multiple linear regression techniques. The main findings were as follows: (1) The consideration dimension of teacher's instructional behavior had more effect than the authority dimension on the personal and social adjustments of elementary school children. (2) School children of warm-restrictive and warm-permissive teachers were better in their personal and social adjustments than children of hostile-authoritarian and hostile-neglectful teachers. (3) The personal and social adjustments of internal locus-of-control students were better than those of external locus-of-control students. (4) All measures of teacher's instructional leadership and student's locus of control together significantly accounted for 53% to 74% of variances in the personal and social adjustments of elementary school children.

2201

Chih, W. H. (1967). [A study of the Brown-Holtzman Survey of Study Habits and Attitudes]. *Psychological Testing, 14,* **416-451.** (In Chinese.)

2202

Chin, L. (1977). [Sex, grade, and testwiseness in examinations]. *Research in Education & Psychology, 1,* **226-227.** (In Chinese.)

2203

Chiou, C. C. (1977). [Educational background, experience, types of study, and the effectiveness of the program for training teachers in counseling in the junior high school in Taipei]. *Research in Education & Psychology, 1,* **233-234.** (In Chinese.)

2204

Chiu, H. H. (1963). [A study on the skill of calculation with abacus in school children]. *Acta Psychologica Sinica,* **No. 2, 106-112.** (In Chinese.)

2205

Chiu, W. C. (1969). [An application of art aptitude tests to high school students]. *Psychological Testing, 16,* **580-583.** (In Chinese.)

2206

Chiu, W. C. (1983). [A follow-up study of the NTNU Art Aptitude Test]. *Bulletin of Educational Psychology, 16,* **29-36.** (In Chinese.)

The Art Aptitude Test has been used to select gifted children to enter the experimental art class of two elementary schools. The present study investigates the validity this test.

2207

Choi, D. P. K. (1979). *Teachers, pupils and schools: A study of social class and school processes in Primary One classes in Hong Kong.* **Unpublished master's thesis, University of Hong Kong.**

The central importance of teachers' evaluation and academic performance in the shaping of pupils' self-perception as well as in pupil interaction was established in this research. Moreover, present findings indicated that teachers' evaluation of pupils is primarily a response to the demands of their occupational roles as disciplinarians and instructors. Hence, it was found that in general, the teachers evaluated their pupils on the criteria of their willingness to comply with orders and their intellectual capacity. The relevance of social class to teachers' perception of pupils was examined. It was found that most teachers invoked the social class factor, not in differentiating among their own pupils, but in distinguishing collectively among pupils of different schools. Great variation in social class background of pupil intake was found to exist among the schools. Moreover, there was indication that the teachers' notions of their pupils' social class might have repercussions on their perception of the demands imposed on them. These findings suggested that social class differences might be perpetuated through the differential teaching processes that take place in local primary schools.

2208

Chou, H. S. (1965). [Analysis of mistakes made in learning resolution of factors by first grade junior middle school pupils]. *Acta Psychologica Sinica,* **No. 3, 223-229.** (In Chinese.)

The results of the present study were that in first grade junior middle school pupils, the comprehension of the concept of factoring was more difficult than the differentiation between various problems of factoring. Some causes of mistakes usually made in factoring were revealed: (1) The configuration of letters and the order of terms; (2) The incomplete comprehension of the law of signs; (3) The incomplete comprehension of basic formulae.

2209

Chou, H. S., Sun, C. H., & Yang, H. C. (1960). [An experiment on teaching seventh-grade school children 'limit' in algebra]. *Acta Psychologica Sinica,* **No. 4, 254-261.** (In Chinese.)

2210

Chou, T. J. (1964). [A study of reading in the junior classes at primary school]. *Acta Psychologica Sinica,* **No. 3, 266-273.** (In Chinese.)

2211

Chou, T. J. (1984). A comparative study of normal, learning disabled and educable mentally retarded students on the quick neurological screening test in Taiwan, the Republic of China. *Dissertation Abstracts International, 44,* **A3348.**

2212

Chu, M. C., & Bai, C. H. (1964). [The thinking process in primary school children solving practical problems in arithmetic]. *Acta Psychologica Sinica*, **No. 4, 361-368.** (In Chinese.)

2213

Chu, M. T., & Wang, M. C. (1962). [Psychological analysis of first grade pupils in comprehending two-step applied problems in mathematics]. *Acta Psychologica Sinica*, **No. 2, 99-110.** (In Chinese.)

Systematic observations of 174 Grade 1 pupils were carried out to test the features of their mental processes of analysis and synthesis, and the periodic nature of their development as they were working out the two-step applied problems. The result indicated that the process of development followed four stages: (1) When proceeding from one-step to two-step problems, they lacked the ability to analyze the objects of the latter. (2) Having overcome the first step, they began to be able to analyze and synthesize some of the explicit features of the two-step problems. However, they were still not able to comprehend fully the subject matter of the problem. (3) In simple type problem exercises, they were able to analyze and synthesize the subject matter of the one type problems, but were unable to do the composite manipulation of the multiple problems. (4) Having comparatively acquired the ability of differentiating and generalizing the subject matter of all types of problem exercises, pupils were able to handle it in dealing with composite problems.

2214

Chu, N. S. (1973). The social context of the elementary classroom and the socialization of national sentiments in Taiwan. *Dissertation Abstracts International*, *34*, **A2155-2156.**

2215

Chu, R. (1971). *Majors of Chinese and Japanese students at the University of California, Berkeley, for the past 20 years* **[Project Report AS 150]. Berkeley, CA: University of California, Asian Studies Division.**

2216

Chuan, S. W. W. (1986). Perceived usefulness of higher education: Major choices and life goal values among Chinese-American students. *Dissertation Abstracts International*, *46*, **B2454.**

2217

Chung, B. J. (1978). [Job satisfaction of the junior high school teachers: An application of the "Motivation-Hygiene Two-Factor Theory"]. *Research in Education & Psychology*, **2, 247-248.** (In Chinese.)

2218

Chung, S. K. (1982). [A study of the joint effects of differential scoring instructions, and criterion referenced and norm referenced testing conditions on state anxiety in a multiple choice achievement test]. *Journal of Education and Psychology*, *5*, **263-280.** (In Chinese.)

This study investigated the joint effects of differential scoring instructions, penalty versus nonpenalty, and criterion referenced versus norm referenced testing conditions on the state anxiety of 722 Chinese junior high school students in Taiwan. The English Achievement Test followed by the A-State Scale of State-Trait Anxiety Inventory were administered to the subjects. The results showed that the penalty scoring instructions affected the students' state anxiety significantly more than the nonpenalty scoring instructions. Tests of the effects of the testing conditions, and for the interaction between scoring instructions and testing conditions yielded insignificant results. A significant, negative relationship was found between the achievement test and state anxiety. There was no significant sex difference.

2219

Coleman, J. S. et al. (1966). *Equality of educational opportunity.* **Washington, DC: U.S. Government Printing Office.**

2220

Coomaraswamy, S. D. (1974). Intellectual development of Malaysian medical students: A follow up study. *British Journal of Medical Education*, *8*, **187-191.**

2221

Dai, L. M. (1977). [Relationships among sex, grade, and intelligence functions]. *Research in Education & Psychology*, *1*, **210-211.** (In Chinese.)

2222

Division of Educational Psychology, Institute of Psychology, Academica Sinica. (1959). [A study of the age of school enrollment]. *Acta Psychologica Sinica*, **No. 6, 357-375.** (In Chinese.)

In order to find out the school enrollment age best suited for children's psychological development, the author set up six experimental classes consisting of 6-year-old children (for comparison, corresponding classes of 7-year-old children were also set up). A summary was given of the psychological characteristics of 6-year-old children in adapting to the school environment, taking responsibility for their own learning, building up their moral quality and studying the major curriculum. One year's study revealed it is feasible to allow children to begin their schooling at the age of six. It was also pointed out the problems to be studied further, if the problem of school enrollment age is to be solved satisfactorily.

2223

Dyer, W. J. (1955). Outside reading interests among Chinese secondary school pupils in Hong Kong. *Journal of Education^ (University of Hong Kong),* **13,** *34-38.*

2224

Fan, D. H. (1979). [A study of the factor structure of the Revised WISC in China and its short form for Chinese subjects]. Bulletin of Educational Psychology, 12, *167-182. (In Chinese.)*

Studied the factor structure of the WISC-R; the contributions of individual subtests to the total scale scores for standardized samples of 8-, 10-, 12-, and 14-yr-old Ss; and the development of a WISC-R form for Chinese children. Extracted factors for the 8-yr-olds were Verbal Comprehension, Perceptual Motor, and Integral Memory; for other age groups, Verbal Comprehension and Perceptual Motor. Among subtests, Arithmetic and Vocabulary had the highest correlation with the total score; Maze and Coding had the lowest. Scores on the short form based on factor loadings were highly correlated with the total scale.

2225

Fan, D. S. (1980). [The effects of teachers' expectation on students' grades of mathematics and deportment]. Bulletin of Educational Psychology, 13, *179-186. (In Chinese.)*

The purpose of the study was to investigate the effects of teachers' expectation on their students' mathematics grades and deportment. The subjects were 205 first and second grade students in a junior high school and four teachers. All students were rated by teachers in terms of expectations on mathematics grades and deportment. An achievement motivation test, a self-expectation rating scale, and an intelligence test were administered. The main findings were: (1) When intelligence was controlled, the high expectation group obtained significantly higher mathematics grades than the low expectation group. (2) Teacher expectations of students' mathematics grades were significantly correlated with students' deportment grades. (3) Teacher expectations were significantly correlated with students' self-expectations in mathematics grades and deportment grades.

2226

Fan, D. S. (1982). [Class-tutor affect in relation to student achievement]. Bulletin of Educational Psychology, 15, *195-203. (In Chinese.)*

Examined the relationship between class-tutor affect and student achievement in Chinese and mathematics. Ss were 7th graders drawn from 8 classes in which a tutor taught either Chinese or mathematics. In 4 of these classes, Ss showed superior scholastic achievement (SA), while in the other 4 classes, Ss had comparatively lower achievement (LA). An intelligence test and the Teacher Affect Questionnaire were administered to Ss. Findings indicate that (1) tutor warmth, as perceived by Ss, had a positive relationship with Ss' achievement in 6 of the 8 classes. An inverse relationship was found with boys' mathematics in the SA group and boys' Chinese in the LA group. After the intelligence factor was controlled, the basic pattern as shown by the simple correlation was still apparent. (2) As to the negative tutor affect (refusal), inverse relationships were found in all 8 classes with Ss' achievement. After the intelligence factor was controlled, the basic pattern was still the same except for girls' in the LA group.

2227

Feldman, D. H. (1971). Map understanding as a possible crystallizer of cognitive structures. American Educational Research Journal, 8, *485-501.*

On the basis of previous research, map understanding was selected for analysis as a school task which may function as a "crystallizer" of cognitive structures. A new instrument, consisting of 25 tasks presumed to be requisite to proper map understanding, was used to test the prediction that ethnic classification would be related to systematic differences in specific sequences of acquisition of the 25 map-test tasks, but that all children would show evidence of similar general cognitive-developmental reasoning sequences. Scalogram and ranked-distractor analyses of the responses of 270 Chinese, Negro, and Caucasian Ss indicated general support for map understanding as a crystallizing task, but limitation of the data restricted the conclusions to hypotheses for future study.

2228

Feng, Z. L. (1982). [On the development of educational psychology]. Acta Psychologica Sinica, 14, *342-350. (In Chinese.)*

2229

Flax, M. H. (1978). Day care services in the People's Republic of China and the United States with a focus upon children's interpersonal aggression. Dissertation Abstracts International, 39, *A2737.*

2230

Fong, M. C. (1970). Conflicts in teaching the emotionally disturbed and the culturally deprived child. Newsletter of the Mental Health Association of Hong Kong.

2231

French, H. P., Jr. (1968). A study of differences in students' learning of Chinese and Japanese culture concepts using lecture and intrinsically programmed methods. Dissertation Abstracts, *29, A1765.*

2232

Fung, Y. W. (1969). Extra-curricular activities as related to some social and personal factors with reference to Hong Kong fifth form students. Journal of Education *(University of Hong Kong), No. 26, 85-106.*

2233

Gimmestad, B. J., & De Chiara, E. (1982). Dramatic plays: A vehicle for prejudice reduction in the elementary school. Journal of Educational Research, *76, 45-49.*

Determined the effectiveness of dramatic plays as a vehicle for the reduction of prejudice among 559 4th, 5th, and 6th graders in 2 public schools in New York City. Ss in an experimental group read 4 plays, focusing respectively on Black, Puerto Rican, Jewish, and Chinese ethnic groups, and participated in post-play activities. Ss in a control group had no contact with the plays but were administered the same knowledge and social distance tests (e.g., Social Distance Scale). ANOVA showed significant differences between the posttest means for the 2 groups on the knowledge tests. A dependent t test indicated a significant gain from pre- and posttesting for the experimental group on the social distance tests and no such gain for the control group.

2234

Godman, A. (Ed.) (1964). The attainment and ability of Hong Kong primary IV pupils: A first study. *Hong Kong: Hong Kong University Press (Hong Kong Council for Educational Research, Publication No. 2).*

2235

Goldman, R. J. (1976). Value and moral education in communist societies. Character Potential, *7, 189-196.*

Reports on moral education in the USSR, Poland, Yugoslavia, and the People's Republic of China after visits to these countries on study leave. Aside from whether or not one is sympathetic to these regimes, it is suggested that the West has much to learn from them in moral education, which is given 1st priority in educational objectives. There are differences among the countries, but all 4 purposively engage in socialization based on Marxist-Leninist social thinking. No firm conclusions concerning the effectiveness of this moral education are offered, but some impressionistic illustrations are given.

2236

Goodman, K. S. (1973). The 13th easy way to make learning to read difficult: A reaction to Gleitman and Rozin. Reading Research Quarterly, *8, 484-493.*

Challenges the bases for the L. R. Gleitman and P. Rozin recommendation that children be taught to read English as a syllabary. The significance of the experiment using Chinese characters with American children and the central Gleitman-Rozin thesis that language is psychoacoustic are challenged. It is noted that the syllable is subject to the complex relationships between morphology and dialect. The contention that children can understand what they can pronounce is also refuted. It is stressed that children are masters of the morpheme and display linguistic competence with words and larger elements more abstract than syllables.

2237

Hamann, J. R. (1974). A study of the relationship between value differences and learning satisfaction in a cross-cultural adult education setting. Dissertation Abstracts International, *35, A155-156.*

2238

Han, Y. H. (1955). [The application of English vocabulary-grammar tests in secondary schools in Taiwan]. Psychological Testing, *3, 195-202. (In Chinese.)*

2239

Hao, P. T. Y. (1955). An analysis of certain learning of Chinese students in New York City. Dissertation Abstracts International, *15, 1551-1552.*

2240

He, J. Q., & Han, L. (1983). [Development of children's conception of the part-whole relationship concerning numbers and arithmetic -- Promotion of children's concept of multiplication and division]. Information on Psychological Sciences, *No. 5, 19-25. (In Chinese.)*

2241

He, T. T., Tu, W. H., Yu, P. Y., & Chia, C. S. (1962). [A preliminary study concerning the formation of conscious discipline in lower grade pupils]. Acta Psychologica Sinica, *No. 1, 57-65. (In Chinese.)*

This paper is the result of a preliminary investigation into the process of formation of conscious discipline in lower grade pupils. Using the method of experimental study under natural conditions, lower grade pupils can, with correct guidance from the teacher, apprehend the meaning of discipline, and conform to conscious discipline. The process of formation of conscious discipline has four different stages, the main one being the conflict between the disciplinary demands of the school and the habitual behavior of the pupil. Consequently, the educator, according to the characteristics at each stage, should organize the pupils to participate in practical activities to establish reachable aims, conduct emulation, and establish training in basic habits of disciplinary behavior.

2242

Henderson, N. K. (1963). Pupils' thinking: Recent research findings and their educational implications. Journal of Education ^ (University of Hong Kong), ***21*, 1-8.**

2243

Ho, C. C. (1977). [A survey of teacher counseling programs in junior colleges and universities in Taiwan]. *Research in Education & Psychology, 1,* **207-209.** (In Chinese.)

2244

Ho, D. S., & Hwang, K. Y. (1974). Characteristics of classroom test items identified by Chinese students as unfair. *Acta Psychologica Taiwanica, 16,* **199-204.**

2245

Ho, D. Y. F. (1970). [Mental stress of examinations on students and parents]. In *Proceedings of the First Annual Mental Health Week of the Mental Health Association of Hong Kong* **(pp. 14-15). Hong Kong: Mental Health Association of Hong Kong.** (In Chinese.)

2246

Ho, D. Y. F. (1979). English language skills and academic performance. In R. Lord (Ed.), *Hong Kong language papers* **(pp. 44-61). Hong Kong: Hong Kong University Press.**

2247

Ho, D. Y. F., & Spinks, J. A. (1984). Intelligence, language, personality, and attitudinal factors as determinants of academic performance by Hong Kong University students. *New Horizons,* **No. 25, 23-42.**

2248

Ho, D. Y. F., & Spinks, J. A. (1985). Multivariate prediction of academic performance by Hong Kong University students. *Contemporary Educational Psychology, 10,* **249-259.**

Verbal intelligence, English-language skills, personality, and attitude scales were used as predictors of academic performance in 230 male and female arts students at the University of Hong Kong. A series of bivariate, multiple, and canonical correlation analyses were performed. The results showed that verbal intelligence and attitudes, excepting study orientation, were not predictive of performance. English-language skills had the most predictive value, accounting for about 10% of the variance of performance measures. Personality variables failed to predict performance when composite criterion measures (GPAs) were used; however, they proved to be of predictive value when results of individual academic subjects were used as criterion measures. The study points to the importance of using noncomposite criterion measures in prediction and of considering the cultural context of achievement.

2249

Ho, E. K. (1983). Maturity and life purpose of Hong Kong Baptist College students: A descriptive study. *Dissertation Abstracts International, 43,* **A2237.**

2250

Ho, H. K. (1984). Vocational maturity among orthopedically impaired and normal students in Taiwan, the Republic of China. *Dissertation Abstracts International, 45,* **A1365.**

2251

Ho, M. K., & Shipley, A. (1974). The culturally different counselor. *Elementary School Guidance & Counseling, 8,* **286-289.**

Presents the particular counseling problems of the "culturally different" counselor. The problems of a Chinese-American counselor mistaken for a "Jap" are presented in a case study format. The process of "working through" cultural differences is outlined.

2252

Ho, Y. F. (1972). Changing interpersonal relationships in education in contemporary China: A report based on first-hand observations. In A. H. Yee (Convenor and Chairman), *Cross-cultural aspects of social interaction in education.* **Free-Discussion Session at the 20th International Congress of Psychology, Tokyo, August.**

2253

Hom, A., & Amada, G. (1977). Overcoming the problem of face-saving: Outreach services to Chinese students. In G. Amada (Ed.), *Mental health on the community college campus* **(pp. 113-129). Washington, DC: University Press of America.**

2254

Hon, Y. L. (1985). [Determination of behavioural instructional objectives in the teaching of Chinese Language in secondary schools]. *New Horizons,* **No. 26, 20-25.** (In Chinese.)

2255

Hou, E. (1964). [Results of four years of intelligence testing of overseas Chinese students]. *Psychological Testing, 11,* **14-19.** (In Chinese.)

2256

Hou, F. (1958). [An analysis of the correlations between school subject scores]. *Psychological Testing, 6,* **402-407.** (In Chinese.)

2257

Hou, F. (1962). [Academic performance of experiment groups in five high schools]. *Psychological Testing, 9,* **618-627.** (In Chinese.)

2258

Hou, F. (1963). [A follow-up study of change of learning interests in school subjects]. *Psychological Testing, 10,* **713-722.** (In Chinese.)

2259

Hsiao, C. Y. (1965). [The characteristics of the thinking process of solving verbal arithmetic problems by first grade children]. *Acta Psychologica Sinica, 30,* **50-56.** (In Chinese.)

The experimental results indicated that the thinking process of solving verbal arithmetical problems by first grade children was of more concrete imagery thinking at the beginning, and that the verbal thinking takes place only at the later stage. During the first school year, the children used less and less concrete imagery for the understanding of verbal problems, and the abstract or verbal analysis developed gradually. In general, the 7 year old children were capable of abstract thinking in certain fields. It was suggested that in the teaching of verbal problems in the first grade, the teacher should consider not only the characteristics of children's thinking, but also the conditions facilitating the development of children's abstract thinking.

2260

Hsiao, W. (1977). [Counseling junior high school students with maladjustment in interpersonal relationships]. *Research in Education & Psychology, 1,* **218-223.** (In Chinese.)

2261

Hsiao, W. (1985). The effects of Chinese culture and locus of control upon Chinese college students' attitudes toward, knowledge about, and perceptions of counseling service in Taiwan, the Republic of China. *Dissertation Abstracts International, 46,* **A614.**

2262

Hsu, C. C. (1975). [A clinical epidemiological study of the absentees in an elementary school. II. A preliminary epidemiological finding of absenteeism and a clinical study of 106 absentees]. *Journal of the Formosan Medical Association, 74,* **775-790.** (In Chinese.)

The entire student population of an elementary school in Taipei City, consisting of 5,605 children attending grade 1 to grade 6 were surveyed for 1 week to obtain preliminary epidemiological data on absenteeism. Altogether 136 children were absent from school for 246 days, yielding 0.73% as the average rate of absence per day. The rate of absence was the lowest among lower graders, the highest among middle graders, and higher for boys than for girls. There was no difference in learning potential between the absentees and the school population, but the academic achievement of the absentees was poorer at all grade levels. The number of children considered maladjusted by the class teachers was significantly higher for the absentees than for the school population. Out of 52 classes randomly selected from 103 classes, 160 children were absent from school for 158 days during a 2-week period which followed the survey. First hand clinical data were gathered on each of these children during home visits in the evening of the day of absence. The data showed that only 1 out of 3 absences was excused, and that 8% of these absences should be considered truancy. Approximately three fifths of the 158 absences were alleged to be due to physical problems; of these, less than 60% were diagnosed as justifiable. Approximately 60% of the absences not due to sickness gave no unjustifiable excuses. Boys tended to be absent more often with unjustifiable physical problems or other excuses. The most frequent reason for sick leaves was upper respiratory infections, followed by gastro-intestinal disorders. The majority of unjustifiable absences not due to sickness reflected the general maladjustment of the absentees and the improper attitudes of their parents toward childrearing and schooling.

2263

Hsu, C. C. (1976). [The learning potential of the first graders in Taipei City as measured by Raven's Colored Progressive Matrices]. *Acta Paedopsychiatrica Sinica, 17,* **262-274.** (In Chinese.)

2264

Hsu, C. C., Lin, T. Y., Ko, Y. H., & Lee, S. S. (1968). Special education for mentally subnormal children in Taiwan. *American Journal of Orthopsychiatry, 38,* **615-621.**

Describes how the mental health professions have participated in the planning, training, and operation of a special education program for the mentally subnormal children of Taiwan.

2265

Hsu, C. C., See, R., & Lin, C. C. (1973). [Assessment of the learning potential of Chinese children with Raven's Standard Progressive Matrices]. *Journal of the Formosan Medical Association, 72,* **658-670.** (In Chinese.)

The learning potential of a group of Chinese 4th and 5th graders was assessed twice, using Raven's Standard Progressive Matrices (SPM). The reliability of the test data was high. No difference in SPM scores was found between boys and girls at either grade level. Family background, as rated by parents' educational level and occupation, was found to be positively associated with the SPM scores for both grades. The correlation between SPM scores and academic achievement at the 4th grade ranged from .49 to .60, the highest being for arithmetic and the lowest for languages.

2266

Hsu, G. L. (1982). Culturally relevant theme and culturally foreign theme: An evaluation of some possible educational effects among Chinese immigrant students. *Dissertation Abstracts International, 43,* **A1426.**

2267

Hsu, P. P. (1983). [The relationships among teacher characteristics, teacher-student interaction, and students' academic achievement]. *Bulletin of Educational Psychology, 16,* **99-114.** (In Chinese.)

This research was designed to investigate relations among teacher characteristics, teacher-student interactions, students' perceptions of teacher behavior, and students' academic achievement. The subjects included 12 female teachers and 573 students. The teachers were given the Self-concept Scale, the Affiliation Scale, the Emotional-stability Scale, and the revised California F Scale. The students were given the Teacher Behavior Rating Scale. Tape recorders were used to record teacher-students verbal interactions in the classroom, which were then categorized by Flanders' Interaction Analysis Category. The data were analyzed by canonical correlation, multiple regression, and path analysis. The major findings were: (1) Among 4 teacher characteristics and 10 categories of teacher-student verbal interaction, teachers' authoritarian personality and teachers' direct influence of language were the most influential variables on students' academic achievement. (2) The data did not support the proposed causal path model that teacher characteristics would first influence teachers' language and then, through teachers' language, influence students' academic achievement.

2268

Hsu, T. C., Moss, P. A., & Khampalikit, C. (1984). The merits of multiple-answer items as evaluated by using six scoring formulas. *Journal of Experimental Education, 52,* **152-158.**

The investigators computed and compared the indices of item difficulty and discrimination, the coefficients of effective length, and the average item information for both single and multiple-answer items, using six scoring formulas and three tests. The subjects were applicants interested in law and business school. The scoring formulas were found to vary in terms of the assignment of partial credit and the correction for guessing. The instruments used were three subtests of the 1979 Joint College Entrance Examination in Taiwan: a Chinese test ($n = 2,647$), a political theory examination ($n = 2,908$), and a history examination ($n = 2,906$). The results showed that items with multiple answers were substantially more discriminating and reliable when partial credit was given. The formulas without correction for guessing seemed to perform at least as well as formulas with correction.

2269

Hu, P. C. (1967). [The revision of the Mooney Problem Check-List and its application on the study of college student problems]. *National Chengchi University Journal* **(Taiwan),** *15,* **55-166.** (In Chinese.)

2270

Hu, Y. P., & Yueh, H. H. (1965). [The effects of silent reading, recital reading with and without expressions on children's memorisation of poetry]. *Acta Psychologica Sinica,* **No. 3, 206-211.** (In Chinese.)

Experiments were carried out to test the effects of and the differences between silent reading, and recital reading with and without expression in memorizing poetry in primary school children. The results indicated: (1) Recital reading both with and without expression were more effective for memorizing poetry than silent reading. (2) Recital reading with expression led to slightly better memorization than recital reading without expression. (3) In primary school children using any kind of reading, those with a higher level of reading ability had better results in memorization. Increasing the level of recital reading in children was, therefore, an important condition for increasing the efficiency of poetry memorization.

2271

Huang, K. L. (1982). [The relationship of teachers' job satisfaction to leadership style, job characteristics, locus of control, achievement motivation and dogmatism]. *Journal of Education and Psychology, 5,* **47-75.** (In Chinese.)

This study investigated the relationship of teachers' job satisfaction to leadership style, job characteristics, locus of control achievement motivation and dogmatism. The subjects were 178 secondary teachers and 247 elementary teachers. The results were: (1) There was a significant negative correlation between job satisfaction and intention to quit. (2) The teachers were more satisfied with their principals and coworkers, and least satisfied with their chances for promotion. (3) Among 19 predictors, consideration had the highest predictive validity for job satisfaction and intention to quit. (4) The higher the principal on consideration and initiating structure, the higher the teacher's job satisfaction and the lower the teacher's intention to quit. (5) The higher the teacher's achievement motivation and his or her disposition to internal control, the higher the teacher's satisfaction with work, promotion, and overall satisfaction.

2272

Huang, M. C. (1978). The effects of the perception and the sex of reading teachers and the sex of students on the reading achievement, attitude, and reading class attendance of junior high school students in Taipei, Taiwan. *Dissertation Abstracts International, 39,* **A1226.**

2273

Huang, P. C. L. (1974). A study of the relationships between the native Chinese speaker's spoken English proficiency and his attitudes, motivation, and backgrounds in learning English. *Dissertation Abstracts International, 34,* **A5481-5482.**

2274

Huang, S. J. (1971). [A study on student's choice of majors in the Joint College Entrance Examination]. *Acta Psychologica Taiwanica, 13,* **196-205.** (In Chinese.)

The present study is an attempt to investigate motivational factors in taking the Joint College Entrance Examination and choice of majors. The subjects were students randomly selected from the freshmen at National Taiwan University. The results showed that the majority of the subjects indicated they took the entrance examination in order to obtain a college education. Male students appeared to be more highly motivated to enter college than female students. With respect to the major subject choice, most students were interested in the same subjects and departments. Hence, only one-third of the students sampled were admitted to the departments of their first choice. More than half of the remaining students intended to transfer to the departments of their first choice or to retake the Joint College Entrance Examination.

2275

Huang, Y. F., Wu, C. H., & Qi, Y. (1985). [On the problem of subjectivity in composition grading]. *Acta Psychologica Sinica, 17,* **46-54.** (In Chinese.)

This article concentrates on the problem of subjectivity in composition grading. It analyzed characteristics of the disparity in composition grading; the reasons causing disparity, arising from different hinting effects; and relationships between hinting effects and the hint giver's age, sex, teaching experience, educational level, and the grade he or she teaches.

2276

Hwang, C. H. (1973). The application of the sentence completion method in junior high schools in Taiwan. *Bulletin of Educational Psychology, 6,* **121-132.**

Investigated the applicability of sentence completion as a personality assessment technique in junior high schools in Taiwan. A Chinese Sentence Completion Test (CSCT) was developed and administered to 449 junior high school students, equally divided by sex. Results show that (a) the interscorer reliability was satisfactory (.82); (b) the test was moderately correlated with teachers' ratings on general adjustment and with the Neurotic scale of the Maudsley Personality Inventory; (c) the mean scores for boys and girls were comparable. Advantages of using the sentence completion method in schools, and suggestions regarding its application, are discussed. Further study is needed to establish a cutting score for the discrimination of the well adjusted and the maladjusted.

2277

Hwang, C. K. (1982). A survey of disabled students in Taiwan, the Republic of China, to assess the need for rehabilitation services. *Dissertation Abstracts International, 43,* **A1426-1427.**

2278

Hwang, J. J. (1982). The determinants and consistency of teachers' expectations: The evidence from Taiwan. *Dissertation Abstracts International, 42,* **A2997.**

2279

Hwang, K. K., & Yang, K. S. (1985). [University disciplinary problems in Taiwan: A conceptual-empirical analysis]. *Chinese Journal of Mental Health, 2,* **53-60.** (In Chinese.)

The authors traced traditional educational thoughts from which the current disciplinary system of universities in Taiwan originated and discussed some relevant student attitudes in connection with major university disciplinary problems. The findings of an empirical research were cited to support the argument that most controversial disciplinary issues resulted from students' resistance to the "arbitrary will" of the authorities in the administrative system.

2280

Hwang, P. O. (1973). Cross-cultural orientation and adaptation: A four-summer program and research. *Dissertation Abstracts International, 33,* **A5492-5493.**

2281

Jiang, S. Y., & Li, B. (1985). A glimpse at reading instruction in China. *Reading Teacher, 38,* **762-766.**

The authors described a Chinese reading instruction program that combines a phonetic writing system (Pingying) with instruction in carefully selected clusters of related Chinese characters. Because of this system, Chinese schools today can start children on productive reading earlier, with texts closer to their cognitive levels. Writing instruction begins up to 2 years earlier, and reading comprehension has been accelerated.

2282

Jing, M. J. (1983). [A study of the relationship between the participation of extracurricular activities and personality trait of Chinese university students]. *Journal of Education & Psychology, 6,* **151-152.** (In Chinese.)

2283

Joe, S. T. (1979). [Diagnostic procedures for guiding activities of Taipei's junior high school students]. *Journal of Education & Psychology, 3,* **219-222.** (In Chinese.)

2284

Katchen, J. E. (1985). Student-initiated question sequences in classes taught by American and Taiwanese teaching assistants. *Dissertation Abstracts International, 46,* **A140.**

2285

Keats, P. M. (1984). Values development and the school. *New Horizons,* **No. 25, 50-65.**

2286

Kippax, S., & Brigden, D. (1977). Australian stereotyping: A comparison. *Australian Journal of Psychology, 29,* **89-96.**

Administered D. Katz and K. W. Braly's adjective check list to 667 Australian university students to investigate their stereotyping of 12 national groups. Results were compared to previous studies of US college students. Results show that the Australian students' stereotyping of the Italians, Germans, and English was remarkably similar to the stereotyping by the US students, whereas the Australian students' stereotyping of the Chinese and Japanese was quite different.

2287

Klein, M. H., Alexander, A. A., Tseng, K. H., Miller, M. H., Yeh, E. K., & Chu, H. M. (1971). Far Eastern students in a big university: Subcultures within in subculture. *Science and Public Affairs: Bulletin of the Atomic Scientists, 27,* **10; 16-19.**

2288

Klein, M. H., Alexander, A. A., Tseng, K. H., Miller, M. H., Yeh, E. K., Chu, H. M., & Workneh, F. (1971). The foreign student adaptation program: Social experiences of Asian students in the U. S. *International Educational and Cultural Exchange, 6,* **77-90.**

2289

Kline, C. L., & Lee, N. (1969). A transcultural study of dyslexia: Analysis of reading disabilities in 425 Chinese children simultaneously learning to read and write in English and in Chinese: A preliminary report. *Bulletin of the Orton Society, 19,* **67-81.**

Ss were 425 Chinese children living in a large Chinese community in Vancouver, British Columbia, and attending grades 1, 2 and 3 in an English speaking public school and also attending Chinese language school. Those with specific reading disabilities in English, Chinese, or both, were singled out and given batteries of tests, for the purpose of attempting an analysis of possible causative factors in their reading disabilities. Findings suggest that "visual perception" is not a significant factor in learning to read. On the Draw-A-Person (DAP) test 72% of Ss with abnormal DAPs had reading disabilities, suggesting a functional neurological disability transient in nature. It is strongly suggested that the most important factor in learning to read is the teaching method. A multisensory phonics approach is most likely to produce a low incidence of reading disability.

2290

Kline, C. L., & Lee, N. (1972). A transcultural study of dyslexia: Analysis of language disabilities in 277 Chinese children simultaneously learning to read and write in English and in Chinese. *Journal of Special Education, 6,* **9-26.**

Tested children in grades 1-3 with a problem in either language (determined by screening tests) to identify the nature of the problem and some characteristics of the reading disabilities. The incidence of reading disability in each language and in both languages is presented. It is concluded that these incidences are no higher than in monolingual children. An analysis is made of such tests as the WISC, Bender-Gestalt and Draw-a-Person in relation to reading disabilities.

2291

Ko, Y. H. (1975). Student mental health problems in two different industrialized cities. *Acta Psychologica Taiwanica, 17,* **25-38.**

The present study examined the hypothesis that industrialization has negative effects on mental health. Based on the hypothesis, it was predicted that the mental health of the dwellers in a large city is poorer than that of the dwellers in a small city. Students in senior high schools in Taipei city and Yi-lan city were used as subjects to represent respectively, large and small city dwellers. Using the scores of the Ko Mental Health Questionnaire, comparison was made between these two groups of dwellers. It was found that: (1) The results of the female subjects, but not the males, supported the prediction. (2) The large city female dwellers were more prone to feeling depressed and hostile. (3) The large city dwellers were less strict about time, money, sex and aggression, and less concerned with the attitude of others toward them.

2292

Ko, Y. H. (1978). The mental health of the overseas Chinese students in the new environment. *Acta Psychologica Taiwanica, 20,* **1-7.**

Tested the prediction that the mental health of the overseas Chinese students studying in Taiwan would be poorer than that of the local students, and that Ss would have no general way of reacting to the new environment. 743 local and 227 overseas Chinese freshmen were tested with Ko's Mental Health Questionnaire (1974). Results confirm the 1st prediction but not the 2nd. It was strongly indicated that becoming more suspicious of others was a generalized way of reacting to the new environment for the newcomer, and becoming depressive and dissatisfied with life were less generalized ways of reacting.

2293

Ko, Y. H., Chang, S. H., Ten, S. C., Huang, H. L., & Yang, M. C. (1980). [Word-number-picture relation inference test]. *Acta Psychologica Taiwanica, 22,* **1-10.** (In Chinese.)

Presents the Word-Number-Picture Relation Inference Test (WNP) designed for the academic guidance of college or university students. The test consists of the following subtests: Number Series, Phrase Analogy, Symbol Series, Spatial Dimension, and Standard Progressive Matrix. The test was administered to 6 groups of Ss, including senior high school graduates and university students. Results show that the WNP is a highly valid and moderately reliable intelligence test, even for the university student with superior intelligence. Suggestions for improving the validity and reliability of the test are discussed.

2294

Kong, D. H., & Zeng, G. H. (1985). [Teachers' expectation of their principals' outstanding traits]. *Acta Psychologica Sinica, 17,* **423-428.** (In Chinese.)

This survey showed that teachers prefer principals who have a high sense of responsibility, keep in close contact with their staff, concern themselves with the teachers' livelihood, choose the right persons for various posts, and are fair and just. Teachers were found to strongly dislike principals who flatter their superiors, cheat their subordinates and are unjust, arbitrary and indifferent to the problems and difficulties of the staff. It is up to the principals to continuously cultivate moral qualities and combat unhealthy tendencies in their conduct so that they can live up to the expectations of the teachers, win their confidence, turn their initiative to good account and, in this way, run the schools well. The study also indicated that a gap existed between what principals expected of themselves and what the teachers expected of their principals. The principals tended to stress the operational requirements of the school and underestimate the importance of human relations. What the teachers expected from a good principal varied according to age and professional status.

2295

Konig, R. (1966). [The teaching of sociology in developed and underdeveloped countries]. *Kolner Zeitschrift Fur Soziologie Und Sozialpsychologie, 18,* **638-670.** (In other language.)

The translation of a manuscript presented at the 6th World Congress of Sociology in Evian, September, 1966 which presents an overview based on the author's experience and on literature accounts about the United States, West Germany, Japan, Taiwan (Formosa), and Hong Kong. Educational level of students is discussed and some data on department sizes, and poststudy activities of the students. A few general remarks are concerned with the status of sociology in some other countries, e.g., Africa, India, and Iran.

2296

Kuo, S. Y. (1979). [Relationships of teachers' professional level to their recognition of formal operations functioning in teaching behavior]. *Bulletin of Educational Psychology, 12,* **157-166.** (In Chinese.)

The assumption that selection of a profession would greatly affect the manifestation of formal operations provided the rationale for the present study. It was hypothesized that degree of professional training would influence recognition of formal operations in teaching. The subjects were 193 secondary school teachers. They were asked to rate two teaching strategies in terms of formal operations after watching two videotapes. The data obtained were analyzed by a two-way multivariate analysis of variance with three professional levels and two levels of cognitive ability. The results indicated that there was no relationship between professional levels and recognition of formal operations in teaching behaviors, and no relationship between teachers' cognitive abilities and recognition of formal operations.

2297

Kuo, S. Y. (1980). [Relationships of teacher expectations with teachers' behavior and students' learning behavior]. *Bulletin of Educational Psychology, 13,* **133-152.** (In Chinese.)

The present study was designed to investigate the effects of teacher expectations, functioning as self-fulfilling prophecies, on students' self-concept, achievement motivation, and academic performance. The subjects were 160 seventh graders and 4 mathematics teachers. Early in the semester the experimenter presented the teachers with information concerning students' home background, IQ, and achievement test scores. After approximately one month, teacher expectations were induced through asking teachers to estimate students' future mathematics achievement. At the end of the semester, the subjects were given a self-concept questionnaire, an achievement motivation questionnaire, and a teacher behavior scale. The data were analyzed by path analysis and multiple regression. The major results were: (1) Teacher expectations acted as self-fulfilling prophecies through determining teacher behavior; in turn, teacher behavior influenced students' achievement motivation through effects on students' self-concept. (2) Nine measures of teacher behavior could serve as powerful predictors for students' self-concept, achievement motivation, and academic achievement. Among these, marmth was found to be the most powerful predictor.

2298

Kuo, S. Y. (1982). [Relationships between teacher expectations and internal-external locus of control in elementary school children]. *Bulletin of Educational Psychology, 15,* **139-147.** (In Chinese.)

Classified 10 teachers and 168 5th graders from an elementary school in Taipei into high expectation and low expectation groups. Classifications were made on the basis of rankings of teacher expectations made after approximately 10 mo of teacher-pupil interaction. Ss completed a locus-of-control test, a self-concept test, and an achievement motivation questionnaire. Intelligence scores were obtained from school records. Data were analyzed by a 1-way analysis of covariance using IQ scores as covariate. Findings indicate that (1) for the teachers' high expectation group, the internal controls were higher in self-concept and achievement motivation than were external controls; and (2) for the teachers' low expectation group, the internal controls scored higher on self-concept than did the external group, but there was no significant difference between the groups on achievement motivation.

2299

Kuo, S. Y. (1983). [Academic achievement of and causal attributions of success and failure by success-oriented and failure-oriented children]. *Bulletin of Educational Psychology, 16,* **47-60.** (In Chinese.)

The objectives of this study were to examine the relationship between academic achievement and achievement motivation, and to investigate causal attributions of success and failure by success-oriented and failure-oriented children. The subjects were 222 fifth and sixth grade children from an elementary school in Taipei. In terms of measures of achievement motivation and test anxiety, the subjects were classified into success-oriented (67 males and 46 females) and failure-oriented (48 males and 61 females) groups. They were given an attributional scale for success and failure and an intelligence test; measures of school achievement were taken from the school record. The data were analyzed by two-way ANCOVA using IQ scores as a covariate. The major results were: (1) Pupils in the success-oriented group had a higher academic achievement than pupils in the failure-oriented group. (2) Pupils in the success-oriented group tended to attribute their success to ability and effort. (3) Pupils in the failure-oriented group tended to attribute their failure to luck.

2300

Kuo, S. Y. (1984). [The relationships between causal attributions of success or failure and achievement-related behavior]. *Bulletin of Educational Psychology, 17,* **51-72.** (In Chinese.)

The present study was designed to explore relations between children's causal attributions of success and failure and achievement-related behavior, including expectancy for future success or failure, achievement motivation, and academic achievement. The subjects were 550 fifth- and sixth-grade children (270 males and 280 females) from an elementary school in Taipei city. They were given an attributional scale for success and failure and an achievement motivation scale; measures of school achievement were copied down from the school record. The data obtained were analyzed by Pearson product-moment correlation, path analysis, and canonical correlation analysis. The major results obtained were: (1) In the case of success attributions, two internal causes (ability and effort) were positively correlated with achievement-related behavior; two external causes (task difficulty and luck) had low correlations with achievement-related behavior. (2) In the case of failure attributions, only luck was found to be positively correlated with achievement-related behavior; however, ability, effort, and task difficulty had positive correlations with the expectancy for future failure. (3) The causal path model proposed, based on Weiner's theory, was not supported by the data. (4) Among four attributions, the two internal causes were more powerful for achievement-related behavior. (5) In the case of failure attributions, all four causes, with the exception of effort for girls, influenced the expectancy for future failure through one canonical factor.

2301

Kuo, S. Y. (1985). [Child perceptions of teacher behaviors in relation to their creativity and academic achievement]. *Bulletin of Educational Psychology, 18,* **57-84.** (In Chinese.)

This study was an investigation of the relationships between direct and indirect teacher behaviors and students' creativity and academic performance. The subjects were 155 sixth-grade students taught by four teachers. Subjects evaluated teachers' behaviors and were tested on creativity. The results were: (1) Five indirect teacher behaviors and three direct teacher behaviors predicted creative thinking adequately; the same numbers of behaviors predicted academic performance in most subjects. (2) For creativity, boys' flexibility, originality, and elaboration were mainly influenced by four teacher behaviors through one canonical factor. Girls' flexibility of thinking was mainly influenced by five teacher behaviors. (3) Boys' Chinese composition and arithmetic performance were mainly influenced through a canonical factor. For girls, two canonical factors were relevant: the first exerted influence on Chinese composition and arithmetic performance; the second influenced composition, arithmetic, and aesthetic and manual work.

2302

Kuo, S. Y., & Spees, E. R. (1983). Chinese-American student life-styles: A comparative study. *Journal of College Student Personnel, 24,* **111-117.**

Compared 2 groups of undergraduates with different cultural backgrounds to determine if differences exist between students reared in different cultures and to provide a profile of Chinese students' culture. Ss were 190 American students enrolled at an American university and 197 Chinese students enrolled at National Taiwan Normal University. Most Ss were aged 17-22 yrs and were in teacher preparation programs. Results indicate that the major academic goal for Chinese Ss was personal knowledge, while the major goal of American Ss was to obtain professional certification. Although approximately 40% of both groups of Ss said that they depended mainly on themselves, twice as many Chinese (40%) as Americans indicated that a parent was the most influential person in deciding their major field of study. In general, Chinese and American Ss' academic life-styles, including learning and study habits, were very similar. It is concluded that Chinese students come from a situation-oriented society and like to be involved with family and friends. When they move to the US, which is individual-oriented, feelings of inadequacy and loneliness are inevitable and are pronounced. Chinese student organizations on the campus not only can provide help with orientation but also can be a continuing support group.

2303

Kwong, J. (1983). Is everyone equal before the system of grades: Social background and opportunities in China. *British Journal of Sociology, 34,* **93-108.**

Discusses how parents' social position influences their children's educational achievement in China. In 1977, the government instituted a 3-tiered examination system to choose students for junior high school, senior high school, and the university. However, the system perpetuates and accentuates inequality be selecting a disproportionate number of students from the intellectual and cadre families. Given the close family units and differences in social stratifications in China, social background influences educational achievements in ways similar and yet different from the West. It is not so much the economic advantage but the encouragement and coaching of the educated parents that give these children the edge. These children do better in the examination than those from the peasant/worker families and, in turn, the examination system gives them further privileges and opportunities, widening the gap between them and others.

2304

Lai, C. K. (1962). [A study of the method of analyzing applied problems in mathematics used by primary school children]. *Acta Psychologica Sinica,* **No. 2, 111-124.** (In Chinese.)

The experimental results of the present study showed the relationship between the methods of analyzing simple and complex applied problems and the structures of such problems; the characteristics and differences in the mastery of various methods by pupils of different academic levels; and the favorable conditions for grasping these methods. Finally, the author pointed out some suggestions for improving the teaching of arithmetics in elementary schools.

2305

Lam, Y. L. J., & Wong, A. (1973). Attendance regularity of adult learners: An examination of content and structural factors. *Adult Education, 1,* **130-142.**

Examined attendance regularity of 70 adult learners enrolled in the Chinese University extramural courses from the perspective of content and structural processes. Correlational analysis of questionnaire data revealed that degree of course understanding, need-fulfillment, approachability of the instructor, and amount of informal and formal interaction were all positively and significantly related to attendance rate, whereas sociability of classmates and attendance rate were negatively and significantly related. F tests from step-wise multiple linear regression analysis indicated that none of these factors made any special contribution in explaining attendance, though their relative contributions could still be detected.

2306

Lampton, D. M. (1978). Thermidor in the Chinese educational revolution. *Theory into Practice, 17,* **367-374.**

Educational policies developed under Mao Tse-tung will be long-lived, but there have been changes in them. From a Mao-inspired policy of emphasizing class origin and practical experience, there has been increased emphasis on standardized achievement testing in admissions. From emphasis on the political and hands-on practical work, there has been a shift to academics, research, and graduate study. Outside classroom laboratory work under the Academy of Sciences has become preferred to manual labor unrelated to the student's area of expertise. Weakening of Mao's egalitarian ideal has led to increased emphasis on achievement in class, more assessment, and the dignity of teachers. "Key schools" are now increasing in favor, and the attempt to keep all schools at the same level is less popular.

2307

Lazure, D. (1972). Education in transition. In *Mental health and urbanization: Proceedings of the 24th Annual Meeting, World Federation of Mental Health* **(pp. 36-42). Hong Kong: Mental Health Association of Hong Kong.**

2308

Lee, E. (1985). Chinese parents' support for the bilingual educational program. *Dissertation Abstracts International, 46,* **A570.**

2309

Lee, K. M., & Hwang, K. Y. (1976). [Relationship between test-taking behavior and classroom test results for elementary school children]. *Psychological Testing, 23,* **63-70.** (In Chinese.)

2310

Lee, L. C. (1975). [An analysis of the English test results of the 1973 University-College Joint Entrance Examination]. *Psychological Testing, 22,* **73-79.** (In Chinese.)

2311

Lee, L. M. P. (1977). An analysis of the problem of grading in the Hong Kong Certificate of Education Examination. *Dissertation Abstracts International, 37,* **A7709.**

2312

Lee, M. K. (1960). [An experimental study on teaching the 1st graders English]. *Acta Psycologica Sinica,* **No. 4, 262-268.** (In Chinese.)

2313

Lee, M. M. (1980). A study of classroom behaviors of Chinese American children and immigrant Chinese children in contrast to those of Black American children and White American children in an urban Head Start Program. *Dissertation Abstracts International, 41,* **A1387-1388.**

2314

Leong, C. K. (1969). Motives for the choice of the teaching profession. *Journal of Education* **(University of Hong Kong),** *26,* **67-84.**

2315

Levitt, J. (1977). An investigation of the learning environment of a student acquiring Chinese as a second language: A case study. *Dissertation Abstracts International, 38,* **A2620.**

2316

Lew, W. J. F. (1983). Personality traits of Hong Kong secondary school teachers. *Chinese University Education Journal, 11,* **36-46.**

2317

Lewis, J. W. (1965). Education and political development: A study of pre-school training programs in Mainland China. In J. S. Coleman (Ed.), *Education and political development* **(pp. 423-429). Princeton, NJ: Princeton University Press.**

2318

Lewis, J. W. (1965). Education and the Chinese polity: Themes in development. In J. S. Coleman (Ed.), *Education and political development.* **Princeton, NJ: Princeton University Press.**

2319

Li, A. K. (1984). Peer interaction and activity setting in a high-density preschool environment. *Journal of Psychology, 116,* **45-54.**

The author conducted a descriptive, field-based observational study of children's peer interactions within the various activity settings in a high-density preschool environment. The subjects were 9 children (aged 2.5-5 years) from three preschool programs in Hong Kong, selected on the basis of observed rate of peer interaction (high interaction positive, high interaction negative, and low interaction). The subjects were observed during all activities throughout the half-day programs on 3 mornings. Patterns of peer interaction indicated an association between level of interaction and variation in activity settings. The data also suggest an association between high spatial density and decreased peer interaction in large muscle activity where space is essential, and provide insights on how size and density might shape program formation.

2320

Li, J. R. (1984). [The effects of student's handwriting, composition ability and grader's characteristics on student's essay-type test scores]. *Journal of Education & Psychology*, *7*, **195-196.** (In Chinese.)

2321

Li, M. C. (1984). [The comparisons of high and low aggressive pre- and adolescent male students on TV-viewing habits, parents' rearing practices, the social status in peer group and academic achievement]. *Journal of Education & Psychology*, *7*, **19-41.** (In Chinese.)

The subjects were 415 male students (fifth to eighth grades), who were scored on the following variables: (1) aggressive behaviors as nominated by the peer group and evaluated by subject himself and self-evaluation of aggressive attitudes, (2) the social status in peer group as measured by a sociometric method, (3) the extent of caring and demanding as showed by subjects' parents, (4) the amount of time spent viewing TV during the week, (5) the kind of TV programs preferred, and (6) academic performance. It was found that, as compared with low aggressive students, the high aggressive students suffered more frustration. Their parents cared for them less but demanded more; they received more physical punishments. Their social status in the peer group was lower; and they had poorer academic performance. The high aggressive students spent more time viewing TV programs of aggressive contents and continuing "soap" operas than documentaries.

2322

Lian, R. (1984). [An experimental study of thought model in solving applied problems of fraction in mathematics in primary school pupils]. *Acta Psychologica Sinica*, *16*, **15-20.** (In Chinese.)

2323

Liang, K. H. (1979). [The effect of ability grouping on junior school students' self-concept: A comparative study of ability grouping by subjects and fixed ability grouping]. *Journal of Education & Psychology*, *3*, **233-235.** (In Chinese.)

2324

Liao, K. L., & Hwang, K. K. (1978). [A contingency model of teaching effectiveness]. *Acta Psychologica Taiwanica*, *20*, **53-66.** (In Chinese.)

2325

Liao, T. S. (1985). A study of article errors in the written English of Chinese college students in Taiwan. *Dissertation Abstracts International*, *45*, **A2017-2018.**

2326

Liaw, H. H. (1978). [Principals' leadership styles, teachers' personality characteristics and their job satisfaction in the elementary school]. *Research in Education & Psychology*, *2*, **230-231.** (In Chinese.)

2327

Lieh-Mak, F., Tam, W. Y. K., & Ng, S. (1979). Husbands of abortion applicants and comparison with husbands of women who complete their pregnancies. *Social Psychiatry*, *14*, **59-64.**

2328

Lim, C. L., & Wong, S. T. (1980). Educational underachievement and emotional and behaviour disorders in children. *Journal of Mental Health of Hong Kong*, *9*.

2329

Lin, C. S. (1974). [Problems of screening by raw scores in the Joint Entrance Examination of Universities and Colleges]. *Psychological Testing*, *21*, **75-77.** (In Chinese.)

2330

Lin, H. T. (1982). A comparison of alternate screening methods for identifying seventh grade students for academically gifted programs in Taiwan. *Dissertation Abstracts International*, *42*, **A3555.**

2331

Lin, K. M., Chen, Y. H., & Kuo, W. F. (1983). The Chinese revision of the Social Learning Curriculum. *Education & Training of the Mentally Retarded*, *18*, **29-33.**

H. Goldstein's (1974, 1975) social learning curriculum (SLC) was translated and modified for use with mentally retarded children in the Republic of China. Some of the major structural and substantive changes are described in relationship to cultural differences. The 1st version of the SLC was field-tested in 51 special classes in 28 schools to validate the translation and to elicit recommendations from teachers for improving the SLC before publication. Reactions of teachers to the SLC suggest that there is a foundation of facts, concepts, and behaviors common to societies with differing cultures that are important to prosocial behavior. Societies may be more alike conceptually than they are different, factually and functionally.

2332

Lin, Y. J. (1981). Cross-cultural construct study of structured role orientation in Taiwan. *Dissertation Abstracts International, 42,* **A2093.**

2333

Ling, F. T. (1963). [A case study on preschool child learning to recite classical poetry and prose]. *Acta Psychologica Sinica,* **No. 2, 98-105.** (In Chinese.)

2334

Liu, C. H. (1960). [A psychological study of experimental teaching of algebra to primary school children]. *Acta Psychologica Sinica,* **No. 1, 13-27.** (In Chinese.)

An experiment was conducted to see whether algebra could be taught to children earlier than is customary. The subjects were 87 children aged 10-11 years from two experimental Grade 5 classes, who would normally not learn algebra for another 2 years. They were taught simple equations in algebra and were tested on using algebra to solve arithmetic problems, understanding and use of formulae, and grasping rules governing the relation between numbers. Within 1 month, with no extra hours of teaching, the children did at least one fifth of all the problems in arithmetic textbooks for primary Grades 5 and 6 and the first year of junior middle school. In the regular municipal examination in arithmetic, the two experimental classes performed much better than average. They also stood out on a test on the rules of arithmetic and the rules governing the relation between numbers. After four months, the experimental classes remained well ahead of two other classes of the same grade in the same school.

2335

Liu, C. Y., Chen, C. H., Chen, Y. H., & Yang, K. S. (1973). [A survey of the everyday behavior of National Taiwan University students]. *Thought and Word* **(Taipei),** *10,* **6-29; 10(6), 1-19.** (In Chinese.)

2336

Liu, H. C. (1974). Media use, academic performance and social-demographic background: A study of Taiwanese children. *Dissertation Abstracts International, 34,* **A3994.**

2337

Liu, H. H. (1970). [The relationship between the social status in the classroom and personality traits among elementary school children]. *Psychological Testing, 17,* **767-789.** (In Chinese.)

2338

Liu, W. T. (1965). Achievement motivation among Chinese youth in Southeast Asia. *Asian Survey, 4,* **186-196.**

2339

Liu, Z. J., & Huang, P. S. (1980). [Preliminary analysis of psychological characteristics of 120 good teachers and model class instructors]. *Acta Psychologica Sinica, 12,* **287-297.** (In Chinese.)

2340

Lo, L. (1982). An investigation of science achievement and its relationships with student characteristics, home background factors and teacher characteristics for junior secondary grades in Hong Kong. *Dissertation Abstracts International, 43,* **A747.**

2341

Lo, M. Y., & Slakter, M. J. (1973). Risk taking and test-wiseness of Chinese students. *Journal of Experimental Education, 42,* **56-59.**

Administered the Standard Educational Intelligence Test which contains measures of risk-taking and test-wiseness to 86 male and 45 female Chinese 12th graders in Taiwan. The reliability (.88) and the mean (.68) of the risk measure were the same magnitudes as that reported for 12th-grade American students. Further analysis of the data indicated that sex and risk-taking, and penalty-experience and risk-taking were not related, but that the test-taking experience and risk were weakly related. The Kuder-Richardson number 20 values for the 4 test-wiseness subscales were low, and, the mean scores were lower for Chinese than for American Ss of all 4 subscales. Furthermore, the mean score for the stem-option scale was essentially equal to chance, and the mean score for the specific-determiner scale was even less than chance. In 2 separate Sex * Test-Experience and Sex * Penalty-Experience multivariate analyses of variance, none of the relationships appeared to be significant.

2342

Lopez, M., Sierra, G. P., & Castro, L. (1978). [Reading comprehension in Chinese without phonetic support]. *Revista Interamericana de Psicologia, 12,* **189-192.** (In other language.)

Examined reading comprehension of introductory Chinese by Spanish-speaking Ss using a visual training task that did not use phonetic referents. Four independent groups of 15 Ss completed a "sensibilization" phase, a general pretest, from 1 to 4 training phases, and a general posttest. The training phases were comprised of study subphases (item observation) and test subphases (Chinese-Spanish or Spanish-Chinese matching to sample). All tests implied reading without phonetic support. Performance was a function of the number of training phases, with the greatest effect occurring in the condition where training was given with illustrative sentences.

2343

Lu, C. H., Mao, Y. Y., Ying, Y. Y., Ma, C. W., & Chang, M. L. (1961). [Some psychological factors in promoting students' grasp of arithmetical knowledge, as found in recent educational reforms]. *Acta Psychologica Sinica*, **No. 3, 190-201.** (In Chinese.)

The present paper sums up 33 psychological studies of mathematics teaching conducted during the past 3 years of the Great Leap Forward. Implications for teaching are discussed.

2344

Lu, C. M. (1974). Personality characteristics of prospective teachers in China. *Dissertation Abstracts International*, *34*, **A4878-4879.**

2345

Lu, C. M. (1978). [An analysis of the language abilities of senior high school students]. *Bulletin of Educational Psychology*, *11*, **49-62.** (In Chinese.)

Administered the Chinese Language Achievement Test and the English Language Achievement Test to 5,197 male and 3,780 female high school seniors, 4,739 majoring in the social sciences and 4,238 in the natural sciences. There were significant Sex * Major interaction effects on test scores. Test scores also significantly correlated with university entrance examination scores.

2346

Lu, C. M., Chen, S. M., & Chen, L. C. (1981). [A study on musical aptitude of Chinese students]. *Bulletin of Educational Psychology*, *14*, **149-159.** (In Chinese.)

The purposes of this study were to develop a standardized musical aptitude test for identifying musically talented students, and to explore the characteristics of musical aptitude. The test battery used consisted of eight subtests: tonal memory, intensity discrimination, tonal movement, rhythm discrimination, pitch discrimination, melodic taste, pitch imagery, and rhythm imagery. The subjects was 4,225 students in Grade 3 to Grade 9 from 13 elementary and 13 junior high schools in Taiwan. The main results were: (1) The mean scores of the musical aptitude test increased with age. (2) There were gradually increasing differences in mean scores between the sexes from the third to the ninth grade. Percentile and T score norms were established; reliabilities and discriminant validities were generally satisfactory.

2347

Lu, C. M., Chien, M. F., & Kuo, S. Y. (1976). [Item types, scoring, and predictive validity of the Joint Examination for Universities and Colleges in Taiwan]. *Psychological Testing*, *23*, **28-45.** (In Chinese.)

2348

Lu, C. M., & Hwang, C. H. (1974). [An analysis of scores on the Joint Entrance Examination of Universities and Colleges, 1973]. *Psychological Testing*, *21*, **87-90.** (In Chinese.)

2349

Lu, C., & Wang, W. C. (1963). [The thinking processes in arithmetical operation in lower-grade school children]. *Acta Psychologica Sinica*, **No. 2, 121-129.** (In Chinese.)

2350

Lu, C., Wang, W. C., & Cheng, Y. T. (1964). [Mastery of reverse operation and flexibility of thinking in arithmetic in school children]. *Acta Psychologica Sinica*, **No. 3, 237-247.** (In Chinese.)

Two instruction methods were used in teaching children of the first and second grades to solve verbal arithmetical problems. The experimental group was instructed with the "contrast method" (the reverse operation of a problem was taught), while the control group was instructed with the "successive method" (only one-way operation of a problem was taught). One year of systematic observation indicated that the former method was better than the latter; it not only promoted the ability to solve verbal arithmetical problems, but also developed the flexibility of thinking. Two types of difficulties in solving verbal problems were revealed. Firstly, the children took only the superficial features and grasped only one or two words in question in the attempt to solve the problems; secondly, they failed to solve the problem because of their limited knowledge and little experience of applying the knowledge in new situations. These difficulties could be overcome by the contrast method of instruction and by increasing the knowledge of the children.

2351

Lu, C. Y. (1968). [Revision of the college qualification test]. *Acta Psychologica Taiwanica*, *10*, **1-21.** (In Chinese.)

2352

Lu, C. Y. (1970). [A study on personality traits of freshmen at the National Taiwan University]. *Acta Psychologica Taiwanica*, *12*, **1-6.** (In Chinese.)

2353

Lu, C. Y. (1973). [An analysis of psychological testing in junior high schools in Taiwan]. *Psychological Testing, 20,* **1061-1066.** (In Chinese.)

2354

Lu, C. Y. (1975). [An application of the DAT to high school students]. *Psychological Testing, 22,* **30-41.** (In Chinese.)

2355

Lu, C. Y. (1976). [Application of the differential aptitude tests in junior high schools]. *Psychological Testing, 23,* **20-27.** (In Chinese.)

2356

Lu, C. Y. (1977). [The development of the high school form of the School and College Ability Test]. *Bulletin of Educational Psychology, 10,* **1-10.** (In Chinese.)

Describes the development of a Chinese version of the high school form of the School and College Ability Test (SCAT) by combining SCAT and the Army Classification Battery. The form was standardized with a sample of 3,429 students from 12 senior high schools and 3 junior high schools.

2357

Lu, Z. H. (1984). [A study of the psychology of learning in raising the effect of self-study]. *Acta Psychologica Sinica, 16,* **349-365.** (In Chinese.)

This is a report on an experiment of guided self-study in mathematics in a 3-year cycle beginning from 1980, involving 23 classes in 7 provinces. The results showed that experimental classes were mostly superior to comparative classes on four indexes, school achievement, growth of ability in self-study, transfer of ability in self-study, and overall development. Results obtained from 77 experimental classes in 16 provinces starting from 1981 and from 70 classes in 22 provinces starting from 1982 also supported the results obtained in 1980. The guided self-study was of benefit to poor students; it also helped to develop the intelligence of superior students, enhancing their initiative and enthusiasm. It can also develop the students' convergent as well as divergent thinking.

2358

Lu, Z. H., Song, T. L. et al. (1980). [A research on the thinking ability in selfstudy of mathematics in middle school children]. *Acta Psychologica Sinica, 12,* **280-286.** (In Chinese.)

2359

Ma, H. H., & Lin, S. L. (1983). [The influence of socioeconomic background on the preschool educational opportunity, and the influence of preschool education on the academic performances of elementary school children]. *Journal of Education & Psychology, 6,* **19-39.** (In Chinese.)

This study investigated the effect of socioeconomic background on kindergarten educational opportunity, as well as the effect of kindergarten education on elementary academic performances. Using stratified random sampling, 2371 first-, third-, and sixth-grade pupils from nine elementary schools in Hsin-Chu Hsien were sampled and their parents were surveyed with questionnaire. Findings included: (1) The higher the socioeconomic background, the greater the chance that the child would have been to a kindergarten; this inequality has improved yearly. (2) Socioeconomic background had a positive effect on the academic performances in Chinese, Mathematics, Science, and Social Study. (3) Kindergarten education had a significant positive effect only on the first-grade academic performances. The growth-rate of the number of kindergarten children and that of the total educational expenditure for kindergarten in Taiwan has risen drastically in recent years. This would contribute to the equality of educational opportunity of the children in Taiwan.

2360

Mair, J. S. (1969). Certain physical and personality characteristics of Hong Kong government secondary school boys in relation to their attitude to physical education. *Journal of Education* **(University of Hong Kong),** *26,* **46-66.**

2361

Maltzman, C. M. (1981). Cross-cultural patterns of response to the WISC/WISC-R and Bender Gestalt Test by Chinese-American, Hispanic-American, and Occidental-American educationally handicapped boys. *Dissertation Abstracts International, 42,* **A658.**

2362

Mao, Y. Y., Ying, Y. Y., & Ma, C. W. (1961). [An experimental study on the processes of learning rational number in algebra by 5-6th grade pupils]. *Acta Psychologica Sinica,* **No. 4, 229-244.** (In Chinese.)

The aim of the research was to analyze the processes of learning rational numbers in algebra by 5-6th grade pupils aged 13-14. Three experiments were performed. The results obtained throw light on the characteristics of the processes of grasping the conception of negative numbers by the pupils, on the interrelation between abstract and concrete thinking, on the ability of verbal accounting and on the speed and accuracy of calculation. The authors concluded it is feasible for 5th grade pupils to learn rational numbers, and suggestions on teaching programs in the educational reform were made.

2363

Matsuda, N., & Robbins, D. (1977). Prototype abstraction and distinctive feature learning: An application to learning Chinese characters. *Journal of Educational Psychology, 69,* **15-23.**

Chinese characters with related meanings often have a common symbol included among their components. In an exemplar-prototype and distinctive feature classification system, the multiple-component characters (the exemplars) can be said to have a common component (the prototype) distinctive to the shared concept. A study was conducted with 60 undergraduates who were administered recognition tests with new and old exemplars and prototypes. Results show that the traditional language learning technique of paired-associate training with exemplars of Chinese characters and specific English translations led to the poorest performance of the 3 methods tested. Learning either the English concept for Chinese exemplars (exemplar-category training) or the English concept for only the distinctive feature (prototype training) produced greatly superior performance. Instructions regarding the nature of Chinese characters had no effect on performance.

2364

Metraux, R. (1953). The Chinese first teacher. In M. Mead & R. Metraux (Eds.), *The study of culture at a distance.* **Chicago, IL: University of Chicago Press.**

2365

Miao, E. S. (1981). Identifying the affectively handicapped among the university freshmen: A cross-cultural approach. *International Journal of Group Tensions, 11,* **81-106.**

Reports on a continuing investigation of 2 mental health indices, the Self-Rating Anxiety Scale and the Self-Rating Depression Scale, which are used to identify the differential status of anxiety and depression among incoming college freshmen. Translated versions of these scales, along with the Mental Health Questionnaire for a correlation study, were administered to 2,121 college students in Taiwan. Cross-cultural comparisons of research in this area, and the goals and strategies of preventive university mental health programs are discussed.

2366

Mickle, K. M. (1985). The cross-cultural adaptation of Hong Kong students at two Ontario universities. *Dissertation Abstracts International, 45,* **A2785.**

2367

Miller, M. H., Yeh, E. K., Alexander, A. A., Klein, M. H., Tseng, K. H., Workneh, F., & Chu, H. M. (1971). The cross-cultural student: Lessons in human nature. *Bulletin of the Menninger Clinic, 35,* **128-131.**

2368

Mitchell, M. H. (1978). International guidance activities. *Viewpoints in Teaching & Learning, 54,* **51-55.**

Briefly examines guidance services for youth in Bermuda, the British Isles, France, Belgium, Holland, Denmark, Greece, New Zealand, Australia, Japan, and Taiwan. Foreign programs tend to be vocational and community based; counselor training programs are rare. The American youth services are still unique.

2369

Mitchell, R. E. (Ed.). (1972). *Pupil, parent, and school: A Hong Kong study.* **Taipei: Oriental Cultural Service.**

2370

Mohd Majzub, R. B. (1984). Differences in priorities for kindergarten goals among parents, teachers, and experts in Malaysia. *Dissertation Abstracts International, 45,* **A406.**

2371

Morris, P. (1983). Teachers' perceptions of their pupils: A Hong Kong case study. *Research in Education, 29,* **81-86.**

24 teachers were shown 3 cards bearing the names of students in their classes and were asked to put together the 2 that were the most alike and explain how they were different from the third. This process was repeated 10 times with each S. Each S was then asked to rank-order the 3 most commonly used constructs according to their importance as influences on a child's success at school. 150 additional teachers were then given a test in which they were asked to write a sentence describing the characteristics of the most and least ideal students they currently taught. Results indicate that both samples of Ss generally used the same set of constructs to distinguish between their students; there was substantial agreement within the samples as to the relative importance of these constructs as influences on a student's educational career. The predominant construct used, in terms of both usage and perceived importance, was the "intelligent-stupid" construct.

2372

Moy, T. (1985). An exploration of the vocational values and needs of Chinese students. *Dissertation Abstracts International, 45,* **B3078.**

2373

Murphy, M. C., Richardson, B. L., & Sims, E. (1976). School desegregation and the role of the urban counselor. *Journal of Black Psychology*, **3, 87-99.**

Examines the role of the urban counselor in the desegregated school system setting; desegregation is seen as an important national goal. It is suggested that (a) urban counselors should promote quality education to all students and implement programs necessary for a better learning experience; (b) cultural differences should be taken into consideration in intelligence testing; (c) career education and curriculum planning are important aspects of the student's academic development, in which the counselor should take an active part; (d) the testing program should employ a measurement specialist who will compose new standardized tests for the multiracial setting; (e) discipline problems should be included in the definition of an urban counselor's role; and (f) the counselor should identify problems arising from the inadequacies of the system. A study revealed that the frequency of expulsions and suspensions of Black, Spanish surnamed, Asian-American, and American-Indian students was nearly twice that of White students, indicating the need for reassessment in this area.

2374

Nelson, T. M., & Ladan, C. J. (1977). Chinese ideograms as intermediaries to reading. *Journal of Reading Behavior*, **9, 167-174.**

Investigated the contributions of visual factors in tasks depending on the use of symbols as intermediary units. It was hypothesized that the perception of Chinese symbols would differ between groups of poor and good readers, with a significant interaction between the visual complexity of ideograms and reading ability. 40 2nd graders of normal visual acuity who scored above 80 on the WISC were evaluated as "better" or "poorer" readers on the basis of their scores on the Metropolitan Tests of Readiness and Achievement. 20 Ss viewed 55 pairs of Chinese ideograms presented simultaneously (SI), and the other 20 Ss viewed the pairs under successive (SU) conditions. Results confirm the hypothesis of a significant difference in perception between groups of poor and good readers; poor readers produced significantly more errors than good readers under both SI and SU conditions. It is concluded that perceptual factors may play an important role in the use of Chinese characters as intermediaries in introducing reading.

2375

[News from regional psychological societies in Honan (Henan), Fuchian (Fujian), Chungching (Chongqing) and other provinces]. (1962). *Acta Psychologica Sinica*, **No. 4, 334.** (In Chinese.)

2376

Ng, M. L. (1986). [Sex education in Hong Kong--current status]. *Bulletin of the Hong Kong Sex Education Association*, **No. 2, 1-9.** (In Chinese.)

2377

North, M. J. (1977). Films in changing ethnic attitudes and behavior in the elementary grades. *Dissertation Abstracts International*, *38*, **A1877-1878.**

2378

Okada, A. (1975). [The effect of legibility and readability on the oral reading of the partially sighted]. *Japanese Journal of Educational Psychology*, *23*, **165-169.** (In other language.)

Studied how size of print, length of line, writing style, contrast between letter and paper, and the ratio of Chinese characters used in Japanese language affected the oral reading of 25 partially sighted 6th graders (visual acuity less than 0.3) from schools for the blind. The oral reading was tape-recorded. 4 types of reading errors were identified. The number of reading errors was negatively correlated with legibility and readability. A positive relationship was found between the number of errors and reading speed.

2379

Okanes, M. M., & Murray, L. W. (1982). Machiavellian and achievement orientations among foreign and American master's students in business administration. *Psychological Reports*, *50*, **519-526.**

Administered the Mach IV Scale and Mehrabian Achievement Scale to 185 graduate business students. An across-countries analysis of scores on both tests was applied to Ss from Algeria, Iran, the Philippines, Taiwan, and the US. An analysis of similarities and differences based on cultural factors is provided. Predictions for Ss from each of the 5 countries derived from hypotheses generated on the basis of cultural background were confirmed more often for Mach scores than for achievement scores.

2380

Ouyang, C. J. (1983). A comparison of two sample groups of elementary science teachers' feelings and attitudes toward the new elementary science curriculum in Taiwan, The Republic of China. *Dissertation Abstracts International*, *43*, **A2952.**

2381

Pao, P. H. L. (1983). Effects of goal setting by Chinese-American children and their parents. *Dissertation Abstracts International*, *43*, **A3873.**

2382

Paul, P. (1985). The use of trivalent verbs of giving by advanced learners of English. *IRAL: International Review of Applied Linguistics in Language Teaching, 23,* **89-115.**

Sixteen university students and professionals in Australia and 30 Hong Kong high school students who spoke English as a 2nd language were given a list of 24 English verbs having to do with the action of giving (e.g., "to donate", "to give") and were asked to produce sentences with them. Subjects were or were not given verb pattern information. According to responses, verbs were classified into 5 patterns. Results indicated that semantic criteria alone cannot, at least for the nonnative speaker of English, satisfactorily explain the difference in verb pattern usage for synonyms like give and donate.

2383

Perkins, C. S., Perkins, M. L., Gulielmino, L. M., & Reiff, R. F. (1977). A comparison of the adjustment problems of three international student groups. *Journal of College Student Personnel, 18,* **382-388.**

Identified some significant differences in the adjustment problems of 210 students representing different national groups (Chinese and Indian) at an American university. The study also investigated significant differences between the groups on particular demographic and social interaction variables. Results suggest a need for more sophisticated statistical analyses in research concerning foreign students.

2384

Peterson, C. C. (1974). Self-selection of vocabulary in reading instruction. *Journal of Educational Research, 67,* **253-254.**

Simulated the child's process of learning to read by teaching 16 undergraduates to associate 30 Chinese characters with spoken words. 15 words were chosen by Ss and the other 15 (E's words) were the 1st 15 words in a basal reader. Learning was more rapid with the words selected by S. Results support the use of self-selection of vocabulary in reading instruction methods (e.g., Ashton-Warner key vocabulary).

2385

Phillips, C. J., & Marvelly, A. (1984). Basic educational skills of Asian children at the end of infant schooling. *Educational Research, 26,* **36-45.**

Presents the results of a longitudinal study of 384 native (UK) and West Indian and Asian (from Pakistan, India, Singapore, and Hong Kong) immigrant children (average age 7 yrs 2 mo) from their urban starting school. Ss were tested individually on vocabulary, spelling, mathematics, and reading. Progress in basic educational skills was compared for the UK and Asian immigrant Ss. Data show that, in reading and spelling, the Asians achieved nearly national norms; their scores were poorer in numerical ability than in literacy. Low scores were more common among the indigenous Ss than the Asians in schools serving socially disadvantaged areas. Results are discussed in terms of the effects of cultural test biases; educational implications are also discussed.

2386

Poirier, J. (1983). Bref historique de l'education des enfants doues et talentueux [A brief history of the education of gifted and talented children]. *Apprentissage et Socialisation, 6,* **137-145.** (In other language.)

Describes the history of selecting and educating gifted children. Biblical, Greek, and Roman references to this question were related to the education of the elite. During the Middle Ages, education was primarily Christian, but during the Renaissance, education of gifted students assumed a secular, literary, and philosophic character. 20th-century education of the gifted has become much more systematic, particularly in the US. It is suggested that, contrary to their doctrine, Soviet and Chinese Marxists select and educate their gifted students by methods similar to the Americans (i.e., offering extracurricular enrichment activities and special classes and schools).

2387

Pope, L. (1982). Reading instruction in modern China. *Reading Teacher, 35,* **688-694.**

The Chinese language, the 1978 Chinese reading primer, Chinese reading methodology, learning problems (hyperactivity and symptoms similar to those of cerebral dysfunction), and specific reading problems are discussed. It is concluded that difficulties in learning to read Chinese are compounded when the learner has constitutional problems or learning disabilities that make it more difficult to concentrate, perceive subtle differences, sequence properly, and understand abstract words and concepts.

2388

Rai, C. K., & Wang, P. D. (1982). [Psychological peculiarities of how primary schools recognize geometrical figures and grasp geometrical concepts]. *Information on Psychological Sciences,* **No. 3, 30-37.** (In Chinese.)

2389

Ray, J. J., & Jones, J. M. (1983). Occupational and educational achievement motivation in Australian and Hong Kong schoolchildren. *Journal of Social Psychology, 120,* **281-282.**

119 Australian 9th graders completed educational and occupational motivation scales that had previously been administered to a group of Hong Kong Chinese students by M. Leung et al (1983). Contrary to common assumptions about the industriousness of the

Hong Kong Chinese and data suggesting that Australian levels of achievement motivation are among the lowest in the world, Australian Ss scored significantly higher on both measures, although the results on the educational motivation measure appeared to be an acquiescence artifact.

2390

Ripple, R., Jaquish, G., Lee, H. W., & Salili, F. (1984). Cognitive and affective costs of bilingual education: A look at the Hong Kong experience. *New Horizons*, **No. 25, 74-81.**

2391

Rodd, W. G. (1959). A cross-cultural study of Taiwan's schools. *Journal of Social Psychology*, *50*, **3-36.**

Analyses of scores of 1,290 students on a battery of tests showed sex and city differences rather than differences attributable to native origin, for example, Taiwan versus Chinese mainland. The ability of the students in senior middle schools in Taiwan was demonstrated to be of a higher caliber when judged against the American norms of individual tests (intelligence, school achievement, and critical thinking).

2392

Rodd, W. G. (1960). [Mathematics and science ability in Taiwan schools]. *Psychological Testing*, *8*, **583-585.** (In Chinese.)

2393

Rogers, C. (1976). Status, ability, encouragement, sex roles, and educational aspirations of adolescents in Taiwan: A replicative study of the Sewell model. *Dissertation Abstracts International*, *36*, **A5955-5956.**

2394

Rozin, P., Poritsky, S., & Sotsky, R. (1971). American children with reading problems can easily learn to read English represented by Chinese characters. *Science*, *171*, **1264-1267.**

Describes a study in which, with 2.5-5.5 yr. of tutoring, 8 2nd grade innercity schoolchildren with clear reading disability were taught to read English material written as 30 different Chinese characters. This accomplishment eliminates certain general interpretations of, e.g., dyslexia, as a visual-auditory memory deficit. The success of this program can be attributed to the novelty of the Chinese orthography and to the fact that Chinese characters map into speech at the level of words rather than of phonemes. It is proposed that much reading disability can be accounted for in terms of the highly abstract nature of the phoneme (the critical unit of speech in alphabetic systems) and that an intermediate unit, e.g., the syllable, might well be used to introduce reading.

2395

Shan, K. M. (1970). The culturally deprived child in Hong Kong: His educational and psychological needs. *Newsletter of the Mental Health Association of Hong Kong*, **May, 2-8. (Available from Mental Health Association of Hong Kong, G.P.O. Box 1534, Hong Kong.)**

2396

Shao, J. C., Shih, J. H., & Chung, C. C. (1965). [The development of the elementary school children's ability of summarizing the contents of paragraphs of prose: A preliminary experimental study on the analyzing and synthesizing activity in the selection of titles]. *Acta Psychologica Sinica*, **No. 1, 28-37.** (In Chinese.)

In order to study the analyzing and synthesizing abilities of school children in selecting a title for a paragraph of a prose, three components of performance were identified and measured. The results showed that: (1) Significant differences in all three aspects existed among three groups of subjects which had high, middle and low scores in reading and arithmetic tasks. (2) The three kinds of organizations of the performance showed different levels of the generalization processes. (3) The characteristics of the selection activity as measured with the method of the present study might be used as a criterion in determining the level of the generalization processes in school children.

2397

Shen, C. H. (1962). [Some problems on the formation of number-conception in 3-4 year children]. *Acta Psychologica Sinica*, **No. 3, 210-218.** (In Chinese.)

This was an experimental study on the formation of number concepts in preschool children. The results were: (1) The development of counting ability was related to the formation of the conception of numbers, but the ability to count numbers was not the same as the formation of number concepts. (2) Children aged 3-4 years could grasp number concepts to a certain extent. (3) The formation of number concepts began in oral number counting and proceeded to the step where children were able to pick the number of objects asked by the experimenter. (4) The processes of the formation of number concepts proceeded from repeating the sounds of sequences of numbers to the understanding of meaning; from discriminating the numbers to the use of them; and from forming the ideas of numbers to the conception of numbers.

2398

Shen, Y. (1959). [Primary school students' vocabulary]. *Acta Psychologica Sinica*, **No. 6, 376-387.** (In Chinese.)

To master a certain amount of vocabulary in everyday use is an important factor in the training of reading and expressive abilities and is also one of the key problems in the overall improvement of the quality of the language teaching. It was revealed in the present investigation that 7- and 8-year-old children could learn Chinese characters more easily if the teachers would improve the method of instruction. The method of teaching in several excellent classes and unsatisfactory ones were analyzed. It was found that the results of teaching depend not only on the teaching of the characters but also on the instruction of the method of learning. The results of a preliminary experiment confirmed that analyzing the structure of characters is an effective method for the mastery of characters. Further studies are necessary for the clarification of the development of the analyzing and synthesizing processes in learning vocabularies.

2399

Sheridan, E. M. (1983). Reading disabilities: Can we blame the written language? *Journal of Learning Disabilities, 16,* **81-86.**

One factor in learning to read is the nature of the script that is used. To understand the particular nature of the English alphabetic script and the specific problems that might arise from it, the following questions are considered: Is it any easier to learn to read through an ideographic, syllabic, or alphabetic writing system? Is there less incidence of reading failure with some "ideal" orthography? Has any particular written language shown itself to be less difficult for beginning reading instruction, especially for particular reading and learning-disabled children? The linguistic nature of Chinese, Japanese, and Korean are examined relative to differences in information processing and cultural factors related to reading disability.

2400

Shiang, B. D. (1979). [Subject matter, grade level, and sex in relation to classroom climate in senior high school]. *Journal of Education & Psychology, 3,* **226-228.** (In Chinese.)

2401

Shih, Y. S. (1985). Determinants of job satisfaction among public special school teachers in Taiwan, the Republic of China. *Dissertation Abstracts International, 45,* **A2837.**

2402

Shu, S. C. (1978). [A comparative study of classroom climates in high-achieving junior high school classes]. *Bulletin of Educational Psychology, 11,* **141-158.** (In Chinese.)

Studied the relationship between classroom climates and gender and achievement in 228 male and 222 female junior high school students, using a Chinese version of the Barclay Classroom Climate Inventory (BCCI). Ss with high achievement scored significantly higher in self-competence, achievement motivation, and vocational interests and earned more teacher approval than low-achievement Ss. Low-achievement Ss showed a greater tendency to associate with peers than did high-achievement Ss. Males and females differed significantly on most BCCI scales.

2403

Shu, S. C. (1979). [Impact of teachers' expectation on teacher-student interaction and students' personal qualities]. *Bulletin of Educational Psychology, 12,* **183-194.** (In Chinese.)

This study investigated relationships between teachers' expectations toward teacher-student interaction and the personal qualities of elementary students. The subjects were 80 students and 4 teachers selected from an elementary school. Systematic observation, tests and questionnaires were means to gather data, which were statistically treated by the chi-square test, multivariate analysis of variance, and multiple regression analysis. The main results were: (1) In the classroom students expected of a high level of interaction indicated more interaction with teachers than students expected of a low level. Teachers tended to accept the former's feelings and used their ideas, but they expressed more criticism toward the latter. (2) Students expected of more interaction had higher mean scores in academic achievement, achievement motivation, peer status, and personal adjustment. (3) Personal qualities together accounted for 69.89% of the variance of teachers' expectations.

2404

Shu, S. C., Chiu, W. C., & Chang, C. H. (1977). [A study of guidance services in junior high schools in Taiwan]. *Bulletin of Educational Psychology, 10,* **83-90.** (In Chinese.)

Studied the status, accomplishments, and problems of the guidance services offered at all 563 junior high schools in Taiwan province and the city of Taipei, using questionnaire surveys of school administrators, teachers, and students. Results indicate emphasis on academic guidance pointed toward higher education, and on eliminating problem behavior by students. Vocational placement advice has been provided by about half the schools.

2405

Siu, P. K. (1973). Relationships between motivational patterns and academic achievement in Chinese and Puerto Rican second, and third-grade students. *Dissertation Abstracts International, 33,* **A3407.**

2406

Smith, N. J. (1982). Reading instruction in Taiwan: A model for using the reader effectively. *Reading Teacher, 36,* **34-37.**

Describes an integrated approach to reading and language arts instruction observed in elementary schools in Taipei, Hwalien, and Taiwan. The reading selection, the instructional sequence for teaching students to write, supplemental activities, and teacher characteristics are discussed.

2407

Solomon, R. H. (1965). Educational themes in China's changing culture. *China Quarterly*, **No. 22, 154-170.**

A content analysis was performed on two sets of Chinese children's texts, one from Shanghai between 1922 and 1929 and the other from Beijing in 1960. It was concluded that there had been an increase in the salience of achievement-oriented activities.

2408

Soong, W. T., & Soong, K. P. (1981). Sex differences in school adjustment in Taiwan. In A. Kleinman & T. Y. Lin (Eds.), *Normal and abnormal behavior in Chinese culture* **(pp. 157-165). Dordrecht, Netherlands: Reidel.**

2409

Sparkes, K. K. (1983). Compliance and noncompliance in preschool centers in Taiwan. *International Journal of Group Tensions*, *13*, **132-145.**

Observed children's compliant and noncompliant behaviors in 10 preschool centers in Taipei, Taiwan, in each of the following settings: large-group instruction or stories, music and movement, art, transitions, and snack and lunch time. Observations indicated that there was a high degree of compliance with basic rules and routines as well as with specific teacher requests. Compliance was typically cheerful and relaxed. Most noncompliant behavior was not disruptive to the central activity of the group. Cultural factors that may account for the good teacher-child relationships in Taiwan were discussed.

2410

Special education in the Republic of China. (1978). *Australian Journal of Mental Retardation*, *5*, **6-9.**

2411

Spinks, J. A., & Ho, D. Y. F. (1984). Chinese students at an English-language university: Prediction of academic performance. *Higher Education*, *13*, **657-674.**

There is a paucity of systematic research on prediction of success at the tertiary education level for Asian students, despite the important role that universities play in Asian communities, and despite the increasing numbers of such students who are coming to the West to study. This study reviews evidence collected over the past ten to fifteen years, which relates to the issue of prediction of academic performance of Chinese students at an English-Language and Western-oriented university - the University of Hong Kong. This review is complemented by an analysis of data collected longitudinally over a five year period, using multiple regression, multiple correlation, path analysis and canonical correlation analyses. The results provide evidence of factors which are important in determining the ability of a student to adapt to the foreign cultural and language barriers that exist at this university. In particular, ability in English language and mathematics provides good and reasonably independent predictors of success. The data show the importance of considering the cultural background of students when assessing their aptitude for study, and offer information for Western universities regarding their admissions procedures for Chinese students.

2412

Spinks, J., & Ho, D. (1983). Prediction of academic success at the University of Hong Kong. *New Horizons*, *24*, **167-183.**

2413

Stevenson, H. W. et al. (1984). Family variables and reading: A study of mothers of poor and average readers in Japan, Taiwan, and the United States. *Journal of Learning Disabilities*, *17*, **150-156.**

Interviewed approximately 160 mothers of poor and average readers in Japan, Taiwan, and the US about their childrearing practices, attitudes, and beliefs as well as their children's current and earlier experiences. 80 poor readers represented the lowest 5th percentile in reading scores; they were matched by classroom, sex, and age with 80 average readers. The groups seldom differed significantly according to environmental variables and parent-child interactions. Maternal ratings of cognitive and achievement variables differentiated both the children in the 2 groups and the mothers themselves. Maternal beliefs and descriptions of how children use time also differed between the 2 groups. Notable was the absence of significant interactions between country and reading level.

2414

Stevenson, H. W. et al. (1985). Cognitive performance and academic achievement of Japanese, Chinese, and American children. *Child Development*, *56*, **718-734.**

A battery of 10 cognitive tasks and tests of achievement in reading and mathematics were given to 1,440 Chinese, Japanese, and American children in Grades 1 and 5. Data showed similarities among children of the three cultures in level, variability, and structure of cognitive abilities. Chinese subjects surpassed Japanese and American subjects in reading scores, and both Chinese and Japanese subjects obtained higher scores in mathematics than American subjects. Prediction of achievement scores from the cognitive tasks showed few differential effects among children of the three cultures. The results suggested that the high achievement of Chinese and Japanese children cannot be attributed to higher intellectual abilities, but must be related to their experiences at home and at school.

2415

Steward, D. S., & Steward, M. S. (1975). Cognitive development and ethnicity: Problems for educational ministry. *Religious Education*, ***70***, **308-316.**

Discusses level of cognitive development and ethnic pluralism as factors to be considered in programs of religious education that recognize the importance of their social context. Research on home learning of preschool children identified 2 components of teaching-learning loops. Giving instructions, a rational component, varied across cognitive levels of the "teachers" in the home more than across ethnic groups studied. Giving feedback, a predominately affective component, varied more among the ethnic groups (Mexican, Chinese-American, and Anglo). Consequent hypotheses regarding church educational programs are suggested.

2416

Stigler, J. W. (1984). "Mental abacus": The effect of abacus training on Chinese children's mental calculation. *Cognitive Psychology*, ***16***, **145-176.**

In 2 studies, 12 Chinese 5th graders (aged 10 yrs 9 mo to 11 yrs 6 mo) at 3 levels of abacus expertise were observed performing both abacus and mental addition. Response times and errors were examined as a function of problem type and mode of computation. Results show that Ss were able to answer correctly--and without using an actual abacus--questions about intermediate states unique to the abacus-based solution of a problem. Response times for answering such questions were a function of the position of the probed state in the sequence required for problem solving. The pattern of response times did not differ according to whether the task was being solved using the abacus or mentally. In a 3rd study, Ss' performance was compared with a group of 4 American adults performing the same mental additions. Analysis of the errors produced by the 2 groups showed that Chinese errors differed from American errors in ways predicted according to characteristics of the abacus. Chinese were also given a task that required them to access intermediate states of mental abacus calculation. Results indicate that abacus training has both quantitative and qualitative effects on children's mental calculation skill and that a "mental abacus" is used by experts.

2417

Stigler, J. W., Lee, S. Y., Lucker, G. W., & Stevenson, H. W. (1982). Curriculum and achievement in mathematics: A study of elementary school children in Japan, Taiwan, and the United States. *Journal of Educational Psychology*, ***74***, **315-322.**

Describes a method for constructing a test of mathematics achievement for use in cross-national study. The mathematics curricula as presented in elementary school textbook series from Japan, Taiwan, and the US were analyzed according to the grade level at which various concepts and skills were introduced. Findings indicate that the Japanese curriculum contained more concepts and skills and also introduced these concepts and skills earlier than the curricula of Taiwan and the US. The curriculum was somewhat more advanced in the US than in Taiwan. Details of the procedure used in constructing the mathematics test are described. The test was administered to 480 1st and 5th graders from 40 classrooms in each of the 3 countries. Results show that Ss from Japan and Taiwan consistently performed at a higher level than their American counterparts. It is concluded that level of achievement in elementary school mathematics appears not to be closely related to the content of the curriculum.

2418

Stodolsky, S. S., & Lesser, G. (1967). Learning patterns in the disadvantaged. *Harvard Educational Review*, ***37***, **546-593.**

2419

Su, C. S. (1986). [A study of present teachers' and future teachers' attitudes toward special education]. *Bulletin of Educational Psychology*, ***19***, **67-84.** (In Chinese.)

This study investigated the cognitive and affective attitudes of present and future teachers in elementary and secondary schools toward special education and exceptional children. Subjects were 179 students from National Taiwan Normal University and 149 elementary and secondary school teachers who were receiving in-service training at the same university. The Special Education Attitudes Questionnaire constructed by the investigator consisted of 14 cognitive items and 9 affective items. Two main findings were: (1) Most of the subjects who had received teacher education revealed attitudes of humanism and role taking toward exceptional students. (2) Teachers who were qualified, female, experienced with the handicapped and had received special education courses possessed more positive attitudes toward special education and exceptional children than those who were disqualified, male, inexperienced with the handicapped and had not received special education courses.

2420

Su, C. W. (1976). [The perceived parental attitudes of high-achieving and under-achieving junior high school students]. *Bulletin of Educational Psychology* **(Taiwan Normal University),** *9,* **21-32.** (In Chinese.)

This study investigated differences in parental attitudes between the parents of high-achieving and underachieving junior high school students matched on the basis of intelligence. The Parent-Child Relations Questionnaire was used to measure parental attitudes as perceived by the students. It was found that, in comparison with underachievers, achieving students perceived their parents as more loving, more accepting (less rejecting), more concerned (less neglecting), using symbolic-love rewards more often and symbolic-love punishments less often. No significant group difference was found, however, on measures of protection, demand, casualness, and use of direct-object rewards or direct-object punishments. Boys perceived their parents as being more demanding and using both reward and punishment more often than girls did. Girls were more likely than boys to perceive their parents as showing more love and care toward them. The subjects' responses to the father-child relations questionnaire and the mother-child relations questionnaire were basically the same, except that mothers were perceived as more rejecting than fathers.

2421

Su, H. Y. (1966). A report on the student counseling center. *Acta Psychologica Taiwanica, 8,* **96-98.**

2422

Sue, D. W., & Kirk, B. A. (1973). Differential characteristics of Japanese-American and Chinese-American college students. *Journal of Counseling Psychology, 20,* **142-148.**

Asked all entering freshmen at a large northern California university to participate in a testing program that included the School and College Ability Test, the SVIB, and the Omnibus Personality Inventory. Results from 106 Japanese-Americans, 236 Chinese-Americans, and all other students were analyzed and compared to 1 another. Findings support the hypothesis that these 2 ethnic groups differ from all other students in the same direction because of similar cultural values. However, Japanese-American Ss consistently occupied an intermediate position between the 2 other groups on all 3 measures. Results suggest some form of differential acculturation due to historical and political circumstances for the 2 ethnic groups.

2423

Sue, D. W., & Kirk, B. A. (1975). Asian-Americans: Use of counseling and psychiatric services on a college campus. *Journal of Counseling Psychology, 22,* **84-86.**

Studied 3,053 Asian-American and non-Asian students in the 1966 freshman class of a large state university over a 4-yr period to determine usage of mental health services. Asian-Americans underutilized the campus psychiatric service but significantly overutilized the counseling center. Possible reasons related to the Asian-Americans' subcultural values explain these findings. Nearly 50% of Chinese-American females utilized mental health services of some kind. This extremely high usage may be due to a domestic vs feminist conflict.

2424

Sue, S., & Zane, N. W. (1985). Academic achievement and socioemotional adjustment among Chinese university students. *Journal of Counseling Psychology, 32,* **570-579.**

The authors examined the academic performance, majors, study habits, and socioemotional adjustment of 177 Chinese and Chinese-American university students. Ninety-four subjects were foreign born, and 83 were 2nd-, 3rd-, or 4th-generation Americans. Data were collected through official university records, questionnaires, and inventories. Subjects were divided into 3 groups, depending on place of birth and length of residency in the US. Results indicated that the image of the high-achieving, well-adjusted Chinese student was tempered when criteria other than grade point average were examined. Although grades received by the 3 groups of subjects exceeded the university average, recent immigrants apparently used certain strategies to compensate for limited English proficiency by taking reduced courseloads, studying more hours, and limiting career majors. There was also evidence that the recent immigrants were less socioemotionally adjusted than were other subjects. Implications for counseling and research were discussed.

2425

Sun, K. K. (1965). [A Diagnostic Arithmetic Test for elementary school children]. *Psychological Testing, 12,* **221-224.** (In Chinese.)

2426

Tang, S. C., & Chang, W. H. (1974). [The application of the differential aptitude tests in Tunghai University]. *Psychological Testing, 21,* **1-10.** (In Chinese.)

2427

Tang, T. C. (1962). [The system of general psychology in pedagogical institutes]. *Acta Psychologica Sinica,* **No. 3, 262-263.** (In Chinese.)

2428

[The collaboration between the Institute of Psychology, Academica Sinica, and Pedagogical Institutions for the development of research work in educational psychology]. (1960). *Acta Psychologica Sinica*, **No. 4, 269.** (In Chinese.)

2429

[The Congress of Educational Psychology held by the Chinese Psychological Society]. (1962). *Acta Psychologica Sinica*, **No. 2, 168-171.** (In Chinese.)

2430

[The Co-operative Research Group on Super-normal Children]. (1979). [A preliminary research of 21 supernormal children]. *Acta Psychologica Sinica, 11*, **118-125.** (In Chinese.)

The purpose of this study is to identify children with superior intelligence, the conditions of their development, and appropriate ways to educate them. Preliminary data on 15 boys and 6 girls aged from 1 to 11 years are presented, including case history, school performance, intellectual faculties, and personality traits. Following-up studies will be conducted.

2431

[The Co-operative Research Group on Super-Normal Children]. (1981). [Summary of a year's research on supernormal children]. *Acta Psychologica Sinica, 13*, **35-41.** (In Chinese.)

Research on superior children was carried out in 14 districts. A total of 29 subjects (18 boys and 11 girls) aged from 4 to 15 years were studied. The methods used included experimentation, observation, interviews, personality assessment, and performance rating. The children were observed to have intellectual curiosity, keen perception and observation, and good concentration, attention, and memory. They showed initiative, and had self-confidence and perseverance. Some were allowed to start primary school aged about 4-5 years; some entered junior high school aged 8-9 years; and some entered the university when only 14 years old.

2432

The Hong Kong Educational Research Association. (1985). *Selected papers on educational research in Hong Kong from The First Annual Conference.* **Hong Kong: Author.**

2433

Thogmartin, C. (1982). Age, individual differences in musical and verbal aptitude, and pronunciation achievement by elementary school children learning a foreign language. *IRAL: International Review of Applied Linguistics in Language Teaching, 20*, **66-72.**

Investigated, in 2 experiments, the ability of monolingual American schoolchildren to learn the pronunciation of 2nd-language speech sounds. In Exp I, 18 children, 3 of each sex from the 2nd, 4th, and 6th grades, were taught to associate a "word" with each of 10 flashcard drawings. Five of the words consisted of an English consonant phoneme plus the vowel a, 3 of a non-English consonant sound plus a, and 2 words were non-English vowel sounds. Results indicate that the effect of age on learning was not significant, and the predicted hypothesis that younger Ss would demonstrate superiority in pronunciation learning was not confirmed. In Exp II, 18 children (aged 5-12 yrs) were participants in a Mandarin Chinese course. Each S was tested on performance in repeating 15 Chinese sentences and in describing 15 posters in Chinese. Results show a tendency for a positive correlation of older age with performance in both production and repetition.

2434

Ting, S. S. (1978). [Effects of cognitive style and incongruity on intentional and incidental learning]. *Research in Education & Psychology, 2*, **242-244.** (In Chinese.)

2435

Tou, L. A. (1974). A study of work orientations of Chinese-American and White-American students of the 7th and 8th grades in Catholic elementary schools. *Dissertation Abstracts International, 35*, **A831.**

2436

Tsai, P. T. (1981). [Principals' leadership styles and teachers' personality traits in relation to school organization and climate in junior high schools]. *Journal of Education & Psychology, 4*, **101-103.** (In Chinese.)

2437

Tseng, L. T. (1966). [Testing of literary and vernacular Chinese and its contribution to the teaching of Chinese in secondary schools]. *Psychological Testing, 13*, **304-310.** (In Chinese.)

2438

Tseng, T. D. (1985). The relationship between principals' leadership style and teachers' professional zone of acceptance in junior high schools of Taipei, the Republic of China. *Dissertation Abstracts International, 46*, **A869.**

2439

Tsu, M. S., & Tsu, Y. Y. (1961). [Psychological analysis of the first year pupils in the understanding of applied problems in mathematics]. *Acta Psychologica Sinica*, **No. 3, 164-179.** (In Chinese.)

The pupils of three sections of a first year class were divided into an experimental group and two control groups (competitive in effect). In the experimental group, systematic observations and experiments were conducted in order to disclose the process and the different levels of understanding of applied problems. On the basis of the characteristics of each individual level, certain methods of instruction were employed in order to promote achievement. Results indicated the process of understanding applied problems could be classified into five levels, which were correlated, yet differentiated. According to the characteristics of each individual level, certain instructional methods were adopted; in consequence, the progression between different levels was accelerated, and the effect of instructions was greater than either of the control groups under general instructional conditions.

2440

Tsung, L. T. (1957). [An analysis of achievement tests data from Hsinchu middle schools]. *Psychological Testing*, *5*, **336-343.** (In Chinese.)

2441

Tsung, L. T. (1967). [The predictive value of aptitude patterns as applied to guidance and counseling]. *Psychology and Education*, *1*, **37-51.** (In Chinese.)

The concept of aptitude and the predictive value of aptitude patterns were discussed in this paper. To illustrate the importance of studies on aptitudes, the views of several prominent scholars were introduced. The author also discussed the development and application of aptitude tests. The use of the High School Comprehensive Aptitude Test Battery in schools in Taiwan demonstrated the possible contribution of such tests to guidance and counseling programs. The need for more aptitude tests to facilitate the Human Resource Actualization Policy was stressed.

2442

Tsung, L. T., & Chiou, W. C. (1962). [A brief report on some tests for secondary school students sponsored by the Ministry of Education]. *Psychological Testing*, *9*, **628-637.** (In Chinese.)

2443

Tuan, H. F., Chao, L. J., & Tsao, J. C. (1964). [Studies on the methods of memorization used by junior middle school pupils: II. Methods for memorizing short classical prose]. *Acta Psychologica Sinica*, **No. 4, 340-351.** (In Chinese.)

A short classical prose, which consisted of 40 sentences was memorized by 63 junior middle school girls. The various methods of memorization used by the pupils were: (1) memorizing sentence by sentence; (2) memorizing sentence by sentence in consecutive order; (3) memorizing by parts of roughly equal number of sentences, (4) memorizing by parts divided according to the content; (5) memorizing with the aid of an outline; (6) memorizing by first analyzing the content and the structure of the prose. The last method was the most effective followed by the fifth method; the first was the least effective method. It seemed that the subjects who used the first three methods mastered the material part by part cumulatively and those using the other three methods first made a framework and then laid out the details step by step. It was suggested that chunking, association with former experiences and outline making were involved, as sub-processes, in memorizing classical prose.

2444

Tuan, H. F., & Tsao, J. C. (1965). [Studies on the methods of memorization used by junior middle school pupils: Vol. 3. Methods and courses of memorizing classical and modern prose]. *Acta Psychologica Sinica*, **No. 1, 10-27.** (In Chinese.)

One classical and one modern piece of prose were memorized each by 30 junior middle school girl pupils. The prose was presented first for 4 minutes and read aloud twice by the experimenter, and then presented sentence by sentence 10 times with each sentence lasting 3 seconds on average. After each presentation the subject wrote down what she remembered. The results showed that the methods used by subjects for memorizing classical prose were the same as in a former study. The analysis of successive dictations by subjects confirmed that the subjects' courses of mastery of the material could be classified into two types: cumulative and schematic. Subjects of the former type mastered the material part by part cumulatively. They could remember the exact order of the sentences of the prose. Subjects of the latter type first made a framework and then laid out the details step by step.

2445

Tze, Y. Y. (1965). [Mathematical thinking in primary school children]. *Acta Psychologica Sinica*, **No. 1, 38-49.** (In Chinese.)

2446

Vernon, P. E. (1982). *The abilities and achievements of Orientals in North America*. **New York: Academic Press.**

2447

Walker, B. M. (1976). Ideological underpinnings of education: China and the West. *Australian & New Zealand Journal of Sociology, 12,* **101-105.**

A consideration of the Chinese educational system allows us to recognize more clearly the ideology that is implicit in our own system. Notions such as the importance of individuality, intelligence, and academic achievement can be identified for what they are: values derived from our cultural tradition, not values in any absolute sense. That they are not necessarily intrinsically "good" or "right" can be seen by comparison of our educational system (and the place of our values therein) with that of the People's Republic of China.

2448

Wang, F. K. (1955). [A comparative study of the reading of literary and vernacular Chinese]. *Psychological Testing, 3,* **150-155.** (In Chinese.)

2449

Wang, J. J. (1978). [The effects of perceptual isolation on reading performance for field-independents and field-dependents]. *Research in Education & Psychology, 2,* **239-241.** (In Chinese.)

2450

Wang, P., Du, W. X. et al. (1980). [An investigation of English learning in children]. *Acta Psychologica Sinica, 12,* **272-279.** (In Chinese.)

2451

Wang, Q. et al. (1986). [Factor analysis of aptitudes for mathematics in primary schoolchildren]. *Information on Psychological Sciences,* **No. 2, 9-15.** (In Chinese.)

2452

Wang, S. S. (1984). [A study of the effects of cross-district placement and its related problems in elementary and junior-high schools]. *Bulletin of Educational Psychology, 17,* **151-176.** (In Chinese.)

The purposes of this study were to investigate the effects of cross-district schooling on the behavior of students in elementary and junior high schools. The relationships between school environments and the performance of students were also studied. The subjects included 863 third-grade students from seven junior high schools. They were classified into the District-Crossing (DC) Group and the Non-district-Crossing (NDC) Group. Six self-devised questionnaires measuring students' experience about school life learning behavior, achievement motivation, self-confidence, social anxiety, and interpersonal relationships, and a basic data inventory to collect information on social-economic status were given to subjects. The intelligence test score at the time of entrance to junior high school was used as an index of intelligence. The total scores of the simulated joint-entrance examinations for senior high school were used as an index of academic achievement. The data were analyzed by analysis of covariance, Pearson product-moment correlation, multiple-stepwise regression analysis, and canonical correlation analysis. The findings were: (1) Students of the DC group showed no superiority in academic achievement, learning behavior, self-confidence, social anxiety, and interpersonal relationships. (2) The achievement motivation of the DC group was inferior to that of the NDC group. (3) School environments explained 11.7% of the total variance of the academic achievement of students. School prestige explained only 0.64%.

2453

Wang, W. S. (1960). [A preliminary study of the age of school enrollment]. *Acta Psychologica Sinica,* **No. 3, 162-170.** (In Chinese.)

After one year's experimental study of the age of school enrollment, the author drew the following conclusions: (1) If children enter school at the age of six, their achievement may be lower than the seven-year-old ones at the beginning, but the difference would gradually diminish. (2) Early school enrollment does no harm to the children's health. First grade instruction may beneficially influence the mental development of six-year-old children. (3) Most of the content of teaching is too simple for the children. (4) Children can enter school at age of six. (5) The content of teaching for seven-year-old children must be promoted, and the organization of teaching materials, especially the teaching method, must be reformed.

2454

Wei, H. Z. (1981). [A research on verbal language memory and finger language memory of the deaf and mute children]. *Acta Psychologica Sinica, 13,* **53-57.** (In Chinese.)

2455

Wong, A. T. (1979). A study of the relationship between the proficiency in English and cultural background of Chinese immigrant students and their educational and social development. *Dissertation Abstracts International, 39,* **A3988-3989.**

2456

Wong, M. J. (1983). The roles of attitude and motivation in second language acquisition among adolescent native Chinese speakers in the United States. *Dissertation Abstracts International, 43,* **A3833.**

2457

Wong, P. C. (1982). Relationship of two field-dependent-independent measures to reading and math achievement of Anglo-American, first-generation Chinese- and Mexican-American elementary school children. *Dissertation Abstracts International, 43,* **A1461.**

2458

Wong, S. L. (1966). [Problems of teaching sociology in Hong Kong]. *Kolner Zeitschrift Fur Soziologie Und Sozialpsychologie, 18,* **753-762.** (In other language.)

2459

Woodson, M. I. (1974). Seven aspects of teaching concepts. *Journal of Educational Psychology, 66,* **184-188.**

7 steps (defining, identifying relevant attributes, identifying irrelevant attributes, listing exemplars, listing nonexemplars, describing the domain of the concept, and using analogies) in the instruction of concepts were isolated, and their relative effectiveness examined by using each to teach verbal concepts (e.g., the "meaning" of Chinese characters) to 14 undergraduates. Ss learned 7 concepts at once in a within-S design. Instructions involving the definition or identification of the relevant attributes were the most effective in terms of errors. Several kinds of generalization errors were isolated, and these were associated with different instructional steps.

2460

Wu, C. S. (1984). [The effects of sex, attitude of discipline and educational background of the junior high school classroom-teachers upon the life adjustment of students]. *Journal of Education & Psychology, 7,* **193-194.** (In Chinese.)

2461

Wu, E. C. (1985). [Test anxiety during the academic term]. *Chinese Journal of Mental Health, 2,* **131-140.** (In Chinese.)

This study examined test anxiety during the school term. Three repetitions of measurements of test anxiety were arranged in each of 12 junior high schools. The timing of the 1st and 3rd measurements was the same for all of the schools, and that of the 2nd measurement was scattered systematically within the term period. The 1st and 3rd measurements were used as covariates. The results showed: (1) The reliability of the tests ranged from .48 to .85. (2) The degree of test anxiety was lower during the first monthly examination than during the 2nd and 3rd monthly examinations. However, the subjective rating by the students was contrariwise. The degree of test anxiety was higher a week before taking a monthly examination than it was a day before taking a monthly examination. Again, the subjective rating of the student was contrariwise. (3) Situations that easily elicit test anxiety, physiological reactions, as well as the behavioral pattern of the anxious state were found to be similar to those reported in a previous study.

2462

Wu, J. S. (1984). Predictors of job satisfaction among elementary school teachers in southern Taiwan, the Republic of China. *Dissertation Abstracts International, 45,* **A721-722.**

2463

Wu, L. C. (1986). [The effects of rational-emotive education on rational thinking, emotional stability and self-esteem of junior high school students]. *Bulletin of Educational Psychology, 19,* **177-218.** (In Chinese.)

The author developed a rational-emotive education (REE) program for junior high school students and investigated its effects on students' rational thinking, emotional stability, and self-esteem. The subjects consisted of 380 eighth graders. In a period of 6 weeks, the experimental group received the REE, while the control group received a general mental health program. Both had ten 50-minute sessions. All subjects were pre- and posttested with the Rational Belief Test (RBT), the Personal Belief Scale (PBS), the Emotional Stability Scale (ESS) and the Self Attitude Scale (SAS). The results were: (1) The REE program increased students' rational thinking, as measured by the content acquisition and irrational ideas scales. (2) The REE program promoted students' emotional stability. (3) There was no significant effect on self-esteem. (4) There were no sex differences. (5) The effects of on rational ideas and emotional stability were more salient for the higher intelligence group than for the lower intelligence group.

2464

Wu, T. H. (1984). [Grade, sex, intelligence, achievement, risk taking, and test-taking skills]. *Bulletin of Educational Psychology, 17,* **121-130.** (In Chinese.)

The purpose of this study was to investigate relations among grade, sex, intelligence, achievement, and risk taking and test-taking skills. The subjects were 279 4th-, 5th-, and 6th-grade elementary school students (147 males and 132 females) and 310 junior high school students (150 males and 160 females). The results were: (1) Intelligence had no relationship with risk taking, but a significant positive correlation with test-taking skills. (2) There was a negative correlation between achievement and risk taking. (3) There was evidence that the higher the grade, the higher the average risk-taking score. Trend analysis indicated the presence of a cubic relationship. (4) There was also a significant relationship between grade and some test-taking skills. (5) No relationship existed between sex and risk taking and test-taking skills.

2465

Wu, T. H. (1985). [Experiment study on junior high students' test wiseness and risk taking]. *Bulletin of Educational Psychology, 18,* **85-96.** (In Chinese.)

2466

Wu, T. H., & Slakter, M. J. (1978). Risk taking and test wiseness of Chinese students by grade level and residence area. *Journal of Educational Research, 71,* **167-170.**

183 Chinese students in Grades 5, 8, and 11 from urban schools and 153 students from rural schools took risk-taking and test-wiseness (TW) tests (Standard Educational Intelligence Test). The reliabilities of the risk measure ranged from .46 to .87 and were of approximately the same magnitudes as those reported for comparable American samples. The Grade by Residence interaction and the simple effects of grade were significant. The residence simple effects only related to risk taking for Grade 8 Chinese and American Ss had the same mean risk score but in the opposite direction. An interaction was found for the Grade by Residence multivariate ANOVA. Additional multivariate simple effect tests indicated there were relationships between grade and TW, and residence (Grades 8 and 11 only) and TW. Chinese students were consistently lower on mean TW than their American counterparts.

2467

Wu, W. T. (1975). Children's sex, locus of control, and academic achievement. *Bulletin of Educational Psychology, 8,* **107-114.**

Studied the relation between locus of control (Intellectual Achievement Responsibility Questionnaire) and academic achievement (average grade in 4 school subjects) in 4th-6th-graders (164 boys and 155 girls). Results indicate that girls relied more on internal factors as explanations for academic failure than boys. Degree of internal control was significantly correlated with school achievement in boys only.

2468

Wu, W. T. (1976). Classroom climates in Chinese and American elementary schools: A cross-cultural study. *Psychological Testing, 23,* **82-94.**

The purposes of this study were: (1) to investigate relationships between selected pupil characteristics and classroom climates within the Chinese cultural setting; (2) to compare the classroom climate in Chinese and American cultures; and (3) to explore the cross-cultural validity of the Barclay Classroom Climate Inventory (BCCI). The BCCI was administered to children in grades 3 to 6 in Taiwan and Indiana. The results showed that: (1) There were complex and meaningful relationships between individual pupil's characteristics and classroom climate indices. (2) The similarities and/or differences between Chinese and American classroom climates were fairly consistent with the respective similar and/or differential cultural transmissions. (3) The BCCI proved to be as effective in the Chinese as in the American cultural context. It appears that Barclay's multiple social interaction model and his multisource-multitrait inventory is appropriate for cross-cultural studies.

2469

Wu, W. T. (1979). [Factor analysis and follow-up study of elementary classroom climates as assessed by the Barclay Classroom Climate Inventory]. *Bulletin of Educational Psychology, 12,* **133-156.** (In Chinese.)

To study the Chinese classroom climate and its stability and variability, the Chinese version of the Barclay Classroom Climate Inventory (BCCI) was administered to 224 boys and 214 girls in Grades 3 to 6 from two elementary schools. Using the multimethod factor analysis procedure, factors for boys and girls were derived separately. The third graders were followed until the sixth grade and were then reassessed with the BCCI. The stability and the significance of mean differences over three years were tested by simple correlational analysis and the t test. Finally, using BCCI factors as predictors and achievement in the sixth grade as the criterion, a multiple regression analysis was performed. The results were: (1) Eight factors emerged for boys, and seven factors for girls. Five factors were equivalent to six American BCCI factors. (2) The BCCI variables were relatively reliable over three years, especially for the multimethod factors and scales of teacher's ratings and peer nominations. The process of schooling tended to be in favor of boys rather than girls. (3) BCCI factors significantly accounted for the criterion variance. It is claimed that the BCCI has cross-cultural validity, conceptually and empirically.

2470

Wu, W. T., & Chen, H. J. (1978). [Teacher leadership behavior as related to students' expectation, achievement and adjustment]. *Bulletin of Educational Psychology, 11,* **87-104.** (In Chinese.)

The study investigated the relationships between teacher leadership behavior perceived by students and the expectation, achievement, and adjustment of the students. A Teacher Leadership Behavior Questionnaire (TLBQ) was designed to assess three types of teacher's behavior, i.e., democracy, authoritarian, and laissez-faire. The TLBQ, along with five adjustment tests, were administered to 13 classes of a junior high school; the subjects consisted of 223 boys and 485 girls. The prominent findings are as follows: (1) Democratic leadership was in general in accordance with students' expectation, while authoritarians produced the greatest "expectation distance". (2) Teacher's democratic behavior correlated positively with the students' academic achievement, their beliefs in internal control, their achievement motivation, and personal and social adjustment, while teacher's authoritative behavior correlated negatively with those variables, except academic achievement. Teacher's laissez-faire behavior also correlated negatively with the students' academic achievement, beliefs in internal control, achievement motivation, and personal and social adjustment. (3) The greater the students' "expectation distance" to teacher leadership behavior was, the poorer was the students' academic achievement, beliefs in internal control, achievement motivation, and personal and social adjustment. (4) Boys differed from girls in many aspects. It can be concluded that how students perceive and expect teacher leadership behavior is significantly related to their behavior in school.

2471

Wu, W. T., & Lin, C. S. (1982). [Family contacts with the school as related to pupils' achievement and adjustment]. *Bulletin of Educational Psychology, 15,* **127-137.** (In Chinese.)

Recorded contacts with schools by families of 86 pupils from 2 classes in Grade 5 in Hualien, Taiwan, for 2 semesters. Ss completed a battery of tests, including the Pupil Academic Achievement Test, the Learning Attitude Inventory, and the Achievement Motivation Questionnaire. Correlational analysis and a 1-way analysis of covariance with intelligence as covariate showed that (1) there were significant positive correlations between family contacts and Ss' academic achievement, learning attitudes, achievement motivation, effort, attitudes toward school, competency, and personality adjustment; and (2) as the intelligence variable was controlled, the higher contact group was superior in the aforementioned variables to the group whose parents had less contact with schools.

2472

Wu, W. T., & Lin, C. S. (1985). [The effects of increasing teacher-parent contacts on children's learning and home climates]. *Bulletin of Educational Psychology, 18,* **97-116.** (In Chinese.)

A two-semester experimental study was conducted on the effects of increasing teacher-parent contacts on pupils' learning and home climates. The subjects were 84 Grade 6 pupils in Taiwan. They were randomly divided into two classes, with pupils in one group receiving about twice as many teacher-parent interactions than those in the other group. A battery of tests was administered to the subjects before and after the experiment. The results showed that, for both sexes, significant group differences were found on 8 of the 14 dependent variables. Increasing contacts with families by teachers resulted in improving the pupils' academic achievement, achievement motivation, attitude toward school, parents' attitude toward education, learning environment at home, verbal interaction at home, and parenting style.

2473

Wu, Y. L., & Li, Z. M. (1966). [An analysis of the aims and purpose of children's study]. *Acta Psychologica Sinica,* **No. 2, 137-145.** (In Chinese.)

2474

Yang, C. J. (1971). Use of the Basic Physical Fitness Test in the Republic of China. *Psychological Testing, 18,* **895-915.**

2475

Yang, C. Y. (1978). The predictive validity of the Scholastic Aptitude Test for Chinese college students. *Dissertation Abstracts International, 39,* **A3538.**

2476

Yang, K. S. (1982). [Causal attributions of academic success and failure and their affective consequences]. *Acta Psychologica Taiwanica, 24,* **65-83.** (In Chinese.)

More than 400 Chinese university students were used as subjects to study the effects of effort and ability attributions of academic success and failure on various positive and negative affects. Forty-eight hypothetical situations of academic success and failure were described and the subjects were required to indicate the attributional and affective responses they would make when placed in the same situations. The major findings were: (1) Although the tendency to attribute academic success to effort was approximately equal to that to ability, the tendency to attribute failure to lack of ability was significantly weaker than that to lack of effort. (2) Effort attributions of success were more or equally productive of morally neutral, positive affects; ability attributions of success were more productive of morally nonneutral, positive affects. (3) Ability attributions of failure were more or equally productive of morally neutral, negative affects; effort attributions were more productive of morally nonneutral, negative affects. (4) The relative effects of effort and ability attributions on all positive affects were different under high and moderate ability assumptions. (5) The relative effects of effort and ability attributions on negative affects, except unhappiness and anxiety, were similar under high and moderate ability assumptions, and no assumption regarding ability. The implications of cross-cultural differences were discussed.

2477

Yang, K. S., & Ou, J. N. (1979). [Psychological reactions to success and failure of junior high school students with different types of problem behavior]. *Acta Psychologica Taiwanica, 21,* **49-59.** (In Chinese.)

Administered a list of 130 problem behaviors to 2,590 male students chosen by stratified cluster sampling from 46 junior high schools in Taipei, Taiwan. Five groups of approximately 30 Ss each were then selected: (a) neurotic behavior (NB); (b) delinquent behavior; (c) learning-difficulty behaviors (LDB); and (d) students with all 3 types of behavior. A control group was also selected. A 5 * 2 factorial design was used to evaluate success and failure conditions to which Ss in each group were randomly assigned. Findings indicate that Ss in all 5 groups displayed more significant differences in the failure condition--LDB Ss showed a significant drop in aspiration level and a tendency to become depressed. However, these Ss showed no change in self-confidence due to failure. NB Ss experienced lower self-confidence, although their aspiration level remained stable during the failure condition. Implications for student guidance and counseling are noted.

2478

Yang, S. H. (1983). A content analysis of elementary school grammar readers in the People's Republic of China and Hong Kong. *Dissertation Abstracts International, 43,* **A2299.**

2479

Yao, E. S. (1971). The efficacy of child development and family life courses for Chinese students in different types of high schools in the Republic of China. *Dissertation Abstracts International, 32,* **A3013-3014.**

2480

Yau, S. H. (1954). [A comparative study of hearing and reading abilities in comprehension]. *Psychological Testing, 2,* **122-134.** (In Chinese.)

2481

Yee, A. H. (1973). Schools and progress in the People's Republic of China. *Educational Researcher, 2,* **5-15.**

Presents descriptions of the methods, types of schools, rationale, facilities, and programs in the educational system of the People's Republic of China, based on the author's 1972 visit. Comparisons between the author's experience in 1947-1948, the present cultural and political contexts of education, and the influence of the collective spirit on education are discussed.

2482

Yee, A. H. (1973). Relating knowledge and application in China. *Educational Psychologist, 10,* **87-89.**

Reports on the activities of educational psychologists in the People's Republic of China. Based on Mao Tsetung's belief that knowledge is meaningless without application, emphasis is placed on solving practical educational problems. Recent developments in promoting Sino-American exchange are also discussed.

2483

Yeh, E. K., Chu, H. M., Klein, M. H., Alexander, A. A., & Miller, M. H. (1979). Psychiatric implications of cross-cultural education: Chinese students in the U.S.A. *Acta Psychologica Taiwanica, 21,* **1-26.**

Discusses the problems encountered by Chinese students in the US through 10 case studies. Traits that are characteristic of these students are noted, including paranoia and depression, personality problems, role conflict, lack of self-confidence, and difficulty in cross-cultural adaptation. Implications for identifying the high-risk student are mentioned.

2484

Yuen, R. K., & Tinsley, H. E. (1981). International and American students' expectancies about counseling. *Journal of Counseling Psychology, 28,* **66-69.**

Investigated whether students from different backgrounds differ in their expectancies about counseling on a university campus. Ss included 40 American, 39 Chinese, 35 African, and 36 Iranian freshmen and seniors who completed a questionnaire measuring college students' expectancies about counseling. Significant differences among the 4 nationality groups were observed on 12 of the 17 expectancy scales. It was found that American Ss expected the counselor to be less directive and protective and expected themselves to be more responsible for improvement. In contrast, the Chinese, Iranian, and African Ss expected to assume a more passive role and expected that the counselor would be a more directive and nurturing authority figure.

2485

Zhang, B. Y. (1982). [The effects of field dependence on programmed instruction and normal instruction in learning achievement]. *Acta Psychologica Sinica, 14,* **50-55.** (In Chinese.)

This study explored the effects of field dependence on programmed instruction and normal instruction in learning achievement. The results showed that: (1) For the field independent group, achievement was not obviously different between children given programmed instruction and those given normal instruction. (2) For in the field dependent group, programmed instruction was obviously better than normal instruction when the materials to be learned were difficult.

2486

Zhang, B. Y. (1985). The psychology of reading in China. *School Psychology International, 6,* **30-33.**

The author discussed recent discoveries made by Chinese psychologists about Chinese reading, neuropsychological differences between Chinese and English reading, and strategies for comprehending Chinese sentences. Two methods of teaching Chinese characters (concentration and dispersion recognition) were also discussed.

2487

Zhang, J. L. (1984). [The comparative study of utilization of models for education]. *Acta Psychologica Sinica, 16,* **27-33.** (In Chinese.)

2488

Zhang, M. L., Liu, J. H., Wang, X. T., He, J. Q., & Chen, S. K. (1983). [A systematic teaching and learning experiment of applying the knowledge of the part-whole relationship with "1" as the underlying basis]. *Acta Psychologica Sinica, 15,* **410-418.** (In Chinese.)

Describes an experiment conducted with 1st graders at a Chinese experimental school to evaluate an arithmetic textbook's effect on Ss' learning of part-whole relationships. Results show that Ss in the experimental class, which used the concept of "one" as underlying the part-whole relationship, learned more and showed a higher learning transition than controls. Implications for the teaching and learning of arithmetic in primary schools are discussed.

2489

Zhang, N. S. (1980). [Characteristics of verbal learning of the deaf children in educational practice]. *Acta Psychologica Sinica, 12,* **390-396.** (In Chinese.)

2490

Zhen Zu. (1982). Preschool education in China. *Early Child Development & Care, 8,* **273-277.**

Describes an experimental preschool education program in China that is based on the premise that the environment exerts the greatest influence on a child's intelligence before the age of 5 yrs. The aim of the program is to develop children's observational, judgmental, and reasoning abilities. The program widens the scope of preschool education to include playing games, observing the environment, and participating in self-service physical labor, as well as studying traditional lessons. Teachers help children master knowledge, store meanings, and form skills through the use of images.

2491

Zhong, M. L. et al. (1983). [Children's concept formation of numbers under 100]. *Information on Psychological Sciences,* **No. 3, 28-34.** (In Chinese.)

The following references are also relevant to this chapter:

21, 139, 163, 202, 203, 219, 284, 287, 301, 539, 590, 638, 639, 678, 733, 763, 833, 834, 892, 914, 941, 946, 1000, 1064, 1130, 1165, 1166, 1199, 1257, 1287, 1300, 1324, 1354, 1367, 1454, 1492, 1521, 1555, 1628, 1783, 1810, 1889, 2044, 2086, 2711, 2729, 2732, 2736, 2740, 2759, 2801.

APPLIED PSYCHOLOGY 11

Frequency data on citations in this chapter, in terms of content classification subcategories, are presented in Table 10.

Table 10: *Number of Citations by Content Classification, Language, and Geographical Area*

Content classification	Total	CL	EL	OL	PRC	T	HK	US
Applied psychology	18	15	3	0	10	4	1	0
Occupational attitudes, interests, and guidance	19	11	8	0	2	12	1	0
Organizational behavior and job satisfaction	15	8	7	0	1	7	1	0
Personnel selection and training	8	8	0	0	2	6	0	0
Personnel evaluation and performance	12	10	2	0	3	9	0	0
Management and management training	14	2	11	1	5	1	4	1
Marketing and advertising	5	2	3	0	2	1	1	0
Human factors engineering	8	7	1	0	6	2	0	0
Environmental psychology and environmental issues	5	2	3	0	0	2	1	0
Total		104	65	38	1	31	44	91

Note: CL = Chinese language; EL = English language; OL = other languages. PRC = People's Republic of China; T = Taiwan; HK = Hong Kong; US = United States (Chinese Americans--according to the frequency of the subject term Asian Americans).

Subject terms used for indexing citations related to applied psychology are grouped according to geographical area, subject population, and topic. These are presented below, in a descending order of frequency. (The frequency of single-word subject terms includes those of compound terms in which the single word appears. Subjects terms used for indexing citations from other chapters may have been included. Terms with a frequency of less than 10 are not shown.)

Geographical area

51	Taiwan
32	Peoples Republic of China
21	Asia

Subject population

19	adults
11	military personnel
10	students

Topic

33	personnel
23	management
23	psychology
15	cross cultural differences
14	industrial psychology
12	adulthood
11	attitudes
10	satisfaction

Clearly applied psychology in China is underdeveloped. Chinese psychologists have yet to apply psychological knowledge to the solution of practical problems on a scale that would make their presence felt in the society as a whole. In particular, they have done almost no research concerning environmental issues which are bound to force their attention on ourselves and our children with increasing intensity.

The reader's attention is directed to a book on Chinese views on management most recently published (Yang and Tseng, 1988).

REFERENCES

Yang, K. S., & Tseng, S. C. (Eds.). (1988). [*Chinese people's views on management*]. Taipei: Kuei Kuan. (In Chinese.)

2492

Aitken, N. D. (1968). Entrepreneurial potential in underdeveloped countries: A test of major hypotheses. *Dissertation Abstracts International, 28,* **A3828.**

2493

Bennett, M. (1977). Response characteristics of bilingual managers to organisational questionnaires. *Personnel Psychology, 30,* **29-36.**

Examined the effects on response bias of presenting questionnaires in English rather than in the first language of respondents. An organizational questionnaire based on R. Likert's 8 organizational variables was completed by 51 Filipino and 71 Hong Kong Chinese bilingual managers who had participated in a management development program. Each group was subjected to conditions designed to induce either an English response set or a Chinese or Filipino response set. For 2 of the 8 variables, communication processes and interaction-influence processes, significant differences between samples were found. Apparently equivalent questions generated negative responses in the English response conditions and positive responses in the Filipino and Chinese response conditions. Methodological implications for comparative management research are discussed.

2494

Bennett, M. (1977). Testing management theories cross-culturally. *Journal of Applied Psychology, 62,* **578-581.**

Administered the Least Preferred Co-Worker Scale (LPC) and the Self-Description Inventory (SDI) to 45 Filipino and Hong Kong Chinese managers working for US-based banks. Results show that high performance was associated with low LPC scores in the Filipino sample and high LPC scores in the Hong Kong sample. Three SDI scales (Self-Assurance, Intelligence, Self-Actualization) were related to high performance in both samples, whereas 2 scales (Working Class Affinity, Maturity) were related to low performance in the Filipino sample and high performance in the Hong Kong sample. An attempt is made to integrate the results in light of known cultural norms.

2495

Bennett, M., & Tiy, F. H. (1976). Psychosocial homeostasis and vocational interest. *Psychologia: An International Journal of Psychology in the Orient, 19,* **35-39.**

Administered the Pacific Vocational Interest Analysis to 177 Chinese 5th formers (11th yr of education) on Hong kong, 89 Chinese 5th formers on Fiji, 170 5th formers of Melanesian origin on Fiji, 212 5th formers of Indian origin on Fiji, and 119 5th formers of Melanesian origin on New Hebrides. Results indicate that occupational values were the same between Chinese groups, but different between all the other groups, thus giving some support to F. Hsu's concept of "psychosocial homeostasis".

2496

Birnbaum, P. H., & Wong, G. Y. (1985). Organizational structure of multinational banks in Hong Kong from culture-free perspective. *Administrative Science Quarterly, 30,* **262-277.**

The culture-free and culture-bound hypotheses used to explain organizational structures were examined by surveying 93 Chinese managerial employees from 20 multinational banks in Hong Kong. The data were obtained from interviews with senior headquarters executives, subjects' responses to the Job Descriptive Index and a demographic questionnaire, and evaluations of subjects' jobs by their supervisors. Work satisfaction was examined with relation to organizational structure (centralization, vertical and horizontal differentiation, and formalization), while controlling for job structure (significance, feedback, variety, identity, and autonomy of the job), and individual attributes (sex, age, tenure, education, and cosmopolitanism). The culture-free hypothesis was supported, except for the managers' preference for centralized decision making.

2497

Chang, S. S., & Lu, C. Y. (1969). [A report on the revision of the Strong Vocational Interest Blank]. *Acta Psychologica Taiwanica, 11,* **1-12.** (In Chinese.)

2498

Chang, W. L. (1975). Primary groups and punishment-based control in an organization: An exploratory study. *Kansas Journal of Sociology, 11,* **29-40.**

Tested the conventional theory that primary groups among the dissatisfied participants in an organization tend to decrease the compliance of the participants. A study of 58 draftees serving in a Nationalist Chinese Air Police company was conducted, using questionnaires and interviews. It was found that primary groups among the dissatisfied actually increased compliance. Possible explanations of the conflicting findings are discussed.

2499

Chen, B. S. (1982). [The contingency model of leadership effectiveness: The empirical study of the meaning of LPC Score and of the validity of model]. *Acta Psychologica Taiwanica, 24,* **111-120.** (In Chinese.)

In this study we studied the meaning of LPC score and then examined the validity of Fiedler's model of leadership effectiveness. To investigate the relationship between LPC scores and judgmental reaction to task success and failure 202 platoon leader and 144 company commanders were used as subjects. It was found that low-LPC persons were more favorable in their attitudes toward the leader behavior, the job, and the group when they (the leaders) were successful on the task than when they were unsuccessful. For high-LPC persons, attitudes of this type were not correlated with task success. These results tended to support Fiedler's concept that low-LPC persons are task-oriented. To examine the validity of the contingency model 13 high performance and 131 low performance company commanders were tested. The results of computing the correlations between LPC scores and task performance in three different control situations (rigid, moderate, and mild control) partially supported the model. Only one correlation coefficient in the rigid control situation (octant I) was negatively significant. The implications of these findings to the leadership research, leadership training, and job satisfaction are discussed.

2500

Chen, L. (1979). [Engineering psychology in marching to the four modernizations]. *Acta Psychologica Sinica, 11,* **144-147.** (In Chinese.)

Summarizes Chinese psychological investigations in the fields of operational rationalization, technological design, and enterprise management from the time of the "Taylor system". It is emphasized that, with the progress of automation, the human role in the automatic system becomes increasingly evident. Human factors in the human-machine system are considered to be decisive.

2501

Chen, S. M. (1985). [A study on multiple aptitude, occupational preference and adjustment between field independents and field dependents]. *Bulletin of Educational Psychology, 18,* **149-168.** (In Chinese.)

This study investigated the relationship between field dependence and multiple aptitude, occupational preference and adjustment. Subjects were 90 field independents and 90 field dependents from one junior high school. A battery of tests was administered to the subjects. The main findings were: (1) There was a relationship between field dependence and multiple aptitude; the field independents showed significantly higher numeral reasoning, perceptual speed and spatial ability than the field dependents. (2) There was a relationship between field dependence and some variables of occupational preference; the field independents had more mechanical and aesthetic preferences. (3) There were no significant differences between the two groups in their personal and social adjustment. (4) There was no significant influence of multiple aptitude on occupational preference and personal and social adjustment.

2502

Cheng, B. S., & Yang, K. S. (1977). [Supervisory behavior, skill level, and interpersonal dominance as determinants of job satisfaction]. *Bulletin of the Institute of Ethnology* **(Academia Sinica), No. 44, 13-45.** (In Chinese.)

The Chinese versions of Fleishman's Supervisory Behavior Description, California Personality Inventory (CPI) Dominance Scale, and Smith's Job Description Index were group-administered to 167 semi-skilled and 58 unskilled factory workers from a big plastic-products manufacturing company in the suburban area of Taipei. The major findings were: (1) The two dimensions of supervisory behavior, consideration and initiating structure, were positively related to the workers' overall job satisfaction. (2) Consideration and skill level had an interactive effect on the workers' satisfaction with respect to work. (3) Initiating structure had a positive relationship with, and skill level and dominance had an interactive effect on, the workers' satisfaction with respect to salary. (4) Skill level and dimensions of supervisory behavior had an interactive effect on the workers' satisfaction with respect to promotion. (5) Consideration was positively related to the workers' satisfaction with respect to coworkers.

2503

Cheng, F. M. (1955). [A study of the mechanical aptitude of workshop trainees]. *Psychological Testing, 3,* **175-184.** (In Chinese.)

2504

Cheng, F. M. (1958). [Measurement of morale]. *Psychological Testing, 6,* **408-417.** (In Chinese.)

2505

Cheng, F. M. (1967). [Revision of Brainard Occupational Preference Inventory]. *Psychological Testing, 14,* **335-345.** (In Chinese.)

2506

Cheng, F. Y., & Yang, Y. W. (1953). [The application of vocational tests in the fifth plant fertilizer company]. *Psychological Testing, 1,* **32-35.** (In Chinese.)

2507

Cheng, P. S., & Chung, C. J. (1981). [A factorial study of the effective leader behavior of low military staff]. *Acta Psychologica Taiwanica, 23,* **97-106.** (In Chinese.)

This study investigated the factor structure of the Chinese revised Subordinate Behavior Description Questionnaire (SBDQ) and assessed relations among subordinates' perception of leader behaviors, leader performance, and leaders' job position. The revised SBDQ was administered to 580 enlisted men who were asked to describe their leaders' behaviors. A factor analysis yielded three factors which accounted for most of the response variance. Two of the factors, named Consideration and Initiative, were the same as those obtained from previous studies, whilst the third factor, named Unselfishness, was new. The results of an ANOVA indicated that Consideration and Unselfishness were positively related to leader performance, whilst Initiative was related to leaders' job position.

2508

Chi, W. H. (1981). [An investigation and prediction of automobile-driver behavior: Relations between anxiety, venturesome, internal-external control, and driver's behavior]. *Journal of Education & Psychology, 3,* **59-81.** (In Chinese.)

This study explored differences in anxiety, riskiness, and locus of control among different kinds and ages of drivers. There were 1,692 subjects, including 179 bus drivers, 755 taxi drivers, 500 drivers who had violated traffic laws, and 258 excellent drivers, who were tested over a period of one and half years. The results were: (1) The riskiness of the excellent drivers was lower than that of the drivers who had violated traffic laws and taxi drivers. (2) The riskiness of drivers aged 41-50 years was lower than that of drivers under 40. (3) There were no differences in anxiety and locus of control among different kinds of drivers and among drivers of different ages.

2509

Chou, S. K., & Chen, H. P. (1936). [The rise of industrial psychology in China]. *Chinese Journal of Psychology, 1,* **140-166.** (In Chinese.)

2510

Chu, P. H. (1975). Cross-cultural study of vocational interests measured by the Strong-Campbell Interest Inventory. *Acta Psychologica Taiwanica, 17,* **69-84.**

This study compared the vocational interests of Chinese and American college students. The Strong-Campbell Interest Inventory (SCII) was administered to 2,178 American and 1,360 Chinese college students to collect data on the standardization of the measure for Chinese subjects. The results showed that: (a) Among females, there were 108 out of 325 items which differentiated between the "Likes" of Americans and Chinese by 15% or more, and among the two male groups, 84 items carried 15% or more response differences; (b) the responses of American females to the SCII were statistically different from those of Chinese females on 255 items, and between the two male groups differences with statistical significance were found on 262 items; (c) differences between American and Chinese subjects indicated that a cultural factor plays an important role in influencing vocational interests.

2511

Chu, T. H. (1961). [Some psychological problems concerning the socialistic competition in industry]. *Acta Psychologica Sinica,* **No. 4, 245-258.** (In Chinese.)

The present study of problems concerning socialistic competition in industry attempted to determine the role played by the production target in socialistic competition. Three problems were discussed: (1) The more definite and more concrete is the way of putting forward the production target, the more marked is its effect on production. (2) The effects of the comparative method of competition in the production process depend to a certain extent upon the degree of similarity of the conditions compared. The more similar are the conditions of comparison, the more marked are the effects of the comparison. (3) The effect of high production targets is different from that of low ones. The targets will have no influence upon production if they are either too high or too low. Advanced and practicable targets exercise bigger influence upon production.

2512

Chuang, C. J. (1979). [Effect of brand preference upon consumers' perceived taste of ice-cream]. *Acta Psychologica Taiwanica, 21,* **99-104.** (In Chinese.)

2513

Chuang, C. J., & Cheng, B. S. (1984). [The psychological meaning of Chinese typographies and its applications to commercial advertisement]. *Chinese Journal of Psychology, 26,* **49-55.** (In Chinese.)

This study explored the psychological meanings of eight Chinese typographies by using forty adjectives on a semantic differential scale. Four factors were derived from a factor analysis, which could explain most of the variances. These four factors were named: Attractiveness (A), Persuasiveness (P), Softness (S), and Elegance (E). The results indicated a significant main effect of typographies, and there were significant main effects on A, P, and S, but no significant effects were found on E. The implications of these findings for commercial advertisements were discussed.

2514

Division of Industrial Psychology, Institute of Psychology, Academica Sinica. (1959). [Some experiences in attempt at promotion of invention and creation]. *Acta Psychologica Sinica,* **No. 1, 36-41.** (In Chinese.)

The present paper is a preliminary attempt to investigate psychological principles in the development of creative thinking in workers. The workers of Hua Tung Switch Factory used a technique of concentrated attacks on a problem, and succeeded in creating 140 sets of automatic and semi-automatic dies. This greatly increased the efficiency of work production. Three conditions must be met to promote invention and creation: (1) the analysis of contradictions and the formulation of problems, (2) the use of a "prototype" to stimulate the solution of contradictions, and (3) the advantageous exploration of the chain-reactive nature of creation and invention. In this paper, actions against obstacles to invention and creation were also proposed. The experiences obtained from Hua Tung Switch Factory also indicate an inventive and creative work can be effected by collective efforts, conceived plans and concentrated attacks.

2515

Division of Industrial Psychology, Institute of Psychology, Academica Sinica. (1959). [Creative thinking as observed in constructing automatic punching and die machinery]. *Acta Psychologica Sinica*, **No. 2, 109-116.** (In Chinese.)

To solve the "bottleneck" problems of production, a shop nuclear sub-group was organized in a factory. This sub-group provided the workers with some oral and written provocative materials, and prototypes such as diagrams and photographs. The workers invented ten sets of automatic and semi-automatic punching and die machinery, thus laying down the foundation for the solution of the "bottleneck" problems. Discussion with the workers and observations of the processes of their creative thinking activities indicated: (1) Creation of new machines was accomplished through a mass movement with well-planned and concentrated efforts of attack. (2) Verbal presentation of problems and prototypes relative to the machinery powerfully provoked and promoted creative thinking of the workers. (3) Creative thinking finds its origin in the necessity of social production. It is produced and developed in the course of practical activities and is the reflective process of objective laws.

2516

Division of Industrial Psychology, Institute of Psychology, Academica Sinica. |1960). [A study of the creative process of technical innovation in machine work]. *Acta Psychologica Sinica*, No. 3, **182-195.** (In Chinese.)

The process of creative thinking of innovators was studied by summarizing their experiences and by controlled experiments in some machine shops. The results indicated that classification of the problems of innovation into appropriate categories may facilitate the process of problem solving. In the course of new tool construction, one of the most important principles for problem solving is to find out the relations between the centers (or axes) of parts and tools. The knowledge of geometry is necessary for the development of creative thinking for workers. If the object of innovation is complex in structure and the relations between space and time in its operation is complicated, a solid model used as a prototype is useful for the worker's imagination. In the course of creative activity, the innovator's cognition of the relations between the object and the tool to be constructed become more and more complete as the creative work goes on. Only under certain conditions would the prototype show its effective result.

2517

Evans, W. A., & Courtney, A. J. (1985). An analysis of accident data for franchised public buses in Hong Kong. *Accident Analysis & Prevention*, *17*, **355-366.**

An analysis of accidents involving franchised public buses in Hong Kong indicated that the city has a high accident rate compared to Japan, the U.K., and the U.S., with particularly high pedestrian involvement rates. Conclusions regarding the most commonly cited cause of accidents; weekly variations in the accident rate; and the relation of accidents to weather conditions, driver characteristics (age, experience, temperament, attitude, and hours on duty) were presented. The reliability of police-reported accident causation data was questioned.

2518

Evans, W. A., & Sculli, D. (1981). A comparison of managerial traits in Hong Kong and the USA. *Journal of Occupational Psychology*, *54*, **183-186.**

Applied E. E. Ghiselli's (1971) work on managerial talent to Hong Kong. His Self-Description Inventory was administered to 49 managers, 45 workers, and 41 engineers, and the results were compared with those obtained on similar groups in the US. The results were broadly similar and indicate that this inventory is potentially useful in cultures other than the US.

2519

Fong, P. L., & Chang, S. S. (1962). [An analytical study of the mentality of factory workers]. *Psychological Testing*, *9*, **656-665.** (In Chinese.)

2520

Furnham, A., & Muhiudeen, C. (1984). The Protestant work ethic in Britain and Malaysia. *Journal of Social Psychology*, *122*, **157-161.**

36 male and 37 female Malaysians (aged approximately 29-30 yrs old) and a control group of 73 British Ss, matched in terms of education, sex, age, and SES class, completed the Protestant Work Ethic Scale, on which high scores indicate strong beliefs in the Protestant work ethic (PWE) and low scores indicate weak beliefs. Although there was no significant difference in scores between the 3 ethnic groups comprising the Malaysian sample (Malay, Indian, and Chinese), there were large significant differences between the British and Malaysians: The former had less belief in the PWE. There were also significant sex differences--females had higher scores than males--and SES dif-

ferences--working-class Ss had higher scores than middle-class Ss. Results are interpreted in terms of the previous studies of the Protestant work ethic in Asia and the social, cultural, and economic differences between Britain and Malaysia.

2521

Gifford, R., & Peacock, J. (1979). Crowding: More fearsome than crime-provoking? Comparison of an Asian city and a North American city. *Psychologia: An International Journal of Psychology in the Orient, 22,* **79-83.**

To learn whether perceptions of personal danger in urban settings might be more closely related to crime rates or to population density, Toronto (4 times greater crime rate) and Hong Kong (4 times denser) were compared. Former residents were queried on numerous crime and security aspects of their urban experience. 40 Toronto residents reported significantly more personal memories of crime, yet felt significantly safer than did 28 Hong Kong residents. In a present, shared environment, the 2 groups felt equally safe. Results suggest that crowding may be more associated with fears for personal safety than crime rates.

2522

Hashmi, H. (1979). A comparison of brand preference amongst different economic systems. *Pakistan Psychological Studies, 3,* **14-24.**

Tested the hypotheses that (1) consumers avoid after-purchase dissonance by adding value to the purchased brand; and (2) the degree of availability of alternative brands in the market may be positively related to the degree of value added to the preferred brand. 10 Ss from the US, 10 from the People's Republic of China, and 10 from Pakistan were used to represent the free enterprise system, controlled economy, and mixed economy, respectively. Ss were asked to name their preferred and nonpreferred brand of soap and to estimate the size of it. Results indicate that only American Ss perceived a difference between the sizes of the preferred and nonpreferred soaps, supporting the hypotheses.

2523

Ho, C. J. (1947). Vocational guidance in China. *Occupation, 26,* **106-107.**

2524

Ho, D. Y. F., & Liao, J. H. (1969). [A study of Chinese attitudes toward various occupations]. *Journal of Sociology* **(National Taiwan University), No. 5, 151-156.** (In Chinese.)

The aim of this study is to understand the ranking of jobs in current Chinese society, and whether or not it is different from that of the western countries. Data was obtained from personal interviews administered during December 1968. There were 100 subjects, divided into four equal groups - Group A, college male students, Group B, college female students, Group C, under college male, Group D, under college female. Based on the results the following conclusions were drawn: (1) The ranking of jobs by present day Chinese youth who have completed at least secondary education is still affected by the traditional culture and the social values of China. Mental work is ranked higher than physical labour. This is the same as in the West except that the Chinese value education more, so teaching is rated as the most important occupation. (2) Under the influence of traditional culture and moral conception, people do not consider the amount of money earned the most significant matter when considering job importance. They consider the nature and reputation of the job and how much good it could do to the community as more important.

2525

Hofstede, G. (1978). *Organization-related value systems in forty countries.* **Paper presented at the Ninth Congress of Sociology, Uppsala, Sweden, August.**

2526

Hong, J. C. (1984). Job satisfaction of Chinese college graduates working in the United States. *Dissertation Abstracts International, 45,* **B708.**

2527

Hsu, C. K. (1977). [Determinants and correlates of Chinese workers' job satisfaction]. *Bulletin of the Institute of Ethnology^ (Academia Sinica), No. 43, 23-64. (In Chinese.)*

This study is part of a larger project which was carried out in a fiber factory. The present article is an exploratory analysis of the determinants and correlates of job satisfaction of Chinese workers. The scale employed is the Smith et al Job Descriptive Index. After putting the Index through item analysis and several tests (validity, reliability and independence), it was found that the Index is appropriate to administer to Chinese industrial workers. The results indicate that among nine personal factors, four (sex, age, educational level and opinion of family) are moderately related to job satisfaction. It was also found that among eight organizational factors, six (work types, position, company policy, organizational identification, feeling of leisure time, and tendency to leave) are strongly related to job satisfaction.

2528

Hsu, C. W. (1958). [The determination and application of aptitude areas of the Army Aptitude Test Battery]. Psychological Testing 6, *418-423. (In Chinese.)*

2529

Hsu, C. W. (1959). [A follow-up study of the Army Aptitude Test Battery (No. 2)]. Psychological Testing *7, 508-511. (In Chinese.)*

2530

Hsu, L. T. (1960). [Strengthening the collaboration between industrial psychology and industrial physiology for service to production]. Acta Psychologica Sinica, *No. 3, 196-198. (In Chinese.)*

2531

Hsu, L. T. (1960). [The process of planning, regulation and control in productive work]. Acta Psychologica Sinica, *No. 4, 235-243. (In Chinese.)*

2532

Hsu, S. C. (1968). [An analysis of the expenditure patterns of the upper-class pupils of Taipei public primary schools]. National Chengchi University Journal *(Taiwan),* **17,** *243-266. (In Chinese.)*

2533

Huang, K. L., & Kuo, W. H. (1984). [Effects of attribution, achievement motivation, dogmatism and demographic variables upon college graduates' job satisfaction]. Journal of Education & Psychology, *7, 43-61. (In Chinese.)*

This study investigated the effects of attribution, achievement motivation, dogmatism and demographic variables upon 187 college graduates' job satisfaction. The results were: (1) There was a significant negative correlation between job satisfaction and intention to quit. (2) The subjects were more satisfied with their supervisors and coworkers, and least satisfied with their opportunities for promotion. (3) In comparison with female subjects and single subjects, male subjects and married subjects were more satisfied with their opportunities for promotion, but less satisfied with their present pay. (4) The higher the subjects' achievement motivation, the higher their satisfaction with work, but the lower their satisfaction with supervision. (5) Among all predictors, attribution variables seemed to have higher predictive validity for job satisfaction and intention to quit. (6) Subjects who were employed by the government agencies were less satisfied with their work than those employed by other organizations.

2534

Huang, T. H. (1973). The interpretation of and the reasons for occupational choice by the rural youth in Taiwan. Journal of Sociology *(National Taiwan University),* **9,** *51-62.*

2535

Hwang, C. H. (1972). [Applied psychology in Taiwan (1950-1970)]. Psychological Testing, 19, *961-966. (In Chinese.)*

2536

Hwang, C. H., & Lu, H. M. (1966). [The selection of candidates for apprentice training at the Taipei Railway Workshop]. Psychological Testing, 13, *264-267. (In Chinese.)*

2537

Hwang, K. K. (1983). [Business organizational patterns and employees' working morale in Taiwan]. Bulletin of the Institute of Ethnology *(Academia Sinica),* **56,** *145-193. (In Chinese.)*

2538

Jin, S. R. (1986). Holland typology: An empirical study on its factorial structure. Bulletin of Educational Psychology, 19, *219-254.*

The construct validity and appropriateness of Holland's hexagonal model were evaluated. Subjects were 880 students from senior, industrial, and commercial high schools. To assess Holland's six career types an adaptation and Chinese translation of the Self-Directed Search (SDS) was used. Based on the data of reliability, convergent and discriminant validity, and construct validity, the Chinese SDS was found to be an equivalent measure of Holland's typology. In general, the results of factor analyses supported the factorial structure of Holland's hexagonal model. By utilizing the Wakefield and Doughtie's spatial analysis, the psychological resemblances among types confirmed Holland's model. However, the hexagon formed was a bell-shaped one, with R and I in the upper portion and A, S, E, C in the lower portion. This implied that the perception of Chinese high school students could be classified into two primary categories, the natural sciences and the humanistic-social sciences. Males were better than females in differentiating the R and I types, while females were better than males in distinguishing the A-S-E-C types, except for the distance between S and E types.

2539

Jin, Z. C., He, Y. R., Cheng, Z. J., & Wang, D. Y. (1986). [Forecast of degree of preference for commodities by using fuzzy mathematics]. Acta Psychologica Sinica, 18, *43-49. (In Chinese.)*

2540

Koo, C. W. (1957). [Psychological tests and army personnel selection]. Psychological Testing, 5, *350-355. (In Chinese.)*

2541

Koo, C. W. (1978). [A study of leadership attitude in industry]. Psychological Testing, 25, *17-28. (In Chinese.)*

2542

Lamal, P. A. (1984). Contingency management in the People's Republic of China. Behavior Analyst, 7, *121-130.*

The author described the behavioral contingencies that have been implemented in the People's Republic of China's attempts to achieve modernization and increased productivity of industry and a significant decrease in the birthrate. Changes from past practices in the industrial sphere, which involved a shift from noncontingent to contingent consequences, were outlined. The use of a variety of consequences as a means of reducing the birthrate was described.

2543

Laurent, C. R. (1982). An investigation of the family life cycle in a modern Asian society. Journal of the Market Research Society, 24, *140-150.*

Interviewed 1,080 residents of Hong Kong (over 18 yrs of age) to investigate the family life cycle within a Chinese culture and how that information can be used for segmenting consumer markets. In comparison with research on US cultures, results show a degree of similarity in terms of the existing stages, but they exhibit considerable differences in the manner in which the stages relate to one another. Differences were also found regarding the incidence of the working housewife, family size and housing type, and the family's net disposable income.

2544

Lee, H. T. (1957). [Ten years of psychological testing of the Chinese police]. Psychological Testing, 5, *373-374. (In Chinese.)*

2545

Lee, H. T. (1967). [The compilation of the aptitude tests for police officers]. Psychological Testing, 14, *371-376. (In Chinese.)*

2546

Lee, P. W. H., Lam, T. H., & Ong, S. G., & Wang, C. M. (1985). A modified version of the general health questionnaire as a measure of occupational mental health in Hong Kong. Chinese Journal of Psychology, 26, *101-106.*

In a survey on occupational health and work stress of 653 Chinese white collar workers in Hong Kong, the 12-item General Health Questionnaire (GHQ) was used to measure the prevalence of mental health problems. The wording of the response scales was changed from the original anchors comparing present state with what was usual to anchors that would be better understood. Two methods of scoring were also investigated. Analyses of the particular response styles of Hong Kong subjects favored the Likert-type scoring (0-1-2-3) over the original GHQ scoring (0-0-1-1) as a more accurate reflection of the prevalence of mental health problems. The use of the GHQ in the Chinese setting of Hong Kong is discussed.

2547

Leong, F. T. (1985). Career development of Asian Americans. Journal of College Student Personnel, 26, *539-546.*

The author reviewed the literature on locus of control, social anxiety, intolerance of ambiguity, and career development among Asian Americans. The following variables were found to be important and relevant to the career development of this population: segregation of occupational choice and interest, occupational values reflecting these cultures, process of acculturation and assimilation, stereotypes, and personality traits characteristic of this group.

2548

Lii, S. Y., & Chen, G. P. (1984). [The researchers' personality and their perception of organizational climate]. Journal of Education & Psychology, 7, *63-94. (In Chinese.)*

Data on work values, achievement motivation, locus of control and perceived organizational climate from 211 researchers showed that: (1) Male subjects emphasized more on social status of job, and showed higher achievement motivation than female subjects. (2) Married subjects put more emphasis on promotion, perceived their company as higher on structure, risk and support variables than unmarried subjects did. (3) College educated subjects showed higher achievement motivation than high school educated subjects. (4) Senior subjects compared with junior subjects, perceived their company as higher on support, fair reward and identification variables. (5) Higher paid subjects perceived their company as higher on responsibility and identification variables than lower paid subjects did. (6) Internal control subjects, compared with external subjects, tended to have a more positive perception of their company. (7) Subjects' locus of control scores were correlated with their perception of organizational climate.

2549

Lin, K. T., Lin, D. L., & Hwang, K. K. (1978). [A study of the functions of facilities for rest: Based on the attitude of visitors to Shih-tou-san scenery area]. Journal of the Chinese Society for Horticultural Science, 24, *105-120. (In Chinese.)*

2550

Lindsay, C. P., & Dempsey, B. L. (1983). Ten painfully learned lessons about working in China: The insights of two American behavioral scientists. Journal of Applied Behavioral Science, 19, *265-276.*

Describes the difficulties encountered in setting up a management training institute in the People's Republic of China. The institute is described in light of the Chinese structural and social variables that influenced its formation. The authors discuss the uncertainty surrounding goals and contracts in China, the importance of political correctness, the importance of participation, and role expectations.

2551

Lindsay, C. P., & Dempsey, B. L. (1985). Experiences in training Chinese business people to use U.S. management techniques. Journal of Applied Behavioral Science, 21, *65-78.*

A training program developed in China and designed to impart U.S. management techniques to Chinese business managers was discussed. Two hundred subjects, most of whom worked as interpreters and/or employees in import-export firms, took part in the 30-week program. The subjects' actions in behavioral exercises and reactions to Western management theories were described. Explanations of these actions and reactions pointed to a combination of influences on modern Chinese organizational behavior. The roles played by traditional Chinese culture and modern socialist development in fostering behaviors currently practiced in Chinese organizations were examined.

2552

Liu, M. T. (1976). [Forced-choice personality tests in personnel classification]. Psychological Testing, 23, *57-62. (In Chinese.)*

2553

Liu, S. N. (1981). [Chinese sports psychology in the making]. Information on Psychological Sciences, *No. 1, 54-55. (In Chinese.)*

2554

Loo, C. (1986). Neighborhood satisfaction and safety: A study of a low-income ethnic area. Environment & Behavior, 18, *109-131.*

The author surveyed 108 Chinese adults living in San Francisco's Chinatown area to test theories related to neighborhood satisfaction and safety and to address planning and policy questions raised by a proposal for controls on development in this area. Findings supported the urban scale, compositional, quality of local conditions, and urban anonymity perspectives as they apply to neighborhood satisfaction. Results revealed a relationship between high population density/commercial development and lowered levels of neighborhood satisfaction and between increased building density and lesser feelings of safety in one's neighborhood. Most subjects liked at least one aspect of their neighborhood. Increased development would be expected to exacerbate undesirable environmental qualities of the area and potentially destroy the ethnic enclave nature of the community. The margin of affordable error was judged to be small given the: (1) lack of alternatives for this Chinese population; (2) low level of neighborhood satisfaction among Chinatown residents; and (3) greater neighborhood satisfaction experienced by some subjects.

2555

Loo, C., & Ong, P. (1984). Crowding perceptions, attitudes, and consequences among the Chinese. Environment & Behavior, 16, *55-87.*

Examined crowding in San Francisco's Chinatown and the attitudes and perceptions of its residents, using interview data from 108 residents (mean age 46 yrs). The objectives of the study were to test the validity of conjectures prevalent in the literature about the Chinese and crowding, to test the theory that crowding is related to psychological stress and social conflict, and to provide a fuller understanding of the nature of crowding and of density. Findings were contrary to beliefs held about Chinese attitudes toward crowding; Ss evaluated crowding as undesirable and harmful. Personal effects of crowding included environmental health problems, social conflict, and psychological stress. Cultural background and environmental referent significantly predicted perceived crowding at the neighborhood level but did not affect perceptions of crowding at the dwelling level. Perceptions of dwelling crowding were instead heavily influenced by objective indices, that is, number of persons and number of rooms. Findings suggest that extended exposure to crowding breeds greater dislike for crowding at the microlevel and that crowding in a primary environment is deemed more undesirable than crowding in a secondary environment.

2556

Lu, C. Y. (1955). [The application of psychological tests in the Chinese Navy]. Psychological Testing, 3, *166-171. (In Chinese.)*

2557

Lu, H. J. (1986). [A tentative study of the situational simulation method in the appraisal and selection of managerial cadres]. Information on Psychological Sciences, *No. 2, 43-48. (In Chinese.)*

A situational simulation method of assessing managerial performance and potentiality suitable to China's conditions was devised and applied on a trial basis to evaluate and select managerial cadres in Beijing and Shanghai. The results showed that this method has high concurrent and predictive validity, and is one of the most valid of various methods of evaluation.

2558

Lun, M. L. (1982). Participative management and the Chinese American: Desires and preferences as a function of acculturation, personality, and work orientation. Dissertation Abstracts International, *42, A3280.*

2559

Mao, K. N. (1985). [Career maturity and youth occupational interests]. Bulletin of Educational Psychology, 18, *229-238. (In Chinese.)*

The purpose of this study was to determine the relationship between the Youth Occupational Interest Survey (YOIS) and Career Maturity Inventory Attitude Scale (CMI). The subjects were 422 freshmen from Taiwan Normal University. The results were as follows: (1) There were significant differences between the two sexes in their occupational interests. (2) Significant canonical correlations were found between YOIS and CMI, one for male subjects and two for females. (3) The high negative loading on female CMI structure coefficients showed that some vocational preferences were related to the uncertainty of their self-concept. (4) The proportion of the redundancy index between YOIS and CMI was small, which indicated that other related factors such as work value, aptitudes, personality, need further exploring.

2560

Nevis, E. C. (1983). Using an American perspective in understanding another culture: Toward a hierarchy of needs for the People's Republic of China. Journal of Applied Behavioral Science, 19, *249-264.*

Analyzes cultural assumptions underlying Chinese management practices in order to construct a Chinese hierarchy of needs. This analysis compares Maslow's hierarchy of needs as applied to the US with the Chinese hierarchy. Outcomes of the Cultural Revolution in China included an emphasis on the group rather than the individual, an emphasis on shared outcomes--regardless of performance, and an emphasis on farming rather than manufacturing. Thus, an important cultural concept underlying Chinese management practices is that being a good member of society and putting group goals before individual needs should govern all practices. In contrast to the group-oriented, central control assumptions of China, American culture has developed out of assumptions stressing individualism and a limited state. While Maslow's hierarchy of needs, from an American perspective, puts self-actualization at the top, followed by self-esteem, belonging (social), safety, and physiology, a Chinese hierarchy puts self-actualization in the service of society at the top, followed by safety, physiology, and belonging. Data from surveys of Chinese workers and graduate students support such a model. The application of a hierarchy-of-needs model to other cultures is outlined.

2561

Peng, J. H. (1961). [A preliminary study of promoting creative thought in technical innovations]. Acta Psychologica Sinica, *No. 1, 13-19. (In Chinese.)*

The difficult problems involved in the different stages of the creative process and the ways of their solutions adopted by innovators were analyzed. Factors which facilitated the process of problem solving included comprehension of relations between the cutting tool of the lathe to be constructed and the object of production, classification of the problems into definite categories, utilization of sketch-representations and models, and mental provocation through group discussion. From analysis of the innovator's experiences, three principles relating to the creative process were suggested: thinking must be associated with tentative activity; perceptual impressions associated with logical thinking and learning associated with actual innovation.

2562

Peng, R. X. (1980). [Thirty years of industrial psychology in China]. Acta Psychologica Sinica, 12, *16-21. (In Chinese.)*

Provides a survey of advances in industrial psychology in the People's Republic. Research is described on railway light signal displays, control room signal design, and the illumination requirements for different visual tasks.

2563

Qiu, Y. J. (1983). [Psychological methods for the selection of qualified athletes]. Information on Psychological Sciences, *No. 2, 24-27. (In Chinese.)*

An attempt was made to develop mathematical models for identifying the psychological characteristics of talented athletes. Available scientific and personality tests were used, together with self-designed testing instruments and devices. After more than two years' study involving a great number of athletes, more than 50 psychological parameters of talented sprinters, gymnasts, swimmers, and volleyball players have been determined; predictive models and selection criteria have been developed.

2564

Qiu, Y. J., & Bei, E. B. (1984). [Research on the operational thinking of volleyball players in class A teams]. Information on Psychological Sciences, *No. 1, 31-37. (In Chinese.)*

The purpose of this study was to investigate the operational thinking of Chinese volleyball players, using V. N. Pushking's Three Number chess. The total number of subjects was 1,506. The results showed that the time used in operational thinking and the number of steps taken decreased with age. The time used by Class A team players was longer, and the number of steps was more than that of players of the same age in college teams and in a control group. Operational thinking appeared to depend on educational level. Duration of training and short-term training had little to do with the time used and the number of steps taken. In conclusion, it is suggested that operational thinking be used as a psychological index for selecting volleyball players, and that intelligence training be emphasized.

2565

Redding, S. G. (1977). Some perceptions of psychological needs among managers in South-East Asia. In Y. P. Poortinga (Ed.), Basic problems in cross-cultural psychology. *Amsterdam, Netherlands: Swets & Zeitlinger.*

2566

Redding, S. G. (1982). Cultural effects on the marketing process in Southeast Asia. Journal of the Market Research Society, 24, *98-114.*

Discusses the Southeast Asian marketing process in the light of the following cultural factors: Asian psychological need structures, Asian interpersonal norms, Asian social relationship patterns, regional business practices, and perceptions of the buying/selling situation. Business practices involve intuitive, immediate decision making; an informal organizational structure; minimal management control over individual performance; and nepotism, cliques, and patronage systems within the firm. Also outlined are some perceptions that a Chinese manager brings to the buying/selling situation: desire for wealth as a source of security, a family consciousness, a heightened sense of nationality, and sensitivity to dignity and "face".

2567

Redding, S. G., & Ng, M. (1982). The role of "face" in the organizational perceptions of Chinese managers. Organization Studies, 3, *201-219.*

Although acknowledged as a human universal, concern for face is seen to be more salient for the Chinese than for most other cultures. In their case it derives from a socialization process that uses shaming techniques to inculcate high sensitivity to group belonging and hence to peer opinion. A survey of 102 Overseas Chinese managers in Hong Kong, using both questionnaires and content analysis of narrated face incidents, produced strong affirmation of the role of face in organizational relationships. Face-related behavior was normally justified in terms of group harmony, and hierarchical perceptions of the social order influenced face transactions. Perceptions of the nature of face are reported, together with face-inducement factors that surround its being given or refused. Its role as an explanatory variable is considered, together with some implications for comparative management.

2568

Saner-Yiu, L., & Saner-Yiu, R. (1984). Confucius say social harmony more important than performance. Training & Development Journal, 38, *28-29.*

In Confucian cultures such as Taiwan, performance appraisals largely reflect the boss-subordinate relationship and are embedded in a sociocultural context characterized by collectivism and large power distance. Appraisals reflect the valuation of social harmony and consensus decision making, and are mostly based on nonperformance criteria. Women, being on the subservient side of the relationship equation, receive lower ratings than men regardless of actual performance.

2569

Schwartzbaum, A., & Tsai, C. L. (1972). The relationship between residence, work attitude & organization commitment in Republic of China. Journal of Sociology *(National Taiwan University), 8, 115-133.*

2570

Shi, J. (1986). [A preliminary study of the psychological training given to table tennis players]. Information on Psychological Sciences, *No. 4, 35-39. (In Chinese.)*

2571

Stening, B. W., & Everett, J. E. (1984). Response styles in a cross-cultural managerial study. Journal of Social Psychology, 122, *151-156.*

Examined the response sets of 1,647 male expatriate and local managers from 9 countries who participated in a study of stereotyping undertaken in American, British, and Japanese firms in Singapore and in Japanese firms in Britain, Hong Kong, Indonesia, Malaysia, the Philippines, and Thailand. Each S completed a questionnaire in his own language that required him to provide an autostereotype (an impression of the typical manager of his own nationality with whom he worked), a heterostereotype (an impression of the typical manager of the other nationality with whom he worked), and a metastereotype (an assessment of how the other nationality would perceive a typical manager of the S's own nationality). However, instead of a metastereotype, Ss in Singapore provided heterostereotypes of the 2 nationalities with whom they did not work. For each stereotype, a set of 18 7-point semantic differential items was used. Results indicate that there were marked differences between various nationalities in terms of their tendency to use extreme responses and midpoint responses. Moreover, age and education had an effect, except among the Japanese Ss: Young (i.e., under 40 yrs of age) and/or graduate Ss tended to use the midpoint, especially if they were from Malaysia, Singapore, the Philippines, or Thailand.

2572

Sun, C. W. (1956). [The relationship between personality and vocational interest]. Psychological Testing, 4, *276-279. (In Chinese.)*

2573

Taiwan Fertilizer Company. (1955). [A study of the intelligence of workmen in the Fifth Plant of the Taiwan Fertilizer Company]. Psychological Testing, 3, *156-162. (In Chinese.)*

2574

Tieh, H. Y. (1963). [Use of the Kuder Preference Record (Form C) for Chinese subjects]. Psychological Testing, 10, *776-780. (In Chinese.)*

2575

Tsai, L. S. (1969). A number-joining test for predicting success of Chinese air cadets. Perceptual & Motor Skills, 29, *623-626.*

Administered a 50-number version of the test to 375 Chinese air cadets. Their time scores are practically normal in distribution, though somewhat positively skewed. 37.07% of those tested failed to graduate from the flying academy. When the cadets were classified into 8 groups according to a 1-min class interval, the percentage of "wash-out" increased directly with time scores. Since the test is of the paper-and-pencil type and can be used as an individual or a self-scoring group test, it is more economical than other time-consuming individual apparatus tests currently employed in the selection of pilots.

2576

Tsao, J. C., & Li, C. C. (1959). [Industrial psychology in China]. Acta Psychologica Sinica, *No. 4, 204-214. (Translated by U.S. Joint Publications Research Service, No. 3,424, pp. 18-35.) (In Chinese.)*

The present paper describes briefly the development of industrial psychology in China and explains its differences from the "Industrial Psychology" and psychotechnology in capitalistic countries. The main results of research obtained by Chinese psychological workers in recent years, concerning the improvement of working methods, the prevention of accidents, the acceleration of technical training and the conditions facilitating new innovations, are presented. It is emphasized that the practice of combining theories with practice and also of utilizing science for production are highly effective. The defects found in the past work of industrial psychology are pointed out, as well as future developments in this field.

2577

Tseng, C. R. (1963). [A case study of an advanced textile worker]. Acta Psychologica Sinica, 1, *75-80. (In Chinese.)*

The purpose of this study was to explore psychological factors for the promotion of productive efficiency. The characteristics of the working skill of a female advanced textile worker were analyzed. The results showed the following characteristics of her working methods: proficient and precise operation skill, accurate observation, efficient distribution of attention, and effective planning of work. In addition, she always checked her work, summarized her experiences regularly, and evenly distributed and rhythmically carried out her operations.

2578

Tsung, L. T. (1956). [A study of the mechanical ability of workmen in the Fifth Plant of the Taiwan Fertilizer Company]. Psychological Testing, 4, *243-252. (In Chinese.)*

2579

Wang, K. L. (1981). [A study of promoting employees' loyalty and job satisfaction]. Journal of Education & Psychology, 4, *83. (In Chinese.)*

2580

Wang, X. H. (1984). [Psychological tests for selecting divers]. Information on Psychological Sciences, *No. 3, 28-32. (In Chinese.)*

2581

Wen, C. I. (1978). [Recreational activities of young factory workers in Taiwan]. In C. I. Wen, I. Y. Li & K. S. Yang (Eds.), Proceedings of Symposium on Youth Problems in a Changing Chinese Society. *Taipei: Academia Sinica, Institute of Ethnology. (In Chinese.)*

2582

Wilson, R. W., & Pusey, A. W. (1982). Achievement motivation and small business relationship patterns in Chinese society. In S. L. Greenblatt, R. W. Wilson, & A. A. Wilson (Eds.), Social interaction in Chinese society. *New York: Praeger.*

2583

Wong, S. L. (1985). The Chinese family firm: A model. British Journal of Sociology, 36, *58-72.*

The author distinguished three aspects of Chinese economic familism (nepotism, paternalism, and family ownership) and discussed, in particular, family ownership and the resultant phenomenon of the prevalence of family firms among privately owned Chinese commercial and industrial enterprises. Four developmental phases of Chinese firms (emergent, centralized, segmented, and disintegrative) were identified and discussed. This pattern was also compared with its Filipino and Japanese counterparts.

2584

Wu, C. Q., Pan, Y. Y., & Ting, H. C. (1980). Internal-external control, job satisfaction and performance. National Chengchi University Bulletin, 41, *61-74.*

2585

Wu, E. C., & Huang, J. T. (1985). [Environmental noise and life stress]. Chinese Journal of Mental Health, 2, *155-164. (In Chinese.)*

This study examined the relationship between environmental noise and life stress. Environmental noise was evaluated in terms of subjective evaluation, recognition of long-term change, and influences of noise upon health. Two studies were conducted. In the first one, 240 residents in a developing rural area were interviewed. The data indicated a significant correlation between recognition of changes in the environment and long-term change in environmental noise. With regard to subjective evaluation, perceived global noise level was significantly correlated with perceived relative noise level. A significant correlation was also found between recognition of environmental changes and variables concerning health and noise. In the second study, 5,131 residents of a metropolitan area in southern Taiwan were studied. The data indicated: (1) Recognition of the sources of environmental noise, the perceived magnitude of each noise source, and the degree of discomfort caused by each noise source were intercorrelated. (2) A change in environmental noise resulted from environmental changes. (3) Recognition of the influences of noise on health was highly correlated with recognition of changes in the environment, causes of disease, and choices of medical behavior.

2586

Wu, W. T., & Hung, J. L. (1981). [Vocational interests of elementary and junior high school students as related to intelligence and sex]. Bulletin of Educational Psychology, 14, *231-240. (In Chinese.)*

The purposes of this study were to investigate and compare the vocational interests of bright, normal, and mentally retarded students, and to identify influential factors in children's career development. The subjects were 192 fifth graders and 288 eighth graders from 10 schools in Taipei city. The Chinese Vocational Interest Inventory was administered. The data obtained were treated by a principle axis factor analysis and two- and three-way analyses of covariance with social-economic status as a covariate. The main results were: (1) The bright and normal students had similar factor structure in vocational preference, whereas the retarded showed less differentiation, with only one factor emerging. (2) Grade-level effects were significant on five types of vocational interests. (3) Boys preferred realistic and investigative occupations, whereas girls preferred artistic and social ones. (4) The retarded showed much fewer vocational interests in all types than the other two intelligence groups. Bright students expressed more interest in investigative and artistic occupations than normal students, in accordance with their abilities and social expectations.

2587

Xu, L. C. (1979). Ergonomics studies in the People's Republic of China. Ergonomics Society of Australia and New Zealand Newsletter, 36, *5-6.*

2588

Xu, L. C., Chen, L., Wang, D., & Xue, A. Y. (1985). [The role of psychology in enterprise management]. Acta Psychologica Sinica, 17, *339-345. (In Chinese.)*

In recent years the focus of economic reform has shifted to enhancing the quality of enterprise management. Chinese psychologists enthusiastically respond to this shift. In the Institute of Psychology, Academia Sinica, a research group is conducting studies on leadership. Modern assessment methods are to evaluate the quality of the leaders as well as situational factors in enterprises and factories. In the present study, a modified PM leadership questionnaire was given to 6,000 respondents in 40 factories and the results were fed back to the leaders and middle-level managers. Workers also participated in the discussion about problems discovered in the survey. The results indicated that this method would benefit economic reform.

2589

Xu, S. X. (1983). [The relationship between operational thinking and action operation in sports psychology]. Acta Psychologica Sinica, 15, *98-105. (In Chinese.)*

This research focused on the relations between operational thinking and assigned task, levels and types of action in various sports. The results showed that operational thinking was closely associated with assigned task and with types of action. Operational thinking was better developed by people concerned with physical training than by learners of other tasks. Sharp differences in developmental level were noticed as long-term training was carried out. Basketball players were better developed in operational thinking; swimmers were the worst. Differences in the development of operational thinking were more significant in terms of speed than of step for various action operation levels or categories of sportsmen.

2590

Xu, X. D. (1986). [Influence of quota-raising on workers' performance]. Information on Psychological Sciences, *No. 2, 36-42. (In Chinese.)*

This was a study of the influence of quota-raising on the performance of workers of a TV factory component workshop. A time series design was adopted. The results indicated: (1) Informal quota-raising resulted in no performance improvement. (2) Formal quota-raising resulted in performance improvement. (3) With quotas raised, there was a rapid increase of production in former low-output workers. (4) With quotas raised, a slow and steady increase in production, which fell behind that of former low-output workers, was made by former high-output workers. The causes of these results were traced.

2591

Yu, P. (1983). [Sex, creativity, and occupational interest]. Journal of Education & Psychology, 6, *153. (In Chinese.)*

2592

Yu, W. Z. (1985). [Social psychological climate in business and the management of teams and groups]. Information on Psychological Sciences, *No. 4, 15-22. (In Chinese.)*

2593

Zhao, J. J. et al. (1985). [Psychological traits of gold miners: Vol. 1. Response test on signalmen and hoistmen at the hoisting system]. Information on Psychological Sciences, *No. 3, 19-25. (In Chinese.)*

2594

Zheng, R. C., & Qiu, Y. J. (1984). [Personality traits of players in first-rate Chinese women's volleyball teams]. Information on Psychological Sciences, *No. 3, 22-27. (In Chinese.)*

The Social Introversion Scale of the Minnesota Multiphasic Personality Inventory (MMPI) was given to 137 players from 12 first-rate women's volleyball teams in China. Based on the results it was concluded that: (1) Most of the players tended to be introverted. (2) The degree of introversion had no linear relation with their sports performance. Usually the players who were moderately introverted were best in performance, and those who were either extremely introverted or extremely extraverted were poor. (3) Personality had nothing to do with the position they played in the game.

2595

Zoulim, S. (1979 - 1980). [Conflict between management models in China]. Bulletin de Psychologie, 33, *497-500. (In other language.)*

Two management models presently vie for acceptance in China: one currently in use and the other proposed as a "radical" solution to problems of industrial organization. The one in use looks back toward economic and social conditions that supported industry as an instrument of political policy. The "radical" solution proposes a more efficient economic model for the organization of industry; it would upgrade production by introducing technological innovations and would institute 3 grades of personnel: manager, technician, and worker. In the face of historical, economic, and demographic conditions, it is difficult to predict the pace of industrial modernization in China.

The following references are also relevant to this chapter:

217, 248, 279, 280, 300, 435, 922, 1695, 2271.

PHYSICAL, PSYCHOLOGICAL, AND PSYCHIATRIC DISORDERS 12

The number of citations in this chapter constitute 14.3% of the total in this book, second only to that in social psychology. Clearly, patterns of abnormal behavior in Chinese society and culture have received much attention from researchers.

Frequency data on citations in this chapter, in terms of content classification subcategories, are presented in Table 11.

Table 11: *Frequency of Subject Terms by Content Classification, Language, and Subject Population*

Content classification	Total	CL	EL	OL	PRC	T	HK	US
Physical and psychological disorders	129	25	101	3	17	26	24	5
Mental disorders	222	83	136	3	79	30	35	7
Behavior disorders and antisocial behavior	59	14	45	0	8	18	18	4
Learning disorders and mental retardation	27	12	15	0	6	7	6	0
Speech and language disorders	9	5	3	1	3	0	0	0
Physical and psychosomatic disorders	61	14	46	1	10	7	13	0
Total		507	153	346	8	123	88	9616

Note: CL = Chinese language; EL = English language; OL = other languages. PRÇ = People's Republic of China; T = Taiwan; HK = Hong Kong; US = United States (Chinese Americans--according to the frequency of the subject term Asian Americans).

Subject terms used for indexing citations related to physical, psychological, and psychiatric disorders are grouped according to geographical area, subject population, specific disorder, and topic. These are presented below, in a descending order of frequency. (The frequency of single-word subject terms includes those of compound terms in which the single word appears. Subjects terms used for indexing citations from other chapters may have been included. Terms with a frequency of less than 10 are not shown.)

Geographical area

138	Asia
132	Peoples Republic of China
101	Hong Kong
90	Taiwan
10	United States

Subject population

67	children
56	Asians
54	adults
31	students
29	patients
26	psychiatric patients
20	adolescents
20	school age children
19	Asian Americans
18	college students

Specific disorder

54	schizophrenia
47	neurosis
32	depression (emotion)
28	psychosomatic disorders
24	suicide
16	mental retardation
15	juvenile delinquency
12	neurasthenic neurosis

Topic

175	disorders
109	mental disorders
63	epidemiology
56	health
45	cross cultural differences
45	psychiatry
39	mental health
35	adulthood
35	case report
34	symptoms
31	sociocultural factors
30	behavior
29	personality
29	sex
27	family
24	history
19	stress
18	psychopathology
17	brain
16	ethnic groups
16	psychodiagnosis
16	sciences

16 transcultural psychiatry
15 Chinese medicine
14 anxiety
14 diagnosis
14 human sex differences
11 adjustment
11 development
10 racial and ethnic differences
10 status

An inspection of Table 11 reveals some noteworthy trends. First, mental disorders (e.g., affective and emotional disturbances, hysteria, mania, neurosis, personality disorders, phobia, and psychosis) have received the most attention (43.8%); speech and language disorders the least (1.8%). Second, English language studies outnumber Chinese language studies by a factor of more than two. This reflects the great interest of foreign investigators in Chinese patterns of abnormal behavior. Third, the number of studies related to Hong Kong is surprising high, surpassing that related to Taiwan. An inspection of the subject terms listed above suggests that there is a remarkably high degree of interest in epidemiological studies among researchers. In this connection, an analysis of publications by the staff of the Department of Psychiatry at National Taiwan University over a 25-year period indicated that epidemiological studies rank first (17 out of a total of 149) among various categories in psychiatry and neurology (Chen and Rin 1975). The frequencies of *cross cultural differences* (together with *ethnic groups* and *racial and ethnic differences*), *sociocultural factors*, and *transcultural psychiatry* are indicative of the importance researchers attach to sociocultural considerations.

As to specific disorders or psychiatric syndromes, schizophrenia ranks first in terms of research attention received; *neurasthenic neurosis* (or *neurasthenia*) is a diagnostic term commonly used by Chinese psychiatrists. Psychoactive substance use, delusional (paranoid), dissociative, sleep, factitious, and impulse control disorders are among those relatively neglected.

Two edited books on mental health and mental disorders in Chinese culture (Kleinman and Lin 1981; Tseng and Wu, 1985) have been published. Another book (Livingston and Lowinger 1983) is devoted exclusively to mental health in the PRC. A review of medical psychology in the PRC is found in Li, Xu, and Kuang (1980).

REFERENCES

Chen, R. C., & Rin, H. (1975). [Editors' remarks: Statistical analysis of presentations and publications by members of the Chinese Society of Neurology and Psychiatry during the past 25 years]. *Bulletin of the Chinese Society of Neurology and Psychiatry*, *1*(1), 2-4. (In Chinese.)

Kleinman, A., & Lin, T. Y. (Eds.). (1981). *Normal and abnormal behavior in Chinese culture*. Dordrecht, Netherlands: Reidel.

Li, X., Xu, S. L., & Kuang, P. Z. (1980). [Thirty years of Chinese medical psychology]. *Acta Psychologica Sinica*, *12*, 135-143. (In Chinese.)

Livingston, M., & Lowinger, P. (1983). *The minds of the Chinese people: Mental health in New China*. Englewood cliffs, NJ: Prentice-Hall.

Tseng, W. S., & Wu, D. Y. H. (Eds.) (1985). *Chinese culture and mental health*. Orlando, FL: Academic Press.

2596

Abbott, K. A. (1968). The use of the California Psychological Inventory in intensive study of family systems. *Psychology and Education*, *2*, **49-60.**

This paper presents some preliminary research findings on Chinese family systems. The subjects were 24 Chinese-American delinquents and their parents, and 22 matched nondelinquents and their parents. The data seemed to support the hypothesis that delinquents tend to have "dominant" mothers in comparison with nondelinquents. The use of the California Personality Inventory as a research instrument in Chinese societies is discussed.

2597

Abbott, K., & Abbott, E. L. (1968). Juvenile delinquency in San Francisco's Chinese-American community: 1961-1968. *Journal of Sociology* **(National Taiwan University),** *4*, **45-56. (Republished in S. Sue & N. N. Wagner (Eds.),** *Asian-Americans: Psychological perspectives*. **Palo Alto, CA: Science & Behavior Books, 1973.)**

2598

Akhtar, S. (1978). Obsessional neurosis, marriage, sex and fertility: Some transcultural comparisons. *International Journal of Social Psychiatry*, *24*, **164-166.**

In a study of 82 obsessional neurotics, it was found that Indian obsessives, unlike their counterparts in other countries, did not display a higher than expected rate of celibacy, bachelorhood, and low fertility. Sociocultural explanations are offered for these findings (e.g., an intention to remain single meets with strong family resistance in India).

2599

Alagaratnam, T. T., & Kung, N. Y. T. (1985). The psychosocial sequelae of mastectomy in Chinese females. *Journal of the Hong Kong Psychiatric Association*, *5*, **39-40 & 42.**

The psychosocial effects of mastectomy were assessed in 23 Chinese patients. Forty-seven percent of the sample was found to be depressed. Loss of femininity and physical disfigurement were not a major concern. Sixty percent of the patients reported difficulties with adjusting to sex after mastectomy. The majority of the patients were able to maintain their previous levels of occupational functioning.

2600

April, R. S., & Tse, P. C. (1977). Crossed aphasia in a Chinese bilingual dextral. *Archives of Neurology*, *34*, **766-770.**

The authors describe a persistent nonfluent aphasia following a right cerebral infarction that developed in a 54-year-old right-handed Chinese man. Computerized axial tomography localized the lesion in the distribution of the right middle cerebral artery. The speech and language dysfunction was greater for performances in Chinese than in English, despite the fact that the patient was born in China, was schooled in Chinese until age 7 years, and spoke Chinese at home and in his business. It is suggested that early learning of Chinese, an ideographic language based on visual spatial percepts, might have been critical for the establishment and maintenance of language dominance in the right hemisphere.

2601

April, R. S., & Tse, P. C. (1979). Crossed aphasia in a Chinese bilingual dextral. *Archives of Neurology*, *36*, **253.**

2602

Arran Street Child Assessment Clinic. (1984). *A study of handicapped children assessed at Arran Street Clinic*. **Hong Kong: Author.**

2603

Bao, Z. C. et al. (1986). [A clinical analysis of 340 cases of war neurosis in comparison with 750 cases of non-war neurosis]. *Chinese Journal of Neurology and Psychiatry*, *19*, **282-284.** (In Chinese.)

The results of a clinical analysis of 340 cases of war neurosis compared with 750 cases of nonwar neurosis were reported. The authors found that hysteria and neurasthenia were common in war neurosis. In wartime hysteria, the common features were convulsive seizure and emotional outburst. There was a higher proportion of neurasthenia and a lower proportion of hysteria in war neurosis than in nonwar neurosis.

2604

Barnett, M. L. (1955). Alcoholism in the Cantonese of New York City: An anthropological study. In O. Diethelm (Ed.), *Etiology of chronic alcoholism*. **Springfield, IL: Thomas.**

2605

Bergman, E. (1972). Autonomous and unique features of American sign language. *American Annals of the Deaf*, *117*, **20-24.**

American Sign Language (ASL) has a syntax, grammar, and rhetoric of its own, along with some unusual features (pronounced polarity, 3-dimensionality). Further, ASL represents a precise and rapid medium of communication capable of expressing abstractions, nuances of meaning, and witticisms, and is a living and growing language as well. Certain parallels between ASL and Chinese are traced, and the effect of the physiological factor is considered. the potential usefulness of ASL as a tool for research into thought processes and for providing a linguistic environment favorable to the growth and maturation of the individual is pointed out.

2606

Berk, B. B., & Hirata, L. C. (1973). Mental illness among the Chinese: Myth or reality? *Journal of Social Issues, 29,* **149-166.**

Examined trends in mental hospital commitments among the Chinese in California over the past 100 yrs. There has been a 2-fold increase for the general population compared to a 7-fold increase among the Chinese; while initially the Chinese were roughly equal to the general population. Rates of increase within the Chinese population were not uniform; males, the aged, and the foreign born experienced substantially greater increases. Changes have also occurred in patterns of diagnosis and length of hospitalization over the century.

2607

Bermann, G. (1968). Mental health in China. In A. Kiev (Ed.), *Psychiatry in the Communist world* **(pp. 223-261). New York: Science House.**

2608

Bott, M. H. (1978). Reactive depression. *British Homeopathic Journal, 67,* **254-262.**

2609

Buhrich, N. (1981). Frequency of presentation of anorexia nervosa in Malaysia. *Australian & New Zealand Journal of Psychiatry, 15,* **153-155.**

Surveyed psychiatrists in Malaysia and determined that primary anorexia nervosa is a rare condition there, especially among Malays compared to Chinese and Indians. The reasons for the racial differences and the apparent infrequency of the condition are discussed with respect to attitudes toward obesity, the medical profession, religious associations, and demographic characteristics.

2610

Buhrich, N., & Haq, S. (1980). Characteristics of first schizophrenic admissions to the General Hospital Kuala Lumpur. *Medical Journal of Malaysia, 34,* **269-272.**

2611

Buhrich, N., Haq, S. M., & George, S. (1981). Profile of alcoholism in a multiracial society. *International Journal of the Addictions, 16,* **1111-1115.**

Demographic characteristics of all patients with a diagnosis of alcoholism or alcoholic psychoses admitted to the Psychiatry Department, General Hospital, Kuala Lumpur, between 1975 and 1978 were examined. The diagnosis of alcoholism or alcoholic psychoses accounted for 2% of the total psychiatric admissions. Males greatly predominated over females; Indians greatly predominated over Malays and Chinese. Reasons for these differences are discussed.

2612

Bullough, V. L. (1976). *Sexual variance in society and history.* **New York: John Wiley & Sons.**

Presents a comprehensive survey of the history of stigmatized sexual behavior throughout Western Culture and in India, ancient China, the Arab world, and primitive groups. Also described are attitudes toward sexual deviance in colonial America and in 19th century America, and trends and assumptions of the 20th century.

2613

Calehr, H. (1976). Acupuncture in psychosomatic medicine: Diagnostic and therapeutic standards. *American Journal of Acupuncture, 4,* **101-129.**

1,052 psychosomatic patients were examined and treated with acupuncture, based upon the Chinese Five Element doctrine and pulse diagnosis. Four phases of human mental evolution, six types of asthenic and six types of neurotic patterns are described in standardized diagnostic and therapeutic parameters in psychosomatosis. Both symptomatic and systematic treatments were applied. The former differentiates between general and specific treatments, whereas the latter makes use of the small and large constitutional treatments.

2614

California Department of Public Health, Bureau of Maternal and Child Health. (1962 - 1967). *Epidemiology of childhood accidents project.* **Berkeley, CA: Author.**

2615

Carpenter, W. T., Bartko, J. J., Carpenter, C. L., & Strauss, J. S. (1976). Another view of schizophrenia subtypes: A report from the International Pilot Study of Schizophrenia. *Archives of General Psychiatry, 33,* **508-516.**

Presents a report, based on sign and symptom data from the International Pilot Study of Schizophrenia, which addresses three questions: (a) Are traditional subtype diagnoses applied similarly across cultures? (b) Are the various traditional subtypes symptomatically distinguishable from one another? (c) Can cluster analytic techniques define a more distinctive set of schizophrenic subgroups? Present State Examination data from 1,202 patients in 9 countries were reduced to 27 psychopathologic signs and symptoms. Profile analysis of variance results indicate that each subtype appears similar, regardless of the center of origin. However, this is based on a lack of distinguishing features between different subtypes. On the other hand, when a cluster analytic technique was used, it showed one large and three small subgroups, each readily distinguishable from the others. These subgroups, labeled ^usual^, ^flagrant^, ^insightful^, and ^hypochondriacal^ , are described clinically. If replicated or validated, such subgroups may prove meaningful in future considerations of subdivisions of the schizophrenia syndrome.

2616

Chakraborty, A., & Banerji, G. (1975). Ritual, a culture specific neurosis, and obsessional states in Bengali culture. *Indian Journal of Psychiatry, 17,* **273-283.**

2617

Chan, C. M., & Tsoi, M. M. (1984). The BDI and stimulus determinants of cognitive-related depression among Chinese college students. *Cognitive Therapy & Research, 8,* **501-507.**

This study examined the relationship between depression and cognitive distortion in 41 male and 41 female Chinese college students. The subjects were given the Beck Depression Inventory and a cognitive distortion measure in which 8 stories described a central character who was involved in negative or unfortunate events. In 4 of the stories, the character's relationship with the events was unambiguous and in the other 4 it was ambiguous. The subjects were given multiple-choice questions pertaining to the central character's feelings, thoughts, and expectations, each of which consisted of 4 response options: depressed-distorted, nondepressed-distorted, depressed-nondistorted, and nondepressed-nondistorted. The results showed general support for A. T. Beck's cognitive theory that depression relates with cognitive distortion in the evaluation of events. However, they demonstrated that this relationship is mediated by the ambiguity level of events and the tone of the options. There were more depressed-distorted responses and nondepressed-nondistorted responses in ambiguous situations than in unambiguous situations. The data suggested that female subjects were more willing to express depressive feelings.

2618

Chan, D. W., & Chan-Ho, M. W. (1983). Stressful life events: Overview and lessons from a Chinese context. *Journal of the Hong Kong Psychiatric Association, 3,* **3-7.**

The current status of life event research was evaluated in an overview, giving specific considerations to some of the central methodological issues concerning measurement. In light of past findings and a study conducted in a Chinese context, issues of event sampling, event clusters, readjustment, undesirability, and uncontrollability as stress-producing features of life events, weighting schemes, event-illness confounding, and mediating variables in event-illness relationships were discussed. Future directions for studies employing causal modelling in the Chinese setting were suggested.

2619

Chan, D. W. O., Chan, T. S. C., & Chan-Ho, M. W. (1984). Occurrence and co-occurrence of stressful life events in a Chinese context. *International Journal of Psychosomatics, 31,* **3-10.**

The authors studied life-event frequencies during the previous year among 201 Chinese university students and staff members (aged 19-60 years) to examine any relationship between the co-occurrence of events and physical illness. The average number of events for a subject was 5.92. Common events included taking a vacation and a minor illness. No differences were found in life-event occurrences between various age, sex, marital status, and student versus staff groups; a few specific events did show a differential occurrence among subjects differing in age, marital status, and staff-student membership. While event interrelationships were generally low, certain events did co-occur to some extent. However, illnesses tended not to co-occur with other events.

2620

Chan, S. K. (1984). An assessment of Chinese-Americans' attitudes toward mental illness and their perceived needs for mental health services. *Dissertation Abstracts International, 45,* **B993-994.**

2621

Chang, B. L. (1985). The comparison of conservation abilities between hearing-impaired students and hearing students in Taiwan, the Republic of China. *Dissertation Abstracts International, 45,* **A3110-3111.**

2622

Chang, L. Y., Wu, E. C., & Hwu, H. G. (1985). [The concept and measurement of life stress]. *Chinese Journal of Mental Health, 2,* **137-151.** (In Chinese.)

We empirically examined major issues of the concept and measurement of life stress based on data collected from 700 respondents from a previous study. Interaction between life cycle and experience of life events, internal structure of the onset of life events, issues on the importance of "change", "emotional response", and "desirability" were studied. Our findings indicated a weak link between life cycle and experience of life events. Age was the only variable which significantly contributed to the accumulation of life events. The onset of life events did not cluster in any particular form. Emotional response and desirability about the experience of life events were fairly independent variables. A method of identifying temporal sequence of life events and mental illness in cross-sectional data was discussed.

2623

Chang, S. S., & Tang, K. Y. (1958). A study of mental disturbance among the retired servicemen tested in the Nuan-nuan Center. *Acta Psychologica Taiwanica*, **No. 1, 64-84.**

2624

Chang, T. H. (1959). [An experimental study of memory disorder in neurasthenics]. *Acta Psychologica Sinica*, **No. 6, 388-401.** (In Chinese.)

This experiment was an investigation of speedy synthetic treatments of neurasthenia. The purpose was to investigate the characteristics of the patients' memory disorder by an objective method and to find out the extent of their recoveries after speedy synthetic treatments. Patients were required to recall and recognize pictures after a short presentation. The patients were also asked about their memory. The result showed that the extent of the patients' memory disorder depended on the severity of symptoms of neurasthenia. Due to individual differences in the effectiveness of treatments, different levels of improvement in memory were observed after treatment. By strengthening the patients' belief in the effectiveness of the treatment, better effects of the treatment were obtained.

2625

Chang, T. H. (1962). [An experimental study of memory disorder in neurasthenics]. *Acta Psychologica Sinica*, **No. 1, 51-56.** (In Chinese.)

This is a continuation of a study of memory characteristics in neurasthenics carried out originally in 1959. The experimental results indicated: (1) Memory impairment of words and pictures is the same; (2) The differences in experimental results between purposeful memorizing and incidental memorizing are not significant; (3) Rote memory is not as effective as meaningful memory; (4) The degree of functional disorder in the cerebral cortex and in memory disorder are correlated.

2626

Chang, W. C. (1985). A cross-cultural study of depressive symptomology. *Culture, Medicine & Psychiatry*, *9*, **295-317.**

Black, white, and overseas Chinese college students were surveyed with the Self-Rating Depression Scale to explore dimensions and configurations of depressive symptomology. With the exception of the symptoms of psychomotor agitation and constipation, there were no quantitative differences of depressive symptoms across groups; however, symptoms clustered in different configurations for the 3 groups. The factors contributing the most variance differed in their item contents: a mixture of affective and somatic complaints characterized the black subjects; existential and cognitive concerns characterized the white subjects, and somatic complaints characterized the overseas Chinese subjects. It was concluded that differences between the American and overseas Chinese in reporting symptoms of constipation and psychomotor agitation may reflect cultural differences in expressing these conditions. It was not clear whether the variation in symptom patterns between black and white Americans is due to cultural or to class differences. The prominence of somatic complaints in the Chinese group suggests that somatic complaints are more indicative of depression for the Chinese.

2627

Chang, Y. H. (1934). [A historial study of the abnormal behavior of Chinese famous men]. *Far Eastern*, *1*, **125-136.** (In Chinese.)

2628

Chao, Y. (1958). [Records on neurology in traditional Chinese medical texts]. *Chinese Journal of Neurology and Psychiatry*, *4*, **122-127.** (In Chinese.)

2629

Chee, K. T. (1974). A case of bestiality. *Singapore Medical Journal*, *15*, **287-288.**

A Chinese male aged 23 years was referred to a psychiatric clinic after admitting he had had sexual intercourse with an old hen 2 months previously. He gave a history of sexual contact with hens for 5 or 6 years and apparently was not worried about it. Some definitions and psychopathological descriptions of sexual perversion are briefly introduced.

2630

Chen, C. H. (1979). [A further study of disturbance of the thinking process in schizophrenia]. *Chinese Journal of Neurology and Psychiatry*, *12*, **7-10.** (In Chinese.)

2631

Chen, C. H. et al. (1986). [Data analysis of an epidemiological study of mental disorders, drug and alcoholic dependence, and personality disorders]. *Chinese Journal of Neurology and Psychiatry*, *19*, **70-72.** (In Chinese.)

Using structured procedures, 38,136 people aged 15 years and over from 12,000 households (6,000 urban and 6,000 rural) in 12 districts were interviewed. The general prevalence rate of psychosis was 1.269%. The prevalence rate of schizophrenia was the highest (0.569%), and that of drug and alcoholic dependence or of personality disorders was less than 0.05%. The general rates varied significantly among different districts, but were not significantly different between the sexes. The current prevalence rates of schizophrenia and cerebrovascular diseases associated with psychotic disturbance in urban districts were higher than those in rural districts; but the prevalence rate of mental retardation in rural districts was higher than that in urban districts.

2632

Chen, C. H. et al. (1986). [An analysis of epidemiological data on schizophrenia]. *Chinese Journal of Neurology and Psychiatry, 19,* **73-76.** (In Chinese.)

An analysis of epidemiological data on schizophrenia gathered from 12 districts in China was reported. The prevalence rate of schizophrenia was 0.569%, which is higher than that reported in the 1970s. The prevalence rate in urban districts was higher than that in rural districts; the prevalence rate was distinctly higher for females than for males. The prevalence rates and outcomes of schizophrenia seemed to be associated with socio-environmental factors, including economic level, occupation, family structure, marital status, relatives' attitude toward the patients, and the social support system.

2633

Chen, C. K. (1962). [On the problems in translating some English psychopathological terms into Chinese]. *Acta Psychologica Sinica,* **No. 1, 83-88.** (In Chinese.)

2634

Chen, C. K. (1963). [Some psychopathological thoughts in the book of ***Tso Chuen*****].** *Acta Psychologica Sinica,* **No. 2, 157-164.** (In Chinese.)

2635

Chen, C. K. (1964). [Psychogalvanic reflex and the subjective states of neurasthenics]. *Acta Psychologica Sinica,* **No. 1, 103-108.** (In Chinese.)

The galvanic skin response (GSR) of 42 neurasthenics and 10 normal subjects was measured. The resting levels of the first 15 minutes were recorded; after this period a stimulus was presented, and followed by an alarm to indicate the end of the experiment. It was found that: (1) neurasthenics with a state of restlessness, emotional anxiety and over-sensitivity showed greater reactivity than normals; (2) neurasthenics with tiredness showed smaller resting scores and greater responsiveness to stimuli than normal subjects; (3) low correlation was found between the degree of self-sensitivity and GSR.

2636

Chen, C. S., & Tang, Y. F. (1956). [Hysterical amnesia]. *Chinese Journal of Neurology and Psychiatry, 2,* **74-78.** (In Chinese.)

2637

Chen, F. P. (1986). [An epidemiologic investigation of neurosis]. *Chinese Journal of Neurology and Psychiatry, 19,* **301-305.** (In Chinese.)

In a population of 75,498 people, 1,011 neurotics were identified in a door-to-door investigation. The prevalence rate was 13.09 per 1,000. From 1976 to 1980, the average annual incidence rate was 0.81 per 1,000. There was a significant difference in prevalence rates between males (3.15 per 1,000) and females (23.45 per 1,000). The highest rates were found among the unemployed, the divorced, widows or widowers, the illiterate, people of middle economic status, and introverts.

2638

Chen, H. B. et al. (1979). [Gilles de la Tourette's Syndrome]. *Chinese Journal of Neurology and Psychiatry, 12,* **213-216.** (In Chinese.)

2639

Chen, S. C. L., & Lau-Yu, P. K. (1982). A study on the phenomenology of depression in the Hong Kong Chinese. *Journal of the Hong Kong Psychiatric Association, 2,* **31-42.**

2640

Chen, Y. H. (1965). [A study of motor and manual skills of feebleminded children]. *Psychological Testing, 12,* **189-202.** (In Chinese.)

2641

Chen, Y. H. (1967). Conditioning of the aplha block in normal and mentally retarded children. *Psychology and Education, 1,* **97-112.**

2642

Chen, Y. H. (1968). Effects of stimulus intensity and duration on alpha block duration of normal and mentally retarded children. *Psychology and Education, 2,* **110-120.**

2643

Chen, Y. H. (1981). [A study of the social-cultural background of mentally retarded children in special classes of junior high schools in Taipei city]. *Bulletin of Educational Psychology, 14,* **41-58.** (In Chinese.)

The present study compared the social-economic status and the home environment of mentally retarded and monretarded children. In addition, the attitude of the family toward retarded children was investigated. Surveys were carried out twice, first in 1973 on 299 retarded children and again in 1980 on 657 retarded children. An equal number of nonretarded students was selected to serve as a comparison group. The main findings were: (1) Parental social-economic status, education, and median income of the retarded group were much lower than those of the nonretarded group; the density per living unit for families of the retarded group was greater than that of the nonretarded group; and more parents of the retarded group had unskilled jobs. (2) The deprivation of social and cultural experiences for the retarded group was more obvious than for the nonretarded group. (3) Only about half of the parents of the retarded group recognized that their children were retarded; about one third hoped that their retarded children could attend senior high school after graduating from special classes. However, a small portion of parents rejected their retarded children. Clearly, the results suggest that specific enrichment or early education programs for disadvantaged children is necessary to reduce the prevalence of cultural retardation in the slum areas of Taipei.

2644

Chen, Z. K., & Zhang, B. Y., Shih, H. Y., Xu, E. T., Chen, Z. L., & Hu, X. F. (1980). [A preliminary research on the arousal level of paranoid and nonparanoid schizophrenics]. *Acta Psychologica Sinica, 12,* **68-74.** (In Chinese.)

This study, utilizing electrodermal activity as an index of arousal level, examined the inconsistency of many previous works on the psychophysiological deficit of schizophrenia. 20 schizophrenics and 10 normal adults were used as subjects. After a 10 minutes "rest" period, 2 series of tones were presented successively as stimulation for an habituation test. The results showed that schizophrenics as a group were overaroused compared with normal adults. There were differences between the two clinical types of schizophrenia: nonparanoid schizophrenics gave the tendency to show higher basal level, greater frequencies of spontaneous electrodermal fluctuations, and slower habituation of response amplitude during repeated stimulations. The concept of arousal continuum was discussed, and further research suggested.

2645

Cheng, F. Y. (1968). Reaction time of introverts vs. extroverts in schizophrenics and normals. *Acta Psychologica Taiwanica, 10,* **45-51.**

The present experiment is designed to test a theory which is a combination of the two theories of Pavlov and Eysenck. According to this theory we can predict that schizophrenics should be extroverted persons and they should have a higher degree of mental illness than introverted persons. The subjects were 33 schizophrenics hospitalized in Jinchi Hospital, and 40 students of National Taiwan University. These students were divided into two groups, extroverted and introverted, based on their extroversion scores on the Mausley Inventory Test. Subjects made 15 reaction time (RT) trials to three tone stimulus intensities, 90, 60 and 30 db. Only the last 10 trials were used for calculating the results. The findings were: (1) The RTs to the tone stimuli when the stimulus intensity decreased were equivalent for the schizophrenics and normals. (2) The RTs of the introverted subjects were significantly shorter than those of the extroverted subjects, but for the schizophrenic subjects this relation was reversed. That is, an extroverted patient has a faster RT than an introverted one. (3) A mentally ill introverted person reacts significantly slower to outside stimuli than a mentally healthy introverted person.

2646

Cheng, S. K. (1985). Cultural explanation of a "psychosis" in a Chinese woman living in Australia. *Australian & New Zealand Journal of Psychiatry, 19,* **190-194.**

The author discussed the case history of a 36-year-old Malaysian-born Chinese woman living in the Australian outback who was diagnosed as psychotic and recovered without drug treatment. An examination into the subject's cultural background revealed several culture-based supernatural beliefs that shed doubt on the assumption that her complaints were psychotic. It was concluded that the case illustrated the importance of adopting a cultural perspective in the understanding and management of psychiatric illness.

2647

Cheng, S. T., Ip, H. Y., & Cheung, F. M. C. (1984). Proclivity to rape: An exploratory study. *Hong Kong Journal of Mental Health, 13,* **45-56.**

Forty Chinese males, aged between 18 and 45 years and belonging to the working class with an education not going beyond the secondary school level, filled out a questionnaire which tapped their self-centeredness, sources of sex information, use of pornography, and attitudes toward rape, sex, and women. The results indicated that proclivity to rape was predicted by promiscuous attitudes toward sex and derogatory attitudes toward women. Implications on the possible means of rape prevention, such as sex education and assertive training for females, were discussed.

2648

Cheng, T. A. (1985). [A study of sociocultural characteristics and adjustment of psychotic patients in Taiwan]. *Chinese Journal of Mental Health, 2,* **117-133.** (In Chinese.)

This study investigated the sociocultural characteristics, conditions of care, and current social function of 1,962 psychotic patients sampled from the general community and mental hospitals. The patients were characterized by low social class, poor education, unemployment, and lack of marital life. Of the community patients, 86.3% lived with their families; the rest were locked in a ward or lived alone. Many patients sought help from traditional healers. One fifth of community patients had never sought psychiatric help; half of all patients did not receive any treatment during the investigation period. Only one third of all patients ever hospitalized had received regular medication after their discharge. Most of the community patients had withdrawn from society, and less than 10% had a job. Fifteen percent of hospitalized patients could work independently, but were unable to return to the community. Most of the patients under custodial care were locked in a ward every day and appeared severely retarded. The need to increase and improve current public mental illness services and welfare was stressed.

2649

Cheng, T. A. (1985). A pilot study of mental disorders in Taiwan. *Psychological Medicine, 15,* **195-203.**

A two-stage case-identification method, using a modified version of the General Health Questionnaire (GHQ) and a Chinese translation of the Clinical Interview Schedule (CIS), was applied to 146 urban residents and 150 comparison individuals from a nearby community in a pilot study of mental disorders in an urban area of Taiwan. The validity of the modified GHQ was proven to be greater than that of the original, with a very high sensitivity and specificity. The Chinese version of the CIS was found to be feasible for community study in Taiwan. The total prevalence rate for all mental disorders was 26%, with a higher morbidity rate among females.

2650

Cheung, F. (1982). Somatization among Chinese: A critique. *Hong Kong Psychological Society Bulletin,* **No. 8, 27-35.**

Reviews the cultural explanations attributed to the phenomenon of somatization, a term that refers to patients' heightened awareness of the body and their presentation of somatic complaints in place of psychological complaints. Complaints are often presented in a dramatic, vague, or exaggerated way or are part of a complicated medical history, but have no physical basis. The cultural explanations are as follows: (1) The cultural trait of withholding emotional expression and avoiding open display of emotions in social interaction is a major reason for the Chinese tendency to somatize their emotional problems. (2) There is a lack of vocabulary and semantic network in the Chinese language for expressing affective states. Chinese mental patients often use physical metaphors instead. (3) There is a lack of differential awareness of affective states among the Chinese. (4) There is an interaction between the mind and the body in the Chinese holistic view of health. (5) Patients often make a situation-appropriate expression of emotions. (6) There is a limited availability and accessibility of psychological treatment in China.

2651

Cheung, F. K. (1979). Mental health problems and services for Asian immigrants in the United States. *Acta Psychologica Taiwanica, 21,* **105-116.**

Presents an overview of mental health in the US, and discusses the types of mental health problems that confront the Asian (Chinese) immigrants and the services that have been provided them. The importance of interaction between ethnic culture and mainstream American values is emphasized. It is concluded that greater efforts are being made toward community education, through the mass media in native languages, to help the total community become aware of and make use of available mental health services.

2652

Cheung, F. K. (1979). Mental health problems and adjustment of Chinese students in the United States. *Hong Kong Journal of Mental Health, 8,* **47-55.**

2653

Cheung, F. M. (1982). Psychological symptoms among Chinese in urban Hong Kong. *Social Science & Medicine, 16,* **1339-1344.**

The responses of 3,925 Ss on the Langner Screening Scale of Psychopathology taken from R. P. Lee's (1976, 1980) Hong Kong Biosocial Survey were reanalyzed in terms of D. L. Crandell and B. P. Dohrenwend's (1967) subscales. Results show that report of psychological symptoms was higher than that of psychophysiological, physiological, and ambiguous symptoms. Significant differences in subscale scores were found among 5 variables: age, sex, education, socioeconomic status, and total number of reported symptoms. Within each subgroup of the variables, scores on the Psychological subscale were significantly higher than scores on the other 3 subscales. Findings dispute the contention that Chinese in general tend to deny their emotions. Somatization among Chinese mental patients in medical settings and report of psychological symptoms by Chinese may not be mutually exclusive phenomena.

2654

Cheung, F. M. C. (1985). [Modes of presentation and help-seeking for psychological problems among Chinese]. *Proceedings of the Conference on Modernization and Chinese Culture.* **Hong Kong: Chinese University of Hong Kong, Faculty of Social Science and Institute of Social Studies.** (In Chinese.)

2655

Cheung, F. M. C. (1985). An overview of psychopathology in Hong Kong: With special reference to somatic presentation. In W. S. Tseng & D. Y. H. Wu (Eds.), *Chinese culture and mental health: An overview* **(pp. 287-304). Orlando, FL: Academic Press.**

2656

Cheung, F. M. C., & Chung, B. J. (1982). An exploratory study on attitudes toward rape. *Hong Kong Journal of Mental Health, 11,* **7-18.**

2657

Cheung, F. M. C., & Lau, B. W. K. (1982). Situational variations of help-seeking behavior among Chinese patients. *Comprehensive Psychiatry, 23,* **252-262.**

Examined the tendency among Chinese to somatize their psychological problems by summarizing explanations for this in terms of 3 attributions: denial suppression or repression of emotions, lack of a vocabulary or mode of expression for affective states, and lack of differentiation between mind and body. Specifically investigated were the presence of situational variations in Chinese help-seeking behavior with 75 patients of an outpatient psychiatric clinic, 80 male prisoners, and 37 Ss in a general outpatient clinic. Patterns of consultation among Ss showed differences in terms of stated intention for consultation, type of symptoms expressed and presented, and the process of help-seeking behavior. These situational variations in help-seeking behavior challenge the simple ascription of somatization to Chinese patients.

2658

Cheung, F. M. C., & Lau, B. W. K. (1982). Cross-cultural perspectives on psychosocial adjustment in Hong Kong. *World Journal of Psychosynthesis, 14,* **6-12.**

2659

Cheung, F. M. C., Lau, B. W. K., & Waldmann, E. (1981). Somatization among Chinese depressives in general practice. *International Journal of Psychiatry in Medicine, 10,* **361-374.**

Depressive illness was a common clinical syndrome found in general practice in Hong Kong. The phenomenon of somatization among Chinese depressives in general practice was investigated. Patients clinically identified as depressed were compared with organic patients in terms of their presenting complaints and responses to a symptom checklist. Sleep disturbances, general malaise, pains and aches, dizziness, and menopausal symptoms were the most frequent disturbances that prompted Chinese depressives to seek help in general practice. When directly asked, these patients admitted having various psychological features including dysphoric mood, self-reproach, loss of interest in social activities and in sex. Subgroup comparisons showed little sex difference in initial complaints and admitted symptomatology among the depressives. Some age differences were observed in the presenting complaints. The discrepancy between the pattern of presenting complaints and admitted symptoms suggested that patients were aware of their emotional disturbance even though they tended to express these disturbances in somatic terms in their help-seeking processes. Distinction between the expression mode and the recognition mode of somatization was discussed.

2660

Cheung, H. K. (1984). Birth rank order in psychiatric in-patients of Hong Kong: A replication study. *Journal of the Hong Kong Psychiatric Association, 4,* **20-25.**

Dr. Edmond Chiu's survey of in-patients of Castle Peak Hospital in 1970 found an excess of last-borns. The present study repeated the survey in 1981 and discovered an excess of first-borns. Such difference in results can be explained in terms of changes in the general population of Hong Kong. The relationship between birth-order and mental illness remains unsettled.

2661

Cheung, H. K. (1986). Psychiatric morbidity of Chinese immigrants in Hong Kong. *Journal of the Hong Kong Psychiatric Association, 6,* **38-40, 42, 44, 46-48.**

Over a period of 16 months, a record was kept of the birth place and native origin of all new attendants to the South Kwai Chung Psychiatric Centre. The results were analyzed against Census statistics. It was found that Chinese immigrants to Hong Kong, when compared with the local-born population, had a significantly higher risk of functional psychoses (mainly schizophrenia) and nonacute organic psychiatric disorders, but a significantly lower risk of mental handicap. The data supported the "selection theory" rather than the "stress theory." Ethnic origin outside the Guangdong Province was associated with a lower incidence of mental handicap in males, regardless of birth place.

2662

Chi, M. (1955). [Records on serious psychiatric disorders in traditional Chinese medical texts]. *Chinese Journal of Neurology and Psychiatry, 1,* **1-5.** (In Chinese.)

2663

Chia, B. H., & Tsoi, W. F. (1974). A statistical study of attempted suicides in Singapore. *Singapore Medical Journal, 15,* **253-256.**

2664

Chien, M. F. (1969). [Patterns of intellectual functioning of prison inmates]. *Psychological Testing, 16,* **680-726.** (In Chinese.)

2665

Chieuh, C. M. (1982). [An analysis of the statistical data on death by suicide and self-inflicted injury in Taiwan]. *Chinese Medical Journal* **(Taipei),** *29,* **36-45.** (In Chinese.)

The standardized death rates (per 100,000) from suicide and self-inflicted injuries in Taiwan from 1960 to 1979 were calculated, using the 1960 Census. Among males, the highest death rate was 33.3 (in 1964); the lowest rate was 12.2 (in 1977). Among females, death rates ranged from 22.3 (in 1963) to 10.1 (in 1975). The change in the death rates seemed to show a similar pattern for both sexes, but the death rate of males was significantly higher than that of females for each year. Deaths from suicide and self-inflicted injuries constituted 2.1%-5.3% of the total annual deaths for males, and 2.1%-4.2% for females. For males, those between 10 to 29 years of age constituted 37.7%; for females, around 49.2%. The females were especially young. Poisoning by solid or liquid substances were the most common method used by both males and females; hanging-suffocation or strangulation and submersion-drowning came next. Firearms and explosives were employed only by males. The younger suicidal deaths resulted predominantly from poisoning; the older suicidal deaths seemed likely to result from hanging-suffocation or strangulation.

2666

Chiu, E. (1977). Fart din: Vol. 1. The plight of the mentally ill Chinese in Victoria, 1867 to 1879. *Medical Journal of Australia, 1,* **541-544.**

2667

Chiu, E. (1977). Fart din: Vol. 2. More about the plight of mentally ill Chinese in Victoria, 1867 to 1875. *Medical Journal of Australia, 1,* **594-597.**

The picture of the conditions for the mentally ill Chinese in Victoria during the 19th century is not a pleasant one. However, it may be said that their colonial counterparts did not fare much better. In such a disadvantaged area of Victoria life, it does not require too much imagination to see what plight beset the Chinese in the asylums. It would have been difficult enough to cope with geographical and social dislocation, poverty, social isolation, discrimination, and struggle for survival without the additional burden of "insanity" and asylum incarceration.

2668

Chiu, E. (1984). Birth rank order and schizophrenia in Hong Kong Chinese. *Journal of the Hong Kong Psychiatric Association, 4,* **10-12, 14-15, 17-19.**

The birth rank of a sample of 890 psychiatric inpatients in Hong Kong was studied. Of the 655 patients with completed sibships selected for analysis, there were 434 schizophrenic and 221 nonschizophrenic patients. The methods of Greenwood-Yule and Slater's Index were used. For the schizophrenic sample, it was found that: (1) Male schizophrenics were more often last born than first born, and last born male schizophrenics were overrepresented in smaller families. (2) The birth-order effect was less significant for female schizophrenics, but last born female schizophrenics from larger families were overrepresented. (3) When compared with the general population, schizophrenics tended to be later born. (4) Schizophrenics from smaller families were overrepresented and those from larger families were underrepresented. For the nonschizophrenic sample, it was found that: (1) There was no significant birth-order effect for the first or the last born, but the intermediate children were underrepresented. (2) The family size of nonschizophrenics also differed from that of the general population, in the same direction as in the case of schizophrenics. (3) No birth-order effect for either sex was found when family size was controlled.

2669

Chiu, E., & Tan, E. S. (1985). Psychiatric pathology among Chinese immigrants in Victoria, Australia. In W. S. Tseng & D. Y. H. Wu (Eds.), *Chinese culture and mental health* **(pp. 251-263). Orlando, FL: Academic Press.**

2670

Chiu, L. P. W., & Yung, C. Y. (1986). A single-session encounter with a patient with a conversion disorder. *Journal of the Hong Kong Psychiatric Association, 6,* **52-54.**

2671

Chou, S. K., & Mi, C. Y. (1937). Relative neurotic tendency of Chinese and American students. *Journal of Social Psychology, 8,* **155-184.**

2672

Chu, C. H. (1961). [Mental development in the child]. *Acta Psychologica Sinica,* **No. 1, 20-32.** (In Chinese.)

2673

Chu, H. M. (1969). The social class factor in psychiatric epidemiology. *Journal of the Formosan Medical Association, 68,* **234-243.**

2674

Chu, H. M. (1972). Migration and mental disorders in Taiwan. In W. P. Lebra (Ed.), *Transcultural research in mental health: II. Mental health research in Asia and the Pacific.* **Honolulu, HI: University of Hawaii Press.**

2675

Chu, H. M., & Rin, H. (1970). [The distribution of psychiatric symptoms in a Chinese community: An application of a modified Cornell Medical Index-Health questionnaire in a psychiatric epidemiological study]. *Journal of Formosan Medical Association, 69,* **87-104.** (In Chinese.)

2676

Chu, L. W., & Liu, M. C. (1960). Mental disease in Peking between 1933-1943. *Journal of Mental Science, 106,* **274-280.**

2677

Chu, T. F., Tseng, N. P., Liu, W. M., & Kuo, Y. C. (1985). [Research on basic living skills of psychiatric patients]. *Chinese Journal of Mental Health, 2,* **47-57.** (In Chinese.)

The Comprehensive Evaluation of Basic Living Skill questionnaire (CEBLS) was given to a group of 340 psychiatric patients, both out-patients and in-patients, and to a group of 60 normal persons in order to determine their functional performance in daily living. Within the patient group, 250 subjects had a diagnosis of schizophrenia, and 90 had a diagnosis of affective disorder. The results showed that 70% of the patients showed mild to severe deficiency in performing basic living skills. Comparisons of scores of the patients from out-patient, day care, acute wards and chronic wards revealed lowest scores for patients from the chronic ward, however the differences in patient scores from out-patient, day care and acute wards were not statistically significant. Outpatients with diagnosis of schizophrenia performed more inappropriately in the basic living skills than those with affective disorders. The average CEBLS score of patients with college education were higher than those with junior or senior high school education. It was recommended that the CEBLS be used to evaluate psychiatric patients as a measure of rehabilitation.

2678

Chuang, S. M. (1979). [A chromosome study of 200 cases of Down's syndrome]. *Journal of the Formosan Medical Association, 78,* **698-705.** (In Chinese.)

A chromosome study has been carried out on 2,039 cases observed during a 10 years period (since 1968) in the cytogenetic laboratory of National Taiwan University Hospital. 200 out of 2,039 cases were found to be Down's syndrome, including 125 males an 75 females in a ratio of 1.67:1. The age varied from newborn to 22 years of age, but most of them (74%) were below 1 year of age. The 10 cardinal signs and symptoms were growth retardation, flat or saddle nose, epicanthus, simian crease, mental retardation, hypertelorism, slanting palpebral fissure, curved and/or short 5th finger, macroglossia and/or protrusion of tongue, and cardiac malformation. Cytogenetically, 180 out of 200 cases (90%) revealed the usual trisomy, 10 cases (55) revealed mosaicism, and 10 cases of translocation included 6 cases of D and G (D/G) translocation and 4 cases of G and G (G/G) translocation. The frequency of structural chromosome abnormalities, excluding chromosome gap, was 1.17% in the males and 0.84% in the females. Single chromatid break was most frequent, followed by fragment, centromere break, isochromatid break and chromatid exchange.

2679

[Control Division of Shanghai Psychiatric Institute] et al. (1980). [An epidemiologic study of mental retardation]. *Chinese Journal of Neurology & Psychiatry, 13,* **19-21.** (In Chinese.)

2680

Cox, D. J., Tsang, K., & Lee, A. (1982). A cross cultural comparison of the incidence and nature of male exhibitionism among female college students. *Victimology, 7,* **231-234.**

Studied 128 female undergraduates in Hong Kong who completed an 11-item questionnaire to estimate the incidence and nature of exhibitionism in an Asian sample and compared these findings to a similar US sample (D. J. Cox and B. McMahon, 1978). Comparisons of the 2 samples revealed no significant differences. The need is suggested for a more extensive and in-depth assessment of the incidence and nature of exhibitionism across multiple cultural samples to clarify its etiology and topography.

2681

Cramer, M. (1980). Psychopathology and shamanism in rural Mexico: A case study of spirit possession. *British Journal of Medical Psychology, 53,* **67-73.**

Reports that the so-called mystical possession of a socially marginal Chinese-Mexican 39-yr-old male of hysterical personality was directly related to the S's psychological conflicts and familial/social standing within his immediate cultural context. The personification of his personal problems in the motif of spirit possessions enabled the S to maintain a measure of self-esteem, social status, and personality integration.

2682

Cunningham, C. (1970). Korean war studies in forensic psychology. *Bulletin of the British Psychological Society, 23,* **309-311.**

The Korean war studies are seen as of doubtful value to forensic science outside the area in which they were applied. These studies did contribute some useful material to penology, clinical psychology, and the understanding of the human thought processes. It is stated that much can be learned from the Chinese use of group dynamics, though doubtless at the risk of being accused of advocating "brainwashing." Penology can profit from the lessons these Korean studies afford concerning the control of the social structure of prisoner groups and the need for extensive segregation facilities within every prison.

2683

Dai, B. (1941). Personality problems in Chinese culture. *American Sociological Review, 6,* **688-696.**

2684

Dai, B. (1958). Science and wisdom: A clinician looks at psychiatry and religion. In R. W. Kernodle (Ed.), *The sixth decade of our century: The developing fabric of American society.* **The Marshall-Wythe Symposium (pp. 35-52). (Also Virginia: Williamsburg, 1959.)**

2685

Dai, B. (1959). Obsessive-compulsive disorders in Chinese culture. In M. K. Opler (Ed.), *Culture & Mental Health* **(pp. 243-255). New York: MacMillan. (Originally published in** *Social Problems,* **1957,** *4,* **313-321.)**

2686

Dai, B. (1965). Culture and delusional systems of some Chinese mental patients. *International Journal of Social Psychiatry, 11,* **59-69.**

2687

Devoy, J. (1972). Hong Kong's runaway girls: Some reflections on the problem. *Hong Kong Journal of Social Work, 1,* **35-37.**

2688

Dominick, J. R., & Stotsky, B. A. (1969). Mental patients in nursing homes: IV. Ethnic influences. *Journal of the American Geriatrics Society, 17,* **63-85.**

Determined the unique features of various ethnic groups which affect social relationships in nursing homes. Detailed examples are given of what was observed in the following geriatric groups during visits to nursing homes: Chinese, Armenian, Roman Catholic, Jewish, predominantly Negro, and Protestant. An example is also given of people who had grown old and were cared for in their own communities by neighbors and relatives. It was evident that loneliness, aimlessness, and monotony tend to dominate the lives of most aged people in institutions. However, those who are strongly bound by ethnic, cultural, and religious ties do not feel isolated, abandoned, and hopeless.

2689

Dunner, D. L., Shen, Q. J., Zheng, Y. P., & Dunner, P. Z. (1984). A study of primary affective disorder in the People's Republic of China. *Biological Psychiatry, 19,* **353-359.**

Symptoms, course, and familial factors relating to depression were ascertained for 40 Chinese patients who had histories of primary affective disorder. In general, the symptoms, course, and familial factors among these patients were similar to findings in equivalent US populations. A high degree of diagnostic interrater reliability was demonstrated in this cross-cultural study. Depression ratings of this population and euthymic controls showed a high correlation between a self-rating scale and the Hamilton Rating Scale for Depression. Many of the currently depressed Chinese showed nonsuppression of serum cortisol after dexamethasone administration. This study suggests that affective disorder (particularly bipolar affective disorder) in China is similar to that seen in the US.

2690

Ede, A. (1976). Koro in an Anglo-Saxon Canadian. *Canadian Psychiatric Association Journal, 21,* **389-392.**

Presents the case of a 21-yr-old unmarried man, a resident of Newfoundland, who suffered from delusions of persecution and from the belief that his penis was shrinking into his abdomen. A year before his psychiatric hospitalization he had been operated on for a coccygeal cyst. He reported that after this operation he "never felt right". This patient's delusion that his penis was shrinking is like the Koro syndrome that has been reported in South China, Indonesia, and Malaya, except that (a) in those places the patients with Koro are neurotic, whereas this patient was psychotic; and (b) the Southeast Asian patients believe they will die when the penis is fully retracted, but this man did not believe he would die.

2691

Eisenbruch, M. (1983). "Wind illness" or somatic depression? A case study in psychiatric anthropology. *British Journal of Psychiatry, 143,* **323-326.**

A 46-yr-old mother with a history of chronic headaches and other symptoms and a clinical diagnosis (in Western terms) of depression ascribed her condition to her nonobservance of a Chinese postpartum ritual. The characteristic features of "wind illness" are described. Western medicine proved useless, but acupuncture was beneficial. The case underlines the importance of understanding the patient's own view of his/her illness and its causes in arriving at a correct diagnosis and intervening effectively, particularly when the gap between the doctor's and the patient's cultures is wide. The value of the distinction between the disease (the pathological process, which may be universal) and an episode of illness (the personal and cultural construction of disease) is emphasized.

2692

Endicott, J. G. (1978). China and mental health. *Canadian Psychiatric Association Journal, 23,* **353.**

2693

Epstein, I. (1985). Juvenile delinquency and reformatory education in Chinese society. *Dissertation Abstracts International, 46,* **A23-24.**

2694

Fahlisch, K. (1967). [On the use of the word "mongolism"]. *Psychiatrie, Neurologie Und Medizinische Psychologie, 19,* **391-394.** (In other language.)

Use of the term "mongolism" seems to have declined since World War II. The term does, however, appear in current Chinese and Japanese medical dictionaries. Use of the term in medical literature is traced back for more than 100 yr. Use of the more specific designation, Down's Syndrome, is recommended.

2695

Fan, Z. S. et al. (1981). [Overinclusive thinking in schizophrenia]. *Chinese Journal of Neurology & Psychiatry, 14,* **65-67.** (In Chinese.)

2696

Fields, A., & Tararin, P. A. (1970). Opium in China. *British Journal of Addiction, 64,* **371-382.**

2697

Flaskerud, J. H. (1984). A comparison of perceptions of problematic behavior by six minority groups and mental health professionals. *Nursing Research, 33,* **190-197.**

Compared the perceptions of problematic behavior and the suggested management of those behaviors by six minority groups and mental health professionals. The 159 minority respondents included Chinese Americans, Mexican Americans, Filipino Americans, Native Americans, Black Americans, and Appalachians. The 68 mental health professional respondents were from Pennsylvania, Louisiana, and California. All subjects were interviewed using a structured interview schedule. Groups were compared on responses to 10 vignettes. There were significant differences between minority and mental health professional groups, both in the labels placed on problematic behaviors and in the suggested management of the behaviors. The relationship of sample variables to response revealed that minority-group status was the strongest descriptor of group response.

2698

Gao, B. L. et al. (1981). [Investigation of cyclic adenosine monophosphate (cAMP) of the blood, urine and CSF in schizophrenics]. *Chinese Journal of Neurology & Psychiatry, 14,* **179-181.** (In Chinese.)

2699

Gao, Z. S. et al. (1981). [A clinical analysis of hallucinations in 70 cases of schizophrenia]. *Chinese Journal of Neurology & Psychiatry, 14,* **219-221.** (In Chinese.)

2700

Gardner, H. (1973). Developmental dyslexia: The forgotten lesson of Monsieur C. *Psychology Today, 7,* **62-67.**

Many children have difficulty learning to read. A 19th century French businessman suffered a stroke which made it impossible for him to read or remember the names of letters, even though he could see and copy them. Current research is making use of early suggestions that a lack of certain interconnections within the brain may be responsible for such disabilities and for the inability of certain children to learn to read. Some workers are convinced that dyslexic children can be taught to read by treating words as designs in the manner of Chinese characters.

2701

Gong-Guy, E. (1986). Depression in students of Chinese and Japanese ancestry: An acculturation, vulnerability and stress model. *Dissertation Abstracts International, 46,* **B2457-2458.**

2702

Goody, M. H. (1981). A comparative study of cross-cultural patterns of intellectual abilities on WISC and WISC-R among Anglo, Chinese, and Hispanic educationally handicapped boys with reading disabilities. *Dissertation Abstracts International, 42,* **A141.**

2703

Grauer, H. (1984). Geriatric depression in the West and the Far East. *Psychiatric Journal of the University of Ottawa, 9,* **118-120.**

In this paper it was contended that depressive illness as it is known in the West is rare in the People's Republic of China. Differences may be accounted for by the role of the family in determining help-seeking behavior; the lower incidence of divorce, alcoholism, and drug abuse; the regulation of marriage, employment, number of children, choice of living quarters, and retirement; standardized mourning rituals and supported grief; disapproval of violent behavior or tantrums in children; and the patriarchal society. Culture may contribute by providing a somatization with complete denial of depression. Neurasthenia; sexual neurasthenia; fear of cold, excess, or death; and "sourness" of heart and body associated with grief may replace depression in the Chinese cultural pattern.

2704

Gui, M. J. et al. (1986). [An investigation of mental retardation and birth defects in county of Jiangxi Province]. *Chinese Journal of Neurology and Psychiatry, 19,* **103-106.** (In Chinese.)

An investigation was made on 11,321 children under 14 years of age to determine the morbidity rates of mental retardation and birth defects. The results showed that 2.5% of the children were suffering from mental retardation and 2% from birth defects. The lower the age of the children, the higher the morbidity rate tended to be; most were mild cases. About 3/5 of the children with birth defects were found to be of school age or in their early childhood. The relation between the two kinds of diseases and population characteristics was analyzed. Practical measures for reducing the morbidity rate and methods of treatment were briefly discussed.

2705

Guo, K. J., Feng, Y. Q., & Dai, C. N. (1982). [Pathological changes in the depths of the left temporal lobe of the brain and language handicaps]. *Information on Psychological Sciences,* **No. 5, 1-6.** (In Chinese.)

2706

Gwee, A. L. (1963). Koro: A cultural disease. *Singapore Medical Journal, 4,* **119-122.**

2707

Gwee, A. L. (1968). Koro: Its origin and nature as a disease entity. *Singapore Medical Journal, 9,* **3-6.**

2708

Gwee, A. L. (1971). Traditional Chinese methods of mental treatment. In N. N. Wagner & E. S. Tan (Eds.), *Psychological problems and treatment in Malaysia.* **Kuala Lumpur: University of Malaysia Press.**

2709

Haq, S. M., & Buhrich, N. (1980). Parasuicides and their determinants in a multiracial society. *Singapore Medical Journal, 21,* **648-651.**

One hundred and forty consecutive case histories of parasuicide admitted to the Psychiatric Department of the General Hospital, Kuala Lumpur, during 1976 were examined. In the three ethnic groups studied, namely Malay, Chinese and Indian, parasuicides were similar to those reported in Western societies in that the majority were young females. They differed from Western societies in the high number of single females who were jilted, the infrequency with which alcohol was consumed and the frequency with which poison was the method chosen to attempt suicide. Reasons for these differences are discussed.

2710

Headley, L. A. (1983). *Suicide in Asia and the Near East.* **Berkeley, CA: University of California Press.**

2711

Hee, L. L. (1978). Attitudes of Chinese-American students toward mental illness: An exploratory study. *Dissertation Abstracts International, 38,* **B5542.**

2712

Hinkle, L. E., Jr., Christenson, W. N., Kane, F. D., Ostfeld, A., Thetford, W. N., & Wolff, H. G. (1958). An investigation of the relation between life experience, personality characteristics, and general susceptibility to illness. *Psychosomatic Medicine, 20,* **278-295.**

2713

Hirasawa, H., Ohashi, Y., & Hagiwara, S. (1982). [Listeners' attitudes toward stuttering -- a study on some illustrative cases in literary works]. *Japanese Journal of Special Education, 19,* **39-46.** (In other language.)

Clarifies what the kanji "kitsu" meant in ancient China and cites examples in which stuttering was used as an object of ridicule in old dramas. The listener's reaction to a stutterer is usually one of criticism, discrimination, or rejection. It is suggested that understanding, patience, and acceptance toward the stutterer would help him/her in social situations.

2714

Ho, D. Y. F. (1979). Psychological assessment and the mentally retarded child. *New Horizons,* **No. 20, 136-141.**

2715

Ho, D. Y. F. (1981). Childhood psychopathology: A dialogue with special reference to Chinese and American cultures. In A. Kleinman & L. Y. Lin (Eds.), *Normal and abnormal behavior in Chinese culture^ (pp. 137-155). Dordrecht, Netherlands: Reidel.*

A dialogue on childhood psychopathology from a cross-cultural perspective between two psychologists, Dr. Relativist and Dr. Universalist. Dr. Relativist's basic position was that the conceptualization, recognition, and treatment of psychopathology are ultimately rooted in the belief systems of a given culture; and to that extent, psychopathology is culture-specific. On the other hand, Dr. Universalist believed that there are certain features instrinsic to psychopathology which are invariant across cultures and which render it recognizable within any cultural context; hence, psychopathology is a universal. The discussion was focused especially on a contrast between the Chinese and the American perspectives. Their dialogue may be divided into four main sections: (a) childhood psychopathology and its relationship with how childhood and the parent-child relationship are conceptualized in different cultures, with respect to both time and space; (b) issues of culture-specificity versus culture-invariance and the conceptualization of psychopathology in general; (c) the problem of how different psychopathological conditions are differentiated and classified, together with a detailed discussion of hyperactivity and aggression in Chinese and American children; and (d) concluding remarks.

2716

Ho, Y. F., & Liu, J. H. (1981). [A critique of "A survey of minimal brain dysfunction"]. Information on Psychological Sciences, *No. 5, 44-45. (In Chinese.)*

This is a critique of the report "A survey of minimal brain dysfunction" (MBD). Methodological, theoretical and ethical issues are discussed: (a) To interpret children's behavioral problems (regarded as clinical manifestations of MBD by the report's authors) solely in terms of self-control deficit leaves out of consideration the importance of environmental conditions; it is also necessary to point out clearly that not all children having this deficit are suffering from MBD; (b) The diagnosis of MBD depends largely on the relative tolerance level of adults (parents, teachers, and doctors) who make judgments of children's behavior; (c) the use of labels, such as MBD, entails professional-ethical implications that cannot be ignored, and (d) an overreliance on drugs in treatment amounts to an evasion of educational responsibilities.

2717

Hock, C. B. (1979). Suicide of the elderly in Singapore. Annals of the Academy of Medicine *(Singapore),* **8,** *290-297.*

2718

Hock, C. B. (1979). A prospective study of suicides among the mentally ill in a specialist practice. Annals of the Academy of Medicine *(Singapore),* **8,** *287-289.*

2719

Hock, C. B. (1979). Suicide of the young in Singapore. Annals of the Academy of Medicine *(Singapore),* **8,** *262-268.*

2720

Holzner, A. S., & Ding, L. K. (1973). White dragon pearls in Hong Kong: A study of young women drug addicts. International Journal of the Addictions, 8, *253-263.*

Interviewed 14 female drug addicts under 25 yrs of age in Hong Kong. Results show poverty, weak family relationships, early school withdrawal, and lack of vocational training as predictors of drug addiction. These factors were reinforced by feelings of loneliness, desire for a stable family life, lack of clear life goals, and perception of an indifferent society. Higher income was the main attraction of occupations which border on the drug subculture (e.g., dance-hall hostess and prostitute). Companionship, enjoyment, and relief from daily problems were cited as reasons for associating with drugs. Social problems peculiar to Hong Kong are considered, as well as economic factors which precipitate drug use.

2721

Hore, B. D. et al. (1973). Male transsexualism: Two cases in a single family. Archives of Sexual Behavior, 2, *317-321.*

Reports the case of 2 Chinese brothers who underwent sex-change surgery to female status. Early life experiences of the 2 siblings differed from those of their nontranssexual brothers and sisters. The pretranssexual Ss were raised primarily by the maternal grandmother, whereas the others were reared by their parents. Feminine role orientation began during childhood and continued through adolescence. Sex-change surgery was performed during adulthood in 2 stages, and both Ss are currently living as females.

2722

Hornstein, H. A., & Mosley, J. L. (1979). Iconic-memory processing of unfamiliar stimuli by retarded and nonretarded individuals. American Journal of Mental Deficiency, 84, *40-48.*

The iconic-memory processing of unfamiliar stimuli was studied using a visually cued partial-report procedure and a visual masking procedure. 11 retarded and 22 CA- and MA-matched males viewed stimulus arrays of 6 Chinese characters arranged in a circular pattern for 100 msec. At variable stimulus-onset asynchronies, a teardrop indicator or an annulus was presented for 100 msec. Immediately upon cue offset, the S was required to recognize the cued stimulus from a card containing a single character. Retarded Ss' performance was comparable to that of MA- and CA-matched Ss. It is suggested that earlier reported iconic-memory differences between retarded and nonretarded individuals may be attributable to processes other than iconic memory.

2723

Hsia, C. Y. et al. (1958). [Clinical analysis and postdischarge investigation of 2,000 cases of schizophrenia]. Chinese Journal of Neurology and Psychiatry, 4, *89-94. (In Chinese.)*

2724

Hsia, C. Y. et al. (1980). [A follow-up study on 704 cases of affective psychosis and a discussion on the classification of its monophasia and biphasia]. Chinese Journal of Neurology & Psychiatry, 13, *151-153. (In Chinese.)*

2725

Hsia, C. Y., & Ling, Y. H. (1957). [Clinical observations of childhood schizophrenia]. Chinese Journal of Neurology and Psychiatry, 3, *145-151. (In Chinese.)*

2726

Hsia, Y. F., & Tsai, N. (1981). Symptomatologie precoce chez 250 patients chinois, atteints de schizophrenie simple [Early symptomatology in a group of 250 Chinese patients with simple schizophrenia]. Psychologie Medicale, 13, *2133-2136. (In other language.)*

250 Chinese patients with simple schizophrenia were divided into the following classifications: apathy, motiveless smiling (56 cases); deterioration of good relation attitude (38 cases); violence toward the surrounding society (36 cases); suicide without particular reasons, free-floating fear and anxiety (8 cases); suspicion (36 cases); erotomania delusion (13 cases); abstract thinking (6 cases); and pathological thinking (6 cases). Retardation and mutism were revealed in 59 cases, apragmatism in 59, and disobedience to rules and regulations in 44. The total amount of clinical symptoms of simple schizophrenia in 250 schizophrenics was 559. From this number, 454 symptoms were directly connected with the disorder.

2727

Hsia, Y. F., & Tsai, N. (1981). Transcultural investigation of recent symptomatology of schizophrenia in China. American Journal of Psychiatry, 138, *1484-1486.*

During the past 15 years a number of new symptoms, rarely seen in the past, have been observed with increasing frequency among Chinese schizophrenic patients. The authors identify the following symptoms: discordant (dissociative) syndrome, denial of lineage, delusion of leadership lineage, delusion of being married, child-bearing delusion, delusion of being despised, delusion of imminent catastrophe, delusion of influence, inferential delusion, delusion of being experimented on, delusion of conducting an experiment, delusion of being cultivated by superiors, delusion of being tested, delusion of being examined, delusion of impending arrest, delusion of being slandered, mirror symptom, and changing dialects.

2728

Hsu, C. C. (1966). A study on "problem children" reported by teachers. Japanese Journal of Child Psychiatry, 7, *91-108.*

This is the report of a mental health survey covering 8,329 children in one of the largest elementary schools in Teipei. The results were: (1) More boys (4.4%) than girls (2.5%) were considered to be problem children by their teachers. (2) The number of problem children reached its peak at the fourth grade for boys and at the fifth grade for girls, resulting primarily from a marked increase in problems associated with acting out and learning attitudes. (3) The overall prevalence rate of 3.5% is much lower than those reported in earlier studies in the United Stated and Britain. A much higher prevalence rate of 12% was obtained from teachers after they attended mental health seminars. (4) The acting-out type of disciplinary problems were reported with the highest frequency, about four times as frequently as behavior problems such as passivity, overdependency, and shyness. (5) No problems related to sex, toilet habits, or obsessive-compulsive behavior were reported by teachers, and even after the seminars these problems were identified only rarely. The question is raised as to whether this reflected an actual low level of psychosexual and psychophysiological urinary problems, or an indifference or reluctance to bring such problems to the open in Chinese culture.

2729

Hsu, C. C. (1973). [A comparative study of well and maladjusted first grade boys in an urban public junior middle school]. Journal of the Formosan Medical Association, 72, *167-183. (In Chinese.)*

2730

Hsu, E. H. (1951). The neurotic score as a function of culture. Journal of Social Psychology, 34, *3-30.*

2731

Hsu, F. L. K. (1952). Sex crime and personality: A study in comparative cultural patterns. American Scholar, 21, *57-66.*

2732

Hsu, L. R. (1984). Loneliness: In foreign students and depressed clients. Dissertation Abstracts International, 45, *B1289.*

2733

Hsu, Y. H. (1955). [Psychopathology in ancient China]. Chinese Journal of Neurology & Psychiatry, 1, *167-174. (In Chinese.)*

2734

Hsu, Y. H. (1956). [A brief introduction to psychopathology in China during the Jin, Southern and Northern, Sui, and Tang dynasties]. Chinese Journal of Neurology and Psychiatry, 2, *14-19. (In Chinese.)*

2735

Hsu, Y. H. (1959). [Introduction to psychiatry from Chin to Sui-T'ang dynasties]. Chung-kuo shen-ching ching-shen k'o tsa-chih, 1, *14-19. (In Chinese.)*

2736

Hu, C. Q. (1986). [Effects of brain damage on the cognitive process of reading]. Acta Psychologica Sinica, 18, *58-62. (In Chinese.)*

2737

Hu, C. Q. (1986). [A study of the effects of reading disability caused by brain damage on the cognitive process of reading]. Acta Psychologica Sinica, 18, *58-62. (In Chinese.)*

On the basis of two typical case studies of different reading disability caused by brain damage, this paper made two inferences: (1) The reading process undergoes two different levels of information processing; the level of word recognition, and the level of sentence comprehension. (2) The psychological activity at the sentence level plays a more active and effective dynamic role in the reading and understanding process.

2738

Hu, H. K., Chang, L. Y., & Wu, Y. C. (1984). [Problems of psychological (psychiatric) illnesses]. In K. S. Yang & C. C. Yeh (Eds.), [Social problems in Taiwan] *(2nd ed.). Taipei: Chu Liu. (In Chinese.)*

2739

Hu, Y. H., & Li, H. C. (1958). [Analysis of cases of the compulsive syndrome]. Chinese Journal of Neurology and Psychiatry, 4, *75-79. (In Chinese.)*

2740

Huang, H. C., Hwang, K. K., & Ko, Y. H. (1983). [Life stress, attribution style, social support and depression among university students]. Acta Psychologica Taiwanica, 25, *31-47. (In Chinese.)*

The purposes of this study were: (1) to investigate the relationship between attribution style and depression; (2) to examine the attribution of "yuan" (natural affinity) in normal and depressive groups; (3) to assess the relationships between objective life stress, and subjective life stress ,and depression, and compare the perception of life events in normal and depressive groups; (4) to find the life events that are correlated with depression; and (5) to examine the relationship between social support and depression and test Ko's formula of mental health. A revised Life Events Scale, Social Support Scale and Depression Scale were administrated to 273 male and 237 female university students. The important findings included: (1) Those subjects who tended to attribute negative life events to internal, stable and global factors were more depressive. Depressive subjects tended to attribute the events to uncontrollable factors. (2) Normal subjects tended to attribute negative events to "yuan" more than depressive subjects did. (3) Objective life stress scores and subjective life stress scores were positively correlated with depression scores. (4) The life events which correlated with depression included frustration in economy, interpersonal relationship and academic achievement. 6) Social support scores were negatively correlated with depressive scores. When the social support scores were used as the index of ego strength, life stress divided by ego strength scores were positively correlated with depressive scores.

2741

Huang, L. J. (1963). The problem child and delinquent youth in the Communist Chinese family. Marriage and Family Living, 25, *459-465.*

2742

Huang, M. H., & Huang, J. T. (1985). [Perceptual distortions in schizophrenics]. Chinese Journal of Mental Health, 2, *23-31. (In Chinese.)*

2743

Huang, R. L. (1981). [A survey of minimal brain dysfunction in children of 11 primary schools and kindergartens in East Hill District Guangzhou]. Chinese Journal of Neurology & Psychiatry, 14, *32-35. (In Chinese.)*

2744

Huang, S. W. et al. (1967). A cytogenetic study of 77 Chinese children with Down's Syndrome. Journal Of Mental Deficiency Research, 11, *147-152.*

Results indicate that the cytogenetic studies are within the ranges found for other ethnic groups in other countries. Maternal age of trisomy g cases in this series was markedly elevated compared to the related general population.

2745

Hung, Y. Y. (1978). [Internal-external locus of control in physically handicapped students]. Bulletin of Educational Psychology, 11, *113-122. (In Chinese.)*

The purposes of this study were to explore the differences in internal-external locus of control between physically handicapped students and nonhandicapped students and to investigate if two different education programs (segregation vs. integration) would affect the locus of control of the physically handicapped students. The Nowicki-Strickland's Locus of Control Scale was given to 240 junior high level students. The subjects included three groups: (1) the physically handicapped students in special school, (2) the physically handicapped students in junior high school, and (3) nonhandicapped students in junior high school. The results indicated that the physically handicapped students, both in special school and in junior high school, were more external than the nonhandicapped students.

2746

Hung, Y. Y. (1982). [Psychological characters among the mentally retarded, and gifted students in junior high schools]. Bulletin of Educational Psychology, 15, *167-193. (In Chinese.)*

Investigated differences in psychological makeup among 240 mentally retarded, normal, and gifted students in the Taipei area. Ss were assessed using the Self-Concept Inventory, Achievement Motivation Questionnaire, General Anxiety Scale for Children, Test Anxiety Scale for Children, and the Intellectual Academic Responsibility Questionnaire. By means of correlation analysis and ANOVA, it was found that (1) the retarded Ss had lower self-concept, achievement motivation, and internal responsibility than the other Ss; (2) males had higher scores in self-identification and lower scores in both general and test anxiety than did females; and (3) males manifested higher self-acceptance and achievement motivation than did females in the normal and gifted groups. It is suggested that mental retardation may lead to a disadvantage in psychological adjustment.

2747

Hwang, C. H. (1956). [Intelligence and criminal behavior]. Psychological Testing, 4, *280-288. (In Chinese.)*

2748

Hwang, C. H. (1959). [A Psychological study of juvenile delinquents in Taiwan]. Psychological Testing, 7, *526-536. (In Chinese.)*

2749

Hwang, C. J. (1966). [A study of new indices of the Rorschach Test for clinical diagnosis]. Acta Psychologica Taiwanica, 8, *69-78. (In Chinese.)*

2750

Hwang, M. T., & Chen, M. J. (1984). [A study of self-concept in persons with schizophrenia]. Chinese Journal of Psychology, 26, *85-93. (In Chinese.)*

The Tennessee Self-Concept Scale was administered to 200 schizophrenic patients treated in four departments of occupational therapy and 189 normal subjects. A comparison of self-concept between the study group and the control group indicated that: (1) The study group had significantly lower Physical-Self, Family-Self, Identity, Self-Satisfaction, Behavior, Self-Criticism, and Total-Self scores. (2) There was no evident difference in Moral-Ethical-Self, Personal-Self, and Social-Self scores. (3) The study group showed no sex difference in self-concept scores, except for the Moral-Ethical-Self score.

2751

Hwang, W. T. (1976). Epidemic hysteria in a Malaysian Chinese extended family. Medical Journal of Malaysia, 31, *108-112.*

The only recorded epidemic hysteria affecting a Chinese extended family over a 13 day period occurred in four nuclear families staying in a rural squatter area seven miles from Kuala Lumpur. Data was collected during personal interviews, home visits, field trips and hospitalization of two of the siblings. On the 1st night, during a religious ceremony for a sister-in-law who had died during puerperium, a brother ran out and screamed that evil spirits were chasing him. By the 3rd day, five siblings and a brother-in-law were involved. A brother was brought to a general practitioner on the 5th night, while the active managements of a bomoh and some spirit mediums were going on the 6th day, friends felt constrained to accept an offer to hospitalize a brother for psychiatric treatment. This brother was subsequently brought for hospitalization on the 13th day, while another brother was hospitalized on the 8th day. Lay and psychiatric diagnoses and management in a Malaysian sociocultural background are discussed.

2752

Ja, D. Y. (1981). The Chinese aged in America: Housing conditions and their effect on health and psychosomatic symptoms. Dissertation Abstracts International, 42, *B1609-1610.*

2753

Jacques, M. E., Burleigh, D. L., & Lee, G. (1973). Reactions to disabilities in China: A comparative, structural and descriptive analysis. Rehabilitation Counseling Bulletin, 16, *206-217.*

Examined the attitudes of Chinese on Taiwan toward disablement and compared them with samples of Danes, Greeks, and Americans. The Taiwan sample consisted of 296 17-41 yr. old Ss, mostly students. Ss responded to the Attitudes Toward Disabled Persons (ATDP), the Feeling Check List (FE), Social Distance Scale (SD), and Social Distance Residence Scale (SDR). The FE and SD are modifications of the ones developed by J. Siller, and the SDR is a modification of SD. The samples of non-Chinese Ss were the ones used by M. E. Jacques et al. Data were analyzed by multivariate analysis of variance. The United States sample ranked first (p .05) on the ATDP, SD, and

SDR followed by Denmark, China, and Greece. A difference between the Chinese and Americans is that disability among the former is a responsibility of the family. The principal components analysis of the SD, SDR, and FE reveals that the attitudinal dimensions toward disability are multidimensional with 2 of the dimensions being level of response and disability type.

2754

Jian, H. L. (1983). [Sex role and socio-economic status differences between delinquents and non-delinquents]. Journal of Education & Psychology, 6, *157-159. (In Chinese.)*

2755

Jiang, Z. N. et al. (1986). [Changes in the admission rate and episode features of hysteria in the past 25 years]. Chinese Journal of Neurology and Psychiatry, 19, *268-271. (In Chinese.)*

The authors analyzed a sample of 179 cases drawn from 2,434 hospitalized hysteric patients over the past 25 years. It was found that since 1967 admission rates have decreased from 6.3-6.6% to 1.4-2.2%. This decrease may be attributable to the steady development of mental health facilities. Outburst of emotion, somatic seizure, twilight state, and possession symptoms were preponderant in the majority of cases. No significant difference over the years was found between the total number of dissociative and that of conversion cases. Typical hysterial personality was found in only one fourth all cases. Conflicts in the family and difficulties in adaptation were causative factors most frequently seen. There were very few cases involving loss in life events.

2756

Jilek, W., & Jilek-Aall, L. (1977). [Mass hysteria with koro symptoms in Thailand]. Schweizer Archiv fur Neurologie, Neurochirurgie und Psychiatrie, 120, *257-259. (In other language.)*

Reports an epidemic of koro, a psychogenic anxiety syndrome interfering with genital body image and sexual functioning, hitherto occurring mainly in isolated cases of South Chinese males. The present outbreaks occurred in northeastern Thailand where within a few days at least 200 patients, most of them Thai and 66% males, were treated at local hospitals. The main presenting symptoms included acute anxiety, (subjective) shrinking of the penis and impotency in men, shrinking and/or itching of the external genitals and frigidity in women; further complaints included nausea, dizziness, abdominal pains, headaches, and facial numbness. All Ss recovered after brief symptomatic intervention. Popular opinion and news media echoed the Ss' paranoid projection of viewing the epidemic as caused by Vietnamese food and tobacco poisoning in an assault against the sexual vitality and general health of the Thai people, in the context of a specific sociocultural and politico-historical situation. It is suggested that an adequate interpretation of koro and of analogous hysterical symptom formation would have to consider the specific sociodynamic factors involved in the pathogenesis of such phenomena.

2757

Jung, S. S., Chen, K. M., & Brody, J. A. (1973). Paroxysmal choreoathetosis: Report of Chinese cases. Neurology, 23, *749-755.*

Reports the 1st documentation of paroxysmal choreoathetosis among the Chinese. In the world literature most cases are familial although sporadic cases have been documented. Inheritance is usually an autosomal dominant trait with incomplete penetrance although autosomal recessive transmission has been reported. 2 sporadic cases and 10 cases in 2 families are described. The mode of inheritance in 1 family was autosomal dominant with incomplete penetrance, while in the 2nd family apparent recessive transmission occurred. In the family with dominant transmission only male members were affected. This has been reported previously and suggests that in some instances expression of the disease in females carrying the gene is reduced. The dramatic attacks observed in these cases do not differ from those described in other series. 1 patient described a type of aura consisting of a peculiar sensation in his mouth hours to days before an attack. This aura has not been previously described and was not present in the other patients.

2758

Kadri, Z. N. (1975). A twelve year survey of schizophrenia in a South East Asian university. Journal of the American College Health Association, 23, *313-317.*

2759

Kadri, Z. N. (1975). Schizophrenia and academic performance. Medical Journal of Malaysia, 29, *250-257.*

2760

Kane, F. D., Richter, P., Hinkle, L. E., Jr., & Wolff, H. G. (1956). Illness, attitudes and behavior patterns in a group of "healthy" Chinese. Archives of Neurology and Psychiatry, 76, *271. (Also in* **Journal of Nervous and Mental Disease,** *1956,* **123,** *408.)*

2761

Kasamatsu, A. (1942). Uber die vergleichend psychiatrische Untersuchung in einem Dorfe bei Cantong. Psychiatria et Neurologia Japonica, 46, *188-194. (In other language.)*

2762

Kau, L. J., Hwang, K. K., & Lin, S. M. (1985). [Relationship between high-risk factors and minimal brain dysfunction in learning disabled children]. Chinese Journal of Mental Health, 2, *107-114. (In Chinese.)*

2763

Khoo, T. P. (Ed.). (1986). Mental health in Hong Kong. *Hong Kong: Mental Health Association of Hong Kong.*

2764

Kim, B. L. S. (1973). Asian Americans: No model minority. Mental Health Digest, 5, *42-46.*

2765

Kinzie, J. D., Ryals, J., Cottington, F., & McDemott, J. F. (1973). Cross-cultural study of depressive symptoms in Hawaii. International Journal of Social Psychiatry, 19, *19-24.*

2766

Kinzie, J. D., & Tseng, W. S. (1978). Cultural aspects of psychiatric clinic utilization: A cross-cultural study in Hawaii. International Journal of Social Psychiatry, 24, *177-188.*

Data were obtained by ethnic status from 411 outpatients at a Honolulu psychiatric clinic and were analyzed according to demographic variables, welfare status, source of referral, primary complaints or symptoms, diagnosis, and duration of treatment received. Clinic utilization was highly related to ethnicity, with Caucasians overrepresented in proportion to the population, and other groups, especially Japanese, being underrepresented. The Caucasians were more likely to be self-referred, to have symptoms of anxiety and depression, and to receive a neurotic diagnosis. The Japanese, and to some extent all other groups, were more often referred after a crisis or severe mental illness, displayed more socially disruptive symptoms, and had a higher percentage of schizophrenic diagnoses. Review of therapist case loads and analysis of duration of treatment revealed no ethnic difference in the clinic's response to patients.

2767

Kitano, H. H. L. (1970). Mental illness in four cultures. Journal of Social Psychology, 80, *121-134.*

2768

Kleinman, A. (1986). Social origins of distress and disease: Depression, neurasthenia and pain in modern China. *New Haven: Yale University Press.*

This book presents an overview of neurasthenia, depression, somatization, and pain, through a discussion of their historical background and current significance in China and North America, as well as cross-culturally. It attempts to understand how culture relates to emotions, mental illness, and human distress generally, and to discuss more specific aspects of illness experience among Chinese patients. The interpretation of distress and suffering by laymen and health professionals in China is examined, compared and contrasted with Western, particularly American, cultures. A number of case studies are presented to illustrate somatization as illness experience and its social causes.

2769

Kleinman, A., & Kleinman, J. (1985). Somatization: The interconnections in Chinese society among culture, depressive experiences, and the meanings of pain. In A. Kleinman & B. Good (Eds.), Culture and Depression: Studies in the anthropology and cross-cultural psychiatry of affect and disorder *(pp. 429-490). Berkeley, CA: University of California Press.*

2770

Kleinman, A., & Lin, T. Y. (Eds.). (1981). Normal and abnormal behavior in Chinese culture. *Dordrecht, Netherlands: Reidel.*

Much of the data presented in this volume came from research in Chinese communities outside of China. Despite this, the volume represents an extensive overview divided into four sections: (a) historical and cultural background, (b) child development and childhood psychopathology, (c) family studies, and (d) psychiatric studies.

2771

Kleinman, A. M. (1977). Depression, somatization and the "new cross-cultural" psychiatry. Social Science & Medicine, 11, *3-12.*

Uses material from field research in Taiwan and data from recent anthropological and clinical investigations to criticize S. Singer's contention that the features of depressive disorders do not exhibit significant cross-cultural differences. The present author contends that such differences do exist and are a function of the cultural shaping of normative and deviant behavior. Somatization among Chinese depressives is used as an illustration. This discrepancy is seen as reflecting substantial changes in the nature of more recent cross-cultural studies by anthropologists and psychiatrists, changes which are giving rise to a new cross-cultural approach to psychiatric issues. Some features and implications of that approach are described.

2772

Kleinman, A. M. (1982). Neurasthenia and depression: A study of somatization and culture in China. Culture, Medicine & Psychiatry, 6, *117-190.*

Reviews conceptual and empirical issues regarding the interaction of neurasthenia (NA), somatization, and depression in Chinese and Western cultures. The historical background of NA and its current status are discussed, along with the epidemiology and phenomenology of somatization and depression. Findings are presented from a combined and anthropological field study of 100 18-56 yr old NA patients. 87 Ss had the DSM-III criteria of major depressive disorder (MDD); diagnoses of anxiety disorders were also frequent. 44 Ss were suffering from chronic pain syndromes previously undiagnosed, and cases of culture-bound syndromes also were detected. For 75% of the Ss the social significance and uses of their illness behavior chiefly related to work. Although 70% of Ss with MDD experienced substantial improvement and 87% some improvement in symptoms when treated with antidepressants, fewer experienced decreased help seeking, and a much smaller number perceived less social impairment and improvement in illness problems (the psychosocial accompaniment of disease including maladaptive coping and work, family, and school problems). It is concluded that NA is most clinically useful when it is regarded as bioculturally patterned illness experience (a special form of somatization) related to either depression and other diseases or to culturally sanctioned idioms of distress and psychosocial coping.

2773

Kleinman, A., & Mechanic, D. (1979). Some observations of mental illness and its treatment in the People's Republic of China. Journal of Nervous & Mental Disease, 167, *267-274.*

The authors discussed the epidemiology of mental illness in China, noting the absence of any reliable data. Also discussed were the delivery of services to the mentally ill and general psychiatric theory and practice.

2774

Knox, V. J., Shum, K., & McLaughlin, D. M. (1977). Response to cold pressor pain and to acupuncture analgesia in oriental and occidental subjects. Pain, 4, *49-57.*

On a no-treatment trial, a group of 24 oriental subjects rated cold pressor pain as significantly more painful and distressing than did a group of 24 occidental subjects. For half of the Orientals and half of the Occidentals, a second trial was conducted after acupuncture analgesia had been induced. The remaining 12 Orientals and 12 Occidentals served as no-treatment controls on trial 2. Regardless of racial group, there was no difference between the pain of those experimental subjects who received acupuncture and the pain of those controls who did not. As they had on trial 1, Orientals reported significantly more pain and distress in response to ice water on trial 2. It is concluded that: if acupuncture does work better for the Chinese than for other racial groups, the likely cause is a more refined patient selection procedure rather than an inherent difference in response to acupuncture; the evidence does not support the stereotyped view of Orientals as stoical in the face of physical pain.

2775

Ko, Y. H. (1962). The discrepancy between the B-G score and the sum of the object-assembly and the block-design test scores as an indicator of organicity. Acta Psychologica Taiwanica, *No. 4, 72-77.*

2776

Ko, Y. H. (1964). The item analysis of the KMHQ Paranoid Scale. Acta Psychologica Taiwanica, 6, *21-27.*

2777

Ko, Y. H., & Sun, L. C. (1965 - 1966). Ordinal position and the behavior of visiting the child guidance clinic (Reports 1 and 2). Acta Psychologica Taiwanica, *1965,* **7,** *10-16 (Report 1); 1966,* **8,** *92-95 (Report 2).*

The present study investigated whether birth order of psychiatric patients is related to the rate of seeking help from psychiatric doctors in Chinese culture. By comparing the case distribution on each of five birth-order categories of the experimental group with that of the control group, it was found that in the patient group, but not the normal group, the only son and the only daughter had much higher percentages than the middle child and the youngest son. The possibilities of influence of family size and parental age on these relationships were dismissed. The proneness hypothesis and the parents' attitude hypothesis were instead proposed. The proneness hypothesis stated that children of certain birth orders were more prone to disturbance; the parents' attitude hypothesis stated children of certain ordinal positions were more likely to be brought by their parents to see a psychiatrist. The case number distribution over various birth-order categories of 146 children who visited the Taipei Children's Mental Health Center because of neurological problems was compared with that of 547 children who visited the same institution for behavioral problems. The results were interpreted as not supporting the parents'attitude hypothesis.

2778

Kok, L. P. (1984). History of incest in a parasuicide population in Singapore. Australian & New Zealand Journal of Psychiatry, 18, *188-190.*

Three cases of suicide attempts occurring in 1982 that involved incest at an earlier age were presented. Subjects appeared to be the helpless young victims of older and more dominant brothers. Certain dialectic

Chinese groups foster an anomalous situation of "sister" wife in their practice of infant betrothal.

2779

Koo, L. C. L. (1982). Nourishment of life: Health in Chinese society. *Hong Kong: Commercial Press.*

2780

Kraft, A. M., & Swift, S. S. (1979). Impressions of Chinese psychiatry, December 1978. Psychiatric Quarterly, 51, *83-91.*

2781

Krcek-Frank, R. (1980). Psychosomatic problems in the People's Republic of China. Journal of Psychiatric Nursing and Mental Health Services, *15-18.*

2782

Ku, Y. C. (1956). [Narcolepsy]. Chinese Journal of Neurology and Psychiatry, 2, *296-299. (In Chinese.)*

2783

Kua, E. H., & Tsoi, W. F. (1985). Suicide in the island of Singapore. Acta Psychiatrica Scandinavica, 71, *227-229.*

A study of suicide in Singapore in 1980 indicated 230 cases and a rate of 9.5 suicides per 100,000 people. Age-specific rates increased steeply after 50 years of age; there was a male preponderance especially in the age group over 60 years. The highest rate of suicide was in the Indians and Chinese, whereas the Malays had the lowest. Fifty-nine of the subjects had mental illness, mainly schizophrenia, and they were generally younger (20-39 years of age).

2784

Kung, Y. H. (1963). [An EEG and clinical study of the cortical function of neurasthenics]. Acta Psychologica Sinica, *No. 1, 65-74. (In Chinese.)*

The electroencephalographic (EEG) responses of 150 neurasthenics were compared with those of 30 normal subjects, and sypmtoms of the neurasthenics were studied. The results indicated: (1) the EEG of patients were different from those of normal subjects in terms of basic rhythms, amplitudes and the reactions to sound and light stimuli; (2) the EEG of the 150 neurasthenics could be classified into 5 groups according to the characteristics of basic rhythms; (3) there was some relationship between the EEG and the symptoms of the patients.

2785

Kung, Y. H. (1965). [An experimental study of the abstraction and generalization processes in schizophrenics: Vol. 1]. Acta Psychologica Sinica, *No. 1, 76-84. (In Chinese.)*

A sorting test was administered to 100 normals and 128 schizophrenics. The test consisted of four sets of materials: 25 pictorial cards; 16 Chinese characters printed on separate cards; 23 wooden blocks of different colors, forms, and sizes; and 10 cards, each showing four meaningful contents, three of which were closely related. Each subject was asked to classify the first three sets of test materials presented in succession and to give reasons for the classifications made. The subject was then asked to point out the outstanding content in each of the 10 cards of the remaining set. The results were: (1) For both normals and schizophrenics, the quality of classification was positively associated with educational level. (2) The percentage of correct classifications for normals was definitely higher than for schizophrenics. (3) Reaction time was shorter for normals than for schizophrenics. (4) Many classifications made by schizophrenics were not only poor in quality but also devious.

2786

Kung, Y. H. (1966). [An experimental study on the abstraction and generalisation processes in schizophrenics: Vol. 2. A comparison of schizophrenics with other patients]. Acta Psychologica Sinica, *No. 2, 124-129. (In Chinese.)*

2787

Kuo, W. H. (1984). Prevalence of depression among Asian-Americans. Journal of Nervous & Mental Disease, 172, *449-457.*

Depression Scale, Chinese- & Japanese- & Filipino- & Korean-Americans. Administered the Center for Epidemiological Studies Depression Scale to 499 Chinese-, Japanese-, Filipino-, Korean-Americans. Findings indicate that the prevalence of depression among Asian-Americans is at least as high as that of the White population and support the interpretation that Asian underutilization of mental health services is not the reflection of a lesser need for services. Factor analysis revealed a pattern of symptoms that was similar among the Koreans, Japanese, and Chinese. Four factors, accounting for 53% of the variance, were identified: Positive Affect, Depressed Affect, Somatic and Retarded Activity, and Interpersonal Problems. Ss tended to express depression through a combination of mood and somatic descriptors. Newer immigrants, notably the Koreans, were more likely to show adjustment problems.

2788

Kuo, W. H., & Gray, R. (1979). Locus of control and symptoms of psychological distress among Chinese-Americans. International Journal of Social Psychiatry, 25, *176-187.*

A sample of Chinese-Americans in the District of Columbia was drawn to examine the relationship between the locus of control, the personality factor, and two indices of symptoms of psychological distress. The findings indicated that externals scored higher on symptomatology than did internals. A multivariate analysis further compared the predictive utility of locus of control with other determinants of psychiatric symptoms, namely, sex, marital status, socioeconomic status, kinship and friendship tie, and amount of life change. The evidence showed that locus of control is an important determinant of Chinese-Americans' symptomatology, accounting for a greater proportion of the variance in the two indices of psychological distress than did the other independent variables.

2789

Kuo, Y. Y. (1973). Identity-diffusion and Tai-Pau gang delinquency in Taiwan. Adolescence, 8, *165-170.*

Discusses the rise of the Tai-pau gangs in 1949 and characterizes their members and group activities. Erikson's theory of self-identity and identity diffusion serves to explain the motivation for the gang activities which were characterized by a strong but unwritten code of loyalty and toughness, assaults (mainly on police), great dependence on group approval, and over identification with leaders or heroes of the gangs. The 5-9 member gangs wore cowboy-like outfits, rode high-seat bicycles, and usually armed themselves with leather belts, chains, and folding knives.

2790

Kwong, B., & Wong, S. W. (1981). Physical presentations of psychological problems among Hong Kong Chinese: Cultural implications. Journal of the Hong Kong Psychiatric Association, 1, *33-39.*

2791

Lai, P. C. (1973). [A relationship between juvenile delinquents' criminal behavior and psychological characteristics]. Bulletin of Educational Psychology, 6, *77-89. (In Chinese.)*

The purpose of this study was to investigate the relationship between juvenile delinquents' criminal behavior and their psychological characteristics. A sample of 239 subjects was chosen from a prison and a reformatory: 96 thieves, 61 robbers, 72 murderers, and 10 cheaters. They were given intelligence and personality tests. The results were: (1) Thieves' IQs were lower than those of murderers and cheaters. (2) The aggression of murderers was not stronger than those of thieves and cheaters. (3) Robbers had a more depressive disposition than thieves, murderers, and cheaters. (4) Thieves had a more social-extravert disposition than robbers and murderers.

2792

Lamont, J., & Gottlieb, H. (1975). Convergent recall of parental behaviors in depressed students of different racial groups. Journal of Clinical Psychology, 31, *9-11.*

Administered to 367 college students a measure of depression and a measure of recall of parental behavior. Ss were 43 Chinese-Americans, 81 Mexican-Americans and 243 Whites. Depression scores were correlated with item endorsement on the recall of parental behavior scale for each race. Seven parental behavior items that produced significant correlations with depression across racial groups were identified, which indicates that depressed Ss recalled their mothers as less positively involved with them and as more guilt-inducing. Results provided cross-cultural confirmation of prior findings in this area.

2793

Lamont, J., & Tyler, C. (1973). Racial differences in rate of depression. Journal of Clinical Psychology, 29, *428-432.*

Administered a 79-item self-report depression questionnaire to 473 American undergraduates of 5 racial groups. Coefficients of congruence computed between 1st factors for each race and the 1st factor of the entire sample were judged satisfactory, and racial groups were compared by means of factor scores on the 1st factor (labeled Depression) produced by the entire sample. It is considered that these procedures avoid problems usually encountered in cross-cultural comparisons. Significant differences were found, and racial groups scored highest to lowest in the following order: Japanese-American, Mexican-American, Chinese-American, Caucasian, and Negro.

2794

Lander, B. (1954). Towards an understanding of juvenile delinquency. *New York: Columbia University Press.*

2795

Lau, B. W. K. (1981). The medical recommendation for psychiatric remands into prison: The Hong Kong scene. Medicine, Science, & the Law, 21, *57-65.*

A review is made of all the remand cases who were referred from the courts to a Government psychiatric unit. Altogether 607 defendants were assessed during a 24-month period. Most of the cases belonged to the 19-39 age group. It is noted that over half of the remands were not mentally disordered, and a psychiatric diagnosis was possible in less than half of the sample. A considerable number had a history of previous psychiatric contacts. The nature of offences varied, involving those against the person, property, and public order. Schizophrenics committing offences against the person of a nonsexual nature formed the largest subgroup. On the whole, the schizophrenics were the most frequently remanded for psychiatric examination, the most likely to be recommended for a medical disposal, and almost certainly allowed to receive the treatment proposed. Factors associated with positive or negative as well as accepted or rejected recommendations were discussed. Special consideration was given to some of the problems concerning treatment orders which are peculiar to Hong Kong.

2796

Lau, B. W. K., Cheung, F. M. C., & Waldmann, E. (1981). Morbidity of depressive illness in general practice. Asian Medical Journal, 24, *518-527.*

2797

Lau, B. W. K., & Chiu, S. H. (1977). A study of effect of economic fluctuation upon patient turnover in a mental hospital. Hong Kong Journal of Mental Health, 6, *19-30.*

2798

Lau, W. K. (1979). Child mental health: Chimera or oblivion. Hong Kong Journal of Mental Health, 8.

2799

Lau, W. K., & Wong, M. H. (1977). A preliminary analysis of mentally subnormal persons requiring admission to a psychiatric hospital. Hong Kong Journal of Mental Health, 6, *11-18.*

2800

Lau, W. M., & Salili, F. (1986). The effect of cue reliability on concept switching ability in children of low mental ability. Psychologia, 24, *235-239.*

2801

Law, S. K. (1978). Urban-rural differences in student mental health: The Hong Kong scene. Australian & New Zealand Journal of Psychiatry, 12, *277-281.*

Assessed the mental health of 481 Hong Kong urban and rural secondary students (5th and 6th formers) by examining their scores on the General Health Questionnaire (GHQ) administered twice. The 1st administration was done soon after commencement of a school term and served as a baseline measure, and the 2nd was done 6 wks before the 5th formers took an important public examination, a significantly stressful event. Results indicate that all 5th formers showed an increase in mean GHQ scores, reaching statistical significance only in urban boys and rural girls. The latter finding is explained in terms of different parental attitudes and expectations of their academic achievement. The 6th formers had no public examination to take and therefore acted as controls. They showed no increase in mean GHQ scores. Lower social class 5th formers also had higher mean scores, and this finding is used to explain urban-rural differences in mean scores. The significance of severe examination distress and its possible late psychiatric sequelae remain unanswered.

2802

Law, S. K. (1979). Common child psychiatric problems in the school setting. Hong Kong Journal of Mental Health, 8, *25-27.*

2803

Law, S. K. (1983). Psychiatric disorders among Vietnamese refugees in Hong Kong: A clinical study. Journal of the Hong Kong Psychiatric Association, 3, *21-24.*

2804

Law, S. K., Chen, W. C., Wong, S. W., Wong, C. W., & Kwong, B. (1986). Mitral valve prolapse and anxiety disorder in Hong Kong. Journal of the Hong Kong Psychiatric Association, 6, *2-5.*

Sixty mitral valve prolapse patients, 43 anxiety disorder patients, and 30 control subjects completed the Minnesota Multiphasic Personality Inventory Hypochondriasis Scale, Eysenck Personality Questionnaire, and Taylor's Manifest Anxiety Scale. The mitral valve prolapse patients and controls had a similar psychological profile, whereas the anxiety disorder patients had higher symptom scores. Clinical examination and echocardiography of anxiety disorder patients showed an 11.6% prevalence of mitral valve prolapse, a rate that was not remarkably higher than that in the general population (8%). The findings suggested that mitral valve prolapse and anxiety disorder are common but not associated conditions.

2805

Lazure, D. (1965). Discussion of J. Cerny's paper, "Chinese psychiatry." International Journal of Psychiatry, 1, *241-245.*

2806

Lee, H. T. (1960). [The effect of recognition in the treatment of neurasthenia]. Acta Psychologica Sinica, *No. 1, 36-45. (In Chinese.)*

Based on the analysis of the results of the group synthetic speedy method of treatment in 117 cases of neurasthenia, this paper was a discussion of the relation between recognition of the nature of the disease by the patients themselves and the clinical dynamics, and the immediate and lasting effects of the treatment. The importance of recognition of the nature of the disease by the patient himself was stressed and several problems which require further investigation were pointed out.

2807

Lee, J. L., & Huang, J. T. (1985). [Syllogistic reasoning and pragmatic inference by schizophrenics]. Chinese Journal of Mental health, 2, *71-84. (In Chinese.)*

The present study investigated differential manifestations of logical inference and pragmatic inference in paranoid and hebephrenic schizophrenics. The performance of syllogistic reasoning in schizophrenics was not significantly different from the normal subjects in the control group. Both types of schizophrenic subjects took longer to respond than normal subjects, and produced more bizarre responses, in pragmatic inference. It was suggested that strange and bizarre inference is characteristic in paranoid and hebephrenic schizophrenics.

2808

Lee, P. K. Y., Ma, K. S., & Lo, W. H. (1973). A note on a study of children with antisocial behaviour. Hong Kong Journal of Mental Health, 2, *11-14.*

2809

Lee, P. W. H., Lieh-Mak, F., Hung, B. K. M., & Luk, S. L. (1983). Death anxiety in leukemic Chinese children. International Journal of Psychiatry in Medicine, 13, *281-289.*

Compared responses to the Children's Apperception Test (CAT) by 13 Chinese 6-10 yr olds with leukemia to those of 15 controls with orthopedic disorders. Leukemic Ss exhibited a distinctly different pattern of psychopathology and psychological defenses. Isolation, detachment, and denial were commonly used to defend against their insecurity, abstract fears, and uncertainties. Themes relating to parental misunderstandings and maltreatment were also elicited. Differences between the 2 groups are illustrated via sample CAT responses, and findings are discussed in relation to the Chinese conception of death as a taboo subject. Recommendations are made for better psychological management of terminally ill children and their parents.

2810

Lee, R. H. (1952). Delinquent, neglected, and dependent Chinese boys and girls of the San Francisco Bay region. Journal of Social Psychology, 36, *35-44.*

A study of Chinese juveniles and delinquency among them based on juvenile court statistics indicates that their overt antisocial activities result from: (a) cultural conflicts between parents of foreign-born or mixed nativity and native-born children; (b) broken homes; and (c) longings for self-expression.

2811

Lee, R. P. L. (1976). Social psychological correlates of psychiatric impairment in Hong Kong. Hong Kong Nursing Journal, 21, *33-49.*

2812

Lee, R. P. L. (1976, July). Sex and social class differences in mental illness: The case of Hong Kong. *Hong Kong: The Chinese University of Hong Kong, Social Research Centre.*

2813

Lee, R. P. L. (1981). Sex roles, social status, and psychiatric symptoms in urban Hong Kong. In A. Kleinman & T. Y. Lin (Eds.), Normal and abnormal behavior in Chinese culture *(pp. 273-289). Dordrecht, Netherlands: Reidel.*

2814

Lee, R. P. L., & Hsu, S. M. (1979). Stress as a function of the inconsistency between education and economic status. Hong Kong Journal of Mental Health, 8, *1-7.*

2815

Lei, C. T., Kuo, T. C., & Chen, Y. C. (1945). [The mental health of Chinese college and secondary school students in war time] *(Report No. 3). Nanking: Central University, Medical Institute, Public Health Section. (In Chinese.)*

2816

Leng, G. A. (1968). Koro -- Its origin and nature as a disease entity. Singapore Medical Journal, 9, *3-6.*

2817

Leng, G. A. (1969). The Koro "epidemic" in Singapore. Singapore Medical Journal, 10, *234-242.*

2818

Leung, E. (1985). Emotional reaction and postnatal adjustment [Selected papers from the 1984 Annual Conference]. Hong Kong Psychological Society Bulletin, *No. 14, 32-46.*

2819

Leung, P. W. L., Lee, P. W. H., Lieh-Mak, F., & Ho, E. K. W. (1985). The psychosocial adjustment of patients with ankylosing spondylitis. Journal of the Hong Kong Psychiatric Association, 5, *31, 33-34, 36-38.*

2820

Leung, P. W. L., Salili, F., & Baber, F. M. (1986). Common adolescent problems in Hong Kong: Their relationship with self-esteem, locus of control, intelligence and family environment. Psychologia, 24, *91-100.*

2821

Leung, S. M., & Carter, J. E. (1983). Cross cultural study of child abuse among Chinese, native Indians and Anglo-Canadian children. Journal of Psychiatric Treatment & Evaluation, 5, *37-44.*

Investigated random samples of child-abusing families among Chinese Canadians (12 abused children, mean age 3 yrs 1 mo), Canadian Indians (20 abused, mean age 2 yrs 7 mo), and Anglo Canadians (46 abused, mean age 2 yrs 10 mo) and established a comparative cultural profile. Findings indicate that in the Chinese group, the mother of a generally stable family was most often identified as the abuser, with superficial facial and neck pinching and hair pulling presenting as the major features in the injured child. The Native Indian group revealed the abusers as both male and female parental figures, with alcohol problems and family neglect as major features. The Anglo-Canadian group had a high incidence of disrupted home life, and the single mother or her male companion was often the abuser, with conventional physical punishment and beating as the major causes of the child's injuries. Four cases are used to illustrate these features and suggest means of early detection and prevention.

2822

Levine, R. V., & Bartlett, K. (1984). Pace of life, punctuality, and coronary heart disease in six countries. Journal of Cross-Cultural Psychology, 15, *233-255.*

Four studies were conducted in a large and a medium city in Japan, Taiwan, Indonesia, Italy, England, and the U.S.. Study 1 indicated that public clocks were most accurate in the most economically developed countries (Japan and the U.S.) and least accurate in the least developed country (Indonesia). Study 2 revealed that walking speed during main business hours was fastest in Japan and slowest in Indonesia, and subjects in smaller cities tended to walk slower than those in larger cities. Study 3 measured average time taken to complete a standardized postal request, and, as predicted, work speed was fastest in Japan. Intercorrelations within cities were high, but findings revealed a lack of cross-cultural generality of relationship between Type A (coronary prone) behaviors and coronary heart disease. Study 4, with 176 undergraduates, found a relationship within the U.S. between self-reports of Type A behavior and attitudes toward punctuality, but results from 36 female Indian undergraduates question the generalizability of this relationship.

2823

Li, W. L. (1972). Suicide and educational attainment in a transitional society. Sociological Quarterly, 13, *253-258.*

Discusses the contradictory sociological evidence on the relationship between suicide and social status. It is postulated that societies in different stages of development may manifest different patterns of etiology of suicide, and thus the suicide rates of different social strata may change over time. Suicide in a transitional society (Taiwan) was examined and educational attainment was used as an indicator of social status, rather than "usual" occupations as in previous studies. It is concluded that the relation between suicide and social status is negative; and, with societal changes, the relation between suicide and social status will also change.

2824

Li, X. T. (1985). The effect of family on the mental health of the Chinese people. In W. S. Tseng & D. Y. H. Wu (Eds.), Chinese culture and mental health *(pp. 85-93). Orlando, FL: Academic Press.*

2825

Li, X. T. et al. (1986). [Speech disorders in patients with cerebrovascular accidents]. Chinese Journal of Neurology and Psychiatry, 19, *112-116. (In Chinese.)*

A clinical study was made on 123 cases of acute cerebrovascular accidents, based on clinical manifestations and findings of CT scans. It was found that, among 57 cases with lesions in the cortical areas, 54 had ischemic lesions; and among 66 cases with lesions in the subcortical areas, 40 had hemorrhagic lesions. Speech disorders and symbolic dysfunction were classified into seven types, taking into consideration the characteristics of the Chinese language. Of the speech disorders, most occurred in patients with lesions in the left cerebral hemisphere; only 22% showed typical aphasic syndromes. Only 29.8% of speech disorders caused by cortical lesions showed typical aphasic syndromes, all the lesions being in the left cerebral hemisphere. No definite correlation was found between the speech disorders and the findings of CT scans.

2826

Li, X. T., Xu, S. L., & Kuang, P. Z. (1980). [Thirty years of Chinese medical psychology]. Acta Psychologica Sinica, 12, *135-143. (Also in U.S. Joint Publications Research Service (Trans.),* **China report: Science and technology, No. 53,** *1980, August, Report No. 76,320, pp. 43-61.) (In Chinese.)*

Reviews the field of psychotherapy, causes and traits of neurosis, psychopathological traits of psychosis, problems in acupuncture anesthesia, and psychological diagnosis of children with mental deficiencies.

2827

Liao, L. Z., Luo, D. H., Ma, M. C. (1984). [Judging the seriousness of offenses by normal young people in Shanghai]. Information on Psychological Sciences, *No. 5, 13-18. (In Chinese.)*

An investigation of attitudes toward the seriousness of 15 offenses was conducted by means of paired comparison among 600 normal young people of ages from 12 to 25 years. All 105 possible paired comparisons were made by each subject. An ordinal scaling of the seriousness of offenses was constructed utilizing Thurstone's Law of Comparative Judgment. The results indicated that such offenses as homicide, rape, counter-revolution, arson, and poisoning were considered more serious, particularly the first two. Offenses against property were judged less serious. Some sex differences were noted. Sex offenses were judged more serious by college students than by middle-school students, whereas offenses against the revolution were judged more serious by the younger than the older people.

2828

Lieh-Mak, F., Chung, S. Y., & Liu, Y. W. (1983). Characteristics of child battering in Hong Kong: A controlled study. British Journal of Psychiatry, 142, *89-94.*

Compared the characteristics of 37 battered children (6 mo to 13 yrs of age) and their families to a control group matched for age of child and social class of family. Results show that the families of battered children had significantly more problems, with a higher prevalence of psychiatric disorder among the parents. The victims were usually the product of unwanted pregnancy and had been separated from their parents in the 1st yr of life. In Hong Kong, older children rather than infants were at risk of being battered.

2829

Lieh-Mak, F., Luk, S. L., & Leung, L. (1979). Gilles de la Tourette syndrome: Report of five cases in the Chinese. British Journal of Psychiatry, 134, *630-634.*

The onset, course, symptomatology, and family psychopathology of these Chinese cases of Gilles de la Tourette's syndrome are similar to those reported in Caucasians. Findings support the hypothesis that the syndrome has an organic substratum subject to psychological influences.

2830

Lieh-Mak, F., & Ng, M. L. (1981). Ejaculatory incompetence in Chinese men. American Journal of Psychiatry, 138, *685-686.*

Reports etiological data on 12 married Chinese men, ranging in age from 22 to 48 yrs, who were referred for ejaculatory incompetence. Masters-and-Johnson-type instruction produced recovery in 7 Ss, improvement in 3, and no change in 2 Ss. In addition to a lack of adequate sexual stimulation, all Ss had a misconception about the relation between a loss of semen and health, reflecting a common belief among the Chinese that sexual intercourse during psychiatric or physical illness will further impair one's health.

2831

Lin, G. X. et al. (1986). [Application of HAMA in the assessment of neurosis]. Chinese Journal of Neurology and Psychiatry, 19, *342-344. (In Chinese.)*

The HAMA was applied to assess the severity of 230 neurotic patients who met the diagnostic criteria previously established in an epidemiological survey. It was found that the total scores of HAMA were substantially correlated with those of GAS and SI. Treatment effectiveness could be measured by HAMA, as indicated by obvious changes in scores before or after treatment. It was suggested that a score of 14 be set as the cut-off point in assessing neurosis.

2832

Lin, H. N., & Rin, H. (1975). [A clinical report on 50 mentally ill offenders]. Journal of the Formosan Medical Association, 74, *280-287. (In Chinese.)*

The clinical pictures and criminal behaviors of 50 offenders are reviewed. Brief histories of 16 cases are presented. Schizophrenia, affective disorder, mental retardation, psychoneurosis, and personality disorder were the main clinical diagnoses among the 50 offenders. There was no significant sex difference among psychotic offenders; among nonpsychotic mentally abnormal offenders, the ratio of male to female was 7:1. Murder and attempted murder were the main offense of the mentally abnormal, most of whom made no attempt to conceal their crimes. Schizophrenic patients showed little emotional change after their offense. Killing their young children before making their suicidal attempt was frequently found among offenders with affective disorders. Most victims of murder or attempted murder by the mentally abnormal were closely related to or were acquainted with the offenders; however, victims of mentally retarded offenders were mainly strangers. There were many more victims than offenders in connection with homicidal behavior by the mentally retarded. Victims of male offenders tended to be adults, but victims of female offenders were usually their own young children.

2833

Lin, K. M. (1981). Traditional Chinese medical beliefs and their relevance for mental illness and psychiatry. In A. Kleinman & T. Y. Lin (Eds.), Normal and abnormal behavior in Chinese culture *(pp. 95-111). Dordrecht, Netherlands: D. Reidel.*

2834

Lin, K. M., & Kleinman, A. (1981). Recent development of psychiatric epidemiology in China. Culture, Medicine and Psychiatry, 5, *135-143.*

The authors review six articles, containing epidemiologic data, published in the 1980 Chinese Journal of Neurology and Psychiatry. The data are based on six samples, covering over 5 million people who were surveyed from 1958 to 1979 (five of the six samples were studied in the 1970s). The surveys were conducted to gather data for mental health service planning, thus only syndromes with significant impact were included. Initial identification of index cases was done by trained local personnel, and final diagnosis was done by psychiatrists. The major findings were: The prevalence rate for schizophrenia was 1.9% (per 1,000 people), with higher rates for females and for urban areas. Mental retardation rates ranged from 1.13% to 2.9% (per 1,000), with a much higher prevalence rate in males.

2835

Lin, K. M., Kleinman, A., & Lin, T. Y. (1981). Overview of mental disorders in Chinese cultures: Review of epidemiological & clinical studies. In A. Kleinman & T. Y. Lin (Eds.), Normal and abnormal behavior in Chinese culture *(pp. 237-272). Dordrecht, Netherlands: D. Reidel.*

2836

Lin, M. C. (1960). General paresis of the insane in Peking between 1933 and 1943. Journal of Mental Science, 106, *1082-1092.*

2837

Lin, M. J. (1978). [A study of menopausal symptoms in Chinese women of various ages]. Research in Education & Psychology, 2, *55 92. (In Chinese.)*

A questionnaire on menopausal symptoms was given to 637 Chinese women of various ages. The results were: (1) Menopausal women were clearly differentiated from other women by the presence of symptoms, such as cold sweats, weight gain, flooding, rheumatic pains, aches in back of the neck and skull, cold hands and feet, tiredness, forgetfulness, and worrying about having a nervous breakdown. (2) Women with a history of severe dysmenorrhea reported significantly more somatic symptoms at menopause. (3) The conditions of dysmenorrhea did not affect postmenopausal women. (4) Menopausal women who had three or more children and postmenopausal women who had no children reported significantly more symptoms than other groups.

2838

Lin, N., Simeone, R. S., Ensel, W. M., & Kuo, W. (1979). Social support, stressful life events, and illness: A model and an empirical test. Journal of Health & Social Behavior, 20, *108-119.*

Examined the effects of social support and stressors (stressful life events) on illness (psychiatric symptoms) in a model with data from a representative sample of the Chinese-American adult population in Washington, DC. 170 Ss were given the Social Readjustment Rating Scale and a psychiatric symptom checklist. The analysis showed that, as expected, stressors were positively related to the incidence of psychiatric symptoms, and social support was negatively related to psychiatric symptoms. Further, the contribution of social support to predicting symptoms was greater in magnitude than that of stressful life events. When marital status and occupational prestige were incorporated into the model, the significant (negative) contribution of social support to symptoms was not reduced. Implications for development of a sociomedical theory of illness are discussed.

2839

Lin, P. C. (1984). [Social desirability, personality traits and juvenile delinquency]. Journal of Education & Psychology, 7, *1-17. (In Chinese.)*

The present study investigated the relationship of social desirability to personality traits and juvenile delinquency. Subjects were 773 juvenile delinquents (aged 14 to 19), 731 middle school students and 2,398 college students. The results were: (1) Juvenile delinquents obtained higher scores on social desirability tests than middle school students. (2) Social desirability was related to juvenile criminal patterns. (3) College students with a high social desirability score obtained lower scores on impulsivity, aggression, and dependence, and higher scores on achievement, affiliation, endurance, cognitive structure, nurturance, order, dominance and understanding on Jackson's Personality Research Form. Implication of these results on test construction and test interpretation were discussed.

2840

Lin, R. Y. (1983). General situation of juvenile delinquency in Taiwan, the Republic of China, and national programs for its prevention and treatment. In Proceedings of the Second Asian-Pacific Conference on Juvenile Delinquency *(pp. 70-95). Seoul, Korea: Cultural and Social Center for the Asia and Pacific Region.*

2841

Lin, S. J. (1961). [On anxiety indices in Rorschach Test]. Acta Psychologica Taiwanica, *No. 3, 115-124. (In Chinese.)*

2842

Lin, T. Y. (1953). A study of the incidence of mental disorders in Chinese and other cultures. Psychiatry, 16, *313-336. (Republished in* **Bulletin of World Federation of Mental Health,** *1955, 7, 56-58.)*

2843

Lin, T. Y. (1958). Tai-pau and Liu-mang: Two types of delinquent youth in Chinese society. British Journal of Delinquency, 8, *244-256. (Republished in M. K. Opler (Ed.),* **Culture and mental health** *(pp. 257-271). New York: MacMillan, 1959.)*

2844

Lin, T. Y. (1983). Psychiatry and Chinese culture. Western Journal of Medicine, 139, *862-867.*

2845

Lin, T. Y. (1985). Mental disorders and psychiatry in Chinese culture: Characteristic features and major issues. In W. S. Tseng & D. Y. H. Wu (Eds.), Chinese culture and mental health *(pp. 369-393). Orlando, FL: Academic Press.*

2846

Lin, T. Y. (1986). Shaping of Chinese psychiatry in the context of politics and public health. In T. Y. Lin, & L. Eisenberg (Eds.), Mental health care for one billion people *(pp. 3-37). Vancouver: University of British Columbia Press.*

2847

Lin, T. Y., & Lin, D. T. (1982). Alcoholism among the Chinese: Further observations of a low-risk population. Culture, Medicine & Psychiatry, 6, *109-116.*

Recent data from the People's Republic of China and Chinese adults living in British Columbia add further support to the suggestion (e.g., T. Y. Lin, 1953) that the Chinese are a low-risk population as far as alcoholism is concerned. Physiological and sociocultural hypotheses regarding the rarity of alcoholism among the Chinese and the effects of "Westernization" on Chinese drinking patterns are discussed.

2848

Lin, T. Y., Rin, H., Yeh, E. K., Hsu, C. C., & Chu, H. M. (1969). Mental disorders in Taiwan, fifteen years later: A preliminary report. In W. Caudill & T. Y. Lin (Eds.), Mental health research in Asia & the Pacific *(pp. 66-91). Honolulu, HI: East-West Center Press.*

2849

Lin, T. Y., Tardiff, K., Donetz, G., & Goresky, W. (1978). Ethnicity and patterns of help-seeking. Culture, Medicine & Psychiatry, 2, *3-13.*

This study reconstructs and analyzes pathways of help-seeking travelled by severely disabled mental patients in the community. Ethnicity is a prime factor in differentiating patterns of help-seeking in that Chinese patients are kept for prolonged periods of time within their families in the beginning of pathways, while Anglo-Saxons and Middle Europeans are referred by their families or themselves to multiple social and mental health agencies. Native Indians are referred by persons other than family members or themselves between social and legal agencies in the community. Eventually all of these pathways lead to psychiatric in-patient intervention. There are major impediments to treatment in these patients, most notably isolation and deterioration of patients within confines of families or lack of coordination of agencies in the community. Recommendations aimed at the improvement of treatment in the community are presented in light of these findings.

2850

Lin, W. J., & Tang, C. M. (1985). [Family environment, attention tests and peripheral adrenaline secretion in hyperactive children]. Acta Psychologica Sinica, 17, *410-417. (In Chinese.)*

2851

Liu, J. Q. et al. (1980). [An epidemiologic investigation of mental disorders in Xuhui District of Shanghai]. Chinese Journal of Neurology & Psychiatry, 13, *1-6. (In Chinese.)*

2852

Liu, X. H. et al. (1980). [An epidemiologic survey of the psychoses in Sizhuan Province]. Chinese Journal of Neurology & Psychiatry, 13, *7-9. (In Chinese.)*

2853

Liu, X. H., Huang, M. S., Zhang, R. S., Zhang, Y. P., & Hu, G. C. (1980). [Survey of psychosis in Sichuan]. China Report: Science and Technology, *No. 53. (Translated by U.S. Joint Publications Research Service, No. 76,320 pp. 24-32.)*

2854

Liu, Z. V. (1985). A cross-cultural study on depression among foreign graduate students from six selected areas. Dissertation Abstracts International, 46, *A1522.*

2855

Lo, M. Y. (1966). A study of juvenile delinquents in northern Taiwan. Psychological Testing, 13, *268-277.*

2856

Lo, M. Y. (1967). [Prediction of the post-institutional adjustment of juvenile delinquents by the Progressive Matrices and the Multiple Choice Rorschach Test]. Psychological Testing, 14, *388-392. (In Chinese.)*

2857

Lo, W. H. (1967). Headache in Chinese psychiatric outpatients. Journal Of Psychosomatic Research, 11, *163-167.*

"45 Chinese psychiatric outpatients with headache as a prominent complaint were studied with respect to the diagnostic entities, and its phenomenological and demographic characteristics". 1/2 the cases were found to be young women forbidden to go out with boys before their arranged marriage.

2858

Lo, W. H. (1967). A follow-up study of obsessional neurotics in Hong Kong Chinese. British Journal of Psychiatry, 113, *823-832.*

2859

Lo, W. H. (1972). Hysterical reaction in children. Hong Kong Journal of Mental Health, 1, *2-8.*

2860

Lo, W. H. (1976). Urbanization and psychiatric disorders: The Hong Kong scene. Acta Psychiatrica Scandinavica, 54, *174-183.*

Used 3 indices (the growth and density of the population, the expansion of the industrial force, and the per capita increase in the gross domestic product) to investigate the rapidity and intensity of urbanization which Hong Kong has undergone in the past 2-3 decades. Preliminary results of a psychiatric survey of mental health in Hong Kong are then presented. Data were obtained from the mental health service to show the increasing demand for psychiatric care for the past 25 yrs. Attempts were made to analyze the basic composition of the new patients attending a psychiatric center during this period. High density living associated with urbanization in Hong Kong was found to generate a high level of emotional strain, and psychiatric ill health was as prevalent as that in New York. Neuroses were on the increase, and psychiatrists were being consulted on a wider variety of problems. Provision of mental health care in future should take the changes in the composition of psychiatric populations into consideration.

2861

Lo, W. H. (1978). Abdominal pain as a psychosomatic manifestation. Hong Kong Journal of Mental Health, 7, *33-38.*

2862

Lo, W. H. (1982). Issues in psychiatric care of the elderly in Hong Kong. Journal of the Hong Kong Psychiatric Association, 2, *6-9.*

2863

Lo, W. H. (1985). Suicide and attempted suicide in Hong Kong: With a note on prevention. Hong Kong Journal of Mental Health, 14, *64-72.*

2864

Lo, W. H., Chan, W., Ma, K. S., & Wong, A. (1971, June). Some Chinese traditional ideas on mental health. Newsletter of the Mental Health Association of Hong Kong, *2-5.*

2865

Lo, W. H., & Lo, T. (1977). A ten-year follow-up study of Chinese schizophrenics in Hong Kong. British Journal of Psychiatry, 131, *63-66.*

133 Chinese schizophrenic patients first seen in 1965 were traced for a follow-up assessment in 1975. 82 patients were fully evaluated, 47 failed to attend, and 4 were known to have died. The course and outcome were graded into 4 categories and it was found that 65% of the fully evaluated group had full and lasting remission or showed no or mild deterioration only, despite some relapses. Intra-group comparison showed that being female, a shorter duration of illness, an acute onset, symptom-groups other than disturbances of emotion and volition, and the presence of a supportive relative were factors affecting the prognosis favorably.

2866

Lo, W. H., & Ong, F. (1984). Suicidal behaviour in Hong Kong: An analysis of Coroners' case-files. Journal of the Hong Kong Psychiatric Association, 4, *4, 6-8.*

2867

Lo, W. H., & Yap, P. M. (1961). Some aspects of thought disorder in schizophrenia. Bulletin of the Hong Kong Chinese Medical Association, 12, *91-97.*

2868

Lu, C. M. (1970). [The prevalence of mentally retarded students in public junior high schools]. Psychology and Education, 4, *41-46. (In Chinese.)*

The main purpose of this research is to determine the prevalence of mentally retarded students in public junior high schools. The sample consisted of 1,000 (596 boys, 404 girls) inhabitants of the northern, middle, and southern part of Taiwan. The Revised AGCT for Chinese people was selected as an instrument to measure the students' IQ. The results indicated that 4.3% of the sample to be mentally retarded. The data suggested that there was no sex difference in the prevalence rate, and that geographic variations were negligible.

2869

Luk, S. L. (1986). Diagnosis and treatment of hyperkinetic syndrome of childhood: Recent advances. Journal of the Hong Kong Psychiatric Association, 6, *28-33.*

2870

Luk, S. L., Lee, P. W. H., & Yu, G. K. K. (1986). Behavior problem in a group of 3 year olds in Hong Kong. Hong Kong Journal of Paediatrics, 1, *14-25.*

2871

Lum, R. (1979). Mental health ideas of Chinese. In E. Jones (Ed.), Minority mental health: A collection of readings. *New York: Holt, Rinehart, & Winston.*

2872

Lum, R. G. (1980). Impact of mental illness in Chinese families. Dissertation Abstracts International, 41, *B356.*

2873

Luo, K. L. (1986). [A study of 31 cases of schizophrenic adoptees]. Chinese Journal of Neurology and Psychiatry, 19, *32-33. (In Chinese.)*

Thirty-one schizophrenic adoptees were compared with a control group of 24 normal adoptees. The psychiatric morbidity rates of the biological parents, adopted parents, and close relatives of the two groups were compared. The environments under which the adoptees grew up were also analyzed. The results showed that the hereditary factor played a more obvious role in the pathogenesis of schizophrenia.

2874

Luo, K. L. et al. (1986). [An epidemiological investigation of mental retardation in 12 districts of China]. Chinese Journal of Neurology and Psychiatry, 19, *83-86. (In Chinese.)*

An epidemiological study of mental retardation in 12 districts was done using standardized sampling methods, instruments, and diagnostic criteria. The data showed that the total prevalence rate of mental retardation was 3.33 per 1,000. The rate for rural districts was higher than that for urban districts. No sex difference was found. An analysis was made of different types of mental retardation in different age groups. Prevalence rates were analyzed in relation to social demographic variables.

2875

Lyman, R. S. (1937). Psychiatry in China. Archives of Neurology & Psychiatry, 37, *765-771.*

2876

Ma, C. C. (1982). [A survey study of parent-child relationship, parental socioeconomic status, family background and school background of juvenile delinquents]. Journal of Education and Psychology, 5, *177-224. (In Chinese.)*

Comparisons were made between 398 delinquent boys from a reformatory or juvenile prison and 996 middle or high school students. The subjects were administered the Parental Disciplinary Attitude Test, Parent-Child Relations Adjustment Scale, Parental Socioeconomic Status Scale, and Family and School Background Questionnaire. The results indicated: (1) The mothers of delinquents with intimidation and sex offences had more rejecting, contradictory and divergent attitudes to their sons than the mothers of delinquents of homicide and unaccomplished homicide offences. (2) The parent-child relations adjustments of the juvenile recidivists were worse than those of the first-time delinquents. (3) The father and mother of juvenile delinquents had more rejecting, overstrict, contradictory and divergent attitudes to their sons than the parents of the students. (4) The parent-child relations adjustment and parental socioeconomic status of juvenile delinquents were worse than those of the students. (5) The family and school background of juvenile delinquents were more unfavorable than the ordinary juvenile.

2877

Ma, C. C. (1984). [The problem of juvenile delinquency]. In K. S. Yang & C. C. Yeh (Eds.), [Social problems in Taiwan] *(rev. ed., pp. 489-521). Taipei: Chu Liu. (In Chinese.)*

2878

Ma, K. S. (1970, December). Emotional development in childhood and its effect on mental health. Newsletter of the Mental Health Association of Hong Kong, *3-5.*

2879

Ma, S. P. (1980). [An epidemiologic investigation of psychoses in Laoshan county of Qingdao]. Chinese Journal of Neurology and Psychiatry, 13, *22-23. (In Chinese.)*

2880

Mak, K. Y. (1983). Mentally handicapped patients in an outpatient psychiatric clinic in Hong Kong. Journal of the Hong Kong Psychiatric Association, 3, *14-15, 17-19.*

2881

Mak, K. Y. (1985). Mental illness among Indonesian Chinese in Hong Kong. International Journal of Social Psychiatry, 31, *119-124.*

Data was presented on the characteristics of 37 Indonesian Chinese psychiatric outpatients who were immigrants to Hong Kong, including age distribution and age of onset, place of onset, marital status, and diagnosis. A majority of the subjects were aged 25-54 years and 65% were schizophrenic, with most of the rest having affective psychoses or neurotic depression. Over half of the male patients developed their illness only after coming to Hong Kong, and 12 of the subjects had a family history of mental illness. Explanations for the high proportion of schizophrenics were considered, and the stresses involved in the double culture shock experienced by the subjects were discussed.

2882

Mak, K. Y., Wong, C. W., & Lo, W. H. (1985). The Capgras syndrome in the Chinese. Journal of the Hong Kong Psychiatric Association, 5, *14-16.*

Twenty Chinese patients with Capgras syndrome were studied. Their demographic data and clinical findings were comparable to that described in the English language literature. The apparent higher prevalence of this syndrome in this study could be partially explained by cultural variables. Low educational attainment, superstition and belief in mystical experience and 'reincarnation' could enable a person to develop and accept the delusion of "doubles" more readily. Psychometric tests and electroencephalogram did not demonstrate any significant organic etiology.

2883

Malinick, C., Flaherty, J. A., & Jobe, T. (1985). Koro: How culturally specific? International Journal of Social Psychiatry, 31, *67-73.*

The authors presented the case of a 51-year-old Black American male with Koro-like symptoms who came to an emergency room extremely anxious with both tachycardia and tachypnea. The subject's history indicated no psychiatric illness, but he maintained a schizoid lifestyle with little contact with family or friends. The Western concept of penis loss was compared to the Chinese or Malaysian concept, and a combined hypothesis for the development of Koro was proposed.

2884

Mao, Y. Y., Gong, W. Y., Fan, C. R., Fang. Y. Y., Zha, Z. X., Ji, C. Q., & Zhou, Z. F. (1979). [A clinical study of mental retardation and a survey of its incidence rate]. Acta Psychologica Sinica, 11, *98-107. (In Chinese.)*

Discusses 2 aspects in mental retardation research. In 1 aspect, a rating scale was developed for diagnosing the intelligent behavior of 150 mentally retarded persons who made monthly visits to 2 clinics to see if any progress was made after taking a certain type of medicine. In another aspect, a survey was conducted in 4 districts in Peking to examine the incidence rate of mental retardation and to analyze the factors that might cause it. The rating scale assessed the behavior in gross and fine motor behaviors, and skills in self-care, language development, and number concepts, each of which was rated on 6 grades; the progress made by the mentally retarded was designated on 3 levels. Such a rating scale was proved to be effective. However, there are many short-comings that should be overcome through further practice. The mean incidence rate of mental retardation in the 4 districts in Peking was 3.4% of the population. This rate is similar to that of other countries.

2885

Marsella, A. J. (1980). Depressive experience and disorder across cultures. In J. Draguns & H. Triandis (Eds.), Handbook of cross-cultural psycology: Vol. 6. Psychopathology *(pp. 237-289). Boston: Allyn & Bacon.*

2886

Marsella, A. J., Kinzie, D., & Gordon, P. (1973). Ethnic variations in the expression of depression. Journal of Cross-Cultural Psychology, 4, *435-458.*

Administered a depression symptom checklist to American college students who evidenced clinical levels of depression and were of Japanese, Chinese, or European ancestry (n = 308, 87, and 112, respectively). Results of a factor analysis show that groups differed with respect to the functional dimensions expressed by the patterns. In general, existential symptoms dominated the patterns of the Japanese and Caucasians, while somatic symptoms were more characteristic of the Chinese. In addition, the Japanese evidenced an interpersonal symptom pattern, and both oriental groups manifested a cognitive symptom pattern. A theory is proposed which suggested that symptoms are related to extensions of the self-conditioned via socialization experiences. The role of individual differences, stress, and cultural definitions of disorder in determining the expression of depression is discussed.

2887

Marsella, A. J., Sanborn, K. O., Kameoka, V., Shizuru, L., & Brennan, J. (1975). Cross-validation of self-report measures of depression among normal populations of Japanese, Chinese and Caucasian ancestry. Journal of Clinical Psychology, 31, *281-287.*

In recent years there has been a proliferation of interest in self report measures of depression; however, there have been relatively few cross validational studies among the different measures. In addition, there has been no study that compared different measures on normal populations or across different ethnic samples. In the present study, 5 self report measures of depression (i.e., Beck Depression Inventory, KAS Hogarty Depression Scale, Minnesota Multiphasic Personality Inventory D Scale, Multiple Affect Adjective Checklist, and Zung Depression Scale) were administered to normal populations of males and females of Japanese, Chinese, and Caucasian ancestry who were residing in Hawaii. Results indicate that the measures yield different levels of depression as a function of ethnicity and gender variables; the different measures correlated highly for certain groups, but not for others. It was speculated that different assessment techniques and ethnic response styles may account for the results that were found. However, both of these factors indicate that alternative self report measures of depression may be differentially sensitive to the detection of depression. New measures need to be developed that consider frequency, intensity, and duration attributes of symptoms as well as the use of varying response styles.

2888

McIntosh, J. L., & Santos, J. F. (1981). Suicide among minority elderly: A preliminary investigation. Suicide & Life-Threatening Behavior, 11, *151-166.*

Notes that in the US, suicide has traditionally been considered a White elderly phenomenon. However, suicide rates have been increasing for non-Whites in recent years, but it is not clear how this may have affected the age distribution, particularly for specific non-White groups. An investigation of official 1976 suicide statistics among minority elderly revealed that suicide rates were highest among the old for Chinese-, Japanese-, and Filipino-Americans. Among Blacks and Native Americans, however, suicide rates were extremely low for the ages. The need for a long term study is indicated.

2889

McIntosh, J. L., & Santos, J. F. (1982). Changing patterns in methods of suicide by race and sex. Suicide & Life-Threatening Behavior, 12, *221-233.*

Examined annual official national statistics for specific methods of suicide by sex and racial groups from 1923 to 1978. Changes were found among groups in the proportions of various suicide methods employed, most notably for women and Asian Americans. Firearm use increased among nearly all ethnic/racial-sex groups, while the use of poisons declined. Although women continue to be more likely than men to use poisons, in recent years firearms have become a more common method. Among Japanese and Chinese Americans of both sexes the most frequently employed method has been hanging, but the use of firearms has increased. Explanations for the changes in method choice include acculturation and changing societal roles.

2890

Metellus, J., Cathala, H. P., Aubry-Issartier, M., & Bodak, A. (1981). Une observation d'aphasie chez une illettree (analphabete). Reflexions critiques sur les fonctions cerebrales concourant au langage [A case of aphasia in an analphabetic woman: Critical reflections on cerebral functions converging with those of language]. Annales Medico-Psychologiques, 139, *992-1001. (In other language.)*

The case of an 80-yr-old right-handed analphabetic Breton woman, hospitalized as a result of a cerebral vascular accident, prompted these questions: (1) What is the impact of not learning written language on the aphasic semeiology of an analphabet? (2) How do physiological mechanisms relate to the production of language in an analphabet? (3) What relationships, if any, can be discerned between an adult analphabet and the aphasia of a child before learning how to write. Patient neurologic and somatic examinations are reviewed as well as those of a language examination in which S attempted to copy (by drawing) letters and digits and to repeat given phrases. Paraphasia, common among aphasiacs, was revealed. However, S was able to use correct word order, grammatical constructions, and tenses with clauses having both a subject and a predicate. The authors also noted opposite cerebral hemispheric difficulties in a case of a Chinese aphasic.

2891

Miao, E. (1976). An exploratory study on college freshmen mental health status. Acta Psychologica Taiwanica, 18, *129-147.*

Investigated the mental health status of 909 undergraduates from 2 institutions, using the Self-Rating Depression (SDS) and Anxiety Scales and Ko's Mental Health Questionnaire. Results show that there was a significant relationship between anxiety and depressive reactions. While differences between Ss from the 2 schools were not significant, some significant within-school differences were found. Results compare favorably with the medium level of mean SDS indices in cross-cultural studies.

2892

Miao, E. (1977). A study on college seniors' mental health status: A sub-cultural and cross-cultural approach to anxiety and depression. Acta Psychologica Taiwanica, 19, *97-110.*

Administered the Self-Rating Depression Scale to 480 senior college students in Taipei to compare the mental health status of freshmen. Ss represented 4 areas of specialization: engineering and physical sciences, arts and humanities, natural sciences and human development, and economics and law. Two school factors -- self-perception of school achievement and satisfaction -- were also compared with the level of anxiety and depression. Both male and female students majoring in agriculture and human development showed significantly lower anxiety and depression levels when compared with those majoring in engineering, humanities, and economics. Self-perception of college achievement was significantly related to differential levels of anxiety as well as depressive reactions.

2893

Miao, E., & Hwang, C. H. (1977). [A study of the mental health of university freshman students]. Psychological Testing, 24, *82-87. (In Chinese.)*

2894

Mok, B. H. (1985). Problem behavior of adolescents in Hong Kong: A socio-cultural perspective *(Occasional Report No. 7). Hong Kong: Chinese University of Hong Kong, Centre for Hong Kong Studies.*

2895

Mok, K. P. (1984). [Mental health thoughts in ancient China]. *Hong Kong: Hong Kong Mental Health Association. (In Chinese.)*

2896

Murphy, H. B. M. (1959). Culture and mental disorder in Singapore. In M. K. Opler (Ed.), Culture and Mental Health. *New York: MacMillan.*

2897

Murphy, H. B. M. (1963). Juvenile delinquency in Singapore. Journal of Social Psychology, 61, *201-231.*

2898

Naeser, M. A., & Chan, S. W. (1980). Case study of a Chinese aphasic with the Boston Diagnostic Aphasia Exam. Neuropsychologia, 18, *389-410.*

Presents the case of a 56-yr-old right-handed monolingual Chinese female aphasic who had suffered a left hemisphere intracerebral bleed and was studied 11/2 and 21/2 yrs post-stroke with a Mandarin translation of the Boston Diagnostic Aphasia Examination and the Token Test. She had a "mixed" aphasia, characterized by moderate-severe deficits in all language modalities.

2899

Nagasima, T. (1972). [The handicapped and showman: The study on the history of dealing with the handicapped]. Japanese Journal of Special Education, 10, *27-35. (In other language.)*

2900

Nanjing Neuropsychiatric Institute. (1980). [An epidemiologic mass survey of mental disorders in Nanjing]. Chinese Journal of Neurology & Psychiatry, 13, *13-14. (In Chinese.)*

2901

Nanjing Neuropsychiatry Hospital. (1981). Nanjing psychiatric survey. Chinese Medical Journal, 94, *622-623.*

A 6-year psychiatric epidemiologic survey of Nanjing resulted in a psychiatric illness rate of 5.4 per million (54.55% female and 45.45% male). Schizophrenia accounted for 34.8%, mental retardation 22.86%, epilepsy 21.58%, and hysteria 15.36%. In the municipal area, 90% of schizophrenics received well-planned care; out of 130 cases, 81.5% achieved good or marked improvement.

2902

Neki, J. S. (1973). Psychiatry in South-East Asia. British Journal of Psychiatry, 123, *257-269.*

Estimates that the mental morbidity rate for the region of South-East Asia is 10/1,000. Mental health has a poor priority and psychiatric services are rudimentary. A vast majority of the population visits folk healers employing charms, magic, and invocation of divine intervention. Clinical patterns vary from culture to culture, but the region tends toward fewer cases of simple schizophrenia, perhaps due to a high social tolerance of seclusion-seeking persons and a large proportion of catatonics among the psychotic. Neuroses tend to be somatized with hysteria, and hypochondriasis is common. Student mental health is a burning issue, with rioting frequent and heroin-opium-alcohol addictions growing. Suicide shows differences, with the female rate being higher than the male in India and highest among the married. Chinese have the highest and Malays the lowest suicide rates.

2903

Ney, P. G. (1977). Depression in children. Hong Kong Journal of Mental Health, 6.

2904

Ney, P., Lieh-Mak, F., Cheng, R., & Collins, W. (1979). Chinese autistic children. Social Psychiatry, 14, *147-150.*

Found that the 14 Hong Kong Chinese autistic children studied had similar backgrounds and symptomatology to their Western counterparts. They differed in being more socialized and more aware of themselves. On a 204-item questionnaire, 10 of 14 parents indicated their child had very sensitive hearing. Auditory hyperacuity might explain an autistic child's apparent aversion to communicating.

2905

Ng, A. (1975). Social causes of violent crimes among young offenders in Hong Kong. *Hong Kong: Chinese University of Hong Kong, Social Research Centre.*

2906

Ngui, P. W. (1969). The koro epidemic in Singapore [Special issue on studies of anxiety]. Australian & New Zealand Journal of Psychiatry, *2, 263-266.*

2907

Ni, L., & Hsiao, S. L. (1958). A study of mental declination with aging among the retired servicemen tested in Nuan-nuan Center. Acta Psychologica Taiwanica, *No. 1, 9-47.*

2908

Nishio, M. R. (1981). Kanji reading by a prekindergarten language-disabled child: A pilot study. Brain & Language, *13, 259-289.*

A 3 1/2-yr-old, severely language-disabled boy was taught 250 words made up of 1-4 Japanese/Chinese kanji. Many kanji words were learned, and some ability to process these in simple sentences was observed. Acquisition of a word for meaning was not dependent on its visual complexity, but on S's ability to grasp the meaning of the word. Results suggest that a whole-word method may facilitate vary early reading acquisition, and a possible neurophysiological correlate of this is proposed. Kanji or whole words may prove useful for language-handicapped individuals unable to process words phonetically.

2909

Niu, D. F. (1981). [Analysis of 35 cases of mental disturbances due to alcoholism]. Chinese Journal of Neurology & Psychiatry, *14, 36-38. (In Chinese.)*

2910

Okada, S., & Kaku, R. (1980). [The relationship between autistic symptoms and Gogi (word-meaning) disturbances]. Japanese Journal of Child & Adolescent Psychiatry, *21, 276-283. (In other language.)*

Analyzed the spoken expressions of 11 autistic children and found symptoms similar to those of adults with disturbances of word meaning (WM). Repetitious speech usually occurs in WM aphasia and Pick's disease, and some of the Ss of this study repeated phrases again and again without paying any attention to what was said to them, or could not stop repeating the last words of questions they had asked, even after they had been answered. The use of Chinese Kanji characters, which are ideomatics, rather than Kana characters, which are phonetic, occurs in aphasia; several of the Ss were interested in writing Kanji characters, even though the characters were meaningless to them. These similarities indicated that the Ss might have a neuropsychological WM disturbance. But while such disturbances in adults are cognitive-intellectual, in children they impair both the development of personality and relations with others. Children with a primary impairment of WM may show autistic symptoms as a secondary impairment.

2911

Ou, L. H. et al. (1986). [An epidemiological survey on affective psychosis in Jieyang County, Guangdong Province]. Chinese Journal of Neurology and Psychiatry, *19, 99-102. (In Chinese.)*

This study applied the method and diagnostic criteria formulated by 12 collaborating psychiatric research units in 1982. A total of 16,111 subjects were examined and 22 cases of affective psychosis were found. The overall prevalence was 1.37 per 1,000 and the morbidity rate was 6/100,000 per year. The highest prevalence rate was found in the 50-54 age group. Social psychosocial factors were the main precipitating cause of the illness. The prevalence, mode of onset, and prognosis of affective psychosis were discussed.

2912

Ovitz, J. M. (1978). Cross cultural comparison of three writing systems with special reference to dyslexia. Dissertation Abstracts International, *39, A3018.*

This thesis compares English, Hebrew and Chinese writing systems with respect to the associated occurrence of dyslexia in children.

2913

Packard, J. L. (1985). A linguistic investigation of tone laterality in aphasic Chinese speakers. Dissertation Abstracts International, *45, A2860.*

2914

Pang, T. C. (1958). Some local beliefs on sexual disorders. Bulletin of the Hong Kong Chinese Medical Association, *10, 109-110.*

2915

Paul, F. M. (1979). The problems of mental subnormality in a developing country. Journal of Singapore Paediatrics Society, *21, 237-243.*

This is a survey of mental subnormality over a 15-year period from 1963 to 1977. The survey showed that 19.5% of children were associated with prenatal, natal, and postnatal conditions; measures were taken to prevent environmental and genetic conditions contributing to mental subnormality, reducing this percentage to 11% in 1971. Singapore glucose-six-phosphate type of kernicterus was prevented by screening all newborn cord blood for this enzyme and by the prevention of trigger factors like drugs and moth balls known to induce haemolysis. Screening of families for this enzyme was also done. Environmental diseases like tuberculous meningitis and Japanese B encephalitis have been prevented by BCG vaccination and by good mosquito control. Epidemics of rubella still exist and this needs to be controlled, although rubella vaccination is offered to young girls. Chromosome studies are done on children and mothers of Down's anomaly, and amniocentesis is carried out for future foetuses and therapeutic abortion advised on eugenic grounds. Active genetic counselling is given for conditions like microcephaly, hydrocephalus and congenital abnormalities. Educational facilities were provided by the Singapore Association for Retarded Children. With limited institutional care, families had to cope with their mentally subnormal child. Families were of the nuclear type centred round the mother and siblings caring for the child.

2916

Pearson, V. (1985). Discussion of papers by Grace Tang, Mona Tsoi and Imogen Sharp [Selected papers from the 1984 Annual Conference]. Hong Kong Psychological Society Bulletin, *No. 14, 28-31.*

2917

Peng, B. W. (1981). Family communication, media behavior and delinquency. Dissertation Abstracts International, 42, *A1840.*

2918

Pollitt, E. (1983). Morbidity and infant development: A hypothesis. International Journal of Behavioral Development, 6, *461-475.*

Data on illnesses during the 1st 6 mo of life for 164 infants in an impoverished rural area of Taiwan were examined in relation to scores on the Bayley Scales of Infant Development obtained at age 8 mo. Gastrointestinal and respiratory illnesses both resulted in lower scores on mental and motor scales. It is suggested that sick, malnourished children seek to reduce activity to decrease energy expenditure, placing them at increased developmental risk.

2919

Pu, J. Y. et al. (1981). [The effect of different cultural backgrounds and religious ideas on the formation of delusions in schizophrenia]. Chinese Journal of Neurology & Psychiatry, 14, *174-175. (In Chinese.)*

2920

Qian, M. Y., & Chen, C. K. (1986). [A comparative study of the physiological responses of hypertensives and coronary heart disease patients in psychological stress situations]. Information on Psychological Sciences, *No. 5, 43-47. (In Chinese.)*

Three matched groups of hypertensives, coronary heart disease patients, and normals were asked to guess two kinds of symbol patterns, one easy and the other difficult. The experimental procedure was: rest (3 minutes), easy task (1 minute), rest (3 minutes), difficult task (1 minute), and rest (3 minutes). Finger pulse volume (FPV) was recorded during the experimental session. The results showed that the FPV of all subjects was weaker during the two task period than during the rest periods. There were no differences between easy and difficult tasks for all three groups. However, the two groups of patients showed greater response variability than the normals. The response amplitude of hypertensives was stronger than that of coronary patients. This result may serve as an indication of the difference in response between the two groups of patients under stress.

2921

Rapport, R. L., Tan, C. T., & Whitaker, H. A. (1983). Language function and dysfunction among Chinese- and English-speaking polyglots: Cortical stimulation, Wada testing, and clinical studies. Brain & Language, 18, *342-366.*

Investigated language functions for 7 23-45 yr old Chinese- and English-speaking polyglots living in a multiracial society, using several methods: the effects of cortical stimulation on object-naming and reading tasks in Ss who required awake craniotomy, lateralization of cerebral dominance for speech by the Wada Test, and the pattern of language loss and recovery following stroke. Data indicate that Ss were all left hemisphere dominant for the languages tested; no consistent evidence for increased participation by the right hemisphere for language functions was found. The cortical stimulation experiments provided data most compatible with the "differential localization" model of cerebral localization in bilingualism. The variable that most influenced performance in all of these investigations was which language was used primarily for speaking as well as reading and writing at the time of the study.

2922

Research Committee, Hong Kong Social Workers Association. (1984). Behavioural problems of mentally handicapped children in schools. *Hong Kong: Author.*

2923

Rin, H. (1961). An investigation into the incidence and clinical symptoms of mental disorders among Formosan Aborigines. Psychiatria Neurologia Japonica, 53, *480-500.*

2924

Rin, H. (1967). A family study of Chinese schizophrenic patients: Loss of parents, sibling rank, parental attitude and short-term prognosis. Journal of the Formosan Medical Association, 66, *461-469.*

2925

Rin, H. (1970). [Twenty years development of psychiatric epidemiological researches in Taiwan]. Journal of the Formosan Medical Association, 69, *123-141. (In Chinese.)*

2926

Rin, H. (1975). Suicide in Taiwan. In N. L. Farberow (Ed.), Suicide in different cultures. *Baltimore: University Park Press.*

2927

Rin, H. (1986). [Mental illness under the impact of social change]. In H. Y. Chiu & Y. H. Chang (Eds.), [Social and cultural change in Taiwan] *(Monograph Series B, No. 16, Vol. 2, pp. 591-616). Taipei: Academia Sinica, Institute of Ethnology. (In Chinese.)*

2928

Rin, H., Chu, H. M., & Lin, T. Y. (1966). Psychophysiological reactions of a rural and suburban population in Taiwan. Acta Psychiatrica Scandinavica, 42, *410-473.*

A brief sketch of epidemiological studies of mental disorder and clinical studies of psychophysiological symptoms in Taiwan is given. Socioenvironmental factors were analyzed to determine distribution of stress as to different milieus of the individual. It was found that the youngest female in a Chinese family showed significantly higher prevalence rates of psychophysiological reactions than other siblings. The need for longitudinal studies is growing in the field of epidemiological and sociocultural studies of mental disorders.

2929

Rin, H., Hsu, C. C., & Liu, S. L. (1958). The characteristics of paranoid reaction in present day Taiwan. Memoirs of the College of Medicine, National Taiwan University, 5, *1-15.*

2930

Rin, H. and Lin, T. Y. (1962). Mental illness among Formosan aborigines as compared with the Chinese in Taiwan. Journal of Mental Science, 108, *131-146.*

2931

Rin, H., Schooler, C., & Caudill, W. A. (1973). Symptomatology and hospitalization: Culture, social structure and psychopathology in Taiwan and Japan. Journal of Nervous and Mental Disease, 157, *296-312.*

2932

Rin, H., Shih, L. Y., Lee, H. S., & Ko, Y. H. (1961). A comparative study of psychiatric symptoms manifested by neurotic patients and college students. Acta Psychologica Taiwanica, *No. 3, 57-72.*

2933

Robinson, N. M. (1978). Mild mental retardation: Does it exist in the People's Republic of China? Mental Retardation, 16, *295-299.*

Posits that the mildly retarded individual in a developing nation like the People's Republic of China is much better able to cope with daily demands than in a complex and technologically sophisticated society. Chinese efforts at prevention, health care, and education are briefly described.

2934

Russell, G. (1982). Writing and dyslexia: An historical analysis. Journal of Child Psychology & Psychiatry & Allied Disciplines, 23, *383-400.*

Hypothesizes that the perfection and simplification of writing over 3,500 yrs and the characteristics of the perfected alphabetical scripts indicate a process adaptive to human linguistic faculties. This process, which is traced from picture writing to hieroglyphics to cuneiform to alphabets, has depended on its becoming increasingly phonetic. The exceptional forms of writing, such as Chinese, remained out of reach of the masses. The hypothesis is put forward that the same process might be maladaptive to a minority of children deficient in the requisite linguistic abilities: In a literate society they would suffer from disorders of reading. Since the process of decoding writing is phonetic, these children are deficient because they do not have ready access to phoneticization abilities.

2935

Sakamoto, Y., & Miura, T. (1976). An attempt to understand Japanese personality from a family psychiatry point of view. Australian & New Zealand Journal of Psychiatry, 10, *A115-117.*

Presents the idea that intrafamilial insight, meaning the recognition of the patient's mental illness by other family members, is lacking among the Japanese. Japanese family relationships emphasize group interaction, and Japanese infants receive less training from their mothers in verbal interaction than do American infants. One basic Japanese personality pattern is described as "helplessness and the desire to be loved," with a corresponding term translated as "fond parent," reflecting the need to love. Failure of the family to recognize that a member is sick may also be related to the Japanese shame or guilt feeling, which is concerned with the family and the society rather than with the individual. Studies are described which compare Japanese with American schizophrenics and the symptomatology of Japanese with Taiwan

Chinese. The Japanese neurosis called "interpersonal phobia" is described. Morita Therapy is discussed in terms of its relationship to Zen Buddhism, and contrasting ideas of the ego in Western psychoanalytic theory and in Japanese thought, as reflected in the Japanese language, are examined.

2936

Salili, F., & Hoosain, R. (1985). Hyperactivity among Hong Kong Chinese children. International Journal of Intercultural Relations, 9, *177-185.*

In the present study 263 male and 243 female unselected 4-15 yr olds and 106 male and 61 female 9-12 yr olds independently diagnosed as hyperactive were tested to study the incidence of hyperactivity in Chinese children. Subjects were administered an abbreviated form of the Conners Teacher Rating Scale by classroom teachers who had known them for at least 3 months. Scores were significantly higher among males than females and among hyperactive than unselected subjects. Sex differences were similar to American findings, although the ratings for Chinese girls were much lower. An overall decrease in hyperactive symptoms toward adolescence was also found. The possible influence of cultural factors such as sex roles and classroom settings is discussed.

2937

Sanua, V. D. (1981). Cultural changes and psychopathology in children: With special reference to infantile autism. Acta Paedopsychiatrica, 47, *133-142.*

Relates the sociocultural changes that have been taking place in the last few decades to the increasing number of children brought to the attention of mental health professionals. Because of the nuclearization of the family in the Western world, particularly in those countries with high technology, many children face greater problems in adapting to society. If the relationship between parents and children is less than optimal, the parties are less likely to obtain parental surrogates to compensate for that deficiency. Present hospital policies seem to affect negatively mother-child bonding immediately after birth. Literature indicates that infantile autism seems to be less frequent among the Italians, Chinese, Hispanics, and Africans and Israeli children living in Kibbutzim. The frequency of infantile autism is rather low among lower class children and minority groups, supporting L. Kanner's (1943) data that illness is more frequent among the upper class. Findings are inconsistent with the theory that autism is of organic origin.

2938

Sasanuma, S., & Monoi, H. (1975). The syndrome of Gogi (word-meaning) aphasia: Selective impairment of Kanji processing. Neurology, 25, *627-632.*

T. Imura (1943) described an aphasic syndrome shown by Japanese patients and designated it as Gogi ("word-meaning") aphasia. Salient features are selective impairment of processing kanji or Chinese characters and difficulty in finding access to the lexicon in both production and reception, with preservation of processing kana or phonetic signs, and fluent oral repetition. The case of a 29-yr-old male patient with his syndrome is presented, with emphasis on the nature of his kanji impairment. Cases of Gogi aphasia in the literature are reviewed and contrasted to cases of Broca's aphasia with selective impairment of kana processing. Implications for a neurolinguistic model of language processing in aphasia are discussed.

2939

Sechrest, L., & Flores, L. (1969). Sibling position of Philippine psychiatric patients. Journal of Social Psychology, 77, *135-137.*

Examined the sibling position of 146 female and 134 male psychiatric hospital patients in the Philippines in the light of previous findings in other cultures. Male patients tended to come from the 1st-born half of a sibling set, especially if the family was large. In the case of females both older children from large families and younger children from small families were over-represented. The findings are at least partially congruent with those for American, Chinese, and Japanese cultures.

2940

Shanming, Y. (1981). Lithium therapy in China. Acta Psychiatrica Scandinavica, 64, *270-272.*

A questionnaire survey among Chinese psychiatrists in June 1980 revealed that lithium treatment is being used in a little over half of the Chinese psychiatric hospitals, mainly for the treatment of mania and schizo-affective patients and only to a limited extent prophylactically. The relatively restricted use of lithium as yet may be due to infrequency of the diagnosis of mania, fear of toxicity, and a lack of laboratory facilities for monitoring serum lithium levels.

2941

Sharp, I. (1985). Sex differences in response to illness [Selected papers from the 1984 Annual Conference]. Hong Kong Psychological Society Bulletin, *No. 14, 17-27.*

Reviews evidence from Hong Kong concerning sex differences in morbidity, vulnerability to disease, perceptions and evaluations of symptoms of illness, and actions taken once symptoms are defined. A model that distinguishes between disease, illness, and illness behavior is presented. Disease refers to a medical conception of pathological abnormality indicated by a set of signs and symptoms; illness refers to a person's subjective experience of ill health; and illness behavior refers to the actions or nonactions that people take once they have interpreted bodily states as being signs or symptoms of illness. Comparisons of these factors among adults in Hong Kong and the West are presented. Sex differences in Hong Kong appear to be related to the type of physicians consulted, rates of consultation, and types of specialists consulted. Twice as many women as men attended government out-patient clinics.

2942

Shen, Q. J. et al. (1979). [Clinical characteristics of graft schizophrenia]. Chinese Journal of Neurology and Psychiatry, 12, *4-6. (In Chinese.)*

2943

Shen, Y. C. et al. (1986). [An epidemiological investigation on mental disorders in 12 regions of China: Methodology and data analysis]. Chinese Journal of Neurology and Psychiatry, 19, *65-69. (In Chinese.)*

This is the first of a series of reports on the investigation of mental disorders in 12 areas. The present paper focused on the methodology used in this epidemiological survey, covering the use of uniform methods, procedures, criteria, and instruments. The results showed that the samples investigated represented the catchment population. A high degree of agreement was found among the 12 areas investigated. A satisfactory result was obtained in the retest on negativeness identified, resulting in false negative rates of 0.4% to 1.0%. The data also revealed a significant difference between urban and rural populations.

2944

Shen, Y. C. et al. (1986). [Investigation of the prevalence of various mental disorders and analysis of the data]. Chinese Journal of Neurology and Psychiatry, 19, *80-82. (In Chinese.)*

This paper presented the prevalence rates of various psychoses, mental retardation, alcoholism, alcoholic dependence, and drug dependence among 38,136 people aged 15 years and over. The three conditions with the highest time-point prevalence rates were schizophrenia, mental retardation, and mental disorder associated with cerebrovascular disease, although the rank order differed between urban and rural districts. The prevalence rate and outcome of schizophrenia were found to be associated with social and familial environments.

2945

Shen, Y. C., Wang, Y. F., & Yang, X. L. (1985). An epidemiological investigation of minimal brain dysfunction in six elementary schools in Beijing. Journal of Child Psychology & Psychiatry & Allied Disciplines, 26, *777-787.*

In order to examine prevalence rates of minimal brain dysfunction (MBD) and its clinical manifestations and psychosocial risk factors, 2,770 children from 6 elementary schools in urban, suburban, and mountain areas of Beijing were screened with a modified version of the Conners Teacher Rating Scale and a children's learning and behavior questionnaire. Each suspected case was interviewed to determine whether diagnostic criteria were met for attention deficit disorder with hyperactivity, with some cultural modification; 160 children were identified as having MBD. Data on parental occupational and educational backgrounds were also obtained. Results showed that the MBD prevalence rate was 3.1% in the urban, 7.8% in the suburban, and 7.0% in the mountain areas. Lower rates were found in the families of scientific and technical professionals and in those with higher education, while the highest rates were in families of peasants and workers. It was concluded that the prevalence rate of MBD may be influenced by social settings as a whole, while the clinical manifestations of MBD may be modified by the cultural and family backgrounds in which the children are brought up.

2946

Shen, Y. C., Zhang, W. X., Shu, L., Yang, X. L., Cui, Y. H., Zhou, D. F., Shi, H. Y., & Su, E. T. (1981). Investigation of mental disorders in Beijing suburban district. Chinese Medical Journal^ (Peking), *94,* **153-156.**

The prevalence and incidence rates of severe mental disorders in the Beijing agricultural Haidian District is investigated. The method of investigation and analysis of the data are briefly described.

2947

Shukla, G. D., & Mishra, D. N. (1981). Koro-like syndrome: A case report. *Indian Journal of Psychiatry,* **23, 96-97.**

This culture-bound syndrome is said to occur almost exclusively among Malay people and Southern Chinese who refer to it as Suk-yeong. However, recently, two cases were reported from Canada. The authors report a case with Koro-like features which appears to be the first of its kind from India.

2948

Singer, K. (1962). Huntington's Chorea in the Chinese. *British Medical Journal, 1,* **1311-1312.**

2949

Singer, K. (1972). Drinking patterns and alcoholism in the Chinese. *British Journal of Addiction, 67,* **3-14.**

Presents a brief review of the literature on the drinking habits of the Chinese. It is noted that while these studies indicate an exceptionally low rate of alcoholism, most were conducted with small samples of expatriate Chinese. The demographic and social characteristics of Hong Kong are outlined and Chinese drinking patterns, behavior, traditional beliefs concerning drinking, and the types of Chinese and Western alcoholic beverages available are described. Data concerning per capita alcohol consumption, alcohol-related arrests, and admissions to a psychiatric hospital for alcoholic psychosis during the 1960s are presented. Results show that while the incidence of alcoholism is substantially less than in Western countries, it is not as uncommon as previously noted and shows a rising trend: 1st admission for alcoholic psychosis increased from 1.2-6.1% between 1962 and 1970. A profile is presented of the Chinese alcoholic which indicates his similarity to the French wine drinker. Possible reasons for the low rate of alcoholism, the narcotic vs. alcohol problem, and treatment and legislation are considered.

2950

Singer, K. (1974). The choice of intoxicant among the Chinese. *British Journal of Addiction, 69,* **257-268.**

Surveys the alcohol and narcotics choices and the prevalence pattern of dependence on these substances among the Chinese, showing that these differ significantly from those in the West. Possible factors responsible for the distinctive pattern in the Chinese are considered. Probably significant are cultural ideology sanctioning acquiescence, moderation, propriety, conformity, and intellectual control; historical events leading to easy availability of opiates over a long period; and a high level of social pathology associated with culture change, economic hardship, and easy accessibility to drugs.

2951

Singer, K. (1975). The role of culture in psychosomatic disorders. *Psychotherapy & Psychosomatics, 26,* **257-264.**

2952

Singer, K. (1976). Gilles de la Tourette's syndrome: A report on three cases in the Chinese. In F. Abuzzahab Sr. & F. Anderson (Eds.), *Gilles de la Tourette's syndrome: Vol. 1. International registry* **(pp. 19-24). St. Paul: Mason.**

2953

Singer, K. (1976). Culture and mental health: Vol. 2. Childhood and family. In W. H. Lo, W. Chan, K. S. Ma, A. Wong & K. K. Yeung (Eds.), *Perspectives in mental health, Hong Kong, 1976* **(pp. 45-48). Hong Kong: Mental Health Association of Hong Kong.**

2954

Singer, K. (1976). Culture and mental health: Vol. 3. Psychodynamics. In W. H. Lo, W. Chan, K. S. Ma, A. Wong & K. K. Yeung (Eds.), *Perspectives in Mental Health, Hong Kong, 1976* **(pp. 49-54). Hong Kong: Mental Health Association of Hong Kong.**

2955

Singer, K. (1977). Somatization and new cross-cultural psychiatry: Reply. *Social Science & Medicine, 11,* **11-12.**

2956

Singer, K. (1981). Some issues in mental health problems in Hong Kong. *Hong Kong Journal of Mental Health, 10,* **2-4.**

2957

Singer, K. (1985). Psychiatric morbidity in university students in Hong Kong: Prevalence, sociocultural and clinical aspects. *Journal of Hong Kong Medical Association, 37,* **117-120.**

This paper discussed the prevalence, sociocultural and clinical aspects of psychiatric morbidity in university students in Hong Kong. In any one year 1 1/2 to 2% of the total student population of the University of Hong Kong were found suffering from severe psychiatric disorder and about 10-20% from milder forms. The findings are broadly similar to those obtained in other countries. Sociocultural influences peculiar to the Hong Kong students and inimical to his mental health were discussed, as well as clinical and treatment aspects.

2958

Singer, K., Chang, P. T., & Hsu, G. L. K. (1972). Physique, personality and mental illness in the southern Chinese. *British Journal of Psychiatry, 121,* **315-319.**

Made anthropometric measurements on 411 schizophrenic, 42 affective, 81 neurotic, and 180 normal Southern Chinese males. All groups were matched for age and socioeconomic status. Findings are in agreement with typical intercorrelations found between body build, personality, and type of mental illness in Caucasians. Neuroticism was negatively related to body size and positively correlated with linearity. The same was true for schizophrenics, particularly those of early onset. Affective disorder showed some positive relation to body size.

2959

Singer, K., Lieh-Mak, F., & Ng, M. L. (1976). Physique, personality and mental illness in Southern Chinese women. *British Journal of Psychiatry, 129,* **243-247.**

Completed several anthropometric measurements (e.g., stature, body weight, and hip circumference) on Southern Chinese women: 317 schizophrenics, 44 with affective disorders, 47 neurotics, and 115 normal controls. All groups and subgroups compared were matched for mean age and socioeconomic status. It was found that the intercorrelations between body build, personality, and type of mental illness were on the whole similar to those reported for Caucasians by Kretschmer.

2960

Singer, K., Ney, P. G., & Lieh-Mak, F. (1978). A cultural perspective on child psychiatric disorders. *Comprehensive Psychiatry, 19*, **533-540.**

Examines similarities and differences between psychiatric disorders of children as encountered in a Hong Kong child psychiatric inpatient setting and those encountered in Western settings. General sociocultural influences in Hong Kong are discussed, including (a) the socioeconomic, political, religious, and demographic aspects of the environment; (b) the folk philosophy regarding human nature, authority, purpose, morality, reality, time, and the universe and man's place in it; and (c) shared belief and value systems concerning the cause and nature of disease and symbolic values attached to body organs and their functions. These influences are illustrated by the case histories of two girls and four boys in Hong Kong. It is concluded, however, that despite cultural factors, in most cases the psychosocial forces seeming to generate abnormal behavior in this Oriental culture, as well as the forms and manifestations of such behavior, are largely similar to those in the West.

2961

Singer, K., & Wong, M. (1973). Alcoholic psychoses and alcoholism in the Chinese: A study of 100 consecutive cases admitted to a psychiatric hospital in Hong Kong. *Quarterly Journal of Studies on Alcohol, 34* **(3, Pt. A), 878-886.**

Compared the histories of 100 consecutive admissions for alcoholic psychoses and alcoholism to a Hong Kong psychiatric hospital during a 1-yr period with those of 100 controls (staff and patients) matched for age and social class. Data concerning social and demographic characteristics and drinking history are presented. Alcoholic psychoses were diagnosed in 69 Ss, alcoholism in 20, and functional disorder associated with alcoholism in 11. Medical complications were present in 45 Ss. According to E. M. Jellinek's classification, 5 were alpha, 27 were gamma, 64 were delta, and 3 were epsilon alcoholics. A Chinese version of the Maudsley Personality Inventory was administered to the 81 alcoholics and 88 controls literate enough to complete the test. The mean scores of the alcoholics on the Extraversion and Neuroticism scales were 18.13 and 18.38 (22.39 and 10.64 in controls). Clinically, the Chinese alcoholics appeared timid, sensitive to stress, lacking in mental vigor, and susceptible to anxiety and depression. One-third of the patients reported a culturally patterned hallucination of a character with the head of a cow and the face of a horse (the traditional guard at the gate of hell). Other differences between Chinese and Western alcoholics are discussed.

2962

Smart, R. G., & Murray, G. F. (1983). Drug abuse and affluence in five countries: A study of economic and health conditions, 1960-1975. *Drug & Alcohol Dependence, 11*, **297-307.**

Examined indicators of affluence (economic and health conditions) and various types of illicit drug abuse in 5 countries (Canada, Hong Kong, Sweden, UK, and US) for the period 1960-1975. Results show that officially recorded measures of drug abuse in each of the countries were related to improvements in economic and health conditions.

2963

Smith, M. E. (1938). A comparison of the neurotic tendencies of students of different racial ancestry in Hawaii. *Journal of Social Psychology, 9*, **395-417.**

College students of Hawaii, of different racial ancestry, when tested by the Thurstone personality schedule and an abbreviation of it, gave larger average scores than those obtained by Thurstone at the University of Chicago, showing a more neurotic group in Hawaii. Those of Korean and part-Hawaiian ancestry showed the highest average scores, Chinese and Portuguese next, with Japanese and other-Caucasians last; none of the differences in average scores between the races were large enough to be statistically significant. The Japanese and other-Caucasians, which average lowest, are the largest elements in the population and the ones with the most prestige.

2964

Smith, S. R., Macht, L. B., & Refsnes, C. C. (1967). Recovery, repression, and art. *Bulletin of Art Therapy, 6*, **103-120.**

A study of "the relationship between a patient's recovery from psychiatric illness and his creativity". A case history of a 30-yr-old Chinese catholic from Formosa hospitalized with acute psychosis is presented. Through the symbolism in his drawings, the therapist was able to see his conflicts and thus bring them out in the open where they could be resolved. It is concluded that art therapy is a very important part of the whole system of psychotherapy. A discussion by Margaret Naumburg follows.

2965

Son, W. C. (1959). [Some characteristics of dynamic processes in the cerebral cortex of neurasthenics as shown by fluctuations in the latency period of discrimination reaction]. *Acta Psychologica Sinica,* **No. 5, 317-328.** (In Chinese.)

Discrimination reactions of 40 normal persons and 78 neurasthenic patients were compared. Before psychotherapy, the wave amplitude of the latency of reaction was greater in the patients than in the normal persons. After therapy, decreases in wave amplitude differed depending on the extent of recovery; the wave amplitudes of completely recovered patients decreased to the same extent as in normal persons, however poorly recovered persons showed only a small decrease in the amplitude. Furthermore, most patients originally showing small wave amplitude recovered completely or basically after the treatment, but only a small percentage of patients originally showing great wave fluctuation recovered well. The wave amplitude of latency of discrimination reaction is one of the indices of the functional states of the cerebral cortex. The pretherapy results demonstrated that functional states of patients' cortex were different from those of healthy persons. The recovery of the functional states of cortex and the improvements in clinical symptoms went together. The patients with severe functional disorder recovered more slowly than those having the lesser disorder. It is concluded that the wave amplitude of the latency of discrimination reaction can be used in diagnosing the severity of illness and the effect of treatment.

2966

Son, W. C. (1962). [Some differences of the functional states of cerebral cortex in patients of neurasthenia, hypertension and peptic ulcer]. *Acta Psychologica Sinica*, **No. 3, 241-247.** (In Chinese.)

This study investigated discriminative reactions in patients of neurasthenia, hyperpiesics and peptic ulcer. The results indicated that the latency period and the fluctuation of discriminative reactions of neurasthenics and hyperpiesics with conspicuous neurasthenic symptoms were significantly larger than those of normal persons. The difference between the discriminative reaction of hyperpiesics without conspicuous neurasthenic symptoms, ulcer gastrics and normal persons was negligible. The results of hyperpiesics without any conscious symptoms and normal persons were similar. This may be due to the fact that their functional disorder was not reflected in this experiment.

2967

Song, M. (1936). [Neurasthenia]. *Tong Ji Yixue Jikan*, *6*, **87-91.** (In Chinese.)

2968

Soong, W. T. (1977). [A clinical epidemiological study of enuresis. First report: The age trend of and factors associated with attaining bladder control among urban Chinese children]. *Acta Paediatrica Sinica*, *18*, **11-23.** (In Chinese.)

2969

Soong, W. T. (1984). [Attention deficit hyperkinetic syndrome: Clinical characteristics]. *Bulletin of the Chinese Society of Neurology and Psychiatry*, *10*, **104-113.** (In Chinese.)

Thirty-six patients, who newly visited a children's mental health center and met the criteria for attention deficit disorder, were studied. In the first study, the results were: (1) 59% percent of the patients were referred by teachers or physicians. (2) The complaints presented by their parents were overactivity, inattention, behavior and disciplinary problems, and learning problems. (3) Inattention, visual-motor incoordination, and relatively low IQ were detected by psychological testing. (4) More than 70% of the children were rated above one standard deviation or at the 85th percentile of the norm on the Chinese version of the Werry-Weiss-Peters Activity Scale. In the second study, samples of urban and rural community children were selected as controls. Sixty-six percent of the patients and 18% of the controls had one or more paranatal risk factors. A greater percentage of the patients had short attention, mirror writing, motor incoordination, poor memory, poor number concept, and speech retardation during early development. The findings of these two studies are similar to those reported in previous studies from Western countries, and support the notion that attention deficit hyperkinesis is a distinct clinical syndrome.

2970

Stevenson, H. W. (1984). Orthography and reading disabilities. *Journal of Learning Disabilities*, *17*, **296-301.**

Disagrees with L. R. Gleitman and P. Rozin (1977) that the English writing system (orthography) plays a role in the development of reading disabilities. The work of O. J. Tzeng et al shows that phonemic recoding occurs in reading Chinese sentences. Although formal studies are lacking, there is evidence that poor readers among elementary school children exist in Taiwan and Japan. It is concluded that it is unlikely that any particular form of writing is conducive to production of severe reading problems.

2971

Stevenson, H. W., Stigler, J. W., Lucker, G. W., Lee, S. Y., Hsu, C. C., & Kitamura, S. (1982). Reading disabilities: The case of Chinese, Japanese, and English. *Child Development*, *53*, **1164-1181.**

Constructed a reading test in English, Japanese, and Chinese to assess the validity of the hypothesis that apparent differences in the incidence of reading disability in Asian and Western languages is related to orthographic factors. 453 American, 956 Taiwan Chinese, and 775 Japanese 5th graders were administered the test and a battery of 10 cognitive tasks. Strong evidence was found that reading disabilities exist among Chinese and Japanese as well as among American Ss. In discriminating between groups of poor and average readers by means of the cognitive tasks, the combined effects of general information and verbal memory proved to be the most powerful predictors in Japan and Taiwan. General information and coding emerged as the most effective predictors for American Ss. Results cast doubt on the crucial significance of orthography as the major factor determining the incidence of reading disabilities across cultures.

2972

Su, H. Y. (1960). [Neurosis and Psychotherapy]. *Acta Psychologica Taiwanica*, **No. 2, 60-62.** (In Chinese.)

2973

Su, H. Y., Chang, S. H., Chang, S., & Hsiao, S. L. (1958). [A study of "Goitrous Personality" from Rorschach Responses]. *Acta Psychologica Taiwanica*, **No. 1, 99-103.** (In Chinese.)

Our interest is to see whether the personality of goitrous patients differs from that of normal people and if so, what the goitrous personality pattern is. Our study was concentrated in Liu-chia, Taiwan, where, in 1956, 95.31% of 1,058 primary school children were suffering from goiter disease. The subjects were 50 goitrous patients of various ages, both sexes, and different levels of education. Comparisons were made among four groups of subjects, classified on the basis of largeness of the swollen neck, and between the goitrous group as a whole and a control group consisting of 20 subjects, all inhabitants of Taipei City, whose education was of primary school level. The comparison among the four goitrous groups revealed no statistically significant difference in Rorschach response patterns; with increase in size of the goitrous tumor, there was no obvious parallel change in personality. The intelligence of the goitrous group was lower than that of the corresponding normal group. The goitrous group showed that their mode of approach belonged to a more detailed and concrete thinking type. They were also less able in ego control. As for the experience type indexes, the goitrous group was poorer in fantasy; the emotional maturation and experience balance of both groups were equal and normal. Associational contents showed many "An" responses, which meant that the goitrous group were very concerned about their health, probably due to their chronic neck disease.

2974

Su, H. Y., & Yang, K. S. (1964). Self-concept congruence in relation to juvenile delinquency. *Acta Psychologica Taiwanica*, *6*, **1-9.**

The present paper reports an investigation of the relationship between the degree of each of three kinds of self-concept congruence and the incidence of juvenile delinquency. The subjects were 36 Chinese male juvenile delinquents and 36 controls. Each subject was individually asked to characterize himself (the actual self), the person he would like to be (the ideal self), and the person his family expected him to be (the family self), by sorting 70 self-referent statements written on separate cards according to the Q-sort method. The discrepancy score, defined as the average of the 70 absolute differences in scale value between two Q-sorts, was taken as the main measure of degree of self-concept congruence. On each of the actual-ideal, actual-family, and ideal-family comparisons, the mean discrepancy score of the experimental group was significantly greater than that of the control. On the basis of these affirmative results we have come to the conclusion that juvenile delinquents were less satisfied with themselves and experienced more conflict between their personal ideals and family expectations.

2975

Su, S. J., Soong, W. T., & Hsu, C. C. (1984). [Dyslexia in Chinese children: The writing errors and WISC-R pattern]. *Chinese Journal of Psychology*, *26*, **41-48.** (In Chinese.)

Twenty Chinese children outpatients (19 males, 1 female; aged from 7 to 13) from the Children's Mental Health Center of the Department of Psychiatry, National Taiwan University Hospital, were used as subjects. Reading disability was defined as a marked delay in reading ability combined with average intelligence. Spontaneous writing samples were collected and the patterns of writing errors were analyzed. Five major patterns were identified: (1) Formal confusions; (2) Phonological confusions; (3) Confusions in the position of a radical in a character; (4) Character order confusions in a phrase; and (5) Mirror writing. The percentages of the five error patterns in the 20 cases were 100%, 85%, 35%, 35%, and 15%, respectively. The analysis of the Chinese form of the Wechsler Intelligence Scale for Children-Revised (WISC-R) of these cases revealed the following findings: (1) Performance IQ was significantly higher than verbal IQ. (2) Block design and object assembly subtests were significantly higher than the other subtests. (3) The perceptual organization factor score was significantly higher than freedom from distractability and verbal comprehension factor scores. The results did not support the notion that reading retardation in Chinese is predominantly related to the impaired spatial relation and perceptual organization ability.

2976

Su, T. P., & Yang, Y. K. (1979). [A follow-up study of inpatients with anxiety neurosis]. *Chinese Medical Journal* **(Taipei),** *26*, **237-245.** (In Chinese.)

63 inpatients seen in the psychiatric section of the Veterans General Hospital in Taiwan met the criteria for the diagnosis of anxiety neurosis, and were followed up for 2 years after their discharge. A brief questionnaire was mailed to all these patients, to understand their present symptoms, neurotic traits, and the level of adjustment in the last half year. The conclusions were: (1) Nearly half of the patients made their first psychiatric visit more than 5 years after the onset of disease. Most of them were advised to seek

psychiatric help by physicians. (2) A less favorable outcome was found in 55% of our patients who were either moderately or severely impaired. But more than 80% had a favorable family adjustment, despite their severity of symptoms and impairment in the physical, interpersonal, social, and vocational areas. It was assumed that the patients' anxiety was induced from extrafamilial stress, and reduced by family support. (3) Patients presented chiefly somatic symptoms during their first hospitalization and increased anxiety symptoms during follow-up. (4) The severity of neurotic traits was positively correlated with the level of overall outcome. (5) Favorable outcome seems to be found among female patients who had onset at an earlier age and asked for psychiatric help before they were 40 years old, patients who made their first psychiatric visit within 1 year after onset, and patients who showed no significant deviant premorbid personality.

2977

Sue, S., & Fung, D. S. (1986). The role of physiological and cultural factors in alcohol consumption among Chinese. *Journal of the Hong Kong Psychiatric Association*, *6*, **6-8.**

The Chinese exhibit low rates of alcoholism and alcohol use throughout the world. Some researchers believe that the low rates of consumption are caused by genetic or physiological factors that place Chinese at low risk for alcoholism. Others believe that Chinese cultural values discourage excessive consumption. This article reviewed the literature on drinking behavior and physiological and cultural factors. It was suggested that alcohol consumption among the Chinese is best understood as a complex phenomenon where physiological and cultural factors interact.

2978

Sue, S., & Sue, D. W. (1974). MMPI comparisons between Asian-American and non-Asian students utilizing a student health psychiatric clinic. *Journal of Counseling Psychology*, *21*, **423-427.**

The MMPI records of a total of 46 Chinese and Japanese students were compared with those of 120 non-Asian students from a university psychiatric clinic. Results indicate that compared to non-Asians, Chinese and Japanese students (a) underutilized the clinic services; (b) possessed more pronounced MMPI scale elevations; and (c) exhibited problems involving somatic complaints, family discord, and social introversion. Findings are discussed within the context of Asian cultural values. It is suggested that rates of psychopathology have been underestimated for Asian-Americans.

2979

Sugg, M. L. (1975). *Adolescent aggression in Hong Kong.* **Hong Kong: Chinese University of Hong Kong, Social Research Center.**

2980

Sun, Z. X., Zhao, J. C., Xia, M. L., Ren, R. Z., Yan, H. J., Yang, L. N., Gao, S., & Wang, S. Z. (1986). [Comparative study on the efficiency of EMG and the thermal biofeedback training the combination of biofeedback and autogenic training in reducing test anxiety]. *Acta Psychologica Sinica*, *18*, **196-202.** (In Chinese.)

This paper compared the efficiency of electromyograph (EMG) and thermal biofeedback and that of the combinations of biofeedback and autogenic training in reducing test anxiety. The subjects were 48 high-school students who were going to join university entrance exams and were selected according to their state-anxiety scores of the State-Trait Anxiety Inventory (STAI). They were assigned randomly to one of the following six groups: EMG feedback plus autogenic training; EMG feedback only; thermal feedback plus autogenic training; thermal feedback only; false feedback; training-delayed. Subjects in the first five groups received four separate 30-minute training sessions everyday. The changes of EMGs and temperatures and the state-anxiety scores of STAI in stressful situations before and after training were recorded and compared. The results showed that both EMG and thermal biofeedback training were effective in reducing anxiety; the combinations of biofeedback and autogenic training seemed to be more effective; false feedback training was no more effective than no training; and the most anxious subjects benefited most from training as far as state-anxiety scores were concerned.

2981

Sung, S. T. (1961). Psychoneuroses in Taiwan and hypothesis of balance-obstacle in the stimulus-reaction systems. *Proceedings of the Third World Congress of Psychiatry*, **Montreal, Canada, June, 1961 (pp. 863-867). Toronto, Canada: University of Toronto Press, McGill University Press.**

2982

Tam, Y. K., Tsoi, M. M., Kwong, B., & Wong, S. W. (1982). Psychological epidemic in Hong Kong: Vol. 2. Psychological and physiological characteristics of children who were affected. *Acta Psychiatrica Scandinavica*, *65*, **437-449.**

A double-blind retrospective study was carried out on 18 elementary school children who were affected in a mysterious gas poisoning epidemic together with controls drawn from the same schools. (Part I of this study (S. W. Wong et al) details an epidemiological study of the phenomenon.) The dependent measures employed were the Junior Eysenck Personality Questionnaire, Hypnotic Susceptibility Scale, heart rate (HR), and skin potential response (SPR). A vigilance task was administered during assessment of the latter 2 variables. No significant differences on the psychological variables were found between the Ss affected in the epidemic and those not affected. However, affected Ss had significantly higher HR together with a marginal increase in SPR. It is proposed that constitutional factors play an important role in determining whether an individual is affected in a hysterical epidemic.

2983

Tan, C. T., Chee, K. T., & Long, F. Y. (1980). Psychiatric patients who seek traditional healers in Singapore. *Singapore Medical Journal, 21,* **643-647.**

This paper analyses some demographic and clinical characteristics of 75 first admissions to the authors' unit in Woodbridge Hospital, all of whom had been to traditional healers prior to hospitalisation. The results suggest that a Chinese with a primary level of formal Chinese education is most likely to seek traditional help. When admitted he is most likely to suffer from schizophrenia and, if neurotic, from a depressive illness with suicidal intent. There is no cultural or religious bias to the types of healers sought, although almost all the Chinese went to the temple mediums and the Malays and Indians to the bomohs. Some probable reasons accounting for the above observations are discussed.

2984

Tan, E. S. (1981). Culture-bound syndromes among overseas Chinese. In A. Kleinman & T. Y. Lin (Eds.), *Normal and abnormal behavior in Chinese culture* **(pp. 371-386). Dordrecht, Netherlands: D. Reidel.**

2985

Tang, G. W. (1985). Emotional reactions to gynaecological surgery [Selected papers from the 1984 Annual Conference]. *Hong Kong Psychological Society Bulletin,* **No. 14, 5-7.**

Presents data from 2 groups of Chinese women who underwent a hysterectomy: 34 who had the operation for benign disease of the genital tract and 18 who had emergency operations because of pregnancy complications. Emotional reactions to the operations varied, but both groups experienced depression, insomnia, doubts and suspicions about the decision to have the operation, anger, and guilt.

2986

Tao, K. T. et al. (1957). [An analysis of 1,600 cases of schizophrenia]. *Chinese Journal of Neurology and Psychiatry, 3,* **134-144.** (In Chinese.)

2987

Tao, K. T. (1959). [Prevention and treatment of childhood psychoneurosis and psychosis]. *Chinese Journal of Neurology and Psychiatry, 5,* **312-315. (Also in** *Collection of theses on achievements in the medical sciences in commemoration of the 10th National Foundation Day of China* **(Vol. 2.), Beijing. Translated by U.S. Joint Publications Research Service, Report No. 14,829, pp. 683-699.)** (In Chinese.)

2988

Teoh, J. I. (1974). Psychological problems among university students in an area of rapid socio-cultural change. *Australian & New Zealand Journal of Psychiatry, 8,* **109-120.**

Conducted a 12-mo study of all students at the University of Malaya referred with psychological problems and symptoms. Data from 308 students treated show that (a) the proportion of students from different ethnic groups agreed with that of the total student population; (b) diagnoses did not differ among students from urban as opposed to rural origins; (c) 56% suffered from symptoms prior to university admission, and a majority of clients were seen during the 1st term of 1st- and 2nd-yr courses; (d) Chinese students had more personality and family problems and more severe acculturation-gap differences from their parents than did Malay students; and (e) 51% of the clients suffered from neuroses and 13% from schizophrenic psychosis.

2989

Teoh, J. I., Kinzie, J. D., & Tan, E. S. (1972). Referrals to a psychiatric clinic in West Malaysia. *International Journal of Social Psychiatry, 18,* **301-307.**

Classified complaints of 200 patients who sought the psychiatric services of the University of Malaya Medical Center. 49% complained of some type of subjective distress, 41% complained of social or interpersonal distress, and 9% came for assessment without specific complaints. Ethnic comparisons showed more Indian patients with subjective complaints and Chinese patients slightly over-represented in the social and interpersonal distress category. There was a tendency for upper social class patients to seek help for subjective reasons. Lower social class patients were more likely to have consulted a native healer prior to admission than other social classes. Data indicate a high degree of acceptance and confidence in western psychiatry in this relatively unsophisticated community.

2990

[The Teaching and Research Group of Psychiatry of Beijing Medical College] et al. (1980). [An investigation of psychiatric disorders in Haidian District of Beijing]. *Chinese Journal of Neurology & Psychiatry, 13,* **10-12.** (In Chinese.)

2991

Tien, L. J., & Soong, W. T. (1984). [Incomplete mourning: A case report]. *Chinese Journal of Mental Health, 1,* **83-89.** (In Chinese.)

2992

Ting, C., & Yu, C. H. (1957). [Prognosis of 200 cases of schizophrenia]. *Chinese Journal of Neurology and Psychiatry, 3,* **152-155.** (In Chinese.)

2993

Touliatos, J., & Lindholm, B. W. (1980). Behavioral disturbance in children of native-born and immigrant parents. *Journal of Community Psychology, 8,* **28-33.**

Examined the mental health status of children whose parents were foreign-born to determine if these youngsters have a special need for mental health services. The incidence of behavioral disturbance was compared in 2,991 kindergarten-8th grade Ss who were native-born and White and 97 children of immigrant parents. General information and ratings on a behavioral problem checklist were obtained from teachers. An ANOVA revealed that Ss of Chinese, Japanese, or Southeast Asian descent exhibited significantly fewer disorders, such as conduct problems and inadequacy/immaturity, than did Ss of native-born parents.

2994

Tsai, M., Teng, L. N., & Sue, S. (1981). Mental health status of Chinese in the United States. In A. Kleinman & T. Y. Lin (Eds.), *Normal and abnormal behavior in Chinese culture* **(pp. 291-310). Dordrecht, Netherlands: Reidel.**

2995

Tsao, P. (1962). [A study of higher nervous activity in normal and abnormal children by the method of combining different connective systems: Pt. I, Pt. II, Pt. III]. *Acta Psychologica Sinica,* **No. 1, 28-41; No. 3, 197-209; No. 4, 265-281.** (In Chinese.)

2996

Tseng, C. C., & Soong, W. T. (1983). [Diagnostic description of speech retardation]. *Acta Psychologica Taiwanica, 25,* **25-30.** (In Chinese.)

Speech retardation is the most frequently observed problem shown by children under 6 years of age visiting the Child's Mental Health Center of the National Taiwan University Hospital. The medical records of 267 speech-retarded children visiting this center in 1981 were reviewed and analyzed systematically. It was found that: (1) The mental retardation group and the multiple handicapped (including speech delay) group were similar in many aspects (including many associated pre- and peri-natal factors), but different from the simple speech delay group. (2) The simple speech delay group showed age-appropriate gross motor, fine motor, and social development, but mildly delayed language development. (3) The birth and developmental history of the simple speech delay group was usually normal. (4) Children with simple speech delay were usually younger, and came from families of higher socioeconomic status. They were taken to the center usually below 3 years of age.

2997

Tseng, W. H. (1971). [Society, culture and the psychiatry]. *Bulletin of the Institute of Ethnology* **(Academia Sinica), No. 32, 279-286.** (In Chinese.)

2998

Tseng, W. S. (1969). A paranoid family in Taiwan: A dynamic study of folie a famille. *Archives of General Psychiatry, 21,* **55-63.**

Reports and discusses a case of folie a famille in Taiwan. 8 persons were involved in a political persecutory delusion. 2 of the 3 adults were hospitalized, and the remaining adult and 5 children and the uninvolved wife of the key person were interviewed. Follow-up of this family group was continued for 4 yr. Emphasis is placed on the personality structure of the family members, on the family situation in the community, and on the dynamics of transmission of the paranoid formation among family members. The total resolution of psychosis in all but the key person was brought about by environmental manipulation.

2999

Tseng, W. S. (1973). The development of psychiatric concepts in traditional Chinese medicine. *Archives of General Psychiatry, 29,* **569-575.**

Traces the development of psychiatric conceptualization in traditional Chinese medicine by reviewing the descriptions of psychiatric maladies appearing in Chinese medical documents of various periods. The theory of mental illness has gone through a sequence of supernatural, natural, somatic, and psychological stages. Psychiatric illness has been recognized in medical literature in the following order: organic mental illness, excited psychosis, hysteria, depression, and minor psychiatric illness. These changes are compared with the development of psychiatric concepts in the West to understand how the perception and interpretation of mental illness have changed and developed through time in different sociocultural environments.

3000

Tseng, W. S. (1973). Psychopathologic study of obsessive-compulsive neurosis in Taiwan. *Comprehensive Psychiatry, 14,* **139-150.**

Studied 10 young Chinese males with obsessive-compulsive neuroses whose parents were living and who had one or more siblings near the same age. It was found that Ss manifested the early personality traits of timidity, obedience, thoughtfulness, etc., which may be constitutionally predetermined. The most outstanding characteristic of the intrafamilial situation was a close, intimate, and prolonged mother-son relationship and the frequent absence of the father or a distant father-son relationship. Through such close mother-son relationships, the mother had pathologically inhibited the child by overprotection, overworrying, and overrestriction. Consequently Ss had become increasingly timid and insecure and had learned to deal with problems by being excessively careful, self-controlling, and rigid. Although the close mother-son relationship is considered the causal condition for the occurrence of such pathology, it is the particular pattern of interaction between them which causes the development of a specific kind of mental illness. Factors intensifying the unusual mother-son relationship are explored and the reason why the mother focuses her attention on a particular child is analyzed.

3001

Tseng, W. S. (1975). The nature of somatic complaints among psychiatric patients: The Chinese case. *Comprehensive Psychiatry, 16,* **237-245.**

Argues that sociocultural factors may help to explain the existence of somatic problems in Chinese persons not fitting into the usual diagnostic groups for psychophysiological disorders (e.g., hysterical conversion or hypochondriasis). Eight case examples are presented to illustrate the influence of (a) the patient's knowledge and concept about his or her problems, (b) socially recognized and accepted signals of illness, and (c) reluctance and/or resistance to explore emotional difficulties on the type of presenting somatic symptom. The characteristics of each case are related to specific Chinese behaviors and attitudes which would help to explain the etiology of the somatic problem.

3002

Tsoi, M. (1985). Psychological contributions to understanding gynaecological problems [Selected papers from the 1984 Annual Conference]. *Hong Kong Psychological Society Bulletin,* **No. 14, 9-16.**

3003

Tsoi, M. M., & Ho, P. C. (1984). Psychological factors related to adjustment after tubal ligation. *Journal of Reproductive & Infant Psychology, 2,* **1-6.**

Interviewed 15 Chinese females (mean age 32.05 yrs) before and 6 months after tubal ligation. Subjects were administered the General Health Questionnaire, the Hypochondriasis scale of the Minnesota Multiphasic Personality Inventory (MMPI), and the Chinese Sex Role Inventory. There was a significant increase in symptomatic complaints at follow-up. There were significant correlations between preoperation hypochondriasis, number of expectations of postoperation changes, and degree of worry and complaints reported after tubal ligation. Contrary to expectation, a high masculinity score in sex-role stereotype tended to relate with more postoperative complaints. Results suggested that reactions to tubal ligation should be investigated within a different perspective.

3004

Tsoi, M. M., Leung, P. W. L., & Chow, S. P. (1982). Psychological reactions to hand injuries among semi-skilled Chinese workers. *Annals of the Academy of Medicine of Singapore, 11,* **214-217.**

3005

Tsoi, M. M., Leung, P. W. L., Chow, S. P., & Lee, P. C. (1985). Short-term reactions to hand injury caused by industrial accidents. *Journal of Hong Kong Psychiatric Association, 5,* **26-30.**

This study examined the psychological reactions of semi-skilled Chinese workers who suffered a hand injury in industrial accidents. The patients were assessed within one month after they had been discharged from hospital, having completed orthopaedic treatment. Although the patient group and the control group did not differ in locus of control, the former scored significantly lower than the latter on self-esteem as related to work. Moreover, severity of injury correlated negatively with self-esteem, and positively with unpleasant mood states. The findings implicated the need for psychosocial rehabilitation when patients are integrated back into society after physical rehabilitation.

3006

Tsoi, W. F. (1985). Mental health in Singapore and its relation to Chinese culture. In W. S. Tseng & D. Y. H. Wu (Eds.), *Chinese culture and mental health* **(pp. 229-250). Orlando, FL: Academic Press.**

3007

Tsoi, W. F., & Chia, B. H. (1974). Suicide and mental illness in Singapore. *Singapore Medical Journal, 15,* **191-196.**

3008

T'sou, B. K. (1978). Some preliminary observations on aphasia in a Chinese bilingual. *Acta Psychologica Taiwanica, 20,* **57-64.**

Presents observations of a 31-yr-old right-handed Cantonese woman literate in English and Chinese. S was hospitalized because of a sudden weakness in her right arm associated with numbness involving the right half of the body. She lost neither consciousness nor memory, but her speech became extremely abnormal. A brain scan indicated a blood clot in her left posterior temporal-parietal area. Data suggest that S had not been adversely affected in her ability to handle rudimentary processing of the semantic aspect of the work, but her ability to handle the acoustic aspect had been impaired. The problem apparently originated with the production (i.e., encoding) rather than the recognition (i.e., decoding) of acoustic images.

3009

Tsuang, M. T. (1971). Abnormality on paternal and maternal sides in Chinese schizophrenics. *British Journal of Psychiatry, 118,* **211-214.**

A family history search revealed 23 schizophrenics with 2 or more abnormal but not necessarily schizophrenic relatives. Analysis of the data shows a significant deviation to the unilateral distribution, supporting the hypothesis of a single dominant major gene in schizophrenic inheritance, as reported by E. Slater and M. T. Tsuang.

3010

Tsuang, M. T. (1972). Psychiatric genetics in Taiwan. *International Journal of Mental Health, 1,* **221-230.**

Reviews the literature on studies of psychiatric disorders in Taiwan, including research on risk of schizophrenia and affective disorders in families, mode of inheritance of schizophrenia, and effects of environmental factors. Cytogenic studies of sex chromosome abnormalities are discussed and projected investigations outlined, including studies of twins, research on sex chromatin in criminals and in normal children, and a psychopharmacogenetic study of drug responses in families containing 2 or more secondary cases of mental disorder.

3011

Tsuang, M. T. (1974). Sex chromatin anomaly in Chinese females: Psychiatric characteristics of XXX. *British Journal of Psychiatry, 124,* **299-305.**

Studied sex chromatin in oral mucosa of large groups of female psychiatric patients and normal girls. Results confirm the previous reports of higher rates of double sex chromatin in these patients. 3 cases of females with double sex chromatin are summarized and the psychiatric characteristics of cases with an XXX chromosome are discussed. These 3 cases exhibited what may be called transient acutely disturbed unspecified psychosis based on personality disorder or borderline mental retardation.

3012

Tsuang, M. T. (1975). Sex chromatin anomaly among Chinese psychiatric inpatients compared to school children. *Acta Psychiatrica Scandinavica, 51,* **88-91.**

In a study of sex chromatin abnormality among Chinese psychiatric inpatients, buccal smears were examined from a total of 639 male and 614 female psychiatric inpatients. One male S(1.6/1000) was chromatin positive (+ ve); 2 female Ss(3.3/1000) were found to have 2 sex chromatin bodies (+ +ve). The lower rate for male inpatients in comparison to a total of 2,157 Chinese schoolboys (2.3/1000) is thought to reflect a higher rate of mental subnormality in primary schoolchildren. This is considered attributable to the special nature of the school system and psychiatric patient facilities in Taiwan. The higher rate for female inpatients in comparison with a total of 2,182 schoolgirls (0.5/1000) indicates a predisposition to mental disorder in favor of psychosis associated with double sex chromatin abnormality in the female.

3013

Tsuang, M. T. (1976). Schizophrenia around the world. *Comprehensive Psychiatry, 17,* **477-481.**

Presents findings of a study sponsored by the World Health Organization on the diagnosis, classification, statistics, and epidemiology of schizophrenia in 9 cities: Aarhus, Denmark; Agra, India; Cali, Columbia; Ibadan, Nigeria; London, England; Moscow, USSR; Taipei, Taiwan; Washington, US; and Prague, Czechoslovakia. 1,202 Ss were interviewed using the Present State Examination Schedule, the Psychiatry History Schedule, and the Social Description Schedule. 811 Ss received a clinical diagnosis of schizophrenia, and the largest single diagnostic subgroup for the 811 schizophrenics was paranoid. The 2nd largest subgroup was schizo-affective schizophrenia.

3014

Tsuang, M. T., & Lin, S. N. (1974). Cutis verticis gyrata in a Chinese mental defective. *Journal of Mental Deficiency Research, 18,* **107-110.**

Presents the history of a case of cutis verticis gyrata in a 20-yr-old Chinese male. The disease was accompanied by strabismus, cerebral palsy, and adiposogenital dystrophy.

3015

Tzeng, O. J. L., Hung, D. L., Chen, S., Wu, J., & Hsi, M. S. (1986). Processing Chinese logographs by Chinese brain damaged patients. In H. S. R. Kao, G. P. van Galen, & R. Hoosain (Eds.), *Graphonomics: Contemporary research in handwriting* **(pp. 357-374). Amsterdam, Netherlands: North-Holland.**

3016

Veith, I. (1955). Psychiatric thought in Chinese medicine. *Journal of the History of Medicine and Allied Sciences, 10,* **261-268.**

3017

Veith, I. (1963). The supernatural in Far Eastern concepts of mental disease. *Bulletin of the History of Medicine, 37,* **139-155.**

3018

Vellutino, F. R., Bentley, W. L., & Phillips, F. (1978). Inter- versus intra-hemispheric learning in dyslexic and normal readers. *Developmental Medicine & Child Neurology, 20,* **71-80.**

Investigated the hypothesis that developmental dyslexia is attributable to dysfunction in inter-hemispheric transfer. 72 dyslexic and normal readers in 2nd and 6th grade were given tachistoscopic presentations of novel visual stimuli (Chinese ideographs), randomly presented to the left and right visual fields and to the central fixation point. Each stimulus was paired with a common English word (spoken), and Ss were asked to associate the two. The transmission deficit hypothesis predicts that poor and normal readers will be differentiated in the case of presentations to the left hemisphere (right visual field). This hypothesis was not supported. Normal readers at both grade levels performed significantly better than poor readers in both visual-field presentations.

3019

Wan, W. P., Yu, W. Y. et al. (1981). [An investigation of psycho-hygiene of the Jinoans--A Chinese minority nationality]. *Acta Psychologica Sinica, 13,* **459-463.** (In Chinese.)

3020

Wang, C. Y., & Tuan, S. C. (1957). [An analysis of the clinical data over four years on patients hospitalized in the Peking Medical College Psychiatric Hospital]. *Chinese Journal of Neurology and Psychiatry, 3,* **162-170.** (In Chinese.)

3021

Wang, H. T. et al. (1959). [Alexia]. *Chinese Journal of Neurology and Psychiatry, 5,* **221-224, 234.** (In Chinese.)

3022

Wang, J. H. (1961). [The role of psychological factors in the genesis, development and speedy-synthetic treatment of hypertension]. *Acta Psychologica Sinica,* **No. 2, 107-116.** (In Chinese.)

This paper analyzes the function of psychological factors in the genesis and development of hypertension, based on 252 cases. The role of psychotherapy in the speedy synthetic treatments of 288 cases of hypertension is also discussed.

3023

Wang, J. H., & Lee, H. T. (1960). [Preliminary study of the etiology of neurasthenia]. *Acta Psychologica Sinica,* **No. 1, 46-53.** (In Chinese.)

Taking "external causes to be the condition of change and internal causes to be the basis of change, external causes becoming operative through internal causes", this paper was an analysis of the etiology of 283 neurasthenics. It was shown that external agents cause overstrain of cortical activity only through the internal characteristics of the patient - the functional state of the cortex and the patient's recognition. The authors drew the preliminary conclusion that the patient's attitude toward his work, study and life has a great effect on the generation and development of neurasthenia. Comments were also made on the problem of the relationship between the patient's recognition and individual characteristics and the characteristics of types of higher nervous activity and on the problem how the two factors interact in causing neurasthenia.

3024

Wang, S. C. (1958). [Postpartal psychosis]. *Chinese Journal of Neurology and Psychiatry, 4,* **494-498.** (In Chinese.)

3025

Wang, S. C. et al. (1981). [An investigation on clinical types of schizophrenia in its chronic stage]. *Chinese Journal of Neurology & Psychiatry, 14,* **215-218.** (In Chinese.)

3026

Wang, X. D. et al. (1986). [Agraphia in Chinese aphasic patients]. *Chinese Journal of Neurology and Psychiatry, 19,* **109-111.** (In Chinese.)

Twenty-five aphasic patients with agraphia following cerebral vascular disease were studied. An aphasic assessment scale designed by the Department of Neurology of Beijing Hospital was used to assess oral and auditory functions, reading, and writing. The results showed that the scores for copying were much higher than those for dictation or filling in blanks. The patients obtained good scores for writing their names voluntarily. Dictation was better for Chinese characters with similar forms than those with similar pronunciations or meanings. Some features such as total agraphia, construction disorder, repetition, overproduction, and mirror writing were described and discussed from a neuropsychological point of view.

3027

Wat, S. (1985). Central Registry of Drug Abuse. *International Journal of the Addictions, 20,* **279-298.**

The background, operation, and findings of the reorganized Central Registry of Drug Abuse, which began operation on September 1, 1976, was described. It serves as an invaluable monitoring device to identify at regular intervals any changes in trends and characteristics that may herald significant changes in the drug abuse patterns in Hong Kong. This marks a major advance in Hong Kong's efforts to improve the database on which realistic antinarcotics policies can be formulated.

3028

Weiner, B. P., & Marvit, R. C. (1977). Schizophrenia in Hawaii: Analysis of cohort mortality risk in a multi-ethnic population. *British Journal of Psychiatry, 131,* **497-503.**

Schizophrenic patients in treatment within the Hawaii state system were followed from 1962 to 1972. The cohort included 1,689 persons: outpatients as well as inpatients; of Japanese, Caucasian, part-Hawaiian, Filipino, Chinese, and other ancestries. After 10 yrs, 60% remain registered with the Hawaii Mental Health Division, 14% were living in the state, 12% were lost to follow-up, and 14% died Morality was analyzed for all causes by comparison with similar ethnic and sex subgroups of the general population.

3029

Wen, C. P. (1974). Secular suicidal trend in postwar Japan and Taiwan: An examination of hypotheses. *International Journal of Social Psychiatry, 20,* **8-17.**

Marked increases in suicide among young adults (ages 15-24) occurred in Japan in the late 1950s and in Taiwan in the early 1960s. In peak years, suicide caused over half of all deaths in this age group. 2-3 yrs after the peak in each country, the rate rapidly declined. Social factors commonly related to suicide are examined as possible causes, but all fail to explain the historical timing or age-specificity of the suicide waves. It is hypothesized that stress caused by World War II in Japan (1942-1945) and the massive immigration of refugees from mainland China into Taiwan (1948-1951) strongly affected children and predisposed them to suicide as young adults, 13 yrs later.

3030

Wen, J. K., & Wang, C. L. (1981). Shen-k'uei syndrome: A culture-specific sexual neurosis in Taiwan. In A. Kleinman & T. Y. Lin (Eds.) *Normal and abnormal behavior in Chinese culture* **(pp. 357-369). Dordrecht, Netherlands: D. Reidel.**

3031

Werner, E. E., & Smith, R. S. (1980). An epidemiologic perspective on some antecedents and consequences of childhood mental health problems and learning disabilities: A report from the Kauai Longitudinal Study. *Annual Progress in Child Psychiatry & Child Development,* **133-147.**

Investigated the interaction effects of perinatal stress and quality of family environment for a multiracial cohort of 660 children born on the island of Kauai, Hawaii, and followed from the prenatal period to age 18 yrs. The subjects included Japanese, Filipinos, Hawaiians, part-Hawaiians, Portuguese, Puerto-Ricans, Chinese, Koreans, and a small group of Anglo-Saxon Caucasians. About half of the subjects came from families in which the fathers were semiskilled or unskilled laborers and the mothers had less than 8 years of education. Antecedents and consequences of childhood mental health problems and learning disabilities illustrate the relationship between social class and vulnerability, the likelihood of persistence of childhood disorders with strong biological and temperamental underpinnings, the pervasive effects of quality of early caretaker-child transactions, the importance of an internal locus of control and communication skills in coping with emotional and academic problems, and the resiliency of most children. Implications of the findings for the child clinical professions were discussed.

3032

White, G. M. (1982). The role of cultural explanations in "somatization" and "psychologization". *Social Science & Medicine, 16,* **1519-1530.**

The "interpretive hypothesis", which explains differences in illness behavior in terms of cultural factors, was explored by eliciting causal inferences about illness and behavioral difficulties from 15 (Caucasian) American and 15 Hong Kong Chinese university students. Comparative analysis gave limited support to the interpretive hypothesis in showing a more "psychologized" American model of illness in comparison with the "situational" explanations given by the Chinese Ss. The contrasts in common sense explanations offered by each sample suggest that these differences are related to implicit cultural modes of interpreting social behavior that have been characterized by other researchers with oppositions such as individual-centered vs situation-centered and internal vs external locus of control. These speculations, however, are tempered by the finding that the Chinese Ss made relatively greater use of personality attributions (a kind of psychological construct) in explaining interpersonal problems. This result indicates that global characterizations of explanatory modes should be limited to specific domains of discourse.

3033

Wittenberg, C. (1977, October). Visitors to China see reduction in illness. *Psychiatric News.*

3034

Wong, C. K. (1986). The case of hysteria as illustrated by a Chinese boy with psychogenic torticollis. *Hong Kong Journal of Mental Health, 15,* **51-55.**

This paper presented a case study of psychogenic torticollis in a 6-year-old Chinese boy. Neither significant physical cause nor deep-seated psychological conflicts were uncovered. It was argued that the boy was actually entrenched in a hysteria process which involved not only himself and his family but also medicine and doctors.

3035

Wong, C. K., & Chan, T. S. C. (1984). Somatic symptoms among Chinese psychiatric patients. *Hong Kong Journal of Mental Health, 13,* **5-21.**

Somatic symptoms in a population of Chinese psychiatric patients were studied, using the somatic scale of the Chinese University Health Questionnaire. Two control samples were included for comparison. It was found that psychiatric patients, especially patients suffering from affective or neurotic disorders, tended to have three or more acute and/or chronic symptoms, whereas only about 10% of the control subjects had the same number of symptoms. The usefulness of the somatic scale in helping to detect psychiatric cases was discussed.

3036

Wong, C. W. (1973). A preliminary study of schizophrenic patients: Chronological age, family size and sibling rank. *Hong Kong Journal of Mental Health, 2,* **8-13.**

3037

Wong, J. W. P., Lau, I. S. Y., & Wong, V. (1984). Work stress among office workers in Hong Kong. *Hong Kong Journal of Mental Health, 13,* **66-73.**

Mental health and work stress among 839 office workers in Hong Kong were studied, using Langner's 22-item scale. Work type, living and working environment, social support factors, and stressful life events were included in a self-administered questionnaire. It was found that 366 of the respondents exceeded the cut-off point of 4 symptoms; the prevalence rate of psychiatric disturbance was thus consided to be 43.6%. Females appeared to have more psychiatric symptoms than males. Social support was an important factor in coping. Respondents who were married, had good relationships with colleagues, and were more active socially seemed to have fewer symptoms. Those with higher education appeared to be more adaptive to stressful situations. Those with job satisfaction and in better living and working environments also seemed to be under less stress. Subjects between 31 to 40 years old tended to be more successful in stress management. Stressful life events were contributing factors to psychological problems; 54% of the "distressed" group had experienced moderate to high clusters of stressful life events.

3038

Wong, M., & Singer, K. (1973). Abnormal homicide in Hong Kong. *British Journal of Psychiatry, 123,* **295-298.**

Reports that from 1961 to 1971 there were 29 suicide-murders and 41 murders by the mentally ill in Hong Kong, in addition to 551 ordinary homicides. This is a total homicide rate 4 times higher than that of the United Kingdom and slightly higher than that of Philadelphia. The rate of murder by the mentally ill in Hong Kong is similar to rates reported elsewhere, but the frequency of suicide-murder is relatively low. Shooting and gas asphyxiation are rare in Hong Kong due to the absence of the means. Chopping weapons are used rather than stabbing points. Age, sex, and social class patterns resemble those elsewhere.

3039

Wong, S. W. (1979). Hypochondriacal complaints among Hong Kong children: A mental health hazard? *Annals of the Academy of Medicine, 8,* **244-251.**

The incidence of hypochondriacal complaints among clinic attenders at a general outpatient clinic is in the region of 51 per 1,000. 33 children were studied in detail. Their age ranged from 1.5-14, with a mode of 8-10 years; females outnumbered males slightly (1.33:1). They usually came from lower socio-economic backgrounds, but a substantial portion also came from a higher social class. Among this latter group, psychological complaints predominate. Pain remained the most frequent complaint. There was also a predominance of complaints confined to the respiratory tract, a tendency which could be explained on a cultural and public-health basis. Very few of the children had previous hypochondriacal traits, a fact which contrasted sharply to those of their parents in whom hypochondriacal traits predominated. Hypochondriacal children, when treated, had good prognostic outcomes.

3040

Wong, S. W. (1981). Culture and psychiatry. *Hong Kong Journal of Mental Health, 9,* **5-15.**

3041

Wong, S. W., & Kwong, B. (1983). Chinese language and hypochondriacal complaints. *Journal of the Hong Kong Psychiatric Association, 3,* **25-29.**

3042

Wong, S. W., Kwong, B., Tam, Y. K., & Tsoi, M. M. (1982). Psychological epidemic in Hong Kong: Vol. 1. Epidemiological study. *Acta Psychiatrica Scandinavica, 65,* **421-436.**

To determine the causes of an epidemic that led to the hospitalization of 413 school-children and that had been thought to be caused by a mysterious gas, interviews were conducted with 684 students who had or had not been affected, their parents, and 89 teachers. No chemical causative agent was found, and findings suggest the role of peer influences and anxiety transmitted unwittingly from teachers and principals. The role of individual response to stress is examined in a 2nd paper by the authors (Y. K. Tam et al).

3043

Woo, E. Y. C., & Hoosain, R. (1984). Visual and auditory functions of Chinese dyslexics. *Psychologia: An International Journal of Psychology in the Orient, 27,* **164-170.**

Thirteen dyslexic Chinese boys were compared to a control group of age-matched boys of normal reading ability on the following tests: a Chinese character recognition test, a Chinese version of the Frostig Developmental Test of Visual Perception, the Auditory Association subtest of the Illinois Test of Psycholinguistic Abilities, and a digit span test. Compared with subjects in the control group, dyslexic subjects made more visual-distractor errors in character recognition but similar phonological-distractor errors. There was a significant difference in all of the 5 subtests of the Frostig Test between the 2 groups, but there was no significant difference in either of the 2 auditory tests. Results indicate the importance of visual processing in the reading of Chinese and suggest that it is the primary cause of dyslexia among Chinese children. Possible orthography differences between Chinese and English are discussed.

3044

Woods, A. H. (1929). The nervous diseases of the Chinese. *Archives of Neurology and Psychiatry, 21,* **542-570.**

3045

Wu, D. Y. H. (1981). Child abuse in Taiwan. In J. E. Korbin (Ed.), *Child abuse and neglect: Cross-cultural perspectives* **(pp. 139-165). Berkeley, CA: University of California Press.**

3046

Wu, W. T., & Liang, C. N. (1978). [Attitudes toward disabled persons: A comparative study]. *Psychological Testing, 25,* **85-93.** (In Chinese.)

3047

Wu, W. Y. et al. (1986). [Application of rating scales in the assessment of depressive neurosis: A preliminary trial]. *Chinese Journal of Neurology and Psychiatry, 19,* **339-341.** (In Chinese.)

The results of a study of 100 patients with depressive neurosis assessed by HAMD, CES-D, GAS, and CGI-SI are reported. The total scores of HAMD, CES-D, CGL-SI, and GAS were highly intercorrelated; responses to HAMD items corresponded to clinical observations. The authors believe that HAMD and CES-D are useful tools for assessing depression.

3048

Xia, Y. F. et al. (1981). [A multivariate study of suicidal behaviors in schizophrenia]. *Information on Psychological Sciences,* **No. 4, 7-13.** (In Chinese.)

Using multiple-variable analysis, an investigation of 75 schizophrenics who had attempted suicide showed that the essential predisposing factors were aggravations of persecutory delusion and delusion of reference. In female patients, the mutual feedback reinforcement between delusions and disorders of association and logical thinking also aggravated committing suicide. In most cases, auditory hallucination was only an intermediate step in the vicious cycle of suicidal attempts. The conclusion was that in most cases of schizophrenia attempting suicide was conscious self-defeating behavior.

3049

Xia, Z. Y. et al. (1979). [A heredofamilial study of schizoaffective psychosis]. *Chinese Journal of Neurology and Psychiatry, 12,* **1-3.** (In Chinese.)

3050

Xia, Z. Y. et al. (1979). [A heredofamilial study of 294 probands of affective psychoses]. *Chinese Journal of Neurology and Psychiatry, 12,* **154-157.** (In Chinese.)

3051

Xiang, D. H. et al. (1980). [Psychogenic factors and schizophrenia]. *Chinese Journal of Neurology & Psychiatry, 13,* **202-204.** (In Chinese.)

3052

Xiang, M. Z. et al. (1986). [An epidemiological investigation of neurosis in 12 districts of China]. *Chinese Journal of Neurology and Psychiatry, 19,* **87-91.** (In Chinese.)

This epidemiological investigation of mental health in 12 districts used a sample of 1,200 families, consisting of 6,754 persons ranging in age from 15 to 59 years. The prevalence rate of neurosis was found to be 22.21 per 1,000. It was higher for females than for males which may be related to females social position in China. The 40 year old group had the highest rate. Compared with those in some Western countries, the prevalence rate in China was relatively low. The author suggested that the stable family structure, the greater importance attached to relatives and friends, and the stronger social supporting system in China may be factors favorable to mental health.

3053

Xu, C. L. et al. (1986). [A trial application of SDSS in Chinese psychiatric patients]. *Chinese Journal of Neurology and Psychiatry, 19,* **92-96.** (In Chinese.)

The social disability screening schedule (SDSS) was used to rate 194 cases of schizophrenia and 153 cases of neurosis. A brief comment on the clinical, familial, and social factors in relation to the SDSS scores was given.

3054

Xu, S. S. (1979). [A special type of psychic infantilism: Disability to manage daily life in coexistence with special talent]. *Chinese Journal of Neurology and Psychiatry, 12,* **207-208.** (In Chinese.)

3055

Xu, Y. (1956). [Brief introduction to psychiatric illness in China during the Six Dynasties, Tsui and T'ang]. *Chinese Journal of Neurology and Psychiatry, 1,* **14-19.** (In Chinese.)

3056

Xum, M. L. (1986). [The problem of birth control in schizophrenic patients]. *Chinese Journal of Neurology and Psychiatry, 19,* **335-338.** (In Chinese.)

3057

Yamamoto, J. et al. (1985). Are American psychiatric outpatients more depressed than Chinese outpatients? *American Journal of Psychiatry, 142,* **1347-1351.**

The assumption was tested that Americans tend to seek psychiatric help for depression, whereas Chinese patients are more likely to have somatic symptoms of emotional disturbance. Ninety-nine Taiwanese and 97 American psychiatric outpatients were given computerized diagnoses based on information obtained in a standard psychiatric interview schedule. It was found that the Chinese subjects scored higher on the measure of somatization and also on the measures of depression. Data did not support the assumption.

3058

Yan, S. M. et al. (1982). Prevalence and characteristics of mania in Chinese inpatients: A prospective study. *American Journal of Psychiatry, 139,* **1150-1153.**

Studied 108 Chinese mania patients (mean index age 31.51 yrs). Ss' clinical characteristics were similar to those reported by R. Abrams and M. A. Taylor for 55 Western patients; their response to treatment was excellent and their course benign. Their 1st-degree relatives had a high morbidity risk for affective disorder and a low morbidity risk for schizophrenia. The authors discuss the implications of their findings in China, where the use of Li is uncommon because of the impression that mania is rare in that country.

3059

Yan, S. M. et al. (1984). The frequency of major psychiatric disorder in Chinese inpatients. *American Journal of Psychiatry, 141,* **690-692.**

Assessed the prevalence of major psychiatric disorder in 268 Chinese inpatients (mean age 31.5 yrs) to whom DSM-III criteria were applied. Nearly a quarter of Ss had affective disorder, one-third had schizophrenia, and, except for 1 S, none had alcoholism or drug abuse. Factors influencing hospitalization in China are discussed.

3060

Yan, S. M. et al. (1985). Torque response in psychotics and normal controls: A study in an Asian culture. *Comprehensive Psychiatry, 26,* **342-344.**

Torque (i.e., drawing circles in a clockwise direction), a putative sign of subtle neurological defect, was assessed in 203 consecutive psychotic Chinese patients admitted to a general adult treatment service in China and 151 normal Chinese controls. Results indicated that, although the proportion of subjects exhibiting torque was greater than that reported in Western samples, there were no significant differences in torque frequency between patients and normals, between schizophrenics and affectively ill patients, or between chronic and nonchronic schizophrenics. It was concluded that torque is not important in the pathophysiology of these psychoses.

3061

Yan, W. W. et al. (1981). [A survey of minimal brain dysfunction]. *Information on Psychological Sciences,* **No. 1, 28-33.** (In Chinese.)

A survey on the prevalence rate of minimal brain dysfunction in school children was conducted. The sample consisted of 402 pupils in an elementary school in Shanghai. Diagnosis was established on the basis of parental reports on the child's behavior, psychological and physical tests. It was found that 13.43% of the pupils had minimal brain dysfunction, 3.43% being severe cases.

3062

Yan, W. W. (1982). [A preliminary study of diagnostic methods for MBD]. *Information on Psychological Sciences,* **No. 5, 7-11.** (In Chinese.)

3063

Yang, D. S. et al. (1980). [An investigation of psychoses in Hunan Province]. *Chinese Journal of Neurology & Psychiatry, 13,* **15-18.** (In Chinese.)

3064

Yang, D. S., & Chen, Y. D. (1980). A survey report on psychosis in Hunan Province. *China Report: Science and Technology,* **No. 53. (Translated by U.S. Joint Publications Research Service, No. 76,320, pp. 32-42).**

3065

Yang, H. G. et al. (1981). [Negative speech and behavior in schizophrenics]. *Chinese Journal of Neurology & Psychiatry, 14,* **39-41.** (In Chinese.)

3066

Yang, J. X. et al. (1985). [Character types of coronary arteriosclerosis patients and dialectic correlation in traditional Chinese medicine]. *Information on Psychological Sciences*, **No. 3, 36-38.** (In Chinese.)

3067

Yang, K. S. (1979). [Mirror-drawing performance under stressful and neutral conditions of junior high school students with different types of problem behavior]. *Acta Psychologica Taiwanica*, *21*, **91-98.** (In Chinese.)

Administered a questionnaire of 130 problem behaviors to 2,509 male Chinese junior high school students. Ss were then divided into 5 groups: (1) Ss with neurotic behaviors (NB), (2) Ss with delinquent behaviors, (3) Ss with learning-difficulty behaviors (LDB), (4) Ss with all 3 types of problem behaviors, and (5) Ss without problem behaviors. Ss then performed a mirror-drawing task, first under a neutral condition for 3 trials and then under a stressful condition for another 3 trials. Results indicate that under neutral instructions the 5 groups did not significantly differ from one another in their average performance. However, under stressful instructions the NB and LDB groups tended to increase their errors, displaying a stronger susceptibility to stress than the other groups. Since the "neutral" condition might not have been completely neutral, the delayed performance drop under the stressful condition seems to suggest an effect of stress immunization.

3068

Yang, K. S. (1981). Problem behavior in Chinese adolescents in Taiwan: A classificatory-factorial study. *Journal of Cross-Cultural Psychology*, *12*, **179-193.**

Obtained anonymous self-ratings of 130 problem behaviors for 2,432 male and 2,723 female students drawn from 14 junior high schools in the Taipei area. Two major unrotated factors emerged with substantial cross-sex invariance and were labeled General Maladjustment and Outward-Inward Orientation. Through oblique rotation, 2 psychologically meaningful factors were identified and named as Delinquent Behavior (further divided into 2 subgroups, Pleasure-Seeking and Rule-Violating Delinquent Behavior) and Neurotic Behavior.

3069

Yang, X. L. (1985). An investigation of minimal brain disorders among primary school students in the Beijing area. In W. S. Tseng & D. Y. H. Wu (Eds.), *Chinese culture and mental health* **(pp. 315-323). Orlando, FL: Academic Press.**

3070

Yap, P. M. (1957). A diagnostic and prognostic study of the schizophrenias in Chinese. *Congress report of the second International Congress for Psychiatry*, **Vol. 1, Zurich, Switzerland.**

3071

Yap, P. M. (1958). Suicide in Hong Kong. *Journal of Mental Science*, *104*, **266-301.**

3072

Yap, P. M. (1958). *Suicide in Hong Kong: With special reference to attempted suicide.* **Hong Kong: Hong Kong University Press.**

3073

Yap, P. M. (1958). Hypereridism and attempted suicide in Chinese. *Journal of Nervous & Mental Disease*, *127*, **34-41.**

3074

Yap, P. M. (1960). The possession syndrome: A comparison of Hong Kong and French findings. *Journal of Mental Science*, *106*, **114-147.**

3075

Yap, P. M. (1965). Koro -- a culture bound depersonalization syndrome. *British Journal of Psychiatry*, *111*, **43-50.**

Koro refers to a state of acute anxiety with partial depersonalization leading to the conviction that a man suffers from penile shrinkage. A series of 19 cases seen over a 15-year period in Hong Kong is discussed.

3076

Yap, P. M. (1965). Phenomenology of affective disorder in Chinese and other cultures (CIBA Foundation Symposium). In A. V. S. de Reuck & R. Porter (Eds.), *Transcultural psychiatry* **(pp. 84-114). London: J. & A. Churchill.**

3077

Yap, P. M. (1967). Ideas of mental health and disorder in Hong Kong and their practical influence. In M. Topley (Ed.), *Some traditional Chinese ideas and conceptions in Hong Kong social life today* **(pp. 73-85). Hong Kong: Hong Kong Branch of the Royal Asiatic Society.**

3078

Yap, P. M. (1972). Mental illness among western expatriates in a plural society: An exploratory study. In W. P. Lebra (Ed.), *Transcultural research in mental health: II. Mental health research in Asia and the Pacific.* **Honolulu, HI: University Hawaii Press.**

3079

Yap, P. M., & Liu, S. (1960). The possession syndrome in Hong Kong and in Catholic cultures. *Bulletin of the Hong Kong Chinese Medical Association*, **53-71.**

3080

Yeh, E. K. (1972). Paranoid manifestations among Chinese students studying abroad: Some preliminary findings. In W. P. Lebra (Ed.), *Mental health research in Asia and the Pacific: Vol. 2. Transcultural research in mental health*. **Honolulu, HI: University of Hawaii Press. (Also paper presented at the Conference on Culture and Mental Health in Asia and the Pacific, March, 1969.)**

3081

Yeh, E. K. (1985). Sociocultural changes and prevalence of mental disorders in Taiwan. In W. S. Tseng & D. Y. H. Wu (Eds.), *Chinese culture and mental health* **(pp. 265-286). Orlando, FL: Academic Press.**

3082

Yeh, E. K., Chu, H. M., Ko, Y. H., Lin, T. Y., & Lee, S. P. (1972). Student mental health: An epidemiological study in Taiwan. *Acta Psychologica Taiwanica*, *14*, **1-25.**

This paper reports some important findings of a 4-year epidemiological study in a university. All the freshmen were studied, by means of questionnaires and individual interviews, from the time of entrance to graduation. Nearly one-third of the freshmen could be classified as "psychiatric cases." Some differences in the prevalence of symptoms among various domicile groups and sexes, and in comparison with the general population, were found. Although the prevalence rates of mental disorders did not, as a whole, change during the later years of college, some changes in symptom manifestation were observed. The social, cultural, and life experience factors related to freshmen mental health and attitudes toward professional help were presented. In addition, academic achievement was found to be correlated with mental health. The value of the Maudsley Personality Inventory and Mental Health Questionnaires, and their correlations with academic achievement were discussed.

3083

Yeh, E. K., Fan, B. Y., & Tien, S. J. (1979). [A statistical study of the discharged patients from the Taipei City Psychiatric Center during 1969-1978]. In *Ten-Years Report of the Taipei City Psychiatric Center* **(pp. 209-240). Taipei: Taipei City Psychiatric Center.** (In Chinese.)

3084

Yen, L. K. (1950). [Amnesia]. *Journal of Internal Medicine*, *3*, **16-23.** (In Chinese.)

3085

Yen, Y. S. (1963). The diagnostic indicators of simple schizophrenia in the Rorschach test. *Acta Psychologica Taiwanica*, **No. 5, 52-56.**

3086

Yen, Y. S. (1983). Deviant verbalization in the Rorschach Test as indices of pathological thinking of schizophrenics. *Acta Psychologica Taiwanica*, *25*, **13-23.**

The hypothesis of the present study was that Watkins and Stauffacher's Delta Scores show a significant correlation with the degree of pathological disorganization. Delta Scores are constituted by 15 types of deviant verbalization. In the present study, four groups (Normal, Neurotic, Borderline State and Schizophrenic) of 100 subjects were investigated. The data indicated that the high degrees of Delta values represented pathological thinking of the clinical groups. The results also showed that among the 15 types of deviant verbalization, "confabulation" was the most autistic, and most clearly a part of schizophrenic thinking. Autistic logic, incoherence, absurd verbalization and deterioration color were also qualitatively significant indicators of unrealistic and disorganized thinking of schizophrenics. The items of fabulized combination, contamination and confusion were very rare occurrences in the psychotic group, although these verbalizations are considered as reliable indicators of pathological thinking. In the Normal group, there was no occurrence of any deviant verbalization. Furthermore, the Borderline State group scored slightly higher than the Schizophrenic group on the items of fabulized responses and relationship verbalization which are characteristics of those clinical groups in which ideation is rich and paranoid preoccupation is indicated.

3087

Yeoh, O. H. (1981). Attempted suicides in Penang. Preliminary observations. *Medical Journal of Malaysia*, *36*, **39-46.**

3088

Yeung, C. Y., & Yang, L. (1976). Down's syndrome with XO/XY mosaicism. *Acta Paediatrica Scandinavica* **(Sweden),** *65*, **391-395.**

A 5 month Chinese infant with combined Down's syndrome and XO/XY mosaicism is presented. The phenotypical features of mongolism are classical and unmodified. The somatic effect of XO/XY mosaicism is that of incomplete masculinization with short phallus, hypospadias, bifid scrotum, urogenital sinus, and bilateral extra abdominal infantile testicles. These features together with the absence of internal female organs and signs of Turner's syndrome in this patient are different from the previous reported cases of mixed gonadal dysgenesis.

3089

Young, D. (1985). In China: Evaluation of social stress as an etiologic factor of mental illness. *Integrative Psychiatry, 3,* **211-213.**

The author discussed problems of qualitative and quantitative assessment of social stress, the role of personal attitude in monitoring response to stress, and the assessment of stress as an etiologic factor of mental illness, based on the author's personal experience in clinical research and with epidemiologic surveys in China. It was suggested that the onset of psychogenic mental illness is probably affected by multiple influences, with one dominant factor and others playing a subordinate role.

3090

Yu, C. H., & Li, S. L. (1958). [Observations on the statistics of manic-depression in the Xian region]. *Chinese Journal of Neurology and Psychiatry, 4,* **288-291.** (In Chinese.)

3091

Yu, H. J. (1981). [Factors influencing the prognosis of schizophrenia in adolescents and children: A report of 118 cases]. *Chinese Journal of Neurology & Psychiatry, 14,* **76-78.** (In Chinese.)

3092

Yu, L. (1985). An epidemiological study of child's mental health problems in Nanjing district. In W. S. Tseng & D. Y. H. Wu (Eds.), *Chinese culture and mental health* **(pp. 305-314). Orlando, FL: Academic Press.**

3093

Yu, T. H., & Chang, W. H. (1986). [An analysis of changes in mental health among university students -- using KMHQ scores at two universities]. In H. Y. Chiu & Y. H. Chang (Eds.), *[Social and cultural change in Taiwan]* **(Monograph Series B, No. 16, Vol. 2, pp. 555-589). Taipei: Academia Sinica, Institute of Ethnology.** (In Chinese.)

3094

Yuan, G. Q. (1980). [The course and outcome of chronic schizophrenia]. *Chinese Journal of Neurology & Psychiatry, 13,* **105-106.** (In Chinese.)

3095

Zhang, B. Y. et al. (1980). [An experimental psychological study on paranoid schizophrenia with different clinical features]. *Chinese Journal of Neurology & Psychiatry, 13,* **102-104.** (In Chinese.)

3096

Zhang, B. Y. (1985). [Psychophysiological reaction in cardiovascular disease: Vol. 2. A study on the behavior pattern of coronary heart disease patients]. *Acta Psychologica Sinica, 17,* **314-321.** (In Chinese.)

Studies on the behavior pattern of coronary heart disease (CHD) patients have begun in China. A survey of 714 CHD patients, 425 normal people and 220 family members of the patients was conducted in 18 provinces and municipalities. The result showed that the scores of Type A behavior pattern (TABP) in CHD patients were significantly higher than in normal people, and the scores of white collar workers were significantly higher than those of physical workers. There was no obvious difference with respect to sex or age.

3097

Zhang, M. Y. (1981). [A survey on the diagnostic criteria of schizophrenia in a number of psychiatrists]. *Chinese Journal of Neurology & Psychiatry, 14,* **176-178.** (In Chinese.)

3098

Zhang, M. Y. et al. (1981). [Symptoms of primary importance in the diagnosis of schizophrenia]. *Chinese Journal of Neurology & Psychiatry, 14,* **72-75.** (In Chinese.)

3099

Zhang, Y. H. et al. (1986). [Genetic investigation of affective psychosis in Shandong province]. *Chinese Journal of Neurology and Psychiatry, 19,* **170-174.** (In Chinese.)

The pedigree of 96 patients suffering from affective psychosis discovered during a psychiatric epidemiological survey was investigated. It was found that the prevalence rate of affective psychosis was 4.84% in the patients' first grade relatives and 1.09% in their second grade relatives. Both were higher than those of the control group and the total population. Analysis of the possible mode of inheritance of affective psychosis showed that it was in accord with the idea of multigenic heredity. The average hereditary degree was higher than that for schizophrenia in the district. Based on a mathematical model, the incidence rates of affective psychosis among second grade relatives under various conditions were calculated, thus providing a scientific basis for hereditary consultation.

3100

Zhao, Y. Z. et al. (1986). [An analysis of epidemiological data on psychosis other than schizophrenia]. *Chinese Journal of Neurology and Psychiatry, 19,* **77-79.** (In Chinese.)

An analysis of the psychiatric epidemiological data gathered from 12 districts showed the lifetime prevalence rate and point prevalence rate (per 1,000) for affective psychosis, paranoid psychosis, reactive psychosis, schizo-affective psychosis, senile dementia, mental disorder associated with physical diseases; and cases of poison, brain trauma, vascular disorders of the brain, intracranial infections, epilepsy, alcoholism, drug abuse, and psychopathy.

3101

Zhao, Y. Z. et al. (1986). [An epidemiological investigation of affective psychosis]. *Chinese Journal of Neurology and Psychiatry, 19,* **97-98.** (In Chinese.)

A collaborative psychiatric epidemiological investigation of affective psychosis was carried out in 12 research districts. The sample consisted of 38,136 people. The prevalence rate was found to be 0.76 per 1,000. The point prevalence rate in 1982 was 0.37 per 1,000 which was higher than those reported in the 1970s, but lower than that for Changshan Islands. The prevalence rate was analyzed in relation to age, sex, educational level, occupation, economic status, and other variables.

3102

Zheng, Y., & Young, D. (1983). [The relationship of life event change and stress to neurosis]. *Chinese Journal of Neurology and Psychiatry, 9,* **65-68.** (In Chinese.)

The following references are also relevant to this chapter:

207, 208, 236, 289, 292, 312, 663, 750, 1143, 1325, 1660, 1667, 1681, 1755, 1781, 2262, 2521, 2546, 3223, 3308, 3317, 3384, 3438, 3441, 3442, 3458, 3472, 3508.

ASSESSMENT, TREATMENT, AND PREVENTION 13

Table 12: *Number of Citations by Content Classification, Language, and Geographical Area*

Content classification	Total	CL	EL	OL	PRC	T	HK	US
Treatment and prevention	189	67	114	8	96	25	16	2
Psychotherapy and psychotherapeutic counseling	47	9	37	1	8	4	10	6
Group and family therapy	7	2	4	1	1	3	0	1
Encounter group, sensitivity, and human relations training	1	0	1	0	1	0	0	0
Behavior therapy and modification	16	6	10	0	4	2	5	0
Drug therapy	13	5	8	0	4	2	0	0
Hypnotherapy	2	0	2	0	0	0	0	0
Speech therapy	0	0	0	0	0	0	0	0
Health care services	46	4	41	1	19	2	11	3
Community services and mental health programs	47	12	34	1	14	11	13	2
Counseling and social casework	8	1	7	0	0	2	0	1
Hospital programs and institutionalization	18	7	10	1	10	0	6	0
Rehabilitation and penology	4	0	4	0	0	0	3	0
Drug and alcohol rehabilitation	9	1	6	2	3	0	2	1
Total	407	114	278	15	160	51	66	16

Note: CL = Chinese language; EL = English language; OL = other languages. PRC = People's Republic of China; T = Taiwan; HK = Hong Kong; US = United States (Chinese Americans--according to the frequency of the subject term Asian Americans).

Frequency data on citations in this chapter, in terms of content classification subcategories, are presented in Table 12.

Subject terms used for indexing citations related to assessment, treatment, and prevention are grouped according to geographical area, subject population, and topic. These are presented below, in a descending order of frequency. (The frequency of single-word subject terms includes those of compound terms in which the single word appears. Subjects terms used for indexing citations from other chapters may have been included. Terms with a frequency of less than 10 are not shown.)

Geographical area

170	Peoples Republic of China
71	Hong Kong
56	Asia
55	Taiwan

Subject population

34	patients
27	Asians
25	psychiatric patients
20	adults
18	children
17	Asian Americans
13	students
10	college students

Topic

123	health
94	psychiatry
68	treatment
64	disorders
48	mental disorders
44	mental health services
33	neurosis
32	Chinese medicine
32	mental health
31	adulthood
31	sociocultural factors
27	psychotherapy
26	case report
26	cross cultural differences
26	psychodiagnosis
21	sciences
20	health care services
20	counseling
19	acupuncture
18	drug therapy
16	attitudes
16	psychology
15	hospitals
15	mental health programs
15	neurasthenic neurosis
14	schizophrenia
14	transcultural psychiatry
13	prevention
12	drug addiction
12	evaluation
10	psychiatric hospitals

Table 12 shows that there is a serious lack or absence of studies in group and family therapy; encounter group, sensitivity, and human relations training; hypnotherapy; speech therapy; rehabilitation and penology. English-language citations outnumber Chinese-language one by a factor of more than two. As to geographical area, the PRC predominates; and Hong Kong surpasses Taiwan.

As indicated by inspecting the subject terms, there is a high degree of attention given to sociocultural considerations and, not surprisingly, to Chinese medicine and acupuncture. Psychotherapy and counseling have received a fair amount of attention. Prevention has not received the attention it deserves.

3103

[*A glossary of psychiatric terms*]. (1935). **Shanghai: Commercial Press.** (In Chinese.)

3104

Abbott, K. A. (1971). Cultural change, psychosocial functioning, and the family: A case study in the Chinese-American community of San Francisco. *Dissertation Abstracts International, 32,* **A1077.**

3105

Abel, T. M. (1962). The dreams of a Chinese patient. In W. Muensterberger, & S. Axeland (Eds.), *The Psychoanalytic Study of Society* **(Vol. 2, pp. 280-309). New York: International University Press.**

3106

Achtenberg, H. (1983). Mental health care in China. *Journal of Psychiatric Treatment & Evaluation, 5,* **371-375.**

Presents an overview of the modern Chinese mental health system, which combines traditional treatment methods, including herbs and acupuncture, with Western chemotherapy and diagnostic concepts. Hospitalization, aftercare, and social reintegration policy are described. It is suggested that the Chinese use of traditional medicine to enhance the effectiveness and minimize the side effects of psychotropic drugs may eventually be helpful to American doctors dealing with the same treatment problems.

3107

Adler, S. S. (1983). Seeking stillness in motion: An introduction to Tai Chi for seniors. *Activities, Adaptation & Aging, 3,* **1-14.**

Describes Tai Chi Chuan, a traditional Chinese exercise, in terms of its potential benefits for older people. Two major philosophical principles underlying Tai Chi exercises are discussed: shen, or spiritual awareness, and seeking stillness in motion. The adaptation of traditional Tai Chi forms for older people is described with detailed instructions on the use of prebirth breathing.

3108

Agren, H. (1975). A new approach to Chinese traditional medicine. *American Journal of Chinese Medicine, 3,* **207-212.**

Argues that traditional Chinese medicine should be analyzed from psychological and anthropological perspectives and according to its subspecialities, levels of knowledge, and sociological and historical divisions. Traditional medicine involves counseling and creation of a milieu of trust; with this in mind, it is possible to understand today's integration of traditional and modern medicine in China.

3109

Ahn Toupin, E. S. (1980). Counseling Asians: Psychotherapy in the context of racism and Asian-American history. *American Journal of Orthopsychiatry, 50,* **76-86.**

Discusses the historical status of Japanese, Chinese, Korean, and Filipino immigrants in the US and the impact of cultural experiences and differences on psychotherapy for Asian-Americans. The major roles of shame and self-discipline in Asian cultures present difficulties for therapeutic work; personal feelings, failures, and weaknesses are discussed in the family or not at all. Attitudes toward mental illness are also connected with shame, because it is regarded as genetic rather than social in origin. Group discussion of such matters is especially distressing for Asians, and group therapy is counterindicated. The well-developed Asian system of nonverbal cues is helpful in psychotherapy, although it differs from European systems. The therapist should be familiar with it so that it can be a help rather than a block to communication.

3110

Alexander, A. A., Workneh, F., Klein, M. H., & Miller, M. H. (1976). Psychotherapy and the foreign student. In P. Pedersen, W. J. Lonner, & J. G. Draguns (Eds.), *Counseling across cultures* **(pp. 227-243). Honolulu, HI: University Press of Hawaii.**

3111

Allodi, F., & Dukszta, J. (1978). Psychiatric services in China or, Mao versus Freud. *Canadian Psychiatric Association Journal, 23,* **361-371.**

Describes the network of mental health services in the People's Republic of China using a sample of 1 mental hospital, 6 general hospitals, and health units in cities, factories, and communes. The basic principles of policy and administration are those of collective socialism with strong central guidelines and considerable local administrative initiative. A review of admissions to the mental hospital in Shanghai revealed that 83% are young, acute schizophrenic cases and that very few are nonpsychotic. Officially, mental illness is not considered a major problem, and it is given very low priority in medical school curricula and in the planning of health services. It is concluded that psychiatric services in China are concerned primarily with cases of psychosis and severe neurosis, that neuroses are viewed as general health problems, and personality and behavior disorders are considered social or community matters.

3112

Anderson, J. (1984). Research on doctor-patient communication in Hong Kong. [Special issue: Psychology and Medicine] [Selected papers from the 1983 Annual Conference]. *Hong Kong Psychological Society Bulletin,* **No. 13, 23-31.**

Reviews problems in communication between doctors and patients, focusing on patient satisfaction, comprehension, and recall of information; and doctor's knowledge about patients' real problems, doctor's interviewing skills, dealing with sensitive topics, and counseling. Two studies examining doctor-patient communication within a behavioral sciences unit are described. In Exp I, doctor-patient communication and compliance in a special outpatient clinic were explored based on interviews with patients before they saw the doctor on their 2nd visit. Findings indicate that most Ss still had unanswered questions after consultations and wanted more information. The most commonly reported information was about diagnosis; the least reported information was about prognosis and effects of medication. Exp II investigated the effects of interview training. First- and 3rd-yr medical students were randomly assigned to either control, self-feedback, or tutor-feedback interview training groups. Results show that there were problems in the ability of doctors and medical students to effectively communicate with patients. Tutor-feedback was more effective than self-feedback.

3113

Atkinson, D. R., & Morten, G. (Eds.). (1979). *Counseling American minorities: A cross-cultural perspective.* **Dubuque: William C. Brown.**

3114

Belgum, D. (1978). Medicine and morals and Mao. *Journal of Religion & Health, 17,* **261-273.**

The article discusses Mao's central beliefs of "put politics in command" and "serve the people" as they relate to medicine. It also deals with the focus on mutual independence, social solidarity, and communal solutions to problems in China. There are some interesting insights on how prostitution and venereal disease were eliminated and on the ability of Mao to use both ancient and modern ways, as well as descriptions of rural health and the education of barefoot doctors.

3115

Bennett, A. E. (1976). Impressions of psychiatry in Singapore, Malaysia, Thailand, and Taiwan. *Biological Psychiatry, 11,* **345-353.**

3116

Bietti, C., & Pietropaoli, D. (1979). [Psychiatric services in Hong Kong]. *Lavoro Neuropsichiatrico, 63,* **329-333.** (In other language.)

3117

Binder, R. L. (1983). Cultural factors complicating the treatment of psychosis caused by B-sub-1-sub-2 deficiency. *Hospital & Community Psychiatry, 34,* **67-69.**

Presents the case of an 83-yr-old non-English-speaking Chinese woman who presented with a vitamin B12 deficiency and psychiatric symptoms prior to the appearance of anemia. Both S and her family resisted S's hospitalization, and S refused to submit to psychological testing. S was successfully treated with haloperidol (20 mg/day) and vitamin B12 (100 mug/day, im), which decreased her agitation and psychotic symptoms, and later, a monthly injection of vitamin B12 alone. S had had no recurrence of symptoms at 40-mo follow-up. The case is discussed in relation to S's cultural values.

3118

Bloomingdale, L. M. (1980). Chinese psychiatry after Mao Zedong. *Psychiatric Annals, 10,* **7-24.**

Describes the development of hospital psychiatry in the Peoples Republic of China, noting that it has recently made rapid progress and is not markedly different from that which existed in the US about a decade ago. Treatment modalities include pharmacotherapy, acupuncture, and acupuncture with ECT. Most hospitalized patients are diagnosed as schizophrenic, and most neurotic disorders, such as hysteria and anorexia nervosa, are not hospitalized. Depressive disorders and suicides are rare. There are no subspecialties in Chinese psychiatry and no concept of legal sanity and its attendant problems. Clinical psychology has been recommended as a specialty only since 1979.

3119

Bos, T. W., & Gorter, R. W. D. (1977). [Acupuncture: real help for addicts]? *Tijdschrift Alcohol Drugs Andere Psychotrope Stoff, 3,* **21-28.** (In other language.)

Acupuncture has its origins in ancient China. The basic principles lend themselves to testing for reliability. Acupuncture is used in the treatment of Western addiction as well. Apart from the more classical methods the treatment of heroin addicts by means of electro-stimulation of the ear has become well-known, especially in the English speaking countries, and is used on a large scale to cure withdrawal symptoms. Prospective (double-) blind controlled trials on this form of treatment are still lacking, and objections that the treatment is based upon hypnosis or suggestion can only be refuted indirectly. Nevertheless knowledge of this treatment is increasing. The authors' experiences with the treatment of addicts by the use of acupuncture are discussed.

3120

Brammer, L. M. (1985). Counseling services in the People's Republic of China. *International Journal for the Advancement of Counselling, 8,* **125-136.**

The author described the status of psychology and counseling in the People's Republic of China, indicating that the principal vehicles for counseling are the neighborhood council and the extended family. The local council offers informal counseling to families and individuals in the neighborhood through peer helpers supplemented by counseling from paraprofessional health care providers in the neighborhood clinics. This council is the 1st level in a 3-tiered health care delivery system. Severe problems are referred to the 2nd level, the district hospital, which usually has a psychiatric unit with medical psychologists able to deal with problems on both in- and outpatient bases. The 3rd level of assistance is provided through specialized institutes that take a few severe psychological problems for treatment, research, and teaching purposes. It was argued that the array of services offered through local councils with a caring neighborly attitude outweighs the disadvantages of loss of privacy and pressures to conform to local behavioral expectations and political demands.

3121

Breger, E. (1984). A child psychiatrist's observations on care of the mentally ill in the People's Republic of China. *Psychiatric Hospital, 15,* **127-132.**

Presents findings from a tour of hospital facilities, schools, and other special youth settings in 6 Chinese cities, including Beijing, Nanjing, and Changsha. Chinese societal attitudes and cultural concepts, such as Yin (negative, feminine, and dark) and Yang (positive, male, and light) are discussed in terms of their effects on psychotherapeutic thought and practice. Therapeutic techniques often feature a blend of Chinese and Western traditions. Facilities for the care of children and delinquents are described.

3122

Bresler, D. E. et al. (1975). The potential of acupuncture for the behavioral sciences. *American Psychologist, 30,* **411-414.**

Discusses the origins of acupuncture in China, the techniques involved, mechanisms of action, and applications to the behavioral sciences. Dangers of acupuncture treatment and the medical-legal status of the techniques are also considered.

3123

Briers, N. (1981). The Emperor's New Clothes. *Hong Kong Journal of Mental Health, 10,* **5-7.**

3124

Brown, L. B. (1980). A psychologist's perspective on psychiatry in China. *Australian & New Zealand Journal of Psychiatry, 14,* **21-35.**

Social and political procedures, which have an important role in Chinese psychiatry, are examined with reference to observations made during visits to hospitals in Shanghai and Tianjin, the available Western literature, and 2 recent Chinese documents.

3125

Brown, T. R., Stein, K. M., Huang, K., & Harris, D. E. (1973). Mental illness and the role of mental health facilities in Chinatown. In S. Sue, & N. N. Wagner (Eds.), *Asian Americans: Psychological perspectives.* **Palo Alto, CA: Science & Behavior Books.**

3126

Calltorp, J. (1981). [Psychiatry in China]. *Lakartidningen, 78,* **3788-3791.** (In other language.)

A report is presented from a study visit to China. Chinese psychiatric care is structured at different levels, where district clinics with their "barefoot doctors" hold pride. At the big psychiatric hospital in Shanghai, the diagnostic panorama is dominated by schizophrenia, while neuroses are conspicuous by their absence--these are usually treated by the barefoot doctors in outpatient care. The dependence-related diseases, that is, addiction to alcohol, narcotics and prescribed drugs, would seem to have been wholly eradicated. The treatment is based on drugs, and the strange encounter between traditional Chinese medicine and Western medical science is also evident within psychiatry. However, social training--in which the patient's family takes an active part--also plays a prominent role in therapy. The existence of a subconscious level in the human mind is denied, and psychoanalysis is not used. The essence is to bring the patient to an understanding of his disease.

3127

Caudill, W., & Lin, T. Y. (Eds.). (1969). *Mental health research in Asia and the Pacific.* **Honolulu, HI: East-West Center Press.**

3128

Cerny, J. (1965). Chinese psychiatry. *International Journal of Psychiatry, 1,* **229-247;** *1,* **648-649.**

3129

Chan, D. W. (1986). Nonverbal communication in gestures: Implications for cross-cultural psychotherapy. *Hong Kong Journal of Mental Health, 15,* **56-64.**

Drawings of ten gestures intended to communicate openness, defensiveness, evaluation, suspicion, frustration, confidence, nervousness, self-control, boredom, and expectancy were presented to two groups of Chinese subjects who judged the frequency of occurrence and meanings of the gestures. Although three gestures rated as relatively more frequent were generally interpreted as intended, multiple meanings were attributed to the other seven. Implications of this lack of relative consensus in gesture interpretation for cross-cultural psychotherapy and the training of therapist skills were discussed.

3130

Chan, D. W. O. (1984). Medication compliance in a Chinese psychiatric out-patient setting. *British Journal of Medical Psychology, 57,* **81-89.**

Investigated the knowledge and attitudes of 19 male and 17 female 17-53 yr old psychiatric outpatients regarding medication by personal interview to examine the extent to which self-report medication compliance was predictable from Ss' sociodemographic and cognitive characteristics. Results indicate that over 80% of the variance of self-report medication compliance was predictable from SES and cognitive variables. Compliers and noncompliers differed in their expectancy and prior experience of beneficial effects of the medication and in their fear of undesirable side effects and addiction. Using causal modeling procedures, self-report compliant behavior was causally linked to favorable attitudes and fear, which in turn were linked to knowledge of name, dose, purpose, and side effects of the medication and the perceived stigma of the illness. Implications for patient education aimed at improving patient compliance are discussed.

3131

Chan, D. W. O. (1985). Psychotherapy: Some practical considerations. *Hong Kong Journal of Mental Health, 14,* **42-46.**

3132

Chan, D. W. O., & Tong, L. (1984). Case identification and classification: An overview of instruments in the two-stage procedure. *Hong Kong Journal of Mental Health, 13,* **22-28.**

3133

Chang, T. H., Lee, J. L., & Vung, H. T. (1961). [The role of 'active consciousness' of neurasthenic patients in the speedy-synthetic treatment]. *Acta Psychologica Sinica,* **No. 3, 155-163.** (In Chinese.)

This paper is a psychological analysis of the role of "active consciousness" displayed by neurasthenic patients during a course of speedy-synthetic treatment. It deals with: (1) Indications of the manifestations of "active consciousness." (2) The part played by "active consciousness" in the genesis, development and course of treatment of the disease. It has been shown that cognition, volitional acts as well as emotional status are indications showing the influence of "active consciousness".

3134

Chang, W. H. (1984). Electroacupuncture and ECT. *Biological Psychiatry, 19,* **1271-1272.**

Comments on the report of D. L. Dunner and P. Z. Dunner that electroacupuncture therapy (EAT) is used extensively as one of the treatments for neurasthenia, depression, and some other mental disorders in psychiatric hospitals in Mainland China. The present author, a former research psychiatrist and chief of the neurochemistry laboratory in the Peking Mental Health Institute, agreed with Dunner and Dunner that EAT is actually a novel variant of electroconvulsive therapy (ECT). Because EAT uses a low-voltage apparatus, it may be much safer than ECT, especially for those antidepressant nonresponders with ECT contraindications.

3135

Chao, Y. C. (1965). [Neurology, neurosurgery and psychiatry in New China]. *Chinese Medical Journal, 84,* **714-742.** (In Chinese.)

3136

Chen, C. C. (1972). Experiences with group psychotherapy in Taiwan. *International Journal of Group Psychotherapy, 22,* **210-227.**

Evaluates the results of 3 projects on group psychotherapy carried out in 3 mental institutions in Taiwan. These projects were (a) group therapeutic approach in a male disturbed ward in a provincial mental hospital as a pilot study for application of group psychotherapy in Taiwan; (b) investigation of cultural implications in group processes engendered in 3 groups 1 all male, 1 all female, and 1 mixed with the same male therapist in a private charity mental hospital; and (c) methodological consideration of group psychotherapy by comparing regularity of patients' attendance at interview group psychotherapy, occupational therapy with group orientation, and didactic group therapy in a psychiatric ward of a general hospital. The universal phenomena in the social structure of patients' subgrouping in psychiatric wards and the applicability of group interview methods in psychiatric treatment of the mentally ill in Taiwan were explored. Cultural implications of group processes, group discussions, intragroup relationships, and communicative tools in group psychotherapy were also studied, and some modifications in therapeutic techniques are suggested.

3137

Chen, C. C. (1974). Group therapy with predelinquent schoolchildren in Taipei. In W. P. Lebra (Ed.), *Youth, socialization, and mental health: III. Mental health research in Asia and the Pacific.* **Honolulu, HI: University Press of Hawaii.**

3138

Chen, C. C. (1984). Group therapy with Chinese schoolchildren. *International Journal of Group Psychotherapy, 34,* **485-501.**

The investigator tested the application of group therapy Taiwanese school children exhibiting problem behaviors. Therapy consisted of two 1.5-hour sessions weekly, arranged to include both a therapist's storytelling and group members' puppet playing. Each activity was immediately followed by a group session in which the contents of the story and puppet play were discussed under the therapist's direction. A behavior rating scale for 20 problem behaviors was used to assess subjects pre- and posttreatment. The experimental groups showed significant improvement in their behavior in comparison with the control groups. A comparison was made between the traditional activity-interview group therapy given in the first phase of the therapy and the storytelling-puppet-play group therapy in the 3rd phase.

3139

Chen, C. C., & Chu, H. M. (1962). [Evaluation of patient attendance in open group psychotherapeutic sessions in a psychiatric ward]. *Journal of the Formosan Medical Association, 61,* **345-351.** (In Chinese.)

3140

Chen, C. C., & Wen, J. K. (1985). [The closedown of the Cafe Cactus: Resistance to the rehabilitation of chronic psychotic patients]. *Chinese Journal of Mental Health, 2,* **11-21.** (In Chinese.)

The authors introduced a rehabilitation program which led to the running of a coffee shop for 10 months. To discover the reasons for the resistance from the community, a questionnaire study was conducted. Among the 257 respondents, there were four demographically different groups: the local community group, the medical college group, members of the Association of Friends for Mental Rehabilitation, and patrons of the coffee shop. The respondents tended to believe that government or other institutions should take care of chronic patients, despite their preference for psychiatric treatment rather than simple custodial care. Those who had some contact or experiences with mental patients tended to be less pessimistic and more realistic about the rehabilitation program.

3141

Chen, C. C., Wu, W. L., & Wen, J. K. (1984). [The story of cafe cactus: A new way for the rehabilitation of chronic psychotic patients]. *Chinese Journal of Mental Health, 1,* **67-73.** (In Chinese.)

To help with the rehabilitation of chronic psychotic patients, the authors cooperated with some ex-patients and their families to establish a self-help program. A coffee shop was opened and sponsored by the families. Twenty-two chronic patients participated in the program for half a year. The authors conducted weekly group psychotherapy sessions for the patients, who also had regular weekly follow-up appointments at an outpatient clinic. A global evaluation of their mental and social condition 6 months later showed that: 6 patients had markedly improved; 7 had mildly improved; 5 had not changed; and 4 had dropped out of the program. The more the families participated in the program, the better the patients' outcome. The importance of the cooperation and interdependence of the supporting systems in a rehabilitation program for chronic psychotic patients was emphasized.

3142

Chen, C. K. (1956). [Preliminary experience in experiments on conditioned reflex using verbal reinforcement]. *Chinese Journal of Neurology and Psychiatry, 2,* **240-244.** (In Chinese.)

3143

Chen, C. S. (1955). [Preliminary results of group psychiatric treatment for neurasthenic patients in Nanking Mental Hospital]. *Chinese Journal of Neurology and Psychiatry, 1,* **104-106.** (In Chinese.)

3144

Chen, H. C., Hsieh, M. T., & Lai, E. (1985). Studies on the Suanzaorentang in the treatment of anxiety. *Psychopharmacology, 85,* **486-487.**

The anxiolytic and psychomotor effects of the ancient Chinese formula of suanzaorentang was studied using 30 patients with sympathetic hyperactivity, motor hypertonicity, and apprehension and with morbid anxiety test scores of 14-30. Subjects received 3-6 250 mg capsules daily for 7 days. Anxiety and psychomotor measures were taken pre- and post-treatment. Findings showed that suanzaorentang improved mood, decreased the accompanying sympathetic symptoms, and improved psychomotor performance during the day.

3145

Chen, J. L., Liu, J. T., & Yeh, E. K. (1985). [Social rehabilitation of chronic psychiatric patients: Evaluation of a half-way house program]. *Chinese Journal of Mental Health, 2,* **59-68.** (In Chinese.)

This study examined the value of half-way house rehabilitation of chronic psychiatric patients, in the areas of social function, family relations, compliance with after-care treatment and self-esteem. Twenty-one patients who had been in a half-way house program for at least 3 months were studied. A control group consisted of 20 patients drawn from the patients discharged from a psychiatric center during the same period. The results showed that the half-way house group were more independent, more autonomous in social adaptation, had better social functioning and interpersonal relationships, better compliance with after-care treatment; and were more satisfied with emotional stability, life arrangements, interpersonal relationships and autonomy. These results indicated the value of half-way house rehabilitation in the treatment of chronic psychiatric patients.

3146

Chen, P. N. (1978). Continuity/discontinuity of life patterns among minority elderly in nutrition programs. *Dissertation Abstracts International, 39,* **A467.**

3147

Chen, P. N. (1982). Eroding filial piety and its implications for social work practice. *Journal of Sociology & Social Welfare, 9,* **511-523.**

Surveyed 82 health and social service practitioners in 6 cities with high concentrations of Asian-Americans (New York, Los Angeles, San Francisco, Chicago, Boston, and Detroit) on their assessment of the effects of compliance/noncompliance with the traditional Asian value of filial piety on Asian-American adult children, aged parents, and the practitioners themselves. Since filial piety is an emotion-laden topic, a projective technique was used in questionnaire design, and Ss were asked questions regarding a hypothetical case. Findings indicate that Ss see a gradual shift of filial responsibilities to health/social service providers with concomitant affective conflicts on the part of Asian-American adult children, aged parents, and practitioners. It is concluded that greater understanding of these conflicts will help to strengthen filial piety and the extended family support system.

3148

Chen, R. C., & Rin, H. (1975). [Editors' remarks: Statistical analysis of presentations and publications by members of the Chinese Society of Neurology and Psychiatry during the past 25 years]. *Bulletin of the Chinese Society of Neurology and Psychiatry, 1,* **2-4.** (In Chinese.)

3149

Chen, R. M. (1986). [A preliminary study of factors affecting treatment and prognosis of schizophrenia]. *Chinese Journal of Neurology and Psychiatry, 19,* **47-48.** (In Chinese.)

A multifactorial clinical analysis of 40 schizophrenics was made in order to predict therapeutic effectiveness and outcome. Criteria for evaluation included the hereditary factor, premorbid personality, speed of remission, degree of improvement before discharge, dosage of drug used for maintenance therapy, and social adaptability before or after hospitalization. The results showed that the criteria were applicable in predicting and evaluating both short-term therapeutic effectiveness and outcome in schizophrenic patients receiving current treatment.

3150

Cheng, A. S. H. (1975). [A comparative study of effectiveness in reducing test anxiety by systematic desensitization and muscle relaxation and electric shock in behavioral counseling]. *Acta Psychologica Taiwanica, 17,* **39-45.** (In Chinese.)

It has been established that systematic desensitization and muscle relaxation in behavioral counseling as well as the technique of electric shock are effective in reducing general anxiety. However, there is still a need to further investigate whether these techniques work in specific test anxiety cases and whether one technique is superior to the others. Eighteen clients were randomly divided into three groups: muscle relaxation group, electric shock group, and control group. The subjects were students at the National Taiwan University who scored higher than normal on the Scale for Test Anxiety. Each client was counseled once a week for four weeks, and each was posttested with the same scale. The results indicated that both techniques were effective in reducing test anxiety, and that there was no significant difference between the results of these two techniques.

3151

Cheng, J. C. C. (1970). Historical note: Psychiatry in traditional Chinese medicine. *Canadian Psychiatric Association Journal, 15,* **399-401.**

3152

Cheng, S. H., & Hsu, L. R. P. (1974). The effectiveness of muscle relaxation and systematic desensitization of behavioral counseling in reducing test anxiety of Chinese students. *Acta Psychologica Taiwanica, 16,* **119-134.**

This study attempts to test the effects of muscle relaxation and systematic desensitization on test anxiety in Chinese culture. Five clients were tested, using the Test Anxiety Rating Scale. The Counseling Service Assessment Blank was administered to measure counseling effectiveness. The results indicated that, generally speaking, the techniques of muscle relaxation and systematic desensitization were effective fo reducing test anxiety.

3153

Cheung, F. M. C. (1976). An integrative view of community mental health. *Hong Kong Journal of Mental Health, 5,* **13-16.**

3154

Cheung, F. M. C. (1979). Care of rape victims. *Hong Kong Journal of Mental Health, 8,* **39-45.**

3155

Cheung, F. M. C. (1981). Opening Pandora's box on counseling: Comments on Norman Briers' article "The Emperor's New Clothes". *Hong Kong Journal of Mental Health, 10,* **10-12.**

3156

Cheung, F. M. C. (1984). Preferences in help-seeking among Chinese students. *Culture, Medicine and Psychiatry, 8,* **371-380.**

Chinese university students were asked to indicate their inclination to seek help and the resources for consultation on the 22 problems listed on the Langner Scale. Results showed that the Chinese students were generally not inclined to seek help and when they did, would most often seek help from medical doctors. However, when items were grouped in terms of clinical content, it was found that friends were predominantly preferred for psychological problems while the doctor was preferred for psychophysiological, physiological, and ambiguous problems. More female than male students tended to rely on friends and family members while the reverse pattern was found in the preference for doctors. The mental health professional was rarely cited as a resource for any of the problems. The results provide some explanation for observations made in previous studies on symptom presentation and help-seeking behavior among Chinese psychiatric patients.

3157

Cheung, F. M. C. (Ed.). (1986). *The Chinese Minnesota Multiphasic Personality Inventory (MMPI): Research and applications* **(Occasional Papers No. 12). Hong Kong: The Chinese University of Hong Kong, Centre for Hong Kong Studies.**

3158

Cheung, F. M. C., Lau, B. W. K., & Wong, S. W. (1984). Paths to psychiatric care in Hong Kong. *Culture, Medicine and Psychiatry, 8,* **207-228.**

The pattern of psychiatric consultation in Hong Kong is examined among 226 patients at a public outpatient clinic and 56 patients at a private psychiatric clinic. The approach to psychiatric services is marked by lengthy delay during which patients get help from their family members or close friends. Arrival at the present psychiatric clinic was diverted through other medical resources, primarily Western-style medical services, and to some extent, traditional Chinese medicine. Individual routes were diverse, characterized by frequent switches among resources especially in the private section. The nature of the patients' presenting complaints as well as the conceptualization of their initial complaints were multifaceted, including both psychological and somatic factors. The overall consultation pattern of patients in Hong Kong is compared with other studies of Chinese and Western patients, and questions are raised for further analysis.

3159

[*Child Health Care in New China*]. **(1973). Beijing: Chinese Medical Association.** (In Chinese.)

3160

China Health Care Study Group. (1974). *Health care in China: An introduction.* **Geneva: Christian Medical Commission.**

3161

Chinese Medical Association. (1973). [*Child health care in New China*]. **Beijing: Author.** (In Chinese.)

3162

Chiu, P. (1980). Group counselling with emotionally disturbed school children in Taiwan. *School Psychology International, 1,* **27-30.**

Results of a study of 29 male Taiwanese emotionally disturbed junior-high-school students indicate that those who received group counseling showed a significant reduction in adjustment problems when compared with those who did not. However, group counseling did not reduce social anxiety or improve personal and social adjustment.

3163

Chiu, P. C. T., & Lin, H. M. (1977). [Evaluation of the effect of group counseling on behavior modification of college males with heterosexual inhibition]. *Acta Psychologica Taiwanica, 19,* **91-96.** (In Chinese.)

Evaluated the effectiveness of a social skills training program for 12 Chinese college males with heterosexual inhibition. Experimental Ss were given 6 consecutive 2-hr weekly social training sessions which consisted of muscle relaxation, group discussion, behavior rehearsal, corrective feedback, and assignment. Ss were evaluated on the Edwards Personal Preference Schedule (EPPS), a survey of heterosexual interaction, a social avoidance and distress scale, and a self-report measure. Results show that experimental Ss made significantly more improvement in social skills than the controls, as assessed by the EPPS and the social avoidance and distress scale. On the self-report measure and the survey of heterosexual interaction, however, the differences of the mean scores of the experimental and control Ss were not significant.

3164

Chu, C. R., Lubin, B., & Sue, S. (1984). Reliability and validity of the Chinese Depression Adjective Check Lists. *Journal of Clinical Psychology, 40,* **1409-1413.**

Data were presented on the translation and reliability and concurrent validity of the Chinese version of the Depression Adjective Check Lists. Thirty-seven subjects were administered versions in which the order of translated adjectives was counterbalanced. The data showed that reliability and validity coefficients were significant and of sufficient magnitude to warrant their use in research.

3165

Chu, Y. M., Lu, S. Y., Tang, T. H., & Wang, T. T. (1983). [Use of the newly abbreviated and revised Denver Developmental Screening Test (DDST-R) in the urban districts of Shanghai]. *Information on Psychological Sciences*, **No. 4, 47-50.** (In Chinese.)

3166

Chungking Mental Hospital. (1959). [Abolition of restraints and isolation]. *Chinese Journal of Neurology and Psychiatry*, *5*, **124-125.** (In Chinese.)

3167

Collins, J. L. (1982). Psychiatry in China. *Journal of the National Medical Association*, *74*, **993-998.**

The author describes his observations of Chinese psychiatry during a 3-wk medical tour in December, 1980. The techniques of treatment in 2 psychiatric hospitals are discussed, with emphasis on the utilization of both Western and traditional Chinese medicine.

3168

Croizier, R. C. (1968). *Traditional medicine in modern China*. **Cambridge: Harvard University Press.**

3169

Deely, P. J., Kaufman, E., Yen, M. S. et al. (1979). The special problems and treatment of a group of elderly Chinese opiate addicts in New York city. *British Journal of Addiction*, *74*, **403-409.**

The Lower Eastside Service Center (LESC) is a social agency which first opened its doors in 1959. The agency's purpose was to rehabilitate narcotic addicts on the lower east side of New York City, which borders on Chinatown. In the summer of 1969, the agency undertook a small out-patient Methadone Treatment Programme in collaboration with the Beth Israel Medical Center. A large number of Chinese addicts applied who were ineligible for methadone because they were older than the maximum allowable age. The workers encouraged the men to try to reach their families and friends in Mainland China or Hong Kong and to send money to their families. Some of them had not been in touch with their families for 20 to 40 years. For them, contacting and sending money relieves guilt and loneliness and enhances self esteem. The success of the program has depended on having two workers who speak their language and share the same cultural background and upbringing as the clients. The workers take an accepting role of their clients' life style, are not judgmental or moralistic, but help them to adjust to the 'New World'. There is no attempt to eliminate drug use, but rather to substitute methadone as a legal drug for the illegal heroin. The fact that their attendance is regular and participation in the group is active suggests that whatever needs they have are being met by the agency. Having another human being who speaks their language and who helps them with concrete services such as housing, welfare, health, and deals with the bureaucracy eliminates some of their tremendous feelings of alienation from society and family.

3170

Department of Medicine, School of Traditional Medicine, Shansi. (1958). [Treatment of hysteria]. *Chinese Journal of Neurology and Psychiatry*, *4*, **434.** (In Chinese.)

3171

Department of Neurology, Peking Medical College. (1958). ["Cupping" done with the aid of bamboo]. *Chinese Journal of Neurology and Psychiatry*, *4*, **499-500.** (In Chinese.)

3172

Department of Psychiatry, the Third Teaching Hospital, Peking Medical College, et al. (1979). [Experiences in the establishment and consolidation of a 3-tier network for the prevention and treatment of psychoses in rural districts]. *Chinese Journal of Neurology and Psychiatry*, *12*, **14-16.** (In Chinese.)

3173

Department of Traditional Medicine, Shenyang Medical College. (1958). [Hysteria: Treatment of 100 cases]. *Chinese Journal of Neurology and Psychiatry*, *4*, **431-432.** (In Chinese.)

3174

Division of Medical Psychology, Institute of Psychology, Academica Sinica. (1959). [Function of psychotherapy in a speedy and synthetic treatment of neurasthenia]. *Acta Psychologica Sinica*, **No. 3, 151-160.** (In Chinese.)

This paper summarizes the experience in the speedy and synthetic treatment of neurasthenia. It is recognized that one of the characteristics of the treatment is the thorough application of psychotherapy based on Materialistic Psychology. A detailed presentation is given of the contents and the methods of psychotherapy and its fundamental difference from the psychotherapy in the past. Problems which require further studies are also pointed out.

3175

Division of Medical Psychology, Institute of Psychology, Academica Sinica. (1959). [A summary of practice in speedy-synthetic treatments of neurasthenics among the steel workers]. *Acta Psychologica Sinica*, **No. 4, 258-263.** (In Chinese.)

This paper summarizes the preliminary experiences obtained in the speedy-synthetic treatment of neurasthenics among steel workers, and clarifies the roles of psychological factors in the genesis, development and therapy of neurasthenia. The three major causes of this disease are hypertension during work and study, an inadequate relationship with other people, and some significant misfortunes in the patient's personal life. The psychotherapy applied here consisted mainly of rational therapy which was undertaken during the state of wakefulness. The results indicated that 81.4% of patients were cured or greatly improved.

3176

Dueng, Q. W. et al. (1980). [Behavior correction therapy in obsessional neurosis]. *Chinese Journal of Neurology & Psychiatry, 13,* **161-165.** (In Chinese.)

3177

Dunner, D. L., & Dunner, P. Z. (1983). Psychiatry in China: Some personal observations. *Biological Psychiatry, 18,* **799-801.**

Observed aspects of psychiatric care at several facilities in China. Observed differences in therapy included laser-beam treatment for schizophrenia, acupuncture modifications of ECT therapy, and lithium and tricyclic therapy that did not include monitoring of levels of the drugs in blood. The overall impression of health care and mental health care in China was on the positive side.

3178

Fantl, B. (1959 - 1960). Cultural factors in family: Diagnosis of a Chinese family. *International Journal of Social Psychiatry, 5,* **27-32.**

3179

Fears, M. (1976). Fighting for freedom: Mental health care in China. *Rehabilitation World, 2,* **21-22, 40.**

3180

Feng, Y. K. et al. (1959). [The immediate effect of acupuncture on the electroencephalograms of epileptic patients]. *Chinese Journal of Neurology and Psychiatry, 5,* **339-345.** (In Chinese.)

Acupuncture was applied to 23 epileptic and 2 non-epileptic patients with moderate degree of stimulation and electroencephalographic tracings were made during insertion, whirling, retention and removal of the needles. In the first group of older subjects (average duration of illness of 6 1/3 years) acupuncture resulted in no alteration in the pre-existing electroencephalogram or only elicited the usual attention phenomena. The second and third groups of respectively, young subjects and children (average duration of illness of 3-4 years), however, responded to acupuncture with the appearance of transient high voltage slow waves, spikes, or spike-and-wave complexes, or with reduction of these waves and better regulation of both frequency and amplitude. It is believed that acupuncture, being a form of arousal stimuli, offers a diagnostic aid in the estimation of liability of cortical activity of epileptic patients and that for early cases of epilepsy, especially petit mal epilepsy, it may have some therapeutic effect.

3181

Fusari, A., & Lorini, G. (1977). [Psychiatry in China: Notes on a visit]. *Rassegna di Studi Psichiatrici, 66,* **1168-1175.** (In other language.)

During a study trip to the People's Republic of China, the authors viewed the relationship between the community and mental patients. One of the main findings was the difference between the morbidity in China and in European countries--not only for neurosis, which was definitely very infrequent, but also for psychosis. Preventive and rehabilitative actions were taken by hospital personnel in close cooperation with the community. A high level in both clinical practice and experimental research was seen in every single hospital, in towns as well as in the countryside.

3182

Garner, T. G. (1978). Rehabilitation of drug addicts in a correctional setting. *British Journal of Addiction, 73,* **205-213.**

Major social problems are always reflected within the prison community, and programs for the rehabilitation of offenders should include provision to tackle them. Drug addiction, particularly to narcotics, is one such problem, and intervention for treatment is appropriate at the time the offender is placed in the custody of the Prison Service. Based on the Hong Kong experience, the period required for treatment, the procedures by which treatment takes place, the treatment program, and the necessity for after-care are discussed. Statistics illustrating the success of the program are included.

3183

Gershman, L., & Stedman, J. M. (1971). Oriental defense exercises as reciprocal inhibitors of anxiety. *Journal of Behavior Therapy & Experimental Psychiatry, 2,* **117-119.**

Describes 2 cases in which kung fu and karate, Chinese and Japanese defense systems, were used to inhibit anxiety. Kung fu was used with a 31-yr-old male with claustrophobia and karate with a 28-yr-old male with fears of flying. Treatment was in vivo for the former and in imagination and in vivo for the latter. Results indicate that the activities are effective counter-conditioners of anxiety.

3184

Goldfield, N. (1984). Trends in adolescent development in the People's Republic of China. *Social Science & Medicine, 18,* **21-26.**

Focuses on changing medical practices toward adolescents in the People's Republic since 1949 indicating the range of medical work on adolescent medicine. The tasks of adolescence as understood in the West, such as individuation, separation from family, and sexual identity, are examined in a Chinese context. Changing patterns in birth control, vocational choice, and youth group organizations are discussed, and attention is drawn to recent Chinese research on adolescence that has appeared in English language journals.

3185

Goldner, V. (1978). The politics of mental health in China. *State and Mind,* **12-16.**

3186

Gouldner, V. (1977, May-July). Mental health treatment in China. *China and the U.S.,* **pp. 6-8.**

3187

Guo, K. J. (1986). [A study of optical illusion of geometric figures in 160 patients with cerebral diseases]. *Information on Psychological Sciences,* **No. 2, 31-36.** (In Chinese.)

The effects of optical illusion of geometric figures designed by Hering and Wundt were studied. It was found that: (1) Pathological changes at different localities in the human brain and obstacles to the visual system at various levels were of no obvious significance to optical illusion effects. (2) No asymetricalness was found in terms of optical illusion effects upon the left and the right cerebral hemispheres. (3) Further studies of the relationships between eye movement and optical illusion effects are needed.

3188

Hagelthorn, C. (1983). Poesi och psykodrama. Om konst och terapi [Poetry and psychodrama: About art and therapy]. *Psykisk Halsa, 24,* **229-239.** (In other language.)

Addresses poets' relationships with their environment, starting in ancient Chinese times when the poet was imagined flying from one world to another on a dragon, up through the epochs of Christian and Western culture. Also discusses the latters' impact on erudition. Emphasis is placed on J. L. Moreno's (1973, 1975, 1977) views on the relationships between the unconscious and the conscious in which he claims the distinction is exaggerated, especially in a continuously creative mind, while western culture tends to separate them. Moreno also believes that psychodrama has more in common with poetry than with theater. Creativity and spontaneity in poetry are qualities to be encouraged among the participants in a psychodrama, perhaps not with the dash of traveling dragons but with the tranquility associated with singing nightingales. This approach shows that it can aid in the solution of problems in life and society. The combination of art and therapy in psychodrama creates a unique tool for the strengthening of human maturity as well as developing society constructively.

3189

Hammer, L. I. (1980). Integrated acupuncture therapy for body and mind. *American Journal of Acupuncture, 8,* **163-169.**

This paper demonstrates the profound interrelationships between different parts and systems of the body. This understanding leads to practical diagnostic and therapeutic procedures now in existence but unknown to Western medical practitioners. A detailed case study demonstrated how Chinese medicine elucidates and uses these systems. The conclusion is that this therapeutic approach offers Western medicine a systematic, practical diagnostic and treatment tool for the large majority of patients with psychosomatic problems.

3190

Hanson, K. J. (1985). Development and preventive health behaviors: The case of Taipei, Taiwan. *Dissertation Abstracts International, 45,* **A3159.**

3191

Hariman, J. (1982). A kung fu derived hypnotic psychotherapy. *International Journal of Eclectic Psychotherapy, 1,* **67-68.ed**

Outlines the procedure for a hypnotic psychotherapy based on the Chinese concept of "ch'i" (vital energy). The technique is effective without the use of a trance state, but because so many clients believe in hypnosis, their expectancy is greatly enhanced when formal hypnotic procedures are used.

3192

Hariman, J. (1982). Clinical hypnotherapy: Transpersonal perspectives. *Australian Journal of Clinical Hypnotherapy, 3,* **37-44.**

Traces the influences of 4 forces on a new form of hypnotic psychotherapy: limsian therapy. As an example of the influences of psychoanalytic psychology, a new age-regression technique, which is an integration of hypnoanalysis, hypnosynthesis, and Rational-Emotive Therapy, is described. As an example of the influences of behavioral psychology, a novel series of suggestions for smoking cessation is discussed. As an example of the influences of existential-humanistic psychology, basic disagreements with M. H. Erickson and E. L. Rossi's (1979) conception of the unconscious are described. The influences of transpersonal psychology are discussed in relation to the following issues: eclecticism, self-transcendence, extraordinary entities, and Chinese hypnosis.

3193

Hariman, J. (1983). The Five Animal Ch'i Kung. *International Journal of Eclectic Psychotherapy, 2,* **1-9.**

Describes the ancient Chinese therapeutic exercises, "ch'i kung". In particular, the 5 animal ch'i kung (FACK) are described. According to tradition, the celebrated surgeon Hua-to of the Han dynasty (2nd century AD) was the first to formulate the exercises. Hua-to experimented with the idea of FACK when he discovered that animals appeared to possess a spontaneous self-healing capacity that they activated and systematically used in rituals and movements. During the FACK, the person not only imitates the movements of the tiger, bear, deer, crane, and monkey, but he/she also assumes each animal's personality in turn. The tiger position is assumed for curing the lungs, the bear for the kidneys, the deer for the stomach, the crane for the heart, and the monkey for the liver. It is claimed that during the process, the person's awareness of self is so heightened that the fingers and hands will automatically and spontaneously manipulate the appropriate acupuncture points.

3194

Hathaway, B. (1982). Psychiatry in China. *Newspaper of the American Psychiatric Association, 17,* **3; 18-19.**

3195

Hendlin, S. J. (1978). T'ai Chi Chaun and Gestalt therapy. *Journal of Contemporary Psychotherapy, 10,* **25-31.**

Discusses T'ai Chi, a Chinese system of integrated exercises, as an effective adjunct to Gestalt therapy. Similarities in the philosophies of Gestalt therapy and T'ai Chi include (a) focusing on the here and now, (b) identification of polar opposites, (c) acceptance of rather than analysis of experience, (d) emphasis on sensation rather than intellect as a way of knowing the world, and (e) development of self-actualization, or being identity, above and beyond ego and existential identity. The use of T'ai Chi in clinical and growth center settings is described.

3196

Hiddlestone, H. J. (1974). Where health is patriotism. Visit of New Zealand Medical Delegation to China: 20 August - 9 September, 1974. *New Zealand Medical Journal, 80,* **509-516.**

3197

Higginbotham, H. N. (1980). Delivery of mental health services in three developing Asian nations: Feasibility and cultural sensitivity of "modern psychiatry". *Dissertation Abstracts International, 40,* **B3934.**

3198

Ho, A. L. (Ed. & Trans.) (1970 & 1972). [The development of the mental health movement in Hong Kong]. *Hong Kong Journal of Mental Health,* **1970, May, 1-3; 1972,** *1,* **4-9. (Original work presented in the 18th Annual Conference of the World Mental Health Association, 1965, November, Bangkok, in English.)** (In Chinese.)

3199

Ho, D. Y. F. (1974). Prevention and treatment of mental illness in the People's Republic of China. *American Journal of Orthopsychiatry, 44,* **620-636.**

This paper traces the development of psychiatry in the People's Republic of China, with special reference to the social aspects of treatment and prevention, and delineates the salient features of the Chinese approach. Implications of this approach for mental health workers in other countries are discussed.

3200

Ho, D. Y. F. (1979). Therapeutic intervention for parents and children in Hong Kong: Problems, frustrations, and reflections from a cross-cultural perspective. *Hong Kong Journal of Social Work, 13,* **15-22. (Republished in C. H. Hwang & E. K. Yeh (Eds.),** *Family, child and mental health: Proceedings of Western Pacific Regional Workshop on Mental Health* **(pp. 162-174). Taipei: Chinese National Association for Mental Hygiene, 1979.)**

3201

Ho, P. (1958). [Active program for the prevention and treatment of mental diseases]. *Chinese Journal of Neurology and Psychiatry, 4,* **343-347.** (In Chinese.)

3202

Ho, S. C., Lun, K. C., & Ng, W. K. (1984). The role of Chinese traditional medical practice as a form of health care in Singapore: III. Conditions, illness behaviour and medical preferences of patients of institutional clinics. *Social Science & Medicine, 18,* **745-752.**

Examined the values and beliefs attached to diseases and health care services by 151 patients seen in clinics in Singapore that provided Chinese traditional medical consultations. The types of illness conditions presented in these clinics, the multi-usage of both modern and traditional health care by these Ss, and the interrelationship between illness behavior and differential preferences of treatment methods for various disease conditions are discussed.

3203

Hoffman, J. et al. (1913). A report of the patients discharged from the John Kerr hospital for insane during 1912. *Chinese Medical Journal*, **369-379.**

3204

Holbrook, B. (1974). Chinese psycho-social medicine-doctor and Dang-Ki: An intercultural analysis. *Bulletin of the Institute of Ethnology* **(Academia Sinica),** *37*, **84-112.**

3205

Hollinrake, J. B. (1974). Treatment and rehabilitation facilities in Hong Kong. *International Journal of Offender Therapy & Comparative Criminology, 18,* **86-92.**

3206

Homma-True, R. (1975). Mental health needs and alternatives in a Chinese American community. *Dissertation Abstracts International, 36,* **B2723-2724.**

3207

Honan Province Mental Hospital. (1958). [Development of occupational therapy in the Honan Province Mental Hospital during the last two years]. *Chinese Journal of Neurology and Psychiatry, 4,* **267-269.** (In Chinese.)

3208

Hong Kong Government, Secretary of Social Services Working Group. (1983). *Report of the working group on ex-mental patients with a history of criminal violence or assessed disposition to violence.* **Hong Kong: Author.**

3209

Hong Kong Psychiatric Association. (1981). Is there a need for a private mental hospital in Hong Kong? *Journal of the Hong Kong Psychiatric Association, 1,* **44-47.**

3210

Hong Kong Psychiatric Association. (1982). The feasibility of having interns in mental hospitals or psychiatric units in Hong Kong. *Journal of the Hong Kong Psychiatric Association, 2,* **43-45.**

3211

Hopkins, J. (1969). Children in hospital: Observations on the reactions of Chinese children to hospitalization with implications for child care practices. *Far East Medical Journal, 5,* **279-284.**

3212

Hou, Y. (1959). [Mental patients should also be politically minded]. *Chinese Journal of Neurology and Psychiatry, 5,* **85-86.** (In Chinese.)

3213

Hou, Y. et al. (1959). [Clinical value of bunched needle acupuncture therapy]. *Chinese Journal of Neurology and Psychiatry, 5,* **91-93.** (In Chinese.)

3214

Hsia, C. Y., & Zhang, M. Y. (1981). History and present status of modern psychiatry in China. *Chinese Medical Journal, 94* **(5), 277-282.** (In Chinese.)

3215

Hsu, C. C., & Lin, T. Y. (1969). A mental health program at the elementary school level in Taiwan: A six-year review of the East-Gate project. In W. Caudill & T. Y. Lin (Eds.), *Mental health research in Asia and the Pacific.* **Honolulu, HI: East-West Center Press.**

3216

Hsu, J. (1976). Counseling in the Chinese temple: A psychological study. In W. P. Lebra (Ed.), *Culture-bound syndromes, ethnopsychiatry, and alternate therapies: Vol. 4. Mental research in Asia and the Pacific.* **Honolulu, HI: University Press of Hawaii.**

3217

Hsu, T. (1959). [Strive for the complete liberation of mental patients]. *Chinese Journal of Neurology and Psychiatry, 5,* **294-296.** (In Chinese.)

3218

Huang, L. N. (1981). A view of psychiatric care in the People's Republic of China. *Journal of the Asian American Psychological Association, 6,* **9-13.**

Presents the author's observations and impressions of the mental health problems, intervention strategies, and service delivery systems from a visit to China's Shanghai Psychiatric Institute and discussions with Chinese psychiatric staff. Chinese explanations of etiology, treatment approaches, environmental interventions, psychological treatment, and aftercare are described. Similarities and differences that emerged between China and the US are discussed.

3219

Hwang, C. H. (1963). [Use of the Multiple Choice Rorschach Test for screening juvenile delinquents]. *Psychological Testing, 10,* **815-828.** (In Chinese.)

3220

Hwang, P. Y. (1957). [The reaction time on the Rorschach of Chinese neuropsychiatric patients]. *Psychological Testing, 5,* **362-366.** (In Chinese.)

3221

Hwu, H. G., & Lin, H. M. (1984). [Screening schedule for psychiatric disorders -- set-up, reliability and validity]. *Chinese Journal of Mental Health, 1,* **27-40.** (In Chinese.)

The screening schedule for psychiatric disorder (SSPD) is an important tool for community mental health service. It is composed of two parts: basic data and screening schedule. The screening schedule has 23 main items to screen 25 categories of psychiatric disorders. This study used nonphysicians to test the interrater reliability and procedural validity of the SSPD. The result showed good interrater reliability. The procedural validity showed that other than the adjustmental disorder, all the psychiatric disorders had a case identification rate between 75% and 100%. All severe psychotic disorders could be screened out. The SSPD was recommended for use in community mental health services.

3222

Jew, C. C., & Brody, S. A. (1967). Mental illness among the Chinese: Hospitalization rates over the past century. *Comprehensive Psychiatry, 8,* **129-134.**

Records of all Chinese male patients admitted to California State Hospitals between 1854 and 1903 were analyzed to determine the hospitalization rate and compared with contemporary 1st-admission rates of Chinese males and with the rates for males of all races for selected yr. The hospitalization rate of the Chinese has gradually increased over the past 100 yr. Chinese males over 40 yr. of age show higher admission rates over the yr. than those under 40. The Chinese males in California have displayed lower rates of 1st admission to mental hospitals than males of all other races combined. Reasons for these findings are discussed.

3223

Jiang, K. D. et al. (1986). [A comparative study of the diagnostic criteria for anxiety neurosis]. *Chinese Journal of Neurology and Psychiatry, 19,* **285-287.** (In Chinese.)

The diagnostic criteria for anxiety designed by the Psychiatric Epidemiological Study Group of China were used to analyse 50 outpatients. Using the Hamilton Rating Scale of Anxiety and Depression, the authors found a significant positive correlation between the scores of anxiety and depression. When patients were treated with tricyclic antidepresants and diazepam, the overall rates of improvement were 72.5% for both drugs. The diagnostic criteria used appeared to have many similarities with those of the DSM-III, with agreement in diagnosis reached in 84.0%. The authors stressed that physical symptoms and symptoms of the vegetative nervous system are crucial in the diagnosis of anxiety.

3224

Johnson, N. K. (1980). Cultural and psychosocial determinants of health and illness. *Dissertation Abstracts International, 40,* **B4235.**

3225

Joos, S. K., Pollitt, E., Mueller, W. H., & Albright, D. L. (1983). The Bacon Chow study: Maternal nutritional supplementation and infant behavioral development. *Child Development, 54,* **669-676.**

294 low-income Taiwanese women (aged 19-30 yrs) were randomly assigned to 2 treatment groups. One group received a high-calorie and protein supplement and the other received a placebo. Infants received no direct supplementation. At approximately 8 mo of age, the mental and motor development of infants was assessed using a research version of the Bayley Scales of Infant Development. There were no sex differences in response to maternal supplementation in either scale, nor were the mental scale scores of infants of supplement mothers significantly higher than infants of control mothers. However, the motor scores of supplement infants were higher than those of control infants, which is consistent with the findings of 2 other large-scale nutritional supplementation studies (M. G. Herrera et al, 1980; and R. E. Klein, 1976).

3226

Jung, M. (1984). Structural family therapy: Its application to Chinese families. *Family Process, 23,* **365-374.**

The author proposed the use of structural family therapy as a treatment model for Chinese individuals seeking therapy from family or mental health agencies. The model emphasizes the social context in which families live, appropriate general boundaries, the joining process, and problem solving, and focuses on the therapist as an authority figure and agent of change. The model can be applied to most problem areas because it is assumed that the presenting problem is reinforced by family structure and repetitive patterns. Consequently, family interactional patterns that reinforce the presenting problems are the major focus of treatment. The theories and practice principles of other clinical approaches can be used in conjunction with this model.

3227

Kagan, L. (1972). Report from a visit to the Tientsin Psychiatric Hospital. *China Notes, 10,* **37-39. (Also published in** *Far East Reporter,* **1973, April, 12-18).**

3228

Kao, C. C. (1976). Maturity and paternalism in health care. *Ethics in Science & Medicine, 3,* **179-186.**

Discusses the relationship between paternalism, maturity, and health care using a cross-cultural comparison between the US and China. Health and maturity are both described as states of readiness for involvement in full living and are characterized by wholeness, balance, and harmony. The application of paternalism to health care necessitates that a distinction be made between paternal (denoting the characteristics of the father in patriarchal society) and paternalistic (domineering, oppressive, dictatorial, and exploitive) figures. It is argued that any form of paternalism in health care which impedes human growth toward health or maturity is undesirable. Physicians dedicated to saving human lives and caring for others in mature ways--expressing their own internal and external harmony--present positive aspects of paternalism which support the patient's integrity. Although the patient-physician relationship is often one of dependence, the emotional relationship is ideally one of mutual respect which fosters the growth of autonomy and self-determination of the patient. It is this relationship of dependence, mutual respect, and emergent autonomy which provides the basis for transference within the psychotherapeutic process. Finally, paternalism in health care is discussed in light of the feminist movement.

3229

Kao, J. J. (1977). Acupuncture therapeutics in the treatment of schizophrenia. *Comparative Medicine East & West, 5,* **181-184.**

Discusses schizophrenia in terms of classical Chinese nomenclature and describes the therapeutic use of acupuncture with schizophrenics. The clinical manifestations of the disorder are examined, and relevant acupuncture methods (auriculo-acupuncture, electroacupuncture, acupuncture, and moxibustion) are described. Acupuncture and moxibustion are viewed as especially effective in the treatment of schizophrenia, but it is noted that it is frequently necessary to combine traditional Chinese methods and Western medications for the effective treatment of the disorder.

3230

Kao, J. J. (1979). *Three millenia of Chinese psychiatry^ [Monograph]. New York: The Institute for Advanced Research in Asian Science and Medicine.*

3231

Karenga, M. R. (1978). Chinese psycho-social therapy: A strategic model for mental health. Psychotherapy: Theory, Research & Practice, 15, *101-107.*

Presents Chinese psychosocial therapy as a valuable strategic model for mental health on both the personal and collective levels. It is argued that the essential merit of this model is its humanistic emphasis which focuses on demonstrating the human capacity for self-comprehension and self-correction. Such an emphasis, it is argued, challenges crass commitments to gimmicks, medicine, machines, and other alternatives to the human factor. Chinese psychosocial therapy is suggested as a reinforcement of the basic humanistic assumption that reality is a human construction and process, and the problems it poses depend on human effort, thought, decision, and daring. This demystifies reality and the problems it poses and places the capacity and responsibility for social and human construction and reconstruction in human hands. Salient features of Chinese psychosocial therapy are identified and discussed: (a) definition of the social dimensions of the problem, (b) definition of the personal dimensions of the problem, (c) posing of a collective solution, (d) collective implementation of therapeutic procedures, and (e) construction and maintenance of supportive relations.

3232

Kas, J. J. (1979). Three millennia of Chinese psychiatry. *New York: Institute for Advanced Research in Asian Science & Medicine.*

The author spent seven weeks in China in 1973 studying Chinese psychiatry. This monograph summarizes his personal experiences and presents an extensive review of the literature. The major portion of the book is devoted to a discussion of Chinese psychiatry since 1949.

3233

Kety, S. S. (1976). Psychiatric concepts and treatment in China. China Quarterly, 66, *315-323.*

3234

Khoo, T. P. (Ed.). (1981). Aspects of mental health care Hong Kong 1981. *Hong Kong: Mental Health Association of Hong Kong.*

3235

Kleinman, A. (1980). A psychiatric perspective from the People's Republic of China. Culture, Medicine & Psychiatry, 4, *15.*

3236

Kleinman, A., & Gale, J. L. (1982). Patients treated by physicians and folk healers: A comparative outcome study in Taiwan. Culture, Medicine & Psychiatry, 6, *405-423.*

Compared the outcomes of 118 patients treated by shamans in Taipei, Taiwan, with those of 112 roughly matched patients treated by physicians. At a 3-4 wk follow-up, more than 75% of the Ss in both groups across 5 distinctive sickness types perceived their health problems as improved and were so evaluated by the research staff. Attributions of source of therapeutic efficacy were more complex and ambivalent. A higher proportion of Ss were dissatisfied with shamanistic treatment than with biomedical care, and this held true even for somatization patients with psychiatric problems. Findings are interpreted with respect to serious limitations on research design and methods in studies of indigenous healing. These limitations call into question certain findings and illustrate why assessments of therapeutic outcome, besides reflecting biological constraints, should be recognized as differential cultural construals of socially constructed reality.

3237

Kleinman, A., Kunstadter, P., Alexander, E. R., & Gale, J. L. (1975). Medicine in Chinese cultures: Comparative studies of health care in Chinese and other societies *(DHEW Publication No. NIH 75-653). Washington: U.S. Department of Health, Education, and Welfare.*

3238

Kleinman, A. M. (1975). The symbolic context of Chinese medicine: A comparative approach to the study of traditional medical and psychiatric forms of care in Chinese culture. American Journal of Chinese Medicine, 3, *103-124.*

Examines the symbolic structure and significance of illness and care in the Chinese context by (a) applying concepts developed in anthropology and the cross-cultural study of medicine and psychiatry; (b) examining recent studies of folk and popular forms of health care in contemporary Chinese communities; and (c) raising questions about the cognitive structure, cultural background, and biosocial significance of traditional Chinese healing beliefs and practices. An attempt is made to place this analysis in a comparative framework, so that Chinese cases can be related to health care systems in other cultural settings.

3239

Kleinman, A. M. (1975). Medical and psychiatric anthropology and the study of traditional forms of medicine in modern Chinese culture. Bulletin of the Institute of Ethnology *(Academia Sinica), No. 39, 107-123.*

This article describes concepts, research approaches, and research problems in the medical and psychiatric anthropological study of traditional forms of health care in Chinese culture. It takes off from specific problems which are found in a recent article by Holbrook, and which set the stage for the presentation of contemporary research by anthropologists and medical researchers, much of it carried out in Taiwan. The article then presents some of the author's theoretical constructs and empirical findings regarding this subject. Basic themes for the future development of medical and psychiatric anthropology in Chinese culture are also discussed. The author attempts to relate such work more generally to the rapidly developing field of comparative cross-cultural medicine and psychiatry. This field appears to be especially important for anthropological teaching and research on Chinese culture.

3240

Kleinman, A. M. (1980). Affects and affective disorders in Chinese culture. In A. M. Kleinman, Patients and healers in the context of culture: An exploration of the borderland between anthropology, medicine and psychiatry. *Berkeley: University of California Press.*

3241

Kleinman, A. M., Ravitz, L. J., & Koran, L. M. (1972). Psychiatry in Mainland China: Additional sources. American Journal of Psychiatry, 129, *482-484.*

3242

Ko, Y. H. (1972). [Validity of the male and female scores on the Ko Mental Health Questionnaire]. Psychological Testing, 19, *967-968. (In Chinese.)*

3243

Ko, Y. H. (1973). [KMHQ norms for university students and the validity of the KMHQ Scales]. Psychological Testing, 20, *1067-1072. (In Chinese.)*

3244

Ko, Y. H. (1974). A study on the effects of psychotherapy. Acta Psychologica Taiwanica, 16, *141-154.*

The present study explored the effectiveness of the author's psychotherapy and whether this effectiveness is limited to certain psychological problems. The Ko Mental Health Questionnaire (KMHQ) was administered to 13 clients both before and after psychotherapy. The KMHQ was also administered, and after five months readministered, to a group of 28 university students. The t ratio analysis yielded 10 significant mean differences between pretherapy and posttherapy KMHQ scores for the client group but only 2 significant differences for the normal group. The finding was interpreted as indicating that the author's psychotherapy is effective and, furthermore, that it is only effective for certain psychological problems.

3245

Ko, Y. H. (1977). [A report on the KMHQ Extraversion, Neuroticism, Psychoneurosis, and Psychosis Scales]. Psychological Testing, 24, *74-81. (In Chinese.)*

3246

Ko, Y. H. (1978). [A validation study of Six Scales of the KMHQ]. Psychological Testing, 25, *29-37. (In Chinese.)*

3247

Ko, Y. H. (1985). [Self-profiting habits in the eyes of psychotherapists]. Chinese Journal of Mental Health, 2, *21-34. (In Chinese.)*

Confucianism and seven theories of psychotherapy were reviewed to see what kinds of habits were deemed good or self-profiting by the propounders of these theories. Theories reviewed included those developed by Freud, Jung, Adler, Erikson, Allport, Rogers, Maslow, and Confucius. Fifty-eight habits deemed to be good or self-profiting by them were discussed and classified into five groups: nature, environment, work, other persons, and the self. It is claimed that such a review will benefit therapists in helping patients to learn self-profiting habits and to facilitate their daily adjustment.

3248

Ko, Y. H., & Liu, M. T. (1974). [Is the Ko's Mental Questionnaire (KMHQ) applicable to junior high school students]? Psychological Testing, 21, *11-17. (In Chinese.)*

3249

Ko, Y. H., Yang, K. S., Cheng, H. H., & Yang-Lee, P. H. (1975). [The relationship between school environment and college student mental health]. Bulletin of the Institute of Ethnology *(Academia Sinica), No. 39, 125-149. (In Chinese.)*

The main purpose of the present study is to examine the relationship between school environment and student mental health. The Ko Mental Health Questionnaire (KMHQ) was administered to 586 male students and 335 female students of the National Taiwan University (NTU). By comparing the older group with the younger one on the KMHQ scores, the authors found, in male and female groups, that the mental health of the older group is significantly better than that of the younger group. The finding was interpreted as indicating that the school environment of NTU is good for student mental health. When the findings with NTU were compared with those obtained in three other colleges, it was clearly seen that different school environments influence the mental health of students in different ways; one environment is good, one is bad, while one is equivocal for student mental health. To help identify important school environmental factors, the authors gave some speculations to six factors which could be used as independent variables in future research.

3250

Koehler, G. K. (1981). [Encounter with Chinese psychiatry: Vol. 2. Communal psychiatry in Shanghai]. Muenchener Medizinische Wochenschiften, 123, *1243-1246. (In other language.)*

The development of communal psychiatry in the city of Shanghai is very advanced. Two large psychiatric hospitals with a total capacity of 2,000 beds, 10 regional and 10 district hospitals with 10,100 beds assume responsibility for the hospital care of local communities. For each 100,000 inhabitants 50 psychiatric hospital beds are available at present. The network of psychiatric and psychosocial services extends beyond special hospitals and psychiatric departments. This is achieved through cooperation with psychiatrically trained and supervised doctors of all hospitals and barefoot doctors, health officers in street committees and in sanitary stations in large factories.

3251

Kohler, G. K. (1981). [Encounter with Chinese psychiatry. I. Traditional medicine and psychiatry in China]. Muenchener Medizinische Wochenschrift, 123, *1239-1242. (In other language.)*

The opening of the People's Republic of China after the cultural revolution also offers an opportunity for German neurologists to become acquainted with Chinese public health organization and the system of psychiatric care in the People's Republic of China. Today, Chinese medicine and psychiatry are faced with the problem of combining traditional diagnostic and therapeutic methods, particularly acupuncture and herbal medicine. With western scientific and psychotherapeutic principles and methods. The example of a Workers' Sanatorium stands for the multiplicity of traditional Chinese methods of treatment and also for psychosomatic disorders and diseases.

3252

Koo, L. C. (1984). The use of food to treat and prevent disease in Chinese culture. Social Science & Medicine, 18, *757-766.*

Interviews of 50 Chinese families in Hong Kong indicated that the proper selection, timing, and preparation of food was the most salient lay method of dealing with the prevention and treatment of 59 common symptoms and illnesses. Food prescriptions and proscriptions were based on the traditional concept of maintaining body homeostasis. Dietary rules filled explanatory and behavioral niches left open in Western medicine, and dietary manipulation was used to complement Western medicine by playing a predominant role at the beginning and end of the period of pathogenesis.

3253

Koran, L. M. (1972). Psychiatry in Mainland China: History and recent status. American Journal of Psychiatry, 128, *970-978.*

Summarizes the English language literature on ancient, modern, and recent Chinese psychiatry for psychiatrists traveling to Mainland China and others interested in cross-cultural psychiatry. Practices and beliefs regarding the etiology, diagnosis, and treatment of mental illness are described, together with manpower and facilities, professional publications, and research directions. A suggested outline for data gathering by psychiatric travelers to Mainland China is also included.

3254

Kroger, W. S. (1973). Acupunctural analgesia: Its explanation by conditioning theory, autogenic training, and hypnosis. American Journal of Psychiatry, 130, *855-860.*

Indicates that acupunctural analgesia seems to work, but better for the Chinese than for other nationalities. Significant antecedent, intervening, and dependent variables indicate that the technique can best be understood within the paradigm of contemporary conditioning theory. It has not been placed in this framework because scientist-observers have not stressed the effects of shaping and modifying behavior by a kind of operant conditioning that brings about compliant behavior without the necessity for overt cooperation. This compliance can account for the broad spectrum of psychobiologic experiences leading to well-known placebo responses. Another factor not generally recognized is the powerful effect of suggestion, which enhances suggestibility and hypnotizability. Neuropsychophysiologic mechanisms involved in acupunctural analgesia are discussed.

3255

Kuang, P. K. et al. (1960). [Evaluation of speedy comprehensive group treatment of 87 ambulatory neurasthenic patients]. Chinese Journal of Neurology and Psychiatry, 1, *12-18. (In Chinese.)*

3256

Kung, Y. H. (1963). [Free association test and its clinical application (I)]. Acta Psychologica Sinica, *No. 2, 130-136. (In Chinese.)*

A free association test with 50 stimulus-words was administered to 496 healthy subjects. The reaction time and the responses were analyzed and discussed in relation to the stimulus words and to the educational level, age, sex, and the types of higher nervous activity of the subjects.

3257

Kung, Y. H. (1963). [Free association test and its clinical application (II)]. Acta Psychologica Sinica, *No. 2, 137-145. (In Chinese.)*

The results of free association test in neurotic patients (neurasthenia, hysteria and obsessional neurosis) and patients of hypertension and peptic ulcer having neurasthenic symptoms were analyzed in relation with: (1) the reaction time and responses of patients of different diseases and of healthy subjects; (2) the effects of significant stimulus words on the cortical activity of the patients; (3) the results obtained under various clinical conditions of the patients in relation with the effects of treatments.

3258

Kuo, S. H. (1983). Forensic psychiatry in Taiwan. International Journal of Law & Psychiatry, 6, *457-472.*

Studied 120 available case records in southern Taiwan that involved a psychiatric examination for 43 Ss suspected of mental disorder and for 77 Ss who had broken the law. Case characteristics were tabulated and comparisons of psychiatric conclusions with court sentences were made. Results show that assessments of schizophrenia, affective disorder, organic brain syndrome, paranoid state, mental retardation, neurosis, and epilepsy were made in relation to acute or active states and severe disability (nonresponsibility), partial remission or moderate disability (partial responsibility), or remission or mild disability (full responsibility). Psychiatric assessments and court dispositions were consistent in 70% of the criminal cases and 74.29% of the civil cases. Taiwan has no specific mental health legislation but outcomes are influenced by social customs and culture. It is concluded that enactment of a comprehensive Chinese mental health act in Taiwan is imperative to provide consistent and conclusive attitudes in the legal system toward insanity.

3259

Kuo, S. S. (1958). [Treatment of excitement]. Chinese Journal of Neurology and Psychiatry, 4, *434. (In Chinese.)*

3260

Kwong, E. (1981). A response to "The Emperor's New Clothes" by Norman Briers. Hong Kong Journal of Mental Health, 10, *8-9.*

3261

Lai, B., & Mak, M. (1986). A study on methods of tracing psychiatric outpatient defaulters. Journal of the Hong Kong Psychiatric Association, 6, *34-36.*

The effectiveness of eight different methods of tracing psychiatric outpatient defaulters was studied. The subjects were 122 psychiatric outpatient defaulters to whom the tracing methods were randomly assigned.

Nurses had significantly higher success rates than doctors in achieving success. The difference appeared to lie in the better use by nurses of phone contact and in tracing only one time. There was no overall significant difference between tracing by phone or by letter, and between tracing once or twice. Tracing once by letter signed by the nurse-in-charge was the preferred method. The overall failure rate of tracing was 40%.

3262

Lam, P. T. C. (1978). The practice of community psychiatry. Hong Kong Journal of Mental Health, *7, 6-14.*

3263

Langsley, D. G., Barter, J. T., & Amir-Moshiri, A. (1983). Psychiatry in Iran and China. International Journal of Social Psychiatry, *29, 39-47.*

Contrasts the development of the health and psychiatric services in Iran (as of 1975) and China: (1) China appears the more committed to total care for the entire population, with the emphasis on prevention and primary care, while Iran's health care system focuses more on a 2-class system of care. (2) Iran is committed to a psychiatric model based on Western training, while China is more devoted to training primary care physicians of whom a few could get a year's specialty training in the treatment of the mentally ill. (3) Both countries hospitalize mostly schizophrenics, treating other conditions as outpatients. (4) Both use Western methods in hospitals, but China uses traditional methods along with Western medicine. (5) Both favor Westernized biological explanations for, and treatment of, mental disorders.

3264

Lau, B. W. K. (1982). Medical help-seeking behaviour in Hong Kong. Hong Kong Journal of Mental Health, 11, *25-30.*

3265

Lau-Yu, P. K. (1974). What a clinical psychologist can offer in the mental health service. Journal of Mental Health of Hong Kong, 3.

3266

Lazure, D. (1964). Politics and mental health in new China. American Journal of Orthopsychiatry, 34, *925-933.*

3267

Lee, D. Y., Sutton, R., France, H., & Uhlemann, M. (1983). Effects of counselor race on perceived counseling effectiveness. Journal of Counseling Psychology, 30, *447-456.*

Predicted that client evaluation of counselor behavior would be significantly influenced by counselor race and that the degree of influence would be a function of a client's racial attitude toward the counselor. Three stimulus interviews, based on an identical script, were videotaped by 3 counselors of different races (i.e., Caucasian, Chinese Canadian, East-Indian Canadian). The stimulus tapes were shown to 195 high school students, and a measure of perceived counseling effectiveness was obtained. Results show that Ss rated Caucasian counselors more favorably than ethnic minority counselors. However, perceived effectiveness of the 2 ethnic minority counselors did not correspond with the Ss' racial attitudes toward these ethnic minority groups.

3268

Lee, E. (1982). A social systems approach to assessment and treatment for Chinese American families. In M. M. Orfanidis, J. K. Pearce, & J. Giordano (Eds.), Ethnicity and family therapy. *New York: Guilford Press.*

3269

Lee, G. G., Li, A. K., & Wright, B. R. (1966). Children with problems: child guidance in Hong Kong. *Hong Kong: Child Guidance Centre, University of Hong Kong.*

Includes chapters on (1) the Hong Kong environment, (2) family situations (cases 1-9), (3) the child guidance center, (4) principles and techniques, (5) case studies (cases 10-20), and (6) sources of referral and analysis of case types.

3270

Lee, H. T. (1963). [The application of psychotherapy in the treatment of chronic schizophrenia]. Acta Psychologica Sinica, *No. 1, 55-64. (In Chinese.)*

A synthetic therapy was devised by combining drug and occupational therapies in treating 60 paranoid schizophrenics, whose duration of disease averaged 5.3 years. The patients were divided into 3 groups of 20 each. Therapy was applied to each group successively for 16 weeks. Three stages of the disease were identified: active delusion, unstable delusion, and disappearance of delusion. At different stages, group psychotherapy in combination with individual psychotherapy were given. At the end of the treatment, 35(58.3%) recovered, 18(30%) much improved, 6(10%) improved, and only 1 case remained unchanged. The patients' responses to psychotherapy at each stage were analyzed, and psychotherapy proved to be an indispensable treatment.

3271

Lee, L. C. (1979). Mental health: A people's project. APA Monitor, 10, *20-21.*

3272

Lee, P. (1984). Medical psychology: Selective review and projections in Hong Kong [Special issue: Psychology and Medicine] [Selected papers from the 1983 Annual Conference]. Hong Kong Psychological Society Bulletin, *No. 13, 7-15.*

Reviews the important contributions of the medical psychologist in his/her role as researcher, clinician, and educator in a medical setting. It is suggested that medical psychologists have an extremely important role as hard-core researchers who are not complacent about well-accepted and dogmatic principles. It is argued that proper research findings can contribute to a more scientifically based foundation in medical practice. The understanding of pain in the clinical setting is presented as an example, focusing on pain sensation, pain-motivated behavior, and the intricate dependency between pain and affect. It is suggested that as a medical educator, the medical psychologist can elicit his/her influence on encouraging a more balanced and comprehensive approach to patients through day-to-day contact with medical colleagues. The need for medical psychologists to have a rudimentary medical knowledge and the importance of their social skills and interpersonal effectiveness are emphasized. Applications of these principles to the author's Hong Kong setting are cited.

3273

Lee, P. W. H., Ho, E. S. Y., Tsang, A. K. T., Cheng, J. C. Y., Leung, P. C., Cheng, Y. H., & Lieh-Mak, F. (1985). Psychosocial adjustment of victims of occupational hand injuries. Social Sciences and Medicine, 20, *493-497.*

3274

Lee, P. W. H., & Hung, B. K. M. (1983). Understanding and improving patient compliance. Hong Kong Practitioner, 5, *553-560.*

3275

Lee, P. W. H., Luk, E. S. L., & Tam, W. Y. K. (1984). Biofeedback treatment of writer's cramp in a twelve-year-old child. Hong Kong Practitioner, 6, *1025-1030.*

3276

Lee, P. W. H., Sharp, I. J., & Fielding, R. (1985). The taming of the devil: The psychologist in the medical setting. Hong Kong Psychological Society Bulletin, *No. 14, 78-83.*

3277

Lee, P. W. H., & Spence, S. H. (1985). Observation and social validation of staff behaviours in a residential care setting. Behavioural Psychotherapy, 13, *43-58.*

3278

Lee, T., Cheng, C. F., & Chang, C. S. (1962). Some early records of nervous and mental diseases in traditional Chinese medicine. Chinese Medical Journal, 81, *55-59. (In Chinese.)*

3279

Lee, T. N. (1977). Lidocaine injection of auricular points in the treatment of insomnia. American Journal of Chinese Medicine, 5, *71-77.*

By combining knowledge in modern medicine and traditional Chinese medicine, auricular points were selected for treatment of insomnia. Instead of the placement of needles, injection of small amounts of Lidocaine into these sites was employed. Fifteen out of 16 patients obtained substantial improvement and one patient received moderate improvement. The therapeutic effect was maintained three months after the end of the treatment series. The physiological and clinical implications of this study in terms of modern medicine and traditional Chinese medicine are also discussed.

3280

Lee, W. S., Yeh, E. K., Liu, J. T., Liu, Y. K., Chang, S. C., & Taipei City Psychiatric Center. (1984). [Assessment of social adjustment of discharged chronic psychotic patients]. Chinese Journal of Mental Health, 1, *41-47. (In Chinese.)*

The social adjustment level of 72 chronic psychotic patients discharged from a rehabilitation ward was assessed using a rating scale. The results showed that most of the patients were at the middle level of the social adjustment scale. The level of social adjustment of the patients in the community was significantly correlated with their self-care ability, social skills, and drug compliance in the ward, and their attitudes to and ability in the sheltered workshop. The level of social adjustment was not correlated with the family attitude to rehabilitation, availability of family resources for occupation in the community and the manifested symptoms of the patients in the ward. Those patients who received government medical financial aid, who had a lower educational level and who were middle aged had better social adjustment in the community. These findings suggested the possibility of establishing a rating scale to predict the patient's level of social adjustment in the community at a very early phase of the patient's admission to a rehabilitation ward.

3281

Lei, B. S. et al. (1986). [A cross-over treatment of obsessive-compulsive neurosis with imipramine and chlorimipramine]. Chinese Journal of Neurology and Psychiatry, 19, *275-278. (In Chinese.)*

3282

Leseth, K. (1974). Psychiatry in China. Tidsskrift for Norsk Laegeforen, 94, *439-441.*

3283

Leung, J. Y. W. (1979). Longstay hostel for chronic schizophrenic patients in Hong Kong. Hong Kong Journal of Mental Health, 8, *19-22.*

3284

Leung, M. T., & Yiu, D. (1986). Day training centre: A community-based resource for the ex-mentally ill. Journal of the Hong Kong Psychiatric Association, 6, *19-23.*

3285

Leung, S. M., Miller, M. H., & Leung, S. W. (1978). Chinese approach to mental health service. Canadian Psychiatric Association Journal, 23, *354-360.*

Reviews health care approaches in the People's Republic of China where lifestyle, political leadership, grass roots health programs, and patriotic zeal are a unified endeavor. Assumptions underlying North American health practices come into particular focus. Specifically, the Chinese experiences raise doubt about the value of a professionally oriented emphasis in health care and deny the worth of health programs that are not woven into the social, economic, political, and ethical activities of society. The Chinese maintain that the key to all health and mental health care advances is social and economic reform, grass roots programs, and most important, self-reliance with an intense personal motivation to produce change in one's way of life. Professional responsibility worthy of public trust would be achieved only insofar as professional efforts facilitate these 3 areas of development.

3286

Leung, S. M. R. (1981). Mental health home care program in the communes of the People's Republic of China. Journal of Psychiatric Treatment & Evaluation, 3, *53-58.*

This paper examines the mental health home care program in a rural community in the People's Republic of China. The program is a pilot project initiated by the Psychiatry Department of Beijing Medical College to provide psychiatric services for the mentally ill in their own commune-homes. The project basically aims for the early detection and treatment of mental patients in their own social milieu with family and community support. The home care program was instituted through the joint effort of the psychiatrists of the Beijing Medical College, the Mobile Mental Health Teams, and the barefoot doctors of the Commune Health Clinic. From July 1974 to February 1977, 12 communes in Haitien District (near Beijing) with a total population of 189,915 were served. The diagnoses were: schizophrenia, retardation, epilepsy, reactive psychosis and manic-depressive psychosis. The innovative project demonstrates the feasibility of a mental health program which combines both prevention and treatment at the community level.

3287

Li, C. H. (1958). ["Chien Nao Wan" in the treatment of neurasthenia]. Chinese Journal of Neurology and Psychiatry, 4, *429-430. (In Chinese.)*

3288

Li, C. K. (1982). Tools for investigating the relationship between the clinical psychologist and the client: A case study. Hong Kong Psychological Society Bulletin, *No. 9, 27-38.*

Presents the case of a 14-yr-old Chinese boy who was institutionalized for committing a burglary and was referred to the author for personality and intelligence assessment. During the only session that the author and S spent together, the author administered the WISC, the TAT, and some projective drawing tests to S. The author also attempted to talk to S about his broken family, his crimes, and sex, but S remained uncommunicative.

3289

Li, C. P. et al. (1959). [Certain etiologic factors in psychoneurosis and a rapid combined method of treatment]. Chinese Journal of Neurology and Psychiatry, 5, *304-307. (In Chinese.)*

3290

Li, C. P., Hsu, Y. H., Keng, C. M., & Wang, M. T. (1959). [Some problems concerning the cause of psychasthenia and attempts to find quick treatments]. In [Collection of theses on achievements in the medical sciences in commemoration of the 10th National Foundation Day of China *] (Vol. 2), Beijing. (Translated by U.S. Joint Publications Research Service, No. 14,829, pp. 652-670.) (In Chinese.)*

3291

Li, C. P., Li, H. T. et al. (1958). [Rapid treatment of neurasthenia]. Chinese Journal of Neurology and Psychiatry, 4, *351-356. (In Chinese.)*

3292

Li, K. C., & Luk, H. (1978). The mental health service to Vancouver Chinese. Hong Kong Journal of Mental Health, 7, *22-29.*

3293

Li, Y. Y. (1976). Shamanism in Taiwan: An anthropological inquiry. In W. P. Lebra (Ed.), Mental health research in Asia and the Pacific: Vol. 4. Culture-bound syndromes, ethnopsychiatry, and alternate therapies. *Honolulu, HI: University Press of Hawaii.*

3294

Lieh-Mak, F. (1979). Parents as behaviour therapists. Hong Kong Journal of Mental Health, 8, *16-20.*

3295

Lieh-Mak, F., Lee, P. W. H., & Luk, S. L. (1984). Problems encountered in teaching Chinese parents to be behavior therapists. Psychologia: An International Journal of Psychology in the Orient, 27, *56-64.*

Problems encountered in training Chinese parents to treat their own children by behavioral methods were discussed. Problems associated with socioeconomic status, traditional patterns of family structure and interaction, the accustomed mode of childrearing practices, the ingrained outlook on childhood problems, and a dependent attitude toward doctors were discussed, along with the cultural and attitudinal backgrounds of Chinese parents in Hong Kong. Chinese parents often fail to recognize the sickness of their children as psychological disturbance, find it difficult to play with or praise their children, and tend to regard problem children as marginal members of the family. Salient sociocultural factors contributing to the difficulties were highlighted, and the ethnocentric bias involved in importing treatment modalities from one culture to another was discussed.

3296

Lin, C. P. et al. (1958). [The speedy treatment of neurasthensia]. Chinese Journal of Neurology and Psychiatry, 5, *351-156. (In Chinese.)*

3297

Lin, E. H. (1983). Intraethnic characteristics and the patient-physician interaction: "Cultural blind spot syndrome". Journal of Family Practice, 16, *91-98.*

Uses case analysis and literature review to present a conceptual framework for analyzing patient-physician interaction in any cultural context. The author's experience as a Western-trained Chinese physician attending to a wide spectrum of Chinese patients challenged the assumption that similarities in backgrounds of physician and patient result in improved outcome. The cultural identity of the Western-trained physician and intraethnic variation among people of a common cultural heritage emerged as key considerations from this analysis of patient-physician interaction. Two cases representing extremes in patient-physician interaction were analyzed with respect to each of 6 essential elements of the interaction. The 1st case concerned a 39-yr-old Cantonese woman who preferred an older White male doctor to a younger Chinese woman. The 2nd case concerned a 29-yr-old Taiwanese housewife who learned to trust her Chinese doctor even while S used Chinese herbal cures. It is concluded that a good match among intraethnic descriptors of patient and physician enhances communication and may thereby improve outcome.

3298

Lin, H. N., & Chen, C. Y. (1980). Tardive dyskinesia in patients treated with antipsychotics in chronic wards in Taipei. Journal of the Formosan Medicine Association, 79, *332-337.*

12 (4.5%) of 268 chronic psychiatric inpatients treated with antipsychotic drugs for at least 6 months were found to have tardive dyskinesia, a condition more frequently associated with older patients. Among these 12 patients, 6 were above the age of 50. Involuntary movement of the tongue is the most frequent sign and in particular an early sign of tardive dyskinesia. This study reveals that involuntary movements are mainly confined to buccolinguomasticatory muscles. No patient has axial involvement. Many drugs have been proposed to treat tardive dyskinesia, but the effects are unsatisfactory. At present, the best way to treat tardive dyskinesia is early diagnosis and early discontinuation of antipsychotic drugs.

3299

Lin, H. Y. (1985). Post-divorce adjustment and post-divorce counselling: A study of counselling effectiveness with divorced women in Taiwan. Dissertation Abstracts International, 45, *A2806-2807. (Also in* **Chinese Journal of Mental Health,** *1985,* **2,** *63-77, in Chinese.)*

The author examined the characteristics of divorced women, effects of counseling on their self-concept, and their postdivorce adjustment. Fifty-three Taiwanese divorced women completed a Psycho-Social Divorce Adjustment Questionnaire. To assess counseling effects, two measures were used: the Tennessee Self-Concept Scale for assessing the self-concept of two groups of 20 divorced women and one group of 20 married women, and the Post-Divorce Adjustment Scale for assessing the postdivorce adjustment of the divorced women. Counseling under the Interpersonal Coping Skills Program was given to the treatment group of divorced women, and the other (control) group of divorced women received no counseling. Both measures were given before and after treatment. It was found that the treatment group made significant improvements in terms of self-concept and postdivorce adjustment. Some improvement was also found in these areas with the control group, due to group experience with women in similar situations.

3300

Lin, M. Y. (1984). Overview of health and services in Taiwan, ROC. Image: Journal of Nursing Scholarship, 16, *101-104.*

The author described health institutions, health organizations, medical facilities and services, health staff, and the current health status in Taiwan. The current health status was defined in terms of communicable disease control, maternal and child health, family planning, adult health, health education, mental health, drugs and cosmetics control, food sanitation, and environmental protection. A recommendation to improve the quality of nursing in Taiwan was also presented.

3301

Lin, T. Y. (1961). Evolution of mental health programme in Taiwan. American Journal of Psychiatry, 117, *961-971.*

3302

Lin, T. Y. (1982). Culture and psychiatry: A Chinese perspective. Australian & New Zealand Journal of Psychiatry, 16, *235-245.*

Proposes that psychocultural interaction influences the normal and abnormal behavior of the Chinese at different levels, including such basic processes as cognition, affect, and communication as well as the perception and management of both universal and culture-specific stresses. Three major areas in Chinese psychiatry are discussed: major psychoses, minor mental disorders, and patterns of help-seeking in Chinese. Longitudinal studies conducted in Taiwan to discover schizophrenics and manic-depressives show that Western psychiatric criteria can be used to diagnose Chinese, but these same criteria may also exclude patients whose behavior is judged to be abnormal in their own culture. Schizophrenic treatment was found to have a higher rate of success in Taiwan than in Western countries. Studies of minor mental disorders among Chinese show that the phenomenology of Chinese depression differs greatly from that in the West and is characterized by somatization. The neurotic and culture-bound syndromes are also predominantly somatic in their manifestation. In most cases of Chinese mental disturbance, sufferers were isolated within their home and family. When the family could no longer cope, a physician was summoned for treatment of a "physiological" ailment. If the patient was sent to a mental hospital, he/she was rejected by the family because of the stigma attached to mental illness.

3303

Lin, T. Y., & Eisenberg, L. (Eds.). (1986). Mental health care for one billion people. *Vancouver: University of British Columbia Press.*

3304

Lin, T. Y., & Lin, M. C. (1978). Service delivery issues in Asian-North American communities. American Journal of Psychiatry, 135, *454-456.*

Describes some of the sociocultural factors (e.g., moralistic, religious, psychological, and familial characteristics) that influence the help-seeking behavior of Chinese psychiatric patients in North America. A replicable approach is proposed for investigating sociocultural patterns relevant to service delivery to Chinese in other communities.

3305

Ling, M. Y. (1946). Psychiatry in China today. National Reconstruction Journal, 6, *20-30. (Reprinted in M. Livingston & P. Lowinger (Eds.),* **The minds of the Chinese people: Mental health in New China** *(pp. 138-148). Englewood Cliffs, NJ: Prentice-Hall, 1983.)*

This article provided a historical setting for the period just before Liberation, and an understanding of traditional Chinese values. Background topics discussed included family ties, attitude toward authority, attitude toward sex, religion, alcohol and drugs, infectious diseases, and industrialization. Present problems, principles of approach, and research were discussed.

3306

Li-Repac, D. (1980). Cultural influences on clinical perception: A comparison between Caucasian and Chinese-American therapists. Journal of Cross-Cultural Psychology, 11, *327-342.*

Compared 5 White and 5 Chinese-American therapists on their conceptions of normality, empathic ability, and perceptions of the same Chinese and White clients seen on a videotaped interview. Results show that (1) the 2 therapist groups basically agreed in their conceptions of normality; (2) White Ss were more accurate in predicting self-descriptive responses of White than of Chinese clients; and (3) there were significant differences between ratings of the same clients given by White and Chinese-American Ss. Ratings given by the 2 groups of therapists were compared on 6 rational clusters. Chinese clients were rated higher on a Depression/Inhibition cluster and lower on a Social Poise/Interpersonal Capacity cluster by White Ss than by Chinese-American Ss. Chinese-American Ss judged the White clients to be more severely disturbed than did the White Ss. Differences are interpreted as reflections of therapists' biases as well as their own world view.

3307

Liu, C. J. (1978). [Rural youth's worries and their guidance in Taiwan]. In C. I. Wen, I. Y. Li, & K. S. Yang (Eds.), Proceeding of Symposium on Youth Problems in a Changing Society. *Taipei: Institute of Ethnology (Academia Sinica). (In Chinese.)*

3308

Liu, H. H. (1959). [Therapeutic effect of sleep therapy on oppressive-compulsive state with various medications]. Chinese Journal of Neurology and Psychiatry, 5, *243-247. (In Chinese.)*

3309

Liu, H. M. (1958). [Treatment of stupor]. Chinese Journal of Neurology and Psychiatry, 4, *432-433. (In Chinese.)*

3310

Liu, J. Q. et al. (1980). [Preliminary study on the effects of short-term hospitalization in 379 cases of schizophrenia]. Chinese Journal of Neurology & Psychiatry, 13, *197-199. (In Chinese.)*

3311

Liu, X. H. (1980). Mental health work in Sichuan. British Journal of Psychiatry, 137, *371-376.*

Discusses such topics as medical services and mental hospitals, the department of psychiatry at the medical college, diagnosis and treatment of psychiatric illness, and psychiatric patients in the community. Recommendations for the future, such as training more medical graduates as psychiatrists, are offered.

3312

Liu, X. H. (1981). Psychiatry in traditional Chinese medicine. British Journal of Psychiatry, 138, *429-433.*

Presents a brief introduction to psychiatry in traditional Chinese medicine by pointing out citations of psychiatric illness dating back to 1100 BC, appearances of psychiatric terminology (781-771 BC), and records of psychiatric symptoms. Also reviewed are descriptions of psychiatric illness in medical classics as well as early (1607, 1739) classification systems, diagnoses, and treatments (e.g., herbal drugs and acupunctures).

3313

Liu, Z. X. (1980). [Clinical observations on 123 cases of psychoses treated by traditional Chinese medicine]. Chinese Journal of Neurology & Psychiatry, 13, *110-113. (In Chinese.)*

3314

Livingston, M., & Lowinger, P. (1983). The minds of the Chinese people: Mental health in New China. *Englewood Cliffs, NJ: Prentice-Hall.*

3315

Lo, M. L. (1976). Folk beliefs of the Chinese and implications to psychiatric nursing. Journal of Psychiatric Nursing, 14, *38-42.*

3316

Lo, W. H. (1973). Social work and psychogeriatrics. Hong Kong Journal of Mental Health, 2, *23-26.*

3317

Lo, W. H. (Ed.) (1976). Perspectives in mental health: Hong Kong, 1976. *Hong Kong: Mental Health Association of Hong Kong.*

3318

Lo, W. H. (1981). Culture and depression with special reference to Hong Kong. Psychopathologie Africaine, 17, *134-142.*

Examined data on 3,577 patients admitted to Hong Kong psychiatric hospitals in 1958 and 1978. It is concluded that depressives constituted an increasing proportion of patients attending psychiatric clinics, but their percentage in psychiatric hospital populations has been decreasing. This trend has been due to various factors (e.g., rapid social changes brought about by industrialization and urbanization, expansion of psychiatric facilities, and advances in psychopharmacology). The manifestation of depression is explained in terms of personality characteristics of Hong Kong Chinese and concepts of traditional Chinese medicines. Discussion of the treatment of depression ranges from indigenous methods to modern treatment.

3319

Lo, W. H., Chan, W., Ma, K. S., & Wong, A. (Eds.) (1971). Aspects of mental health in Hong Kong. *Hong Kong: Mental Health Association of Hong Kong.*

3320

Lo, W. H., & Kwok, I. (1981). History of psychiatry in Hong Kong. Journal of the Hong Kong Psychiatric Association, 1, *14-17.*

3321

Loo, C. (1982). Chinatown's wellness: An enclave of problems. Journal of the Asian American Psychological Association, 7, *13-18.*

Data obtained from 100 Chinese-American women shows that Ss exhibited low self-esteem and assertiveness and were frequently dissatisfied with their traditional roles in marriage and with their quality of life. Most desired a larger social support network, but a majority felt uncomfortable dealing with those from outside their ethnic group. A high prevalence of mental health problems was found, particularly depression, anxiety, and psychosomatic disorders, but service utilization was low. The need for expanded provision of psychological support services is stressed.

3322

Loong, S. C., & Ong, Y. Y. (1973). Paroxysmal kinesigenic choreoathetosis: Report of a case relieved by L-dopa. Journal of Neurology, Neurosurgery & Psychiatry, 36, *921-924.*

Describes a case of paroxysmal kinesigenic choreoathetosis in a 21-yr-old Chinese male. A hitherto unreported response to levodopa was recorded and its possible relevance to the pathophysiology of the disorder is discussed.

3323

Lorenzo, M. K., & Adler, D. A. (1984). Mental health services for Chinese in a community health center. Social Casework, 65, *600-609.*

This paper described the present author's experience in providing mental health services to Chinese patients in a community health center in Boston's (Massachusetts) Chinatown/South Cove community. A description of the population served and a summary of the cultural issues encountered were presented. A profile of the group of patients treated and the modifications in clinical practices that were adopted to meet the mental health needs of this group were discussed. Several case histories were included to illustrate the issues presented by the Chinese patients.

3324

Lorini, G., & Fusari, A. (1977). [Acupuncture and psychiatry]. Minerva Medica, 68, *711-715. (In other language.)*

Personal experience with acupuncture as a therapeutic technique in psychiatry is presented. Its effects on the patient and the taking of drugs are discussed. The results, like those reported by Chinese and other Italian workers, were encouraging and indicate that the technique may be more widely adopted in this field.

3325

Louie, T. T. (1977). The pragmatic context: A Chinese-American example of defining and managing illness. Dissertation Abstracts International, 38, *B140-141.*

3326

Lowinger, P. (1973). How the People's Republic of China solved the drug abuse problem. American Journal of Chinese Medicine, 1, *275-282.*

Discusses the history of narcotics use in China and the various efforts to combat it. In the present People's Republic, narcotic addiction is considered a health and political problem to be dealt with by action of the entire society. Treatment, provision of meaningful alternatives, and legal restrictions are described.

3327

Lowinger, P. (1977). The solution to narcotic addiction in the People's Republic of China. American Journal of Drug & Alcohol Abuse, 4, *165-178.*

Examines the success of the People's Republic of China in dealing with a 200-yr-old problem of opium addiction. The treatment of addiction as a political problem is discussed, including replacement of poppy growing with food crops, imprisonment of large opium distributors, value changes among the youth, and the offering of new educational, social, and vocational opportunities.

3328

Lu, Y. C. (1978). The collective approach to psychiatric practice in the People's Republic of China. Social Problems, 26, *2-14.*

Describes and analyzes the effects of changes in 4 social values (the value of collective responsibility, the application of the value of sharing and "serving the people" to methods of psychiatric therapy, the value of "minimization of elitism" as practiced in the role relationships among members of different categories in mental hospitals, and the reaffirmation of faith in human ability to conquer difficulties) in China on the approach to treatment of the mentally ill since the 1949 revolution. Attention is focused on the effects of these social values on psychiatric practice.

3329

Luk, S. L., & Lieh-Mak, F. (1979). Difficulties encountered in training parents as behavioural therapists. Hong Kong Journal of Mental Health, 8, *9-14.*

3330

Lum, D. (1982). Toward a framework for social work practice with minorities. Social Work, 27, *244-249.*

Presents case histories of 2 women, a 35-yr-old Mexican American and a 63-yr-old Chinese American, to show how a psychosocial framework can be used to identify problems specific to the individual (cognitive, affective, or behavioral) and the environment (economic, cultural, or institutional). It is noted that social workers need to develop demographic profiles of major ethnic groups, become aware of world views of minorities, and develop theories applicable to minority groups.

3331

Lyman, R. S., Maeker, V., & Liang, P. (Eds.) (1939). Social and psychological studies in neuropsychiatry in China. *Peking: Peking Union Medical College.*

3332

Ma, J. (1986). Mutual aid group as a practice model in working with the family members of psychotic patients. The Hong Kong Journal of Social Work, 20, *40-46.*

3333

Mak, D. K. Y. (1984). The 'safeness' of psychiatric half-way house residents. Hong Kong Journal of Mental Health, 13, *74-77.*

3334

Mak, K. Y. (1986). Why do residents in psychiatric halfway houses relapse? Hong Kong Journal of Mental Health, 15, *72-75.*

3335

Martgetts, E. T. (1972). Hong Kong mental health services in November 1971, with particular reference to services for drug addiction. *Report to World Health Organization, 1972.*

3336

Masserman, J. H. (1980). Psychiatry in China: Background, theory, and practice. Current Psychiatric Therapies, 19, *195-206.*

This report is an overview that covers not only psychiatric concerns, but scenery, travel, and general health. Psychiatric topics were discussed in the context of a historical-geographical panorama, with careful attention paid to such aspects as the cost of hospital care and hospital routines.

3337

Masunaga, S. (1969). Diagnosis and treatment in Oriental medicine. Psychologia: An International Journal of Psychology in the Orient, 12, *74-80.*

In Japan, Western medicine and Oriental medicine differ. The latter is based mainly on medicine organized in China 2000 yr. ago. It is at 1st glance like Greek and Roman medicine. In Oriental medicine, "diagnosis means selection of therapy according to the patient". Kampo (Oriental medicine) uses 4 kinds of diagnosis: watching, listening, questioning, and feeling. Psychotherapy is now thought to be a necessary addition to physical therapy. No medicine exists without some psychotherapy. The most suitable therapy "gives the most basic and agreeable sensation to the patient".

3338

Matsumoto, K., Tsujimoto, T., Morishita, H. et al. (1975). A variation of acupuncture used in the sedation of hyperactive children. American Journal of Acupuncture, 3, *43-46.*

Twenty hyperactive children were divided into 2 equal groups at random. All children were given monosodium trichlorethyl phosphate for a EEG examination. One group underwent modified acupuncture therapy without needles in addition to medication, while the other served as a control group. The time from the administration of the drug until onset of sleep was 69.5 min in the acupuncture treated children, while in the control group the average was 247.5 min. Although the theory of Chinese medicine may not necessarily be enough to explain the results of this study, it is suggested that acupuncture may be an effective adjunct for the sedation of hyperactive children.

3339

McCartney, J. L. (1926). Neuropsychiatry in China: A preliminary observation. Chinese Medical Journal, 40, *617-626.*

3340

McCoy, M., & Kvan, E. (1979). Attitudes towards punishment: A repertory grid study of young offenders in Hong Kong *[Working paper]. Hong Kong: University of Hong Kong, Center of Asian Studies.*

3341

Mechanic, D., & Kleinman, A. (1980). Ambulatory medical care in the People's Republic of China: An exploratory study. American Journal of Public Health, 70, *62-66.*

The authors visited the People's Republic of China and spent considerable time in rural medical facilities. This article is based on brief interviews with 138 patients. The Chinese medical care system does not recognize and deal with psychosocial issues in illness, and the stigma of mental illness is still prevalent.

3342

Mental Diseases Hospital, Peking Medical College. (1958). [The therapeutic effect of artificial hibernation treatment of mental diseases]. Chinese Journal of Neurology and Psychiatry, 4, *436-454. (In Chinese.)*

3343

Miao, E. (1978). Diagnosing how children think as an approach to preventive mental health for children. Acta Psychologica Taiwanica, 20, *15-28.*

This paper examined preventive clinical psychology in relation to the development of cognitive abilities. Children's thinking was investigated through a search for the simultaneous occurrence of cognitive and affective abilities. The subjects were drawn from a public school in the suburb of Taipei, Taiwan.

3344

Miller, M. F. (1978). Psychiatry in the People's Republic of China. World Studies of Psychiatry, 2.

3345

Millikin, D., & Rothchild, M. (1982). What Hong Kong doesn't know about psychosurgery. Asia 2000, *37-41.*

3346

Miskel, J. F. (1973). Religion and Medicine: The Chinese opium problem. Journal of Historical Medicine, 28, *3-14.*

3347

Mu, K. M. (1959). [A review of the work of Canton mental hospital in past ten years]. Chinese Journal of Neurology and Psychiatry, 5, *310-311. (In Chinese.)*

3348

Muensterberger, W. (1982). Versuch einer transkulturellen Analyse: Der Fall eines chinesischen Offiziers [A transcultural analysis: The case of a Chinese officer]. Psyche: Zeitschrift fur Psychoanalyse und ihre Anwendungen, 36, *865-887. (In other language.)*

The case history of a former officer of the Kuomintang, now living in the US, shows that the universal human conflicts discovered by psychoanalysis as well as the forms of their elaboration assume specific configurations in different cultures. Subjected to a transcultural analysis, they can only be understood by reference to the mother tongue and the habits, manners, and common mythologies of the patient's culture of origin.

3349

Muensterberger, W. (1984). Transcultural psychoanalysis: The case of a Chinese army officer. Journal of Psychoanalytic Anthropology, 7, *3-21.*

The author discusses his experience as a transcultural psychoanalyst with a Chinese male in his 30's. S presented with unresolved oedipal-fraternal antagonism, castration fear, and a sense of sinfulness associated with masturbation. The case shows a relation between symptom formation, life experiences, and defense patterns. S's manifest symptoms can be viewed as an elaboration of archaic experiences linking sociocultural criteria and adaptation modes.

3350

Nanking Mental Hospital. (1958). [Preliminary experiences in the prevention and treatment of mental illness]. Chinese Journal of Neurology and Psychiatry, 4, *263-266. (In Chinese.)*

3351

Neurasthenia Treatment Unit, Peking Traditional Hospital. (1959). [Traditional Chinese medicine in treatment of neurasthenia: Report of 115 cases]. Chinese Journal of Neurology and Psychiatry, 5, *87-90. (In Chinese.)*

3352

Neurath, P. (1980). [Chinese and other methadone patients in New York's Chinatown]. Wiener Zeitschrift Suchforsch, 3, *23-26. (In other language.)*

At a methadone maintenance clinic in New York's Chinatown, most of the Chinese patients are between 60 and 80 years old; other patients (mostly Negroes and Puerto Ricans, and a few Whites) are mostly between 20 and 35, just as in all other methadone clinics in New York. Differences in social environment, the history of addiction, the distribution system, and ways of taking the drug are discussed.

3353

Neurology-psychiatry in the People's Republic of China (No. 74-56, pp. 71-95; trans.). (1973). Bethesda, MD: DHEW (NIH). (Reprinted in M. Livingston & P. Lowinger (Eds.), The minds of the Chinese people: Mental health in New China *(pp. 169-192). Englewood Cliffs, NJ: Prentice-Hall, 1983.)*

3354

Newman, R. G., Lee, E. I., & Wu, P. M. (1982 - 1983). Reporting history to an addict registry before and after admission to methadone treatment in Hong Kong. American Journal of Drug & Alcohol Abuse, *9, 251-261.*

Determined the likelihood of being reported to an addict registry before and after admission to a methadone treatment program in Hong Kong for 1,908 patients (the majority aged 20-50 yrs) who enrolled during May and June in 1978. In the 6 mo before enrollment, 2 out of every 5 Ss had contact with at least 1 reporting source, and 10% of all Ss had contact with a criminal justice system agency. Cohorts grouped according to retention in treatment did not differ with respect to preadmission reporting experience. Following enrollment, however, these cohorts demonstrated a strong association between continued treatment and a decreased likelihood of contact with a reporting system. 13% of continuously active patients were reported during the 6 mo after enrollment compared to 68% of those who dropped out of treatment within 2 mo; the corresponding reporting history from criminal justice system agencies was 6 and 23%, respectively. The association between retention and decreased contact with reporting agencies was observed for each age group studied.

3355

Ng, H. S. (1978). The first two years of the Tuen Mun Hostel. Hong Kong Journal of Mental Health, *7, 15-19.*

3356

Ng, M. L. (1980). Music therapy and its use in psychiatry. Hong Kong Journal of Mental Health, *9, 21-33.*

3357

Ng, M. L. (1983). Experiences with non-directive psychotherapeutic techniques for Chinese in Hong Kong. Journal of the Hong Kong Psychiatric Association, *3, 35-36, 38-39.*

3358

Ng, M. L. (1985). Psychoanalysis for the Chinese -- applicable or not applicable? International Review of Psycho-Analysis, 12, *449-460.*

The major problems that have bothered Chinese psychiatrists and prevented them from doing the psychoanalytic types of psychotherapy were reviewed. Opponents argue that psychoanalysis is not applicable to the Chinese because the Chinese have a particular concept of psychiatric illness, their psychosexual development is still not completely understood, they do not disclose their personal problems easily, and they are used to authoritative and directive approaches. The validity of these problems was addressed, and possible ways to overcome these problems were suggested, based on the author's understanding of psychoanalysis and Chinese culture, his experiences of using psychoanalytic psychotherapy, and experimental data. It was recommended that more of the psychoanalytic type of psychotherapy should be implemented with Chinese patients.

3359

Ng, M. L. (1986). Sex therapy in the Hong Kong University Psychiatric Unit. In T. P. Khoo (Ed.), Mental Health in Hong Kong^ (pp. 279-283). Hong Kong: The Mental Health Association of Hong Kong.

3360

Ng, M. L., & Lin, T. Y. (1985). Some views on psychoanalysis for the Chinese. *Journal of the Hong Kong Psychiatric Association*, *5*, **2-5.**

3361

Ng, M. L., Tam, Y. K., & Luk, S. L. (1982). Evaluation of different forms of community meeting in a psychiatric unit in Hong Kong. *British Journal of Psychiatry*, *140*, **491-497.**

Assessed the therapeutic value of doctor-directed, nurse-directed, and nondirective community meetings in an inpatient psychiatric unit attached to a teaching general hospital in Hong Kong. In the retrospective study, the rates of ward incidents and discharge rates of inpatients before and during the 3 stages were compared. In the prospective study, an ABA design was used with 10-wk blocks of regular nondirective meetings, cessation of meetings, and then resumption; ward incidents, discharge rates, and ward atmosphere during these blocks were compared. Nurses and patients completed the Ward Atmosphere Scale. Both the nondirective and nurse-directed forms were equally associated with a reduction in ward incidents, with aggressive incidents showing the greatest tendency to change. Ward atmosphere and patient discharge rates did not change with community meetings.

3362

Ngan, Y. S., & Tang, G. W. (1984). Needs and emotional states in cancer patients: A study of 21 Chinese women with carcinoma of the ovary. *Journal of Psychosomatic Obstetrics & Gynaecology*, *3*, **223-231.**

The authors studied 21 Chinese women (aged 18-75 years) suffering from carcinoma of the ovary who had received surgery and chemotherapy. Their needs and emotional states related to their disease and treatment were observed. Factors studied included marital relations, family, social activity, knowledge about disease and treatment, information seeking, doctor-patient relations, and mood changes. Only half of the subjects admitted that they realized that they had cancer and only two knew exactly what kind of cancer they suffered from and the reasons for receiving chemotherapy. It appeared that most subjects did not want to seek information about their illness and the therapy they received. They seemed to be content to leave all decisions to their attending doctors. Implications for management strategies were proposed.

3363

Nielsen, S. K. (1975). Letter: Research on Chinese health care. *American Journal of Psychiatry*, *132*, **688-689.**

3364

Norman, J. (1971). *How to cure drug addicts*. **London: Tom Stacey.**

3365

O'Hoy, K. M., & Tang, G. W. (1985). Sexual function following treatment for carcinoma of cervix. *Journal of Psychosomatic Obstetrics & Gynaecology, 4,* **51-58.**

The changes in sexual functioning were evaluated in 103 Chinese females who were treated for cervical cancer. Comparisons were made between 10 subjects who underwent radiation treatment, 40 subjects treated by surgery, and 53 subjects who received both surgery and radiation. Results revealed changes in sexual function in all 3 groups. Combined treatment produced the most marked changes in coital frequency and delay in resumption of sexual activity. Subjects who had undergone a major operation were reluctant to resume sexual intercourse because of cultural beliefs and erroneous ideas regarding sex, surgery, and cancer. While the value of radiotherapy as the best treatment for cervical cancer remains to be determined, it was concluded that it may be a better form of treatment for some Chinese patients because it is less physically and psychologically traumatic for them.

3366

Ong, S. B., & Leng, Y. K. (1979). The treatment of an obsessive-compulsive girl in the context of Malaysian Chinese culture. *Australian & New Zealand Journal of Psychiatry, 13,* **255-259.**

Reports the case history, treatment, and followup of a 13-yr-old girl with obsessive-compulsive neurosis of 6 mo duration. Behavior modification techniques were effective, although a 2nd course of treatment was required. Her illness and its treatment by behavior therapy in relation to the Malaysian Chinese culture is discussed.

3367

Panas, K. (1983). Therapist perceptions of cultural factors in therapeutic relationships: The Mexican American: I and II. *Dissertation Abstracts International, 43,* **B2714.**

3368

Pao, B. (1985). Mental health implications of the Chinese linguistic concept of "hsin" (heart). *Dissertation Abstracts International, 46,* **B1509.**

3369

Parsons, M. (1984). Psychoanalysis as vocation and martial art. *International Review of Psycho-Analysis, 11,* **453-462.**

In a paper presented at a meeting of the Independent Group of the British Psychoanalytical Society in November 1983, the author discussed the relationship between psychoanalysis and the traditional martial arts of China and Japan. Both were described as examples of a vocation. The author argued that psychoanalysis, like martial arts, is not only something the analyst does; it is also an expression of his or her being. It was concluded that analysis as a mode of being can only be achieved by constantly grounding oneself in technique and basic principles.

3370

Patterson, C. H. (1986). Culture and counseling in Hong Kong. *The Chinese University of Hong Kong Education Journal, 14,* **77-81.**

Questions are raised concerning Ho's (1985) paper on cultural values and professional issues in clinical psychology. The author basically agrees with Ho's conclusion that a creative synthesis of individualist and collectivist values holds an exciting promise for the future of clinical (and counseling) psychology. However, this synthesis does not differ from the self-actualization that humanistic psychologists have long extolled, as Ho maintained. Rather, humanistic psychologists include in their goals of counseling and psychotherapy the development of society and its institutions. The implications of this understanding for counseling in Hong Kong are discussed.

3371

Pederson, P., & Draguns, J. (Eds.) (1976). *Counseling across cultures.* **Honolulu, HI: University of Hawaii Press.**

3372

Pillsbury, B. L. (1978). "Doing the month": Confinement and convalescence of Chinese women after childbirth. *Social Science & Medicine, 12,* **B11-22.**

Discusses the traditional custom in China which stipulates that a woman should be confined to home for one full month of convalescence after giving birth. The specific rules and rationale are examined from the ethnomedical folk perspective of those who do the month, analyzed according to the logic of classical Chinese medicine, and appraised in light of Western medical and nutritional knowledge. From the latter perspective, some of the practices are efficacious, while others appear dysfunctional. From the Chinese perspective, the practices taken together are considered efficacious for curing the body's imbalance but especially as preventive therapy against ailments in later years. A direct bearing on mental well-being and familial relationships is also recognized. The original data on which the study is based were gathered in interviews in Mandarin Chinese with laypersons, herbalists, and physicians in Taiwan and with physicians and laypersons from the People's Republic of China.

3373

Potkin, S. G. et al. (1984). Haloperidol concentrations elevated in Chinese patients. *Psychiatry Research, 12,* **167-172.**

After 6 weeks of fixed-dose oral haloperidol treatment, Chinese schizophrenic patients had 52% higher plasma haloperidol concentrations than US non-Asian schizophrenic patients. The Chinese and US patients were matched for sex and body weight, resulting in 6 pairs of female and 11 pairs of male patients. The difference in plasma drug concentrations may explain why Asians are reported to require smaller dosages of neuroleptic drugs than non-Asians and why they may be more sensitive to neuroleptic-induced side effects. When prescribing haloperidol to persons of Asian ancestry, physicians should consider that higher-than-expected plasma haloperidol concentrations and an increased sensitivity to haloperidol may occur.

3374

Potter, J. M. (1974). Cantonese Shamanism. In A. P. Wolf (Ed.), ***Religion and ritual in Chinese society.*** **CA: Stanford University Press.**

3375

Priestley, K. E., & Wright, B. (1956). ***Mental health and education in Hong Kong.*** **Hong Kong: Hong Kong University Press.**

3376

Provencher, R. (1984). "Mother Needles": Lessons on inter-ethnic psychiatry in Malaysian society. ***Social Science & Medicine, 18,*** **139-146.**

Discusses social and cultural bases of medical pluralism in Malaysia, which is defined as a circumstance in which a number of different health care systems coexist in the same society without sharing a significant number of health care practitioners, patients, or therapies. In Malaysia, cosmopolitan, Malay, Chinese, Indian, and Aboriginal systems coexist. It is suggested that those aspects of the systems other than the cosmopolitan that are most closely related to what might be called folk psychiatry and psychosomatic medicine are likely to persist until cosmopolitan medicine develops less Western-centric and more cultural-specific therapies for illnesses. Mak Jaruni, a local healer whose name is crudely translated as "Mother Needles", is presented as an exemplar of the complex ways that different health care systems may overlap in a single society. Mak Jaruni attracts a large and diverse clientele, including many non-Malays, with a number of different personalities that are available to her as a curer. Each personality, in effect, comprises a different curer with whom some patients can experience the process of "transference" and other psychological processes that relate the "repressed" social traumas of the patient to the symbolism in the curing ritual.

3377

Pryde, N. A. (1985). Psychologists in primary care settings. ***Hong Kong Journal of Mental Health, 14,*** **5-8.**

3378

Pryde, N. A., & Jachuck, S. J. (1985). Clinical psychologists in general practice: Data and observations. ***Public Health, 99,*** **89-97.**

3379

Rathbun, C., & Kolodny, R. L. (1967). A groupwork approach in cross-cultural adoptions. ***Children, 14,*** **117-121.**

Concerns 5 sets of adoptive white parents of 5 preadolescent Chinese girls from Hong Kong. The primary concern of all of them was having to "prepare their oriental child for the status accorded a member of a minority group while simultaneously attempting to help . . . (Her) become emotionally a part of a family that is part of the dominant majority". There was also concern over the conflicts of the children's dual culture and racial background. The group discussion approach, however, enabled all the parents to discuss their problems with people with the same or similar problems and thus be better able to cope with them.

3380

Ratnavale, D. N. (1973). Psychiatry in Shanghai, China: Observations in 1973. ***American Journal of Psychiatry, 130,*** **1082-1087.**

Describes the structure and organization of the Shanghai Psychiatric Institute, a therapeutic community in which the staff and patients work together in a classless social organization. Brief general information on acupuncture is presented, and its use in psychiatry is described. However, the preeminence of group activities in the therapy of mental illness is stressed.

3381

Raveau, F. H., Chiche, J., & Hibou, F. (1984). Don du sang et determinants socio-culturels: Le cas de Macao [Gift of blood and sociocultural determinants: The case of Macao]. ***Cahiers d'Anthropologie et Biometrie Humaine, 2,*** **1-32.** (In other language.)

The authors discussed the fear and acceptance of blood donation in different cultures based on a survey of 1,757 adolescents and young adults aged 14-22 years from the multicultural population of Macau, a Chinese territory administered by Portugal. Levels of fear in the sample did not seem high enough to interfere with the operation of a blood transfusion center. Free blood donation was accepted by the majority of the population as the best way to collect blood.

3382

Redick, L. T., & Wood, B. (1982). Cross-cultural problems for Southeast Asian refugee minors. ***Child Welfare, 61,*** **365-373.**

Presents a composite case example of a 17-yr-old Chinese-Vietnamese male to illustrate cultural misunderstandings likely to be experienced by refugee minors and their American foster families. Resolution of misunderstandings involved the S's overt adoption of American customs, acceptance of the S's cultural customs by his American family, compromise by persons in both cultures, and a peaceful coexistence of the 2 cultures.

3383

Rifkin, S. B. (1973). Health care in China: Put prevention first. *Assignment Children*, *23*, **35-45.**

In every country the most precious possessions of parents are their young children. We now have the technical knowledge and the means needed to reduce the mortality among children in most developing countries by half within a few years. This would be the most effective way of winning the co-operation of the people which can in turn be used to promote developments in medical and other disciplines.

3384

Rin, H. (1976). [A psychopathological study of the criminal responsibility of mentally ill offenders]. *Journal of the Formosan Medical Association*, *75*, **175-182.** (In Chinese.)

The main purpose of this paper is to draw criteria to determine criminal responsibility of the mentally ill through psychopathological studies. A total of 60 mentally ill offenders were referred from various courts for psychiatric examination during the years 1950-1974. The present law adopts two statuses of insanity defense using the terms of testamentary capacity and criminal responsibility. The former indicates total incompetency, either temporary or permanent, to which compulsory hospitalization must be applied; the latter indicates partial incompetency with a reduced penalty for the criminal behavior. Psychiatric terms, especially when written in Chinese, are difficult to understand and are sometimes misinterpreted by court personnel, causing a considerable amount of confusion during judicial proceedings. In this study the author classified 60 cases into five clinical groups: schizophrenia, non-schizophrenic psychoses, psychoneurosis and personality disorder, mental retardation, and organic brain syndrome, and illustrated specific psychopathologies for each category of diagnosis corresponding to the legal criteria of incompetency. An evaluation of the consequences of 28 judicial precedents found that the court would impose a heavier penalty if the psychiatric examiner did not participate in the decision of incompetency.

3385

Rin, H., Schooler, C., & Caudill, W. A. (1973). Culture, social structure and psychopathology in Taiwan and Japan. *Journal of Nervous & Mental Disease*, *157*, **296-312.**

Reports 3 major findings of an analysis of the symptomatology of 866 Japanese and 890 Taiwan Chinese mental patients. Factor analysis of the symptom patterns showed both cross-culturally applicable and culturally specific symptoms factors. While the Japanese were likely to have disorders in arousal levels, to turn against themselves, and to see the source of their problems as being within themselves, the Taiwanese were much more likely to direct their symptoms outward, to turn against others, and to perceive the outside world unrealistically. Women in each culture were more likely than men to show more severe symptomatology and to have a higher incidence of culturally-specific symptom patterns.

3386

Rosner, S. (1976). Treatment in China. *MH (Mental Hygiene)*, *60*, **5-9.**

Reports impressions of mental health care in China and a visit to Peking Psychiatric Institute. Since the 1949 revolution, the Chinese have built 60 mental hospitals, each with a 1,000-bed capacity, and trained close to 3,600 psychiatrists, plus psychiatric nurses and other mental health workers. Community involvement is seen as an important factor in reducing hospital admissions. Recognition is given in research and training to both social and biochemical causes of mental illness.

3387

Ryan, A. S. (1985). Cultural factors in casework with Chinese-Americans. *Social Casework*, *66*, **333-340.**

Confucianism, Taoism, Buddhism, and Chinese-American family relationships were reviewed to provide information on how these influences may affect a client's way of life, thinking, and communicative behavior. Cultural factors and psychosocial assessment, particularly as they relate to depression, suicide, the experience of Chinese immigrants, and implications for treatment were discussed. A case example of family service was included to illustrate the case worker's responsibility to understand cultural factors that predispose a client.

3388

Sainsbury, M. J. (1974). Psychiatry in the People's Republic of China. *Medical Journal of Australia*, *1*, **669-675.**

An account of psychiatry is given as observed in the People's Republic of China in October 1973. The incidence of psychiatric disorders and their treatment, including the use of acupuncture, is described. Aspects of training of workers in psychiatry, the delivery of mental health care and the effects of the Great Proletarian Cultural Revolution on psychiatric management are mentioned and two psychiatric facilities are described.

3389

Saito, K., Maruyama, S., & Otsuka, T. (1983). [Survey on psychiatric problems in senior nursing institutions]. *Journal of Mental Health*, **No. 30, 103-132.** (In other language.)

The current state of 64 institutions in a Chinese prefecture were reported. Six institutions have resident psychiatrists, and most mental disorders are treated in the institutions.

3390

Saner-Yiu, L., & Saner-Yiu, R. (1985). Value dimensions in American counseling: A Taiwanese-American comparison. *International Journal for the Advancement of Counselling, 8,* **137-146.**

The authors discussed value conflict between the American and Taiwanese-Chinese cultures, arguing that basic differences in values influence the perception, cognition, and behavior of American and Taiwanese culture bearers and result in predictable cross-cultural conflicts. The impact of American individualism on counseling theory and how the strong American belief in the universality of individualism can lead to an inability to validate collectivist cultures were described.

3391

Schuhl, P. M. (1967). [Musical therapy in ancient Greece]. *Annales De The1rapeutique Psychiatrique, 3,* **67-77.** (In other language.)

Examines the role of music in ancient Greece, where, as in China, it attained a high degree of development. Music played an important role in charms, incantations, the ecstatic exaltation of collective frenzy, and mystical and ascetic movements such as the Pythagoreans, who believed in the transmigration of souls (metempsychosis) and used the lyre to help in reminiscences of previous lives, and, before sleep, to exercise the irrational and passional elements of the soul. It is in this sense that Pythagoras spoke of Katharsis, i.e., purification or purgation.

3392

Schultz, S. L. (1982). How Southeast-Asian refugees in California adapt to unfamiliar health care practices. *Health & Social Work, 7,* **148-156.**

Interviewed 14 Southeast Asian refugees to determine their adjustment to Western medical care and to further illuminate the Vietnamese, Laotian, Cambodian, and Chinese health systems. It was noted, for example, that Buddhist monks treat mental health problems and ease family problems but are called upon only as a final recourse. The author stresses the role of the social worker in helping to resolve conflicts experienced by such clients over their adaptation to Western practices.

3393

Shan, H. H. et al. (1986). [A preliminary evaluation on relaxation treatment of anxiety]. *Information on Psychological Sciences*, **No. 3, 32-35.** (In Chinese.)

According to traditional Chinese medicine and Jacobson's relaxation theory, a set of relaxation exercises was designed to treat eight patients suffering from anxiety. Electroencephalogram, galvanic skin response, rate of respiration and heart beat, and oxygen consumption were recorded before and after the exercises. The patients' anxiety and depression were evaluated by the Hamilton Rating Scale. The results showed that, after 1 month's treatment, five patients were cured and two improved, but one failed to respond.

3394

Shen, Y. C. (1983). Community mental health care within primary care in the People's Republic of China: The home care program in the Beijing countryside. *International Journal of Mental Health, 12,* **123-131.**

Describes the establishment and evaluation of a community-oriented home-care program for the mentally ill in a rural area outside Beijing (Peking). The success of the program is attributed to the importance placed on social activities and family support for the patients, the beneficial effects of patients' participation in the social life of the commune, and the contributions of properly trained primary health care workers under the direction of psychiatrists.

3395

Shen, Y. C. (1985). The mental health home care program: Beijing's rural Haidian district. In W. S. Tseng & D. Y. H. Wu (Eds.), *Chinese culture and mental health* **(pp. 357-366). Orlando, FL: Academic Press.**

3396

Shen, Y. T. (1958). [Prevention of mental diseases must have political guidance and follow the mass line]. *Chinese Journal of Neurology and Psychiatry, 4,* **348-349.** (In Chinese.)

3397

Shen, Y. T. (1959). [Application of artificial hibernation in practice]. *Chinese Journal of Neurology and Psychiatry, 5,* **297-303. (Also in** *Collection of Thesis on Achievements in the Medical Sciences in Commemoration of the 10th National Foundation Day of China,* **(Vol. 2), Beijing. Translated by U.S. Joint Publications Research Service, Report No. 14,829, pp. 618-641).** (In Chinese.)

3398

Shu, T. H. et al. (1959). [Ten years of psychiatric work in Shanghai]. *Chinese Journal of Neurology and Psychiatry, 5,* **308-309.** (In Chinese.)

3399

Shum, P. S. (1981). Hospital-based community work and aftercare in the rehabilitation of chronic schizophrenic patients. *Journal of the Hong Kong Psychiatric Association, 1,* **27-32.**

3400

Shum, P. S., Iu, P. C., & Chiu, F. K. (1986). KCH 2000 experience of consultation psychiatry from Kwai Chung Hospital. *Journal of the Hong Kong Psychiatric Association, 6,* **72-78.**

3401

Shum, P. S., & Lee, E. I. (1980). A profile of the drug problem in Hong Kong with special reference to treatment and rehabilitation. *Hong Kong Journal of Mental Health, 9,* **13-20.**

3402

Sidel, R. (1972). Social services in China. *Social Work, 17,* **5-13.**

Describes methods being used to train and utilize paraprofessionals on the community level. A sketch of social and political life is presented and illustrations given of the diffusion of social services into every aspect of life. Implications and possible benefits for western societies are discussed under 4 headings: deprofessionalization, mass participation, mutual help, and self-help.

3403

Sidel, R. (1972). *Women and child care in China: A firsthand report.* **New York: Hill & Wang.**

3404

Sidel, R. (1973). The role of revolutionary optimism in the treatment of mental illness in the People's Republic of China. *American Journal of Orthopsychiatry, 43,* **732-736.**

Reports observations made during 2 recent trips to the People's Republic of China which indicate that psychiatric patients are encouraged to feel part of a force larger than themselves-the revolution. They are urged to take an optimistic view of their problems, and to understand and overcome their illness, not only for their own benefit but also for the sake of the revolution.

3405

Sidel, R. (1973). Mental diseases and their treatment. In J. R. Quinn (Ed.), *Medicine and public health in the People's Republic of China* **(HEW Publication 72-67). Washington, DC: U.S. Government Printing Office.**

3406

Sidel, R., & Sidel, V. W. (1972). The human services in China. *Social Policy, 2,* **25-34.**

3407

Sidel, V. W., & Sidel, R. (1973). *Serve the people: Observations on medicine in the People's Republic of China.* **Boston, MA: Beacon. (Republished New York: Josiah Macy, Jr. Foundation, 1973.)**

Based on the author's visits in 1971 and 1972, the philosophy, development, methods, and facilities of the health care system in China are described. Health care in the cities and in the country, the role of the community and the patient in health care, medical education, the treatment of mental illness, and health administration and research are examined.

3408

Simmons, R. J. (1983). Observations of child psychiatry in China. *Canadian Journal of Psychiatry, 28,* **124-127.**

Discusses child and adolescent psychiatry in the People's Republic of China. The Chinese practice of psychiatry is the same for adults and children and primarily involves the treatment of severely disturbed patients in psychiatric hospitals. There is also a trend toward movement into the community and the schools as a result of the Chinese focus on attention deficit disorders. Antisocial and delinquent behaviors, developmental problems, relationship and family problems, and reactions to illness and hospitalization are not handled by psychiatrists but by others in the local communities. These problems are managed, however, and with the shortage of child psychiatrists the arrangement may be appropriate.

3409

Singer, K. (1974). Society and rights of the mentally ill: A historical perspective of the Chinese. *Mental Health & Society, 1,* **49-55.**

Describes the treatment of the mentally ill from a historical perspective within Chinese culture. The effects of the culture, values, and public programs of particular eras in time on the rights of the mentally ill are examined.

3410

Singer, K. (1975). Psychiatric aspects of abortion in Hong Kong. *International Journal of Social Psychiatry, 21,* **303-306.**

Examines cultural and legal aspects of abortion in the United Kingdom colony of Hong Kong from cultural, legal, and current practices. While traditional Chinese social attitudes encourage large families, they do not place religious restrictions on abortion. Nevertheless, the current law is moderately prohibitive, making abortion legal only to lessen risk to the life or health of the mother. For those who can afford it, there is no difficulty in obtaining the abortion. Guidelines for translating the law into clinical practice are offered.

3411

Singer, K. (1976). Cross-cultural dynamics in psychotherapy. In J. H. Masserman (Ed.), *Social psychiatry: Vol. 2. The range of normal human behavior* **(pp. 115-148). New York: Grune & Stratton.**

3412

Sommers, V. S. (1960). Identity conflict and acculturation problems in Oriental-Americans. *American Journal of Orthopsychiatry, 30,* **637-644.**

3413

Spinetti, G. (1980). [Acupuncture in psychiatric therapy]. *Minerva Psichiatrica, 21,* **167-170.** (In other language.)

Experiences with acupuncture as a therapeutic technique in psychiatry is presented. Like those reported by Chinese and other Italian workers, the results are encouraging and indicate that acupuncture may be more widely used in this field.

3414

Stevens, R. L. (1985). Nonverbal components of first impression formation in cross-cultural counseling. *Dissertation Abstracts International, 46,* **A355-356.**

3415

Streltzer, J., & Wade, T. C. (1981). The influence of cultural group on the undertreatment of postoperative pain. *Psychosomatic Medicine, 43,* **397-403.**

Analyzed the variance in postcholecystectomy narcotic requirements (meperdine, morphine, pentazocine, and levorphanol) accounted for by 85 Whites, 30 Chinese, 53 Japanese, 34 Filipinos, and 51 Hawaiians (ages 20-90 yrs) in a clinical setting. Results indicate that Whites and Hawaiians received significantly more analgesics than Filipinos, Japanese, or Chinese. Race and its interactions with age and sex accounted for 11% of the variance. It is concluded that while individual factors are probably of greatest importance in the treatment of postoperative pain, cultural factors do contribute to the variability.

3416

Su, F. et al. (1986). [Psychological counseling for neurotics]. *Chinese Journal of Neurology and Psychiatry, 19,* **311-313.** (In Chinese.)

This is a report on 130 neurotic cases seen as outpatients receiving psychological counseling in the Shanghai Mental Health Centre. Most of the patients were neurotics (58.6%), including 36 obsessive-compulsive neurotics, 31 depressive neurotics, 27 anxiety neurotics, and 11 neurathenics. These data differed to some extent from those reported in this country and abroad. Some concepts and practice of psychological counseling were suggested.

3417

Su, R. V., & Chen, C. C. (1979). [Diagnostic and therapeutic implications of Chinese calligraphy in psychiatric occupational therapy]. *Journal of Formosan Medical Association, 78,* **419-432.** (In Chinese.)

3418

Sue, D. W., & Sue, S. (1972). Counseling Chinese-Americans. *Personnel and Guidance Journal, 50,* **637-644. (Republished in P. Pedersen, Ed.,** *Readings intercultural communication: Vol. 4. Cross-cultural counseling.* **Pittsburgh: Regional Center for International Education, 1974.)**

3419

Sun, M. C., Yen, Y. Y., Shiau, T. E., Lee, S. L., Chen, F. L., Yeh, E. K., Yang, Y. Y., & Hwu, H. G. (1984). [A study of the acceptance of follow-up service by public health workers and patients' families]. *Chinese Journal of Mental Health, 1,* **49-55.** (In Chinese.)

Follow-up care service of discharged patients has been a major integral part of the whole community mental health services developed by the Taipei City Psychiatric Center. The main characteristics of operation is to integrate this service into the daily public health services of public health nurses and social workers in Taipei City. This study reports the attitudes of public health workers and the patients' families toward this model of service. Around 90% of public health workers considered that follow-up care of discharged patients was an important part of the public health service and could be meaningfully integrated into their daily services. About 75% of the patients' families considered that the service was helpful to their daily care of the patients. Some differences in attitudes between the public health nurses and social workers were revealed and discussed. In general, the public health workers and the patients' families favored the service provided by this model.

3420

Sun, Z. X. et al. (1986). [Treatment of writer's cramp by means of combination of biofeedback with brush-writing]. *Information on Psychological Sciences*, **No. 1, 28-31.** (In Chinese.)

This paper reports a treatment of a 30-year-old female patient with 20-years writer's cramp by means of biofeedback combined with Chinese brush-writing. The authors maintain that with suitable methods writer's cramp can be cured. It is most likely that the combination of biofeedback with brush-writing is an effective cure for writer's cramp.

3421

Taipale, V., & Taipale, I. (1973). Chinese psychiatry: A visit to a Chinese mental hospital. *Psychiatria Fennica*, **79-85. (Also** *Archives of General Psychiatry*, **1973,** *29*, **313-316.)**

Describes changes in Chinese psychiatry since 1949 when psychoanalytical theories were abandoned and American influence declined, while Pavlovian theory and biological psychiatry developed. The expansion of mental health services, the rarity of psychiatric disturbances in children and suicide, and attitudes toward mental illness are discussed.

3422

Talbot, P. S. (1978). Chinese approach to mental health. *Australia's Nurses Journal*, *7*, **31-32.**

3423

Tan, H. (1967). Intercultural study of counseling expectancies. *Journal of Counseling Psychology*, *14*, **122-130.**

200 students from the united states, England, and 5 Asian countries and 62 graduate counselors in training in 2 American universities were given a 36-item questionnaire. The Asian cultures, selected on the assumption that they were similar in their authoritarian orientation, e.g., respect to elders and authority figures, tighter family ties, submission, and nurturance, were found to be similar in their counseling expectancies. They, as a group, tended to differ from the United States group. When the American and foreign student groups were compared to the professional group, both student groups appeared to be rather alike and authoritarian in their counseling expectancies. Those foreign students who have been in the United States longer were found most similar to the American students. A follow-up study needs to be carried out with comparable groups in their native countries.

3424

Tang, G. (1983). Knowledge about reproductive organs in Chinese women: Some overlooked "common sense". *Journal of Psychosomatic Obstetrics & Gynaecology*, *2*, **256.**

Findings of M. M. Tsoi et al (1983) regarding the necessity of finding out how Chinese patients feel about their body before receiving advice about gynecological operations are considered to be in agreement with the present author's results. However, the author does not agree that erroneous traditional beliefs should not be corrected because they could arouse undue emotional stress and anxiety in the patients. Thus when a gynecological operation is necessary, a Chinese woman should be thoroughly informed, her thinking explored, and her erroneous beliefs rectified.

3425

Tao, K. T. (1956). [Problems in the prevention of mental disorders]. *Chinese Journal of Neurology and Psychiatry*, *2*, **67-73.** (In Chinese.)

3426

Teoh, J. I. (1973). Chinese spirit-mediumship: Its socio-cultural interpretation and psychotherapeutic aspects. *Singapore Medical Journal*, *14*, **55-61.**

3427

The Cooperation Group for the Construction of "The Clinical Memory Test". (1986). [The Construction of "The Clinical Memory Test"]. *Acta Psychologica Sinica*, *18*, **100-108.** (In Chinese.)

A battery called The Clinical Memory Test was constructed to meet the need for memory assessment in practice and research. It consists of 5 subtests: directed memory, paired-association learning, free recall of pictures, recognition of meaningless figures, and recall of the connection between portraits and their characteristics. Two matched forms, A and B, are available. For standardization, a literate sample of 2,161 subjects and an illiterate sample of 1,149 subjects were used. All subjects were between 20-89 years of age. The test scores of the two standardization samples showed normal distribution. The correlation ratio between forms A and B was .85. The relationship between memory assessment and learning performance, or between memory assessment and age, is consistent with expectations based on experience. The application of this test to patients with brain tumor patients showed that the recognition of meaningless figures was related with the function of the right hemisphere, and paired-association learning with that of the left hemisphere. These results indicate the satisfactory reliability and validity of the test constructed.

3428

The National Mental Illnesses Prevention Work Plan (1958 - 1962). In U.S. Joint Publications Research Service (Trans.), *Compendium of Laws and Regulations in the People's Republic of China* **(No. 14,335, pp. 562-575). (Reprinted in M. Livingston & P. Lowinger,** *The minds of the Chinese people: Mental health in New China* **(pp. 149-154). Englewood Cliffs, NJ: Prentice-Hall, 1983.)**

This document is the first national plan put forward by the profession of psychiatry in the People's Republic of China. The topics discussed included the basic conditions and principles for the prevention of mental illness; a 5-year plan for prevention was outlined.

3429

Tien, J. L. (1984). Do Asians need less medication? *Journal of Psychosocial Nursing & Mental Health Services, 22,* **19-22.**

This author reviewed the limited research on comparisons of psychotropic drug responses of Asians and non-Asian-Americans and concluded that Asians can easily develop adverse reactions or side effects even with smaller dosages of psychotropic drugs than are normally prescribed. Illustrative case studies of Asian patients were presented. It was suggested that to prevent further misuse and abuse, psychopharmacology should be included in the curriculum for psychiatric professionals and that additional research be done on the effects of psychotropic drugs on Asians and other groups.

3430

Ting, T. (1956). [Develop the work of medical psychology in our country]. *Chinese Journal of Neurology and Psychiatry, 2,* **322-325.** (In Chinese.)

3431

Tinloy, M. Y. (1978). Counseling Asian-Americans: A contrast in values. *Journal of Non-White Concerns in Personnel & Guidance, 6,* **71-77.**

Suggests that Chinese-Americans require different counseling techniques from those currently used with Whites since the two cultural groups have different values. It is also suggested that since White counselors are not generally familiar with many of the customs and values of Chinese-Americans, they are less likely to be effective in counseling individuals from this group. It is concluded that Chinese-American counselors are more appropriate for counseling members of their culture.

3432

Tom, J. C. (1982). Psychological treatment in the mental health system of the People's Republic of China. *Dissertation Abstracts International, 43,* **B268-269.**

3433

Tousley, M. M. (1985). China: Psychiatric nursing in the People's Republic. *Journal of Psychosocial Nursing & Mental Health Services, 23,* **28-35.**

The present author described mental health services in China, based on her experience as a participant in bilateral exchange of mental health nurses between the US and China. Chinese mental health services were viewed in the context of the cultural revolution between 1966 and 1976. Basic Chinese nursing programs, grades of care, staff nursing, methods of treatment, children's services, admission, diagnosis, psychotherapy, family role, patient participation, charting, recording, and follow-up and discharge were described.

3434

True, R. H. (1975). Mental health services in a Chinese American community. In W. H. Ishikawa & N. H. Archer (Eds.), *Service delivery in Pan-Asian communities.* **San Diego: Pacific Asian Coalition.**

3435

Tsai, J. H. (1985). [Group counseling with transactional analysis]. *Chinese Journal of Mental Health, 2,* **79-101.** (In Chinese.)

3436

Tseng, C. C., Shiau, S. J., & Cheish, C. F. (1984). [Intervention techniques of leaders in a didactic therapy group]. *Chinese Journal of Mental Health, 1,* **75-82.** (In Chinese.)

3437

Tseng, W. S. (1975). Traditional and modern psychiatric care in Taiwan. In A. Kleinman, P. Kunstadter, E. R. Alexander & J. L. Gale (Eds.), *Medicine in Chinese culture: Comparative studies of health care in Chinese and other societies* **(pp. 177-194). Washington, DC: U.S. Department of Health, Education and Welfare.**

3438

Tseng, W. S. et al. (1986). Diagnostic pattern for neuroses in China, Japan, and the United States. Regional Symposium of the Transcultural Psychiatry Section of the World Psychiatric Association (1985, Beijing/Nanjing, China). *American Journal of Psychiatry, 143,* **1010-1014.**

To investigate the diagnostic patterns for neuroses in China, Japan, and the U.S., videotapes of clinical interviews and brief written case histories of 6 Chinese patients were shown to 60 psychiatrists and psychiatrists-in-training in Beijing, Tokyo, and Honolulu. The results showed that in cases with a well-distinguished clinical picture, the diagnoses were congruent in the three countries. Diagnostic disagreement occurred in cases with symptoms of decline in mental function and complaints of mental and physical fatigue, which were overwhelmingly diagnosed as neurasthenia by the Chinese clinicians and as adjustment reaction, anxiety, or depressive disorder by their Japanese and American colleagues. Cases with situational stress were diagnosed as adjustment reaction by the Americans but not by the others. The findings illustrate that different professional concepts and classification systems are used in different countries.

3439

Tsoi, M., Chan, R., Ho, E., Lee, P., Leung, P., & Tsang, A. (1982). A behavior modification training course for the helping professionals in Hong Kong. *Hong Kong Journal of Mental Health, 11,* **19-27.**

3440

Tsoi, M. M. (1982). A three-tier model to optimize resources in the services for the mentally handicapped. In K. Bayes et al. (Eds.), *Developing resources for mentally handicapped persons.* **Proceedings of the 5th Asian Conference on Mental Retardation.**

3441

Tsoi, M. M., Ho, P. C., & Poon, R. S. (1984). Pre-operation indicators and post-hysterectomy outcome. *British Journal of Clinical Psychology, 23,* **151-152.**

Interviewed 20 40-50 yr old Chinese females before their hysterectomy operations and administered a general health questionnaire, the Hypochondriasis Scale of the MMPI, and a sex-role inventory to them. 18 Ss were interviewed postoperatively and were readministered the health questionnaire and the Hypochondriasis Scale. Ss who expected changes to be brought about by hysterectomy tended to complain more at follow-up, but the difficulties they experienced (e.g., hot flush and vaginal dryness) were genuine physical symptoms that had not been anticipated by them. It is suggested that more information be given to patients preoperatively and that further investigation is needed on the link between personality factors and perceived outcome of hysterectomy.

3442

Tsoi, M. M., Poon, R. S., & Ho, P. C. (1983). Knowledge about reproductive organs in Chinese women: Some overlooked "common sense". *Journal of Psychosomatic Obstetrics & Gynaecology, 2,* **70-75.**

Investigated woman's knowledge of the shape, size, and functions of the female reproductive organs. Ss were 80 gynecological patients who were divided into 2 age groups--mean ages 46.48 and 31.03 yrs. Results show that the ovaries were the least understood organs in terms of shape and size and the vagina in terms of functions. Compared with younger Ss, older Ss only knew less about the vagina. Assessment of relationships between gynecological knowledge and pre-operative anxiety in 20 hysterectomy Ss showed that although gynecological information was not correlated with the number of anticipated postoperative changes, Ss who understood less about their body tended to believe that a hysterectomy would have certain effects, which in fact lacked any medical basis. Results are discussed with reference to Chinese health beliefs, and the implications for the preparation of Chinese women for a gynecological operation where the Western biomedical model and the traditional non-Western cultural beliefs might play a role are highlighted.

3443

Tsu Tang Shan Correctional Sanatorium. (1958). [How psychiatric patients are managed in the Tsu Tang Shan Correctional Sanatorium]. *Chinese Journal of Neurology and Psychiatry, 4,* **259-262.** (In Chinese.)

3444

Tsui, A. M. (1979). Transcultural perceptions of mental health: Culture of the patient as a consideration in treatment. *Dissertation Abstracts International, 39,* **B3543-3544.**

3445

Tully, B. (1984). Clinical psychology and mental health services in the People's Republic of China. *Bulletin of the British Psychological Society, 37,* **120-122.**

The author discusses his observations on clinical psychology and mental health services in the People's Republic of China following a 1983 visit as a member of a study group. Two broad areas seemed of particular interest to the Chinese psychologists and some of their students: basic physiological psychology and the application of behavioral methods to health problems. The overall impression was one of (1) a small but dedicated service attempting to deal with large numbers of people and (2) the desire of the Chinese psychologists to learn and to make use of knowledge and techniques wherever they could be found.

3446

Tung, M. (1981). On being seen as a "Chinese therapist" by a Caucasian child. *American Journal of Orthopsychiatry, 51,* **654-661.**

Describes the reactions of a 10-yr-old White male to his Chinese therapist and his use of this racial difference to express his acute alienation. Stages included S's initial projection of aggression and evil onto the "Chinks", subsequent ambivalence and anxiety as attachment to the therapist increased, and eventual trust and alleviation of his loneliness. Aspects of the therapist's countertransference are explored.

3447

Tung, M. (1984). Life values, psychotherapy, and East-West integration. *Psychiatry, 47,* **285-292.**

Examines Eastern and Western lifestyles and values and notes apparent differences and underlying commonalities relevant to psychotherapy and clinical issues. Psychiatry in the People's Republic of China is briefly summarized and concluded to be oriented to the public and community, to the pragmatic and the rational, and to conformity and dependence, in contrast to the US orientation toward privacy, the theoretical and psychodynamic, and the individualistic.

3448

Veith, I. (1972). Acupuncture: Ancient enigma to East and West. *American Journal of Psychiatry, 129*: **333-336.**

3449

Veith, I. (1978). Psychiatric foundations in the Far East. *Psychiatric Annals, 8,* **275-289.**

Discusses traditional practices in the treatment of mental illness in Japan and China, the concepts and customs on which these treatments are based, and how they have been modified as a result of Westernization. Both countries have traditionally given overwhelming importance to the family, filial piety, ancestor worship, and the concept of "face". In China the concept of balance between the forces of yin and yang and the philosophy of Taoism, and in Japan Zen Buddhism, were powerful influences on attitudes toward mental illness and its cure. In both countries respect for tradition has led to the persistence of folk medicine, which is practiced alongside Western psychiatric methods. Psychoanalysis has little appeal in countries that lay such stress on reverence for parents. Japan, much influenced by German scholars, emphasizes neuropsychiatry; Morita therapy, based on Zen Buddhism, is unique to Japan. In China preventive medicine, community medicine and psychiatry, and group therapy are practiced. Acupuncture, moxibustion, meditation, and breathing therapy are also accepted methods of treating mental illness.

3450

Visher, J. S., & Visher, E. B. (1979). Impressions of psychiatric problems and their management: China, 1977. *American Journal of Psychiatry, 136,* **28-32.**

The authors, who visited the People's Republic of China in October 1977, describe the treatment methods used there, particularly in the Shanghai Mental Hospital, a 1,000-bed hospital for acutely ill patients. Psychiatric treatment there appears to be a blend of Western pharmacology, traditional Chinese medicine, and group therapy. The possible cultural sources of stress-related and interpersonal problems are examined, and a review of the literature regarding psychiatry in modern China and the history of psychiatric treatment there is presented.

3451

Walsh, N. (1978). Psychiatry in the People's Republic of China. *Psychiatric Annals, 8,* **290-295.**

The author, one of a team of Irish physicians visiting China to observe health practices, reports on the Shanghai Mental Hospital. According to statistics based on clinical practice, 70% of the patients had been diagnosed as schizophrenic. Affective disorders, alcoholism, drug addiction, and psychoneurosis were also under treatment. Drug therapy is utilized, but dosages of many drugs would be considered non-therapeutic in Western hospitals. ECT, psychosurgery, insulin therapy, and behavior therapy are not practiced. Acupuncture is used to treat a wide spectrum of psychiatric disorders. Community and social psychiatric efforts concentrate on the prevention of mental illness. Political concepts exert considerable influence on treatment methodology and strategies.

3452

Wang, B. (1986). [Observations on the effects of traditional Chinese medicine to invigorate blood and relieve stasis in treating schizophrenia]. *Chinese Journal of Neurology and Psychiatry, 19,* **44-46.** (In Chinese.)

Twenty schizophrenic patients were treated with traditional Chinese medicine to invigorate blood and relieve stasis or antipsychotic drugs, and were observed by the rating methods of BPRS, TESS, CGI. The results showed that traditional Chinese medicine had an effect on schizophrenic patients with less side reaction, and was superior to antipsychotic drugs in the effects of anti-anxiety-depression and anti-psychomotor inhibition. It was less effective in controlling psychomotor excitement, hallucination, delusion, and disrupted thinking as compared with antipsychotic drugs.

3453

Wang, C. F. et al. (1959). [Neurasthenia treated by bunched needle acupuncture therapy: Report of 58 cases]. *Chinese Journal of Neurology and Psychiatry,* *5,* **94-96.** (In Chinese.)

3454

Wang, C. K., Chang, C. N., & Kuo, M. S. (1961). [Some psychological problems in speedy-synthetic treatments of neurasthenia]. *Acta Psychologica Sinica,* **No. 2, 101-106.** (In Chinese.)

3455

Wang, J. H. (1961). [The role of psychotherapy in speedy-synthetic treatment of chronic diseases]. *Acta Psychologica Sinica*, **No. 1, 44-50.** (In Chinese.)

This paper summarizes the experiences obtained in the speedy-synthetic treatment of the chronic diseases of neurasthenia, peptic ulcer and hypertension in the last two years by the division of medical psychology, Institute of Psychology, Academia Sinica. The author points out that applications of the knowledge of medical psychology to mobilize the conscious activity of patients in their struggle against diseases is a new method of psychotherapy, playing an important role in speedy treatment of the chronic diseases. The author also gives an outline of the theory of psychotherapy.

3456

Wang, J. H. (1961). [The influence of some personality traits on the psychotherapy of neurasthenia and hypertension]. *Acta Psychologica Sinica*, **No. 4, 267-279.** (In Chinese.)

Nineteen neurasthenics and 16 hypertensive patients were cured with controlled treatment. The course of treatment was divided into two stages: re-education, and synthetic treatment. Forty patients cured by synthetic treatment one year before were also investigated in order to study the influence of some psychological factors on the strengthening effect of the therapy. It was found that some personality traits, such as the inclination to anger and to depression, remarkably affected the temporary and the lasting effects of therapy.

3457

Wang, M. J. (1965). [Size of Bender-Gestalt test figures and manifest anxiety]. *Acta Psychologica Taiwanica*, *7*, **67-72.** (In Chinese.)

3458

Wang, X. Y. et al. (1986). [A clinical analysis of 79 cases of neurosis in general hospitals]. *Chinese Journal of Neurology and Psychiatry*, *19*, **288-290.** (In Chinese.)

The authors rediagnosed 79 cases of neurosis from departments of medicine in general hospitals. It was found that there were 24 cases of endogenous depression; the rate of misdiagnosis was 30.4%. The main cause of misdiagnosis seemed to be the lack of familiarity with the symptoms of somatization in depression by doctors in general hospitals. The authors suggested that diagnostic criteria of neuroses should be established as soon as possible, to reduce misdiagnosis in clinical practice.

3459

Wen, H. L. (1977). Fast detoxification of heroin addicts by acupuncture and electrical stimulation (AES) in combination with naloxone. *Comparative Medicine East & West*, *5*, **257-263.**

Detoxification can be accomplished more rapidly by first 'flushing' the opiates from the receptor sites. Naloxone, a short acting antagonist, displaces opiates from the receptor sites and such displacement precipitates an abstinence syndrome. Recently, a method of using acupuncture and electrical stimulation (AES) in combination with naloxone for fast detoxification was reported. This technique was applied to 50 cases of heroin addicts. Forty-one were detoxified. There were nine failures. Of the 41 cases, 18 patients were sent to rehabilitation centers and did not experience abstinence symptoms. Six were sent out of Hong Kong where heroin is not available, and two others did not go to a rehabilitation center but still abstained. The other 15 were presumed to be on the drug. It is advocated that AES increases endorphin and relieves abstinence syndrome, but also at the same time inhibits the autonomic nervous system, mainly the parasympathetic nervous system. The technique does not stop the craving, therefore after detoxification, the patients should be sent for psychosocial rehabilitation, or alternatively be put on long acting antagonist.

3460

Wen, J. K. (1985). [Mental disorders and help-seeking behavior: problems and strategies]. *Chinese Journal of Mental Health*, *2*, **36-45.** (In Chinese.)

The fact that chronic mental patients do not receive proper and adequate mental health care in Taiwan was addressed, and the reasons behind it were elucidated in terms of the help-seeking behavior of the patients and their families. A review of the literature was made with particular reference to five articles written by the author and his associates. A three-dimension approach in accordance to the bio-psycho-social model was adopted to analyze and formulate the associated problems as well as the pertinent strategies with reference to the findings of the literature review. The chronicity of mental disorders, the popularity of folk healing, the unique role played by the family, and other characteristics in the help-seeking process in Chinese culture were depicted. Cultural accommodation and indigenization of modern psychiatry to the community were emphasized and discussed.

3461

Westbrook, C. H. (1953). Psychiatry and mental hygiene in Shanghai. *American Journal of Psychiatry*, *110*, **301-305.**

3462

Williams, J. (1957). Child health and psychiatry in China today. *Medical Journal of Australia, 44,* **630-631.**

3463

Wolfe, J. C. (1980). Special report: Community mental health in China. *Community Mental Health Journal, 16,* **241-248.**

The author's 2-wk visit to China provided a basis for comparing that country's community mental health system with that of the US. The Chinese value the group and mental health treatment reflects group goals as determined by the government. Confidentiality (vis-a-vis family and work associates) is not an issue when working with the patient. The family makes the final decision regarding hospitalization.

3464

Wong, C. W. (1978). Contributions of a clinical psychologist in rehabilitation. *Journal of Mental Health of Hong Kong, 76.*

3465

Wong, E. Y. (1982). A validation study of non-verbal eye pattern strategies related to language and therapeutic processes. *Dissertation Abstracts International, 42,* **A4729.**

3466

Wong, K. C. (1950). [A short history of psychiatry and mental hygiene in China]. *Chinese Medical Journal, 68,* **44-48.** (In Chinese.)

3467

Woon, T. H. (1978). A history of psychiatry in peninsular Malaysia, 1830-1975. *Medical Journal of Malaysia, 32,* **258-263.**

3468

Wray, J. D. (1975). Child care in the People's Republic of China. *Pediatrics, 55,* **539-736;** *55,* **723-734.**

3469

Wu, C. Y. (1959). [Psychiatry in past ten years]. *Chinese Journal of Neurology and Psychiatry, 5,* **286-293. (Also in** *Collection of theses on achievements in the medical sciences in commemoration of the 10th National Foundation Day of China* **(Vol. 2), Beijing. Translated by U.S. Joint Publications Research Service, Report No. 14,829, pp. 594-617).)** (In Chinese.)

3470

Wu, D. (1982). Psychotherapy and emotion in traditional Chinese medicine. In A. J. Marsella & G. M. White (Eds.), *Cultural conceptions of mental health and therapy* **(pp. 285-301). Dordrecht, Netherlands: D. Reidel.**

3471

Wu, W. T. (1976). Saying "hello" first: A self-change experiment. *Bulletin of Educational Psychology, 9,* **95-102.**

Established a cognitive set in a self-change study to induce an S to use more "say hello first" behavior. Five weeks of training resulted in a significant increase in the rate of "saying hello first" when encountering friends.

3472

Wu, W. Y. et al. (1986). [A trial application of the self-report symptom inventory (SCL-90) in the evaluation of neurosis]. *Chinese Journal of Neurology and Psychiatry, 19,* **291-293.** (In Chinese.)

The self-concept symptom inventory (SCL-90), global assessment scale (GAS), and severity of illness (SI) were used to assess 245 cases of neurosis. The results showed that the main symptoms found in the SCL-90 were concordant with clinical findings. The total scores, positive total scores, average positive scores, numbers of positive items, and factor scores were significantly different before and after treatment, suggesting that clinical efficacy can be measured by the SCL-90. The total scores of the SCL-90 were correlated positively with SI scores and negatively with GAS scores. In differential diagnosis, the SCL-90 appeared capable of reflecting the characteristics of different types of neurosis. In conclusion, the SCL-90 seems to be a valid and useful instrument in evaluating neurosis.

3473

Wu, Z. Y. et al. (1979). [Psychiatric progress in China during the past 15 years]. *Chinese Journal of Neurology and Psychiatry, 12,* **149-153.** (In Chinese.)

3474

Wu, Z. Y., & Zhang, J. Z. (1979). [The last fifteen years of progress in our country's treatment of mental diseases]. *Chinese Journal of Neurology and Psychiatry, 12,* **149-153. (English translation in M. Livingston & P. Lowinger (Eds.),** *The minds of the Chinese people: Mental health in New China* **(pp. 203-211). Englewood-Cliffs, NJ: Prentice-Hall, 1983.)** (In Chinese.)

This recent summary of Chinese work in mental health is not otherwise available in English. Dr. Wu has given his permission for us to use the article.

3475

Xia, Z. Y. (Ed.). (1981). [*English-Chinese psychiatric glossary*]. **Beijing: People's Hygiene Press.** (In Chinese.)

3476

Xia, Z. Y. (1985). The mental health delivery system in Shanghai. In W. S. Tseng & D. Y. H. Wu (Eds.), *Chinese culture and mental health* **(pp. 341-356). Orlando, FL: Academic Press.**

3477

Xia, Z. Y., Yan, H. A., & Wang, C. H. (1980). [Mental health work in Shanghai]. *Chinese Medical Journal, 93,* **127-129.** (In Chinese.)

3478

Xia, Z. & Zhang, M. (1981). [*History and present status of modern psychiatry in China*]. *Chinese Medical Journal, 94,* **277-282.** (In Chinese.)

In this article the development of Chinese psychiatry in the 1900s was outined. Attention was focused particularly on developments that occurred after the establishment of the People's Republic of China in 1949.

3479

Xu, L. et al. (1986). [Evaluation of persistent and interrupted treatments for schizophrenics]. *Chinese Journal of Neurology and Psychiatry, 19,* **175-178.** (In Chinese.)

The regularity of taking medicine by schizophrenics was investigated in this field study. A highly significant relationship was found between degree of regularity and the patients' social environments. Taking medicine regularly at home has definite curative effects. Understanding the reasons for stopping to take medicine and considering suggestions from patients and their relatives can strengthen preventive work outside the hospital and mental health services.

3480

Xu, Y. X. et al. (1986). [Preliminary results of a clinical study of four types of neurosis]. *Chinese Journal of Neurology and Psychiatry, 19,* **264-267.** (In Chinese.)

A 30-item schedule for the examination of four types of neurosis was developed through a modification of Present State Examination (PSE) items. The method of use and the principles of symptom rating were the same as those of the PSE. An acceptable level of reliability (71%) and efficiency (98.4%) was attained in clinical trials. The diagnoses made by four psychiatrists were the same in 42 out of 50 cases, among which there were 25 cases of neurasthenia, 5 of anxiety neurosis, 5 of hypochondriacal neurosis, and 7 of depressive neurosis. Some viewpoints regarding symptom assessment and differential diagnosis were discussed.

3481

Yamamoto, J., & Acosta, F. X. (1982). Treatment of Asian Americans and Hispanic Americans: Similarities and differences. *Journal of the American Academy of Psychoanalysis, 10,* **585-607.**

Discusses how characteristics, language, and social-class issues affect the therapy of Asian Americans (AAs) and Hispanic Americans (HAs). Therapy of AAs is discussed with regard to Confucius; various ethnic differences among Japanese, Koreans, and Pacific Islanders; familialism vs individualism; hierarchical vs egalitarian psychotherapist roles; therapist activity vs therapist passivity; and brief vs long-term therapeutic considerations. A brief case history of a 38-yr-old Japanese-American woman referred for depression, insomnia, and weight loss is presented. Therapy of HAs is discussed with regard to sociocultural variables, language, family networks, religion, trust, intra- vs extrapsychic stress, the applicability of behavior therapy, the utility of pharmacological therapy, and the impact of brief and environmental interventions.

3482

Yan, S. (1981). Lithium therapy in China: Brief communication. *Acta Psychiatrica Scandinavica, 64,* **270-272.**

A questionnaire survey of 60 Chinese psychiatrists revealed that Li treatment is being used in a little over half of the Chinese psychiatric hospitals mainly for the treatment of mania and schizo-affective illness and only to a limited extent prophylactically. The relatively restricted use of Li may be due to infrequency of the diagnosis of mania, the fear of toxicity, and the lack of laboratory facilities for monitoring serum Li levels.

3483

Yang, Y. Y. (1985). Prophylactic efficacy of lithium and its effective plasma levels in Chinese bipolar patients. *Acta Psychiatrica Scadinavica, 71,* **171-175.**

One hundred and one Chinese patients with bipolar affective disorders (aged 12-46 years at the onset of illness) with at least two episodes during the successive 2 years prior to the present study received continuous Li treatment for 2 years to investigate the prophylactic efficacy of Li and its plasma levels. The prophylactic efficacy of Li increased from 60 to 73% when subjects with individual standard deviations of plasma Li of more than 0.2 mM/1 were excluded. Most good responders showed individual mean plasma Li levels ranging from 0.5 to 0.79 mM/1.

3484

Yang, Z. L., Cai, T. W., & Wu, J. L. (1984). Psychological aspects of components of pain. *Journal of Psychology, 118,* **135-146.**

The present investigation employed psychophysical and electrophysiological methods to study the compound action potential induced by square pulse stimulation on the saphenous nerve. The first experiment was to establish an emotional scale of pain by observing the emotional states of nine subjects under various pain stimulation conditions. The second experiment applied electro-acupunture on the same nerve and recorded the changes of the sensory as well as the emotional components of pain during and after electro-acupuncture processes. The result indicated that electro-acupuncture had differential inhibitory effect on the sensory component and the emotional component of pain. This suggests: (1) Pain involves two related but different components (the sensory component and emotional component of pain). (2) Electro-acupuncture has stronger inhibitory effect on the emotional component of pain. This result provides a new outlook for the improvement of clinical effect of acupuncture and for further studies of the pain mechanism.

3485

Yap, P. M. (1971). Traditional Chinese medicine. *Canadian Psychiatric Association Journal, 16,* **99-101.**

3486

Yap, P. M. (1974). *Comparative psychiatry: A theoretical framework.* **Toronto: University of Toronto Press.**

This monograph examined the common etiology of mental disease within cultural diversity, and presents a theoretical framework for transcultural psychiatry.

3487

Yeh, E. K. (1971). [Mental health conditions in Taiwan and an examination and outlook on solutions]. In E. K. Yeh & W. S. Tseng (Eds.), *[Modern life and mental health]* **(pp. 209-234). Taipei: Buffalo.** (In Chinese.)

3488

Yeh, E. K. (1984). [Establishment of a mental health care network in Taiwan: A proposal]. *Chinese Journal of Mental Health, 1,* **1-10.** (In Chinese.)

This paper presents a proposal for the establishment of a mental health care network as an integral part of the nationwide medical care delivery system. Fourteen administrative prefectures and 2 special cities should be divided into 6 catchment areas. It was proposed that the public mental hospitals, psychiatric units of teaching general hospitals and provincial community mental health centers be assigned as main area treatment centers; while all government general hospitals and some private mental hospitals under social welfare funds be assigned as affiliating treatment centers. Main treatment centers in each catchment area should extend their treatment to the community by establishing various service programs between each of the agencies in the community related to mental health. To develop a nationwide mental health care network, it was recommended that a relevant institute and/or administrative unit be established with the Department of Health of the Executive Yuan and a special committee be appointed within the governments of Taipei city and Kaoshiung city.

3489

Yeh, M. H., Ko, Y. H., & Hwang, K. K. (1981). [Life stress and mental health]. *Bulletin of the Institute of Ethnology* **(Academia Sinica), No. 52, 173-210.** (In Chinese.)

The main purpose of this study was to investigate the influence of life stress, ego strength, and individual modernity on mental health. The major results were: (1) Life stress was found to be positively correlated with nonadapative habits and uncorrelated with adapative habits. (2) Stimulus tolerance and problem solving ability were both positively correlated with adapative habits and negatively correlated with nonadapative habits. (3) Individual modernity failed to have a significant correlation with adaptive as well as nonadaptive habits. (4) When problem-solving ability, stimulus tolerance, and individual modernity were all low, the correlation between life stress and mental health was significant; when they were all high, the correlation was nonsignificant. (5) The level of mental health decreased with life stress and increased with ego strength.

3490

Yen, Y. S. (1970). On the modified BRS. *Acta Psychologica Taiwanica, 12,* **101-111.**

Describes a modification of the "basic Rorschach score" (BRS) of C. Buhler, K. Buhler, and D. W. Lefever, for use in Taiwan. Ss were 100 schizophrenics (Group S), 50 neurotics (Group P), and 50 normals (Group N). The modified BRS was established by computing the X2 differences between the S-N, S-P, and P-N groups. The weight and positive and negative values of the items were determined by the level of significance of statistical results with reference to the diagnostic consequence of each item, the BRS of Buhler, the modified BRS of Y. Kataguchi, and clinical experience.

3491

Yip, Y. M. (1986). Custodial remands for psychiatric reports in men. *Journal of the Hong Kong Psychiatric Association, 6,* **59-65.**

Three hundred and sixty-three male adult offenders remanded into custody for psychiatric reports were studied. The results indicated that the remand population were inclined to be more socially ineffective, educationally underprivileged, and maladjusted in their background. Violent crimes appeared to alert the courts to the need for psychiatric reports under custodial remand more often than other offense categories. Remanded sexual offenders had the lowest rate of being found to be mentally disordered. The concurrence rate of the courts in accepting recommendations for hospital treatment was high (90%). Psychiatrists tended to recommend treatment mainly for those offenders suffering from formal mental illness with active symptoms, particularly schizophrenics. The problems and significance of communication and liaison among court, psychiatrists, and other disciplines were discussed.

3492

Yiu, L. C. R. (1979). Degree of assimilation and its effect on the preference of counseling style and on self-disclosure among Chinese-Americans in Hawaii. *Dissertation Abstracts International, 39,* **A5340-5341.**

3493

Young, D. (1980). The relationship between etiology and symptomatology in psychiatry. *Culture, Medicine and Psychiatry, 4,* **17-23.**

3494

Young, D., & Chang, M. (1983). Psychiatry in the People's Republic of China. *Comprehensive Psychiatry, 24,* **431-438.**

Discusses the forces that have shaped Chinese psychiatry from the preliberation period through the cultural revolution to the present. Today, the dominant theoretical and practical orientation to psychiatry in the People's Republic of China is descriptive and biological. Its psychiatry continues to be influenced by the psychiatric schools of Germany, Russia, Britain, and America. The prevalence of mental illness and diagnostic conceptualizations in China are discussed.

3495

Yu, C. H. (1958). [Methods and results of treatment of mental diseases in the Autonomous Region of Inner Mongolia]. *Chinese Journal of Neurology and Psychiatry, 4,* **435.** (In Chinese.)

3496

Yu, S. J. (1974). [Development of psychiatry in South Korea]. *Kyushu Neuro-psychiatry, 20,* **138-150.** (In other language.)

Presents a history of South Korean psychiatry, which has been influenced by 4 major factors: (a) superstitions, (b) Chinese medicine, (c) humanistic psychiatry, and (d) modern medical psychiatry. In 1945, Korean psychiatric medicine was still underdeveloped; e.g., there were only about 10 psychiatrists in the country, and about 200 hospital beds for mental patients. In 1950 there were 20 psychiatrists, who began to apply clinical psychological techniques, shock treatment, the Freeman-Watts transorbital method, etc. Since the 1950 Korean conflict, South Korean psychiatry has been greatly influenced by the neuropsychiatric methods applied by US military psychiatrists. Currently, South Korea has over 200 psychiatrists and approximately 3,000 hospital beds for mental patients. However, there are probably about 230,000 mentally disturbed persons in the country, and the immediate problem of Korean psychiatrists is to reach and treat these patients and to further the development of psychiatric techniques.

3497

Yu, Y. H. et al. (1986). [Treatment of 61 cases of neurosis with traditional Chinese medicine]. *Chinese Journal of Neurology and Psychiatry, 19,* **309-310.** (In Chinese.)

Reported are the results of treating 61 cases of neurosis, classified into three types from the perspective of Chinese medicine: irritability stasis (32 cases), excited depression (22 cases), and deficient and weak function of the vital energy (7 cases). Treatments were based on a consideration of the characteristics of these types. The overall therapeutic effective rate was 82.0%, and the rate of marked improvement was 77.1%. The results of follow-up study showed that long-term effects were stable. The authors regarded their method of treatment to be of value.

3498

Zhang, C. X. (1980). [*Chinese medical treatment of psychiatric illness*]. **Hupei, China: Hupei People's Publishers.** (In Chinese.)

3499

Zhang, M. Y. (1986). [The diagnosis of neurasthenia]. *Chinese Journal of Neurology and Psychiatry, 19,* **261-263.** (In Chinese.)

Forty patients diagnosed as neurasthenic in an outpatient department of a psychiatric hospital were rediagnosed according to ICD-9, PSE/CATEGO, DSM-III, and DIS/DSM-III. The main findings were: (1) According to these diagnostic systems (except DIS/DSM-III), the majority of the patients were rediagnosed as having certain types of neurosis. (2) Most of them were reclassified in the category of anxiety or depressive neurosis. (3) A considerable number of them could be rediagnosed as depressives. The authors suggested that China should develop its own system of diagnostic criteria and examination instruments for neurosis.

3500

Zhang, Y. L. et al. (1986). [A study of hysteria treated with systematic desensitization]. *Chinese Journal of Neurology and Psychiatry, 19,* **297-300.** (In Chinese.)

The effectiveness of systematic desensitization in the treatment of hysteria was investigated. The subjects were 58 hysterics, randomly assigned into two groups: the experimental group treated with systematic desensitization, and the control group treated with suggestion therapy. Therapeutic effectiveness was assessed with objective indicators, self-rating scales, and physiological records. Follow-up results indicated that systematic desensitization was effective in reducing the patients' physiological reactivity, and that its long-term effects were significantly superior to those of suggestion therapy.

3501

Zhao, J. C., & Tang, S. Q. et al. (1982). [A primary study of the MMPI in Shanghai]. *Information on Psychological Sciences,* **No. 6, 22-28.** (In Chinese.)

A study of the Minnesota Multiphasic Personality Inventory (MMPI) was carried out, using 98 normals and 120 schizophrenics in the Shanghai area as subjects. Generally speaking, the result was concordant with those of studies conducted in Beijing and Tienjin. The mean scores of both normal males and females on the D scale and the mean score of normal males on the Sc scale were greater than 70. The mean scores of schizophrenics on the Ss scale and the Pa scale were significantly greater than those of the normal group. It was considered that the MMPI may be applied to clinical assessment in psychiatry, but that it would be necessary to modify some items to conform to the society and culture of China and improve the acceptability of the inventory.

3502

Zhao, J. C., Xia, M. L., Yan, H. Q. (1984). [Results of Halstead-Reitan Test among schizophrenics]. *Information on Psychological Sciences,* **No. 5, 19-21.** (In Chinese.)

This study investigated use of the Halstead-Reitan Battery for groups of acute schizophrenics and chronic schizophrenics. The results showed that 68.18% of the patients were suffering from moderate or above-moderate brain damage. This brain damage may be connected with abnormality of brain morphology. The poor outcomes on certain items might have been affected by antipsychotic drugs or fluctuation of attention.

3503

Zhao, K. Y. et al. (1986). [An analysis of 1,500 counseling cases]. *Chinese Journal of Neurology and Psychiatry, 19,* **325-328.** (In Chinese.)

This is a report on 1,000 outpatients who received psychological counseling in the OPD of a general hospital and 500 clients who received counseling through correspondence. It was found that most of the clients were males. Outpatients in the hospital were young workers, college or middle school students, cadres, intellectuals, and farmers; about half were neurotics. Psychosexual problems were encountered in 6.4% of the outpatients and in 11.4% of the corresponding clients.

3504

Zheng, J. L., & Luo, B. W. (1986). [An investigation into the mental health of young children]. *Information on Psychological Sciences,* **No. 4, 24-29.** (In Chinese.)

The present paper studied the mental health problems of 851 children (aged 5-7) in terms of age, sex, emotion and character with an inquiry into the causes of the problems. The results indicated: (1) There were considerable occurrences of mental health problems in young children, which merits attention. (2) A child's mental health may be affected by the mother's health, nutrition and emotion during pregnancy, the age and process of the mother's parturition, the diseases in the early stage of the child's growth, and how the child is fostered and instructed.

3505

Zhenyi, V., & Mingfyuan, Z. (1981). History and present status of modern psychiatry in China. *Chinese Medical Journal* **(Peking),** *94,* **277-282.**

3506

Zhou, K. et al. (1981). [Periodic psychoses and its treatment by promoting blood circulation and relieving stasis]. *Chinese Journal of Neurology & Psychiatry, 13,* **114-115.** (In Chinese.)

3507

Zhou, K. et al. (1986). [A study of the treatment of neurasthenia with combined Western and traditional Chinese medicine]. *Chinese Journal of Neurology and Psychiatry, 19,* **306-308.** (In Chinese.)

The common symptoms of neurasthenia were studied. Clinical cases were classified into the following clinical types based on diagnostic criteria in traditional Chinese medicine: heart dysfunction, overactivity of yang in the liver, stagnation, insufficiency of yin, insufficiency of yang, monosymptom, and unclassified type. Diagnostic classification into these types was established on the basis of two major symptoms, or one major symptom with two minor symptoms. The prescriptions for different types were regularized but could be modified according to the patient's condition. The results in 50 cases treated by combined traditional Chinese and Western medicine were compared with those of another 50 cases treated by Western medicine alone. Better therapeutic effects were observed in the former group.

3508

Zhu, C. M. et al. (1986). [Results of rating 271 neurotics with symptom scales]. *Chinese Journal of Neurology and Psychiatry, 19,* **294-296.** (In Chinese.)

The HAMD, CGI-SI, and GAS were applied to 271 neurotics before treatment; the total rating scores obtained were 17.19, 3.49 and 60.97 respectively. The scores were quite different among four subtypes of neurotics. However, there was no significant difference in mean scores between cases of depressive neurosis and anxiety. There were no significant differences among the subtypes on 17 symptoms, such as guilt, retardation, agitation, and loss of body weight. High correlations were obtained among 3 indices of treatment effects, suggesting that the three ratings scales have satisfactory validity.

3509

Zuo, C. Y., Yang, L. L., & Chu, C. C. (1985). Patterns of psychiatric consultation in a Chinese general hospital. *American Journal of Psychiatry, 142,* **1092-1094.**

In this study of patterns of psychiatric consultation in a Chinese general hospital, it was revealed that 75 inpatients aged 5 to 92 years (0.74% of the patients in the hospital) were referred to the psychiatry service by other services over a 1-year period. Internal medicine referred 32 subjects, the highest number of a service, and organic brain syndromes were the most common diagnoses. Depression was not a frequent diagnosis, but 9 subjects were diagnosed with schizophrenic disorder, and an additional 9 subjects suffered from neurasthenia; 7 subjects were found to have no mental disorder. None of the referred patients had a diagnosis of alcoholism, drug abuse, or personality disorder. A comparison was made of these data with those of Western studies, and factors influencing psychiatric consultation in China were discussed.

The following references are also relevant to this chapter:

39, 150, 210, 258, 488, 571, 1478, 1491, 1492, 1740, 1741, 1944, 2607, 2610, 2620, 2639, 2651, 2688, 2692, 2693, 2735, 2773, 2780, 2849, 2901, 2964, 3022, 3524, 3526, 3541.

PROFESSIONAL PERSONNEL AND PROFESSIONAL ISSUES 14

The number of citations in this chapter rank last among the 13 chapters in the present volume, amounting to only 39 or 1.1% of the total (see Table 1). Most citations are in English and slightly more than half pertain to Hong Kong.

Only four subject terms used for indexing citations related to professional personnel and professional issues (including any from other chapters) have frequencies of 10 or more: *Hong Kong* (23), *psychology* (22), *education* (11), and *Peoples Republic of China* (10).

What is revealed is a lack of attention given to research or discussions on professional development.

3510

Andry, R. G. (1984). The current status of the psychologist as an expert witness in criminal trials. *Bulletin of the British Psychological Society, 37,* **236-237.**

Contends that a forensic psychology option should be included within the clinical psychology course in lieu of forensic courses in their own right and that a Division of Criminological and Legal Psychology within the British Psychological Society should be established. It is suggested that the forensic field, which spans such disciplines as law, education, and biology, is highly subspecialized and requires hard work. Sound criminological and penological policy enacted in Hong Kong has resulted in impressive nonrecidivist rates and can serve as a model for the UK.

3511

Blowers, G. H. (1981). [Psychology in Hong Kong: The growth of professionalism]. *China Forum, 12,* **16-18. (Republished in** *Hong Kong Economic Journal Monthly,* **1982,** *58,* **97-98.)** (In Chinese.)

This paper is intended to provide a sketch of some historical developments that have taken place in psychology in Hong Kong as they affect the teaching of students and their subsequent training to professional levels. It is not meant to be an exhaustive search through nor compendium of all activities carried out under the umbrella of psychological practice but tries to illustrate how expansion and alteration of academic practices and changes in Government policy have shaped the growth of professional psychology. It thus reveals something of the structure and functioning of academic teaching, the edition of "expertise" and how "professionalism" has been used as a term to promote psychology as a growth industry. The particular focus is on clinical psychology since it is the most well developed. However, there is every reason to believe that educational psychology (to be offered as a postgraduate training course for the first time in September 1981) will develop along similar lines. There is not at present postgraduate training in industrial psychology in Hong Kong.

3512

Brammer, L. M. (1967). Counselor education abroad: Republic of China. *Counselor Education & Supervision, 6,* **293-296.**

Briefly surveys the structure and goals of the counselor education efforts in Taiwan, noting the university programs, the professional associations, i.e., the Chinese Guidance Association, the Counselor Seminar Programs, and the developing counseling traditions.

3513

Carlos, C. (1983). Politics and mental health: With some reference to Hong Kong. *Hong Kong Psychological Society Bulletin,* **No. 10, 35-39.**

Presents an incident involving a World War II Filipino veteran who hijacked an airplane to have various political demands met. This case is used to illustrate that using the label of "mentally ill" as a convenient excuse for the shortcomings of the political system masks the real issue. The role of the mental health practitioner in "subverting the individual" by engaging in such labeling is discussed.

3514

Chan, H. (1982). Presidential address 1981/82. *Hong Kong Psychological Society Bulletin,* **No. 9, 47-48.**

3515

Chen, C. N. (1984). Behavioral sciences: Plural or singular? *Bulletin of the Hong Kong Psychological Society,* **No. 13, 41-47.**

It was asserted that, because behavioral sciences (BHSs) have only recently begun to be taught in medical schools, their role in the preclinical curriculum has not yet been established. The structure and content, as well as the problems, of BHS courses were reviewed. The future of the BHSs in medicine was discussed, and it was suggested that professionals such as psychologists, sociologists, and neuroscientists should be included in the BHS discipline to help develop an integrated study of human behavior in health and in disease.

3516

Chen, C. N. (1985). Psychiatry in transition. *Journal of the Hong Kong Psychiatric Association, 5,* **11-13.**

3517

Chen, T. P. (1976). The acceptability of behavioristic and phenomenological schools of counseling psychology in Chinese higher education. *Dissertation Abstracts International, 36,* **A7286.**

3518

Dawson, J. L. M. (1970). Psychological research in Hong Kong. *International Journal of Psychology, 5,* **63-70. (Also** *Australian Psychologist,* **1970,** *5,* **59-68.)**

Describes the facilities for psychological research and teaching at the University of Hong Kong, a multicultural, multilingual university setting. Funding for cross-cultural research, with an emphasis on biological and sociological effects on cognitive and perceptual variables, is anticipated.

3519

Ho, D. Y. F. (1971). The role of psychologists in mental health in Hong Kong. In W. H. Lo (Ed.), ***Aspects of mental health in Hong Kong*** **(pp. 39-45). Hong Kong: Mental Health Association of Hong Kong.**

3520

Ho, D. Y. F. (1985). Cultural values and professional issues in clinical psychology: Implications from the Hong Kong experience. ***American Psychologist, 40,*** **1212-1218.**

The author discussed the growth of clinical psychology as a profession in Hong Kong despite the difficulties and barriers, including traditional cultural forces antagonistic to clinical psychology (i.e., the moralistic-authoritarian orientation). It was argued that there are also ideological biases underlying clinical psychology in the West, traceable to individualism. A creative synthesis of collectivism and individualism was suggested as a direction for the future of clinical psychology in the East and in the West.

3521

Hong Kong Psychiatric Association. (1983). Views: The Un Chau Estate incident. ***Journal of the Hong Kong Psychiatric Association, 3,*** **42-46.**

3522

Kao, J. J. (1974). Psychiatry in the People's Republic of China: A prospectus. ***American Journal of Chinese Medicine, 2,*** **441-444.**

Discusses the nature and evolution of psychiatric theory and practice in China since 1949. The practice of Chinese psychiatry combines both Western and traditional Chinese medicine with contemporary Chinese political ideology. A marked decline in mental illness since 1949 is reported. Psychiatric theories appear to use an inductive method closely related to the culture's contemporary social development. The goals of Chinese therapy are indistinguishable from the goals of society - to attain a state of maximal productivity and contribution to the growth of Chinese society.

3523

Kuo, Y. Y. (1971). Psychology in Communist China. ***Psychological Record, 21,*** **95-105.**

Outlines the theory and development of psychology in Communist China emphasizing the differences between Western and Communist Chinese psychology. Mainland Chinese psychologists are described as seeking a psychological basis for communism. Psychology is defined as the brain's reflection of reality, determined by the contradictions that exist in objective reality and the ideology of the social class to which the individual belongs. Western psychology is blamed for helping the capitalists to suppress the workers' class struggle. Research on the development of brain function in children is being conducted with the EEG instead of intelligence tests, while Piaget's theory is being used to study cognitive development. Research is also described as emphasizing the traditional Chinese interest in moral development. Research and professional organizations and publications are noted.

3524

Lai, B., & Tsoi, P. T. K. (1985). The psychiatrist in a general hospital: The role in consultation psychiatry. ***Hong Kong Journal of Mental Health, 14,*** **9-21.**

Consultation-liaison psychiatry develops from the extension of the practice of psychiatry in mental hospitals to general hospitals with the establishment of general hospital psychiatric units, the development of psychosomatic medicine, and the biopsychosocial approach to medicine. The differences between consultation and liaison psychiatry were explained. Both in theory and in practice psychiatry is important for general hospital patients with their high rate of, often undetected, psychiatric morbidity. The preliminary data of consultation cases seen in one hospital were presented, and comparisons among three hospitals were made. Differences found in the rates of referred psychotic and nonpsychotic conditions between two hospitals may indicate regional variation in the prevalence of psychiatric illnesses or different admission and referral policies. There were low rates of psychiatric referral in all three hospitals. Research into the problems, education of the public and professionals, and the inclusion of consultation psychiatry in the planning and provision of psychiatric services are needed.

3525

Lau, B. W. K. (1982). Mental health aspects of leprosy patients. ***Journal of the Hong Kong Psychiatric Association, 2,*** **24-30.**

3526

Lebensohn, Z. M. (1978). Private practice of psychiatry: Future roles. ***American Journal of Psychiatry, 135,*** **1359-1363.**

The impact of national health insurance on the future character of the private practice of psychiatry and the thorny problems to be resolved are discussed and compared with the experiences of England, USSR, and China. Future trends will most likely include increased emphasis on adjuvant techniques, greater emphasis on resident training in general psychiatry, briefer forms of therapy, and psychiatry's return to the medical model.

3527

Lee, R. P. L. (1975). Interaction between Chinese and western medicine in Hong Kong: Modernization and professional inequality. In A. Kleinman, P. Kunstadter, E. R. Alexander & J. L. Gale (Eds.), *Medicine in Chinese culture: Comparative studies of health care in Chinese and other societies* **(pp. 219-240). Washington, DC: U.S. Department of Health, Education & Welfare.**

3528

Lethbridge, H. (1981). The expert and the inexpert. *Hong Kong Psychological Society Bulletin*, **No. 7, 35-45.**

3529

Li, E., Chan, M., Lau Ng, H. Y., & Lai, L. (1981). Issues in the practice of clinical psychology in Hong Kong. *Hong Kong Psychological Society Bulletin*, **No. 6, 7-21.**

This paper discusses the work setting and its limitations, the clientele, territorial integrity, and public image of the clinical psychologist in Hong Kong. The comments of three other clinical psychologists of the area are also included.

3530

Lowe, B. (1984). Preparation for work with young pre-primary children in Hong Kong. *Early Child Development & Care*, *17*, **291-306.**

Some training opportunities available to adults working with or desiring to work with young children in Hong Kong were described. Courses were considered that prepare staff for daycare centers and kindergartens. Although all kindergartens are privately provided by profit-making or nonprofit-making individuals or organizations, there is increasing involvement by the government; and the relevant proposals of a policy paper on primary education and preprimary services were considered.

3531

Matsuyama, Y. (1978). A visit with Chinese psychologists at Beijing University. *Psychologia: An International Journal of Psychology in the Orient*, *21*, **177-178.**

Reports observations by a Japanese university president of educational and research work in psychology in the People's Republic of China. The offerings and orientations in psychology at Peking University and Peking Teacher's College are listed. In the Chinese Science Academy, research groups are functioning in the areas of perceptional, abnormal, developmental, and theoretical psychology.

3532

Ney, P. G., & Jones, L. S. (1985). Psychiatry in the medical curriculum. *Canadian Journal of Psychiatry*, *30*, **586-592.**

3533

Ng, B. P. (1985). A descriptive study of Chinese American psychotherapists and their attitudes toward psychotherapy. *Dissertation Abstracts International*, *45*, **B3953.**

3534

Pan, S. (1979). [Chinese psychology in the new period of development]. *Acta Psychologica Sinica*, *11*, **1-9.** (In Chinese.)

Presents an address delivered at the 2nd annual meeting of the Chinese Psychological Society. Three main problems that face Chinese psychologists are discussed: (a) the modernization of psychology and its implications, (b) how to modernize psychology, and (c) how to resolve the contradiction between the arduous tasks facing Chinese psychologists and the present meager conditions.

3535

Patterson, C. H. (1986). Culture and psychology in Hong Kong. *American Psychologist*, *41*, **926.**

The author comments on a discussion of clinical psychology in Hong Kong by David Ho. It is argued that Ho's otherwise admirable article is marred by the misidentification of Maslow and Rogers as "modern prophets of individualism," as both would have accepted Ho's synthesis of Western individualism and Chinese collectivism.

3536

Sata, L. S. (1977). Asian psychiatric resources in the United States. *Psychiatric Annals*, *7*, **29-35.**

Discusses preliminary data that identify Asian psychiatric resources within the US, assembled by the Ad Hoc Committee on Asian Psychiatrists (later a Task Force of the American Psychiatric Association). From the Association's 1973 directory, 243 psychiatrists were of Asian origin (73 Chinese, 72 Filipino, 66 Korean, and 32 Japanese). Tables show census data, the ratio of Asian population to Asian psychiatrists by state, and comparisons of census data and psychiatric resources.

3537

Shek, D. T. L., & Lam, L. K. H. (1985). Mental health education in Hong Kong: A critical review of the formal curriculum. *Hong Kong Journal of Mental Health*, *14*, **22-33.**

3538

Sue, S. (1973). Training of "third world" students to function as counselors. *Journal of Counseling Psychology, 20,* **73-78.**

Provided more responsive counseling services to ethnic minority students by selecting 20 minority undergraduates (Chicanos, Asian-Americans, blacks, and American Indians) to function as counselors for other minority individuals. Ss were chosen from among 70 who successfully completed a pilot minority-counseling project course at the University of California, Los Angeles. Despite initial difficulties in developing trust and in defining the goals of the program, it is concluded that the training and use of minority-group paraprofessionals are feasible alternatives to current mental health services on campuses.

3539

Tang, G. W., & Whyte, P. M. (1985). Teaching human sexuality to Chinese medical students: Curriculum and difficulties. *Journal of Psychosomatic Obstetrics & Gynaecology, 4,* **129-135.**

The authors presented the modifications made over 5 years in the presentation of a human sexuality course (first given in 1980) to Chinese medical students in response to subjects' evaluations of the course.

3540

The Chinese Psychological Society. (1981). [The Chinese Psychological Society joins the International Union of Psychological Science]. *Information on Psychological Sciences,* **No. 1, 56-58.** (In Chinese.)

3541

Walls, P. D., Walls, L. H., & Langsley, D. G. (1975). Psychiatric training and practice in the People's Republic of China. *American Journal of Psychiatry, 132,* **121-128.**

Improved political relations between the United States and the People's Republic of China have led to closer contact in many areas. The authors trace the development of psychiatric training and practice in China with emphasis on the years after 1949. Since then, China has expanded psychiatric services to meet the needs of a vast population and has developed a theoretical approach to psychiatry that emphasizes sociopolitical factors. Additional information given to the authors in 1973 by psychiatrists in Nanking and Shanghai is presented and correlated with reports by other recent visitors to the People's Republic of China.

3542

Weinman, J. (1984). Priorities in psychology teaching in medicine. *Bulletin of the Hong Kong Psychological Society,* **No. 13, 17-21.**

The author discussed key issues in planning effective psychology teaching for medical students, emphasizing the notion of effective teaching. It was suggested that there is abundant evidence that the majority of medical students find it difficult to appreciate the relevance of psychology to medicine. It was contended that three key issues need to be attended to with considerable thought and planning: (1) the provision of an adequate preparation for the psychology course, (2) careful planning and presentation of the course, and (3) proper follow-up in the clinical curriculum to ensure that the course has an enduring effect.

3543

Whittaker, J. O. (1970). Psychology in China: A brief survey. *American Psychologist, 25,* **757-759.**

Discusses evidence that psychology still exists as a viable profession within China. 3 specialities appear to predominate: medical (or clinical), educational, and industrial. Graduate training is available in these specialities at a few universities including Peking. Research is carried out mainly at the Chinese Academy of Sciences in Peking and Peking University, although educational research in psychology is probably conducted more widely. Although professional psychology is quite limited, perhaps as many as 40,000-50,000 students are enrolled in lower-level psychology courses.

3544

Wong, C. W. (1985). 10 years at Castle Peak Hospital: Some personal reflections and propositions. *Journal of the Hong Kong Psychiatric Association, 5,* **43-44.**

3545

Xu, L. C. (1979). [Psychology in the realization of the Four Modernizations]. *Acta Psychologica Sinica, 11,* **22-28.** (In Chinese.)

Discusses the 4 main tasks of Chinese psychologists. First, to make China a modern socialist country, there is a need to educate and train many experts. To this end, psychologists should make their contributions to education. Second, psychologists should make every effort to increase labor productivity. Third, psychological tasks in medicine are examined within the context of pollution, environment, and family changes. Behavior modification and counseling are also emphasized. Fourth, social psychology studies should help to resolve questions of how to mobilize the initiative of the broad masses; more effective measures should be taken in the investigation of public opinion, social feeling, and attitudes toward various policies and events. Finally, the importance of the fundamental theoretical research of psychology is emphasized.

3546

Xu, L. T. (1978). Some psychological investigations in the People's Republic of China. *Australian Psychologist, 13,* **359-367.**

Describes some of the research being conducted by the Institute of Psychology of the Chinese Academy of Sciences. Topics examined include sensory and perceptual processes, physiology, genetic psychology, and psychological problems in acupuncture anesthesia.

3547

Yee, A. H. (1981). Psychology in China: Perspectives of 1972, 1980, and 1981. *Journal of the Asian American Psychological Association, 6,* **14-17.**

Presents the author's observations and impressions of Chinese psychology after visiting the country in 1972, 1980, and again in 1981. As a result of the Cultural Revolution, the author, in 1972, was able to contact only 5 Chinese psychologists, who conducted no teaching or research and were secretive about their situation and the fate of their colleagues, especially those who were educated in the US and Europe. However, in 1980 and 1981 1,000 psychologists were met who were enthusiastic about learning and promoting psychology in China.

3548

Yee, J. K. (1986). The stress buffering effects of social support: A retrospective and intervention study of Chinese American and Anglo American nurses. *Dissertation Abstracts International, 46,* **B2830.**

The following references are also relevant to this chapter:

8, 3112, 3210, 3430, 3435.

AUTHOR INDEX

This index refers, not to page numbers, but to the number of each relevant citation.

SUBJECT INDEX

This index refers, not to page numbers, but to the number of each relevant citation.

ABOUT THE EDITORS

DAVID YAU-FAI HO received his doctoral training in psychology and logic in the United States. In 1968, he returned to his birthplace Hong Kong, where most of his time has been devoted to the introduction and development of professional clinical psychology. Presently he is Reader in the Department of Psychology at the University of Hong Kong. Dr. Ho is committed to the development of an Asian psychology with indigenous roots in the cultural heritage of Asia. His research interests have focused on personality development, psychopathology, and social behavior in Chinese culture. Dr. Ho has had multicultural clinical experience in North America, Hawaii, and the Far East. He has been elected President of the International Council of Psychologists (1988- 1989).

JOHN A. SPINKS was born in the U.K. and graduated from the University of Newcastle-Upon-Tyne there in 1973. After obtaining his Ph.D. in psychophysiology at the University of Southampton, he joined the University of Hong Kong, where he is now Senior Lecturer. His research interests lie primarily in the areas of cognitive and medical psychophysiology, with recent work in psychoneuroimmunology, but he has devoted a great deal of his time to computer software development. He has been particularly involved in the development of psychology in Hong Kong, from both a professional and a research perspective, being President of the Hong Kong Psychological Society from 1985-86, and now External Examiner in Psychology at the new City Polytechnic of Hong Kong.

CECILIA SIU-HING YEUNG was born and educated in Hong Kong. Although the training she received in college was in economics, in recent years her interests have turned to psychology. She has served as Research Assistant in the Department of Psychology at the University of Hong Kong for a number of years.

www.ingramcontent.com/pod-product-compliance
Ingram Content Group UK Ltd.
Pitfield, Milton Keynes, MK11 3LW, UK
UKHW051933150926
475560UK00005B/370